Rowan Hillson, MD, FRC[ ] a special interest in dial[ ] [ ]ngdon Hospital, Middlesex. She wrote her first book about diabetes while working in Oxford, where she completed several diabetes research projects. Now she shares the care of several thousand people with diabetes with other members of the Hillingdon Diabetes Team. Dr Hillson has a particular interest in helping people with diabetes to learn more about their condition. She is the author of *Late Onset Diabetes*, *Diabetes: A Young Person's Guide*, *Diabetes: A Beyond Basics Guide* and *Thyroid Disorders*, all published by Vermilion.

DIABETES UK

Diabetes UK (formerly known as the British Diabetic Association) has been helping people with diabetes for over 60 years. Since it was set up in 1934 by RD Lawrence and the author HG Wells, both of whom had diabetes, Diabetes UK has concentrated on care and research.

Diabetes UK has a very active branch network with over 400 voluntary groups nationwide. These include specialist groups for young people, parents and Asian people. In June 1994, they opened their first regional office in Glasgow and they now have offices in Warrington, Walsall, Darlington, Cardiff and Belfast. A further six are planned across the UK. National and Regional offices aim to help improve the provision of health care through the NHS at local level, support the local Area Co-ordinators and voluntary groups, and provide information and a presence on a regional basis.

Diabetes UK is dedicated to fighting prejudice and the myths that surround diabetes. They do this by increasing awareness of the condition through advertising and the media. They also work to influence government policy, act as the voice of diabetes and campaign for the best care, the best quality of life, an end to unfair discrimination, and much more.

Diabetes UK's Careline offers help and support on all aspects of diabetes. It provides a confidential service which takes general enquiries from people with diabetes, their carers and from health care professionals. The specialist staff can give you the latest information on topics such as taking care of your diabetes, diet information and information on children with diabetes, their parents and families.

Diabetes UK is one of the largest funders of diabetes research in the UK. If you would like to contact Diabetes UK or become a member, you can telephone on:

**020 7323 1531 between 9am and 5pm Monday to Friday or write to them at:
10 Queen Anne Street, London, W1G 9LH.**

DIABETES

The Complete Guide

The essential introduction to managing diabetes

Dr Rowan Hillson
MD FRCP

Illustrated by
Maggie Raynor

Vermilion
LONDON

For those who live with diabetes

First published by Macdonald Optima in 1992

5 7 9 10 8 6

This edition published in the United Kingdom in 2001 by Vermilion, an imprint of Ebury Press

Random House Group Ltd
Random House
20 Vauxhall Bridge Road
London SW1V 2SA

Random House Australia (Pty) Ltd
20 Alfred Street, Milsons Point, Sydney,
New South Wales 2061, Australia

Random House New Zealand Limited
18 Poland Road, Glenfield,
Auckland 10, New Zealand

Random House, South Africa (Pty) Limited
Box 2263, Rosebank 2121, South Africa
www.randomhouse.co.uk
The Random House Group Limited Reg. No. 954009

A CIP catalogue record for this book is available from the British Library.

ISBN 0 09 182701 9

Printed and bound in Great Britain by Mackays of Chatham, plc

Papers used by Vermilion are natural, recyclable products made from
wood grown in sustainable forests.

CONTENTS

	Foreword	viii
	Introduction	ix
1	Symptoms of diabetes	1
2	The diagnosis of diabetes	7
3	Assessing a person with diabetes	16
4	What is diabetes? Why me?	27
5	Getting started	38
6	Blood or urine glucose testing	46
7	Healthy Eating	55
8	Glucose-lowering pills	73
9	Insulin treatment	85
10	Hypoglycaemia or low blood glucose	108
11	Hyperglycaemia or high blood glucose	122
12	Diabetic tissue damage	129
13	Preventing diabetic tissue damage	157
14	Living with diabetes	164
15	The diabetes team and the diabetes service	178
16	Pregnancy	186
17	Sport and exercise	193
18	Travel	207
19	Setting goals	220
	Glossary	243
	Contacts	250
	Index	253

ACKNOWLEDGEMENTS

This book would not have been written without the constant stimulus and enthusiasm of the people with diabetes I have known over the years. I thank them for sharing their experience of diabetes with me.

I am very grateful to the following for their help, ideas, comments, encouragement and support:

Kate Adams, Jayne Booth, Diabetes UK (formerly the British Diabetic Association), Brenda Cox, the Hillingdon Diabetes Team, Sinead Dunne, Kay and Rodney Hillson, Simon Hillson, Margaret Hounslow, Richard Hourston, Hugh Mather, Richenda Milton-Thompson, David Perkin, Suzanne Redmond, Gill Ruane, Kate Smallman, Yvonne Stawarz, Peter Thomson, Clare Wallis.

Maggie Raynor converted my drawings into illustrations. Photography is by Yvonne Hollis.

I would also like to thank the following for their permission to use material reproduced in this book:

Cohn Duncan and *MIMS* for the tables on pages 50 and 90, taken from the August 2001 edition (n.b. this chart is up-dated in each month's issue of *MIMS*); the *Journal of the Royal College of Physicians of London* for the table shown on page 72 taken from Volume *17*, no. 1 of January, 1983; Diabetes UK for 'What diabetes care to expect' on pages 224–32 and 'What care to expect if your child has diabetes' on pages 232–9; International Diabetes Federation (Europe) and the editor and publishers (John Wiley and Sons Ltd) of *Diabetic Medicine* for The St Vincent Declaration (*Diabetic Medicine* 1990: *7*: 360) and the European Patients' Charter (*Diabetic Medicine* 1991: 8: 782–3); University of Toronto Press for extracts from *Living with Diabetes* by Heather Maclean and Barbara Oram, 1988 (page 177).

*To maintain your health it is not enough that your
doctor should put you on the proper lines of treatment.
You must learn to follow it and carry it out yourself
in your own home. This alone will insure your health
and give you a mastery over the disease and liberty to
carry on your usual life.*

R.D. Lawrence, 1935
(Co-founder of the British Diabetic Association – now Diabetes UK)

FOREWORD TO SECOND EDITION

The diagnosis of diabetes hits people with an awful force. Suddenly no longer a person but a 'patient', life is suddenly filled with questions. Will I need injections every day? Must I stop eating my favourite foods? Can I have children? Am I now a sick person? Dare I go on holiday? And, always, who or what's to blame? Is there a cure? Is life going to be worth living?

While these questions crowd in most of all on the newly diagnosed person, they also besiege parents, partners, relatives and friends. They are questions that must be answered for life to be as full and complete, as gratifying and productive as it was before. This book aims to answer these questions.

This is a helpful and hopeful book. It tackles all the key questions fully and frankly and in a way that all of those with, or living with, diabetes can understand. It will be a valuable aid to the essential process of understanding and coming to terms with diabetes, a process in which doctors, nurses, members of the diabetes care team and other people with diabetes all play an important part.

The book opens with a quotation from perhaps the most remarkable diabetic patient of them all, the redoubtable Dr R D Lawrence. He not only wrote a classic book *The Diabetic Life* – he also lived it to the full. His major memorial is Diabetes UK, formerly the British Diabetic Association which he founded and which offers its support and a welcome to all members of this club that nobody wanted to join.

Sir Michael Hirst
Diabetes UK

INTRODUCTION

This book is for people who have just learned that they have diabetes, for their relatives and carers, and for people who have had diabetes for some time but would like some revision.

Two in one hundred people have diabetes and know it. We all know someone who has diabetes – someone in the family, a friend, someone at work. One person in a hundred has diabetes and does not realise that they have it. People will have diabetes without you being aware of it – for people with diabetes look no different from anyone else, and can work and have fun just like anyone else.

But having it yourself is different. Until it has been treated it can make you feel off colour or very ill. And it is always frightening when you discover that something is wrong with you. It is especially frightening if you do not know anything about this new condition. As a small child I was always told to be very, very careful with electricity. If I wasn't, 1 would get a shock. Everyone kept telling me how careful I must be. So I thought that a shock must be very, very dangerous. Then one day, as I plugged in the iron, I had a small electric shock. I was terrified! I ran upstairs crying 'I've had a shock, I've had a shock!' I was convinced I was going to die there and then. I stood, panting melodramatically, waiting to die. But nothing happened. I can laugh at my terror now. But, of course, electricity can injure if not treated with respect.

Diabetes is obviously rather more serious than a minor electric shock. But if you learn about the condition, what caused it, what is happening in your body, and, most importantly, how to look after yourself and keep fit, it need not be frightening. You can carry on doing the things you enjoy with very few limitations. If you ignore it and hope it will go away, it may cause you trouble.

This book is an introduction to diabetes – what it can feel like to have it and what the doctor may ask and may look for on examination. There is a section on the tests your doctor may do. A chapter discusses what you need to know straightaway and there is further information to help as you continue in your diabetic career. Diet and other treatments for diabetes are detailed. The rest of the book is about keeping fit and enjoying life with diabetes.

The sequence in which this book is written is designed to be easy for someone with newly diagnosed diabetes to follow. However, those of my readers who are experienced in diabetes may wish to go straight to the sections relating to enjoying life with diabetes (travel, sport and so on), specific aspects of treatment, self-monitoring or tissue damage. Each chapter can be read on its own.

I use proper medical terms throughout this book, always with explanations, so that you can interpret any 'Medspeak' you encounter in the surgery or clinic. There is also a glossary at the end. To enliven the book I have included stories about people with diabetes. These stories are based on real life but have been altered to protect the participants.

Throughout the book I have assumed that your doctor is male, your nurse and dietitian female and so on. This is to save writing he/she throughout the book. But your doctor may be a woman – as I am – and indeed your nurse or dietitian may be male. No offence is intended to those of the opposite sex.

This book is one doctor's description of some of the ways of assessing and helping people with diabetes. But there are many people with diabetes (over 150 million worldwide) and tens of thousands of doctors with a special interest in diabetes. The people who know most about *your* diabetes are you and the diabetes team who help you to care for it. It is to your own doctor that you must go for advice about your personal condition. If you have questions about what you have read in this book or about other aspects of your diabetes, please contact your diabetes team straightaway. Remember, diabetes care is a rapidly moving field. Ask your diabetes team to help you to keep up-to-date with new ideas.

All comments about medications, their effects and doses must be checked with your doctor. Do not alter your medication without having checked that your doctor is happy for you to do so.

I could not have written this book without the support and encouragement of thousands of people with diabetes who have shared their experiences and their friendship with me over the years. One of them, who attended a British Diabetic Association/Outward Bound course with a group of other people with diabetes said, 'I feel more confident about being diabetic. It is not going to stop me doing anything in life I want to do. Being diabetic has made me a stronger person. I am happy and optimistic about my future as a diabetic.' Another said, 'Diabetes isn't the problem people think it is. It's not the end. It's a beginning.'

SYMPTOMS OF DIABETES

Symptoms are unusual feelings or body changes you notice yourself. How do you know you have diabetes? What do you feel?

WHAT ARE THE SYMPTOMS OF DIABETES?

Nothing at all

Many people feel nothing at all. They go to a doctor for a routine check-up and are astonished to discover that there is glucose in their urine and, subsequently, to be told they have diabetes. 'But how can I be diabetic? I don't feel ill', they say. Some of them may look back and realise that they have, after all, been feeling below par. But some people are not aware of chemical imbalance in their bodies. Unfortunately, even though you do not feel unwell you must still take your diabetes seriously.

Thirst

Thirst, or polydipsia *(poly* – much, *dipsia* – thirst), is a classic diabetes symptom. Your mouth may feel like the Sahara desert and many pints of fluid may fail to quench your thirst.

Joe was 23 when he developed diabetes. In the week before it was diagnosed he would wake up and have a glass of water, then have three cups of tea for breakfast. He works hard on a building site and he would take two big bottles of Pepsi with him in the morning. But by lunchtime they were drunk and he had to buy other drinks from the corner shop – six little boxes of juice and four cans of shandy to last the afternoon. At home he drank six or seven cups of tea and half a dozen beers, and he still had to take a jug of water to bed with him for the night.

Not everyone is as thirsty as Joe, but many people get into the habit of having extra drinks at their breaks or mealtimes.

Polyuria

This means passing a lot of urine (*poly* – much, *uria* – urine). You may need to urinate often and pass big volumes each time. Where is it all coming from? Most people think it is because they are drinking so much. But it is the other way round. The high glucose levels in the blood of someone with diabetes spill over into the urine making it syrupy. This draws water out of the body producing large volumes of urine and making you thirsty.

Miss Green looked after her 84-year-old mother who was rather shaky and had had a weak bladder for some years. Her mother usually slept well but one night she woke up her daughter. 'I'm so sorry dear,' she said, 'I've wet the bed. I wanted to go so badly and I just couldn't get out to the toilet in time.' 'Never mind, mother,' said Miss Green, as she got a fresh sheet out of the cupboard. But this went on for several nights, so Miss Green called the doctor. Since her mother's diabetes has been treated there have been no more wet beds.

If you have diabetes the polyuria continues night and day. In frail, elderly people or in small children this can occasionally lead to bed-wetting. Polyuria is inconvenient for everyone – you have to learn where all the toilets are at train stations and in shopping precincts.

Weight loss

Glucose, the simple form of sugar we can eat directly or derive from digesting sweet or starchy foods, is the body's main fuel. People with untreated diabetes cannot use this glucose properly. It overflows into the urine and is passed out of the body – wasted. So body tissues are broken down in an attempt to provide fuel for the body. Gradually you lose weight.

Doris, aged 56 years, had been feeling rather under the weather lately. She was thirsty, and it was irritating having to get up to go to the toilet in the middle of the night. But she was eating well so there could not be much wrong. One weekend she decided to clear out her wardrobe. That blue suit, too tight for years, just try it once more before giving it to Oxfam. The suit fitted perfectly – in fact, it was a bit loose if anything. Doris was delighted. It was not until she went for her blood pressure check at her doctor's some months later that she discovered she had lost some 20 pounds in weight over the past year. Then the doctor found her to have diabetes.

Diabetes is one of the causes of weight loss despite a good appetite. Some people actually have a craving for sugary foods.

Constipation

As you pass more and more urine, it becomes harder and harder to keep up with your fluid loss. Your body starts to dry out (become dehydrated). This can lead to constipation.

Tiredness, malaise, no energy

Malaise is uneasiness or a non-specific feeling that all is not well. Diabetes can make you feel tired and lacking in energy. You may feel that your get-up-and-go has gone. You may be so tired that you go straight to bed on your return from work.

Tingling

The chemical changes of diabetes can alter the function of the nerves, the cables that carry the electric signals between your brain and your body. This can produce tingling or pins and needles in hands or feet. These usually improve with treatment of the diabetes.

Infections

Mrs Bibi is 42 years old and works in the family greengrocer's shop. One evening, helping to unload the van, she scratched her foot on a crate of apples. She washed the wound and soon forgot all about it as she hurried around the shop. Two days later her foot began to hurt. On inspection the wound was oozing pus and the foot was red and swollen. Her doctor said she had an

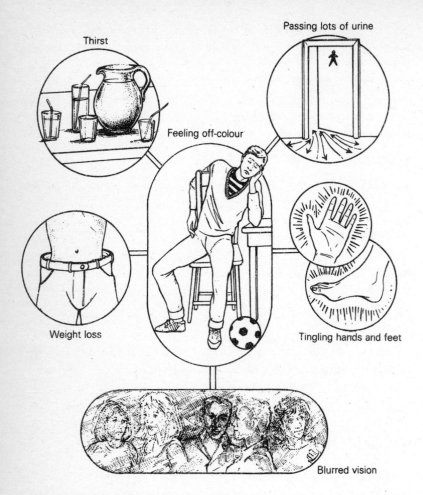

Thirst

Passing lots of urine

Feeling off-colour

Weight loss

Tingling hands and feet

Blurred vision

Symptoms of diabetes

infection and gave her antibiotics. But the infection was very slow to heal and further tests revealed diabetes. Once that was treated the foot infection healed.

All our body's defence mechanisms work best in a normal chemical environment. If the body's chemistry is awry, you may not be able to fight infection properly. In uncontrolled diabetes, the white blood cells which seek out and destroy bacteria, do not move as well as usual and the bacteria multiply.

Common infections in previously undiagnosed diabetics include boils or carbuncles, other abscesses, chest infections, urinary tract infections (e.g. cystitis) and thrush. Thrush can cause discharge, itching (pruritus) and soreness around the vagina in women (vulvitis or vaginitis) and the penis in men (balanitis). Once the diabetes is under control, antifungal cream will cure thrush. Any infection may be worse or take longer to resolve in people with high blood glucose levels due to diabetes.

Blurred vision

Just as stirring sugar into water makes it thick and syrupy, glucose in the blood alters its consistency. The body can equalise this to some extent but high glucose levels throughout can alter function of some body components. This includes the lens of the eye. Its focusing properties are disturbed and the vision may become blurred or hazy. Wait until your diabetes has been treated and your vision is stable before buying new glasses.

> Austin was fed up with his glasses. He could not see the paper clearly and reading was a real strain. He clearly needed a new pair – something stronger. He went to an optician who gave him a new prescription. He chose some sophisticated new frames as well. It was very expensive but he was pleased with the result – for about two weeks. Then his vision changed again. His diabetes was diagnosed after an insurance medical check. Once it had been treated the blurring of vision settled and his old spectacles were fine.

THE PATTERN OF SYMPTOMS

How many symptoms?

Everyone is different. Do not expect to have all these symptoms. Some people have none of them. Usually thirst and polyuria occur together. Once your diabetes is treated your symptoms will settle.

How fast do the symptoms come on?

In younger people the symptoms may come on over days or weeks. They may be severe. It is usually very obvious that something is wrong. In older people the onset of diabetes can be very subtle. It may take weeks or months for anyone to realise that something is wrong. One man had had classic, albeit mild, symptoms of diabetes for 14 years before he sought medical help and the diagnosis was made. What is sadly more common is for people to have a gradual increase in blood glucose which they don't notice. It is obvious from large research studies thet many people have diabetes for years before it is diagnosed. Over a third of peoplewith newly diagnosed Type 2 diabetes (see page 33) already have evidence of diabetic tissue damage. If you or family members have any suspicion at all that you may have diabetes see your doctor for a blood glucose test straight away.

SUMMARY

- A symptom is something unusual you notice about yourself.
- Symptoms of diabetes include thirst (polydipsia), polyuria, weight loss, constipation, infections which are severe or slow to resolve, tingling in the hands or feet and blurred vision.
- Some people have no symptoms at all.

2

THE DIAGNOSIS OF DIABETES

THE INITIAL CONTACT

There are many paths to the diagnosis of diabetes. Often the person who suspects that you may have diabetes is not the person who will care for your diabetes long-term. However, with the advent of increased health screening by general practitioners (GPs) in Britain it is becoming more likely to be your GP who finds that you are diabetic and who subsequently treats your diabetes in part or completely.

A routine check of a well person

Testing the urine for glucose forms part of most 'well man' and 'well woman' checks. Urine or blood glucose testing is also part of company or insurance medical tests. Most people with untreated diabetes will have glucose in their urine. (But not everyone with glucose in his or her urine has diabetes – see page 8–9.) Any doctor who does not usually care for your general health will almost certainly return you to your GP for further tests.

Going to your doctor because of symptoms of diabetes

If you have some of the symptoms described in Chapter 1, especially thirst and polyuria, your GP will probably check for diabetes. If he confirms the diagnosis he will then either refer you to a diabetes specialist clinic for further advice, or, if he has had training in diabetes care, will give you the help you need himself. Either way, he should give you some initial explanation about what diabetes is and how to start looking after yourself.

Going to a doctor for another reason

Some people discover they are diabetic because of the initial screening which doctors or hospitals perform in people who come to them for help with some other condition. I have seen people with diabetes who were initially referred as outpatients to urologists (specialists in urinary tract disease) with frequent urination, ophthalmologists (eye doctors) with blurred vision, dentists with dry mouths, dermatologists (skin doctors) with recurrent boils and so on. Patients may be admitted through casualty with severe infections and be found to have diabetes by the casualty officer. Sometimes people are first seen because of the tissue complications of diabetes (see chapter 12). The problem is that all the symptoms of diabetes bar the thirst and polyuria are non-specific and some are common. Most people who feel tired are not diabetic.

DIAGNOSING DIABETES

The point at which the diagnosis is confirmed varies. The formal diagnosis relies on one or more blood tests taken from a vein in your arm and tested by a laboratory. Until this has been done you do not know for certain that you have diabetes. Most doctors would not refer a patient to a diabetes specialist clinic until the diagnosis has been confirmed in this way.

Keeping the blood glucose normal

Normally, the blood maintains the blood glucose level at around 3.5 to 7.8 millimols (a unit of measurement) of glucose in every litre of blood. This is usually written as 3.5–7.8 mmol/l. For simplicity I will use 4–8 mmol/l in most of the book. In America, they measure the blood glucose concentration in milligrams per decilitre (mg/dl). 18 mg/dl equals 1 mmol/l and their normal range is about 60–140 mg/dl.

The body strives to maintain normality. If something goes wrong many mechanisms are brought into play to return everything to a normal state. This process is called homeostasis.

GLUCOSE IN THE URINE

The kidney filtering system is one of the ways in which the body attempts to maintain a normal blood glucose level. In most people the kidneys do not allow glucose to enter the urine if the blood concentration is below 8 mmol/l. If you have diabetes the blood glucose rises. The reasons for this are discussed in Chapter 4. As the glucose level rises above 8 mmol/l and then 10 mmol/l and upwards, glucose starts to leak into the urine. The blood glucose at which this occurs is called the kidney threshold or renal threshold (renal = kidney). This threshold is usually 10 mmol/l. The higher the blood glucose, the more glucose there is in the urine. On its way through the kidney filtering system this syrupy urine draws water with it.

Urine flows down the tubes draining the kidneys (called ureters) to collect in the bladder. When the bladder is full its walls stretch and you feel the desire to pass urine. The large volumes produced by someone with diabetes fill and stretch the bladder repeatedly.

You can already see that the concentration of glucose in the urine depends on many factors. At what point does the kidney begin to allow glucose into the urine? How much water is drawn in with the glucose? How long is the urine in the bladder before voiding? The amount of glucose filtered by the kidneys may fluctuate from hour to hour.

The kidney threshold for glucose

If someone has a low threshold for glucose, it will appear in the urine at a blood glucose concentration of, say, 6 mmol/l. This person is not diabetic but his or her urine will give a positive result on glucose testing. This condition is called renal glycosuria (renal – kidney, *glycos* – glucose, *uria* – in the urine). These people can be wrongly labelled as diabetic. This is one reason why it is essential to confirm the diagnosis of diabetes on blood testing.

If someone has a high threshold for glucose, say 16 mmol/l, their urine will be free from glucose until that level is reached. Thus, in them, a negative urine test does not mean that they are free from diabetes.

The blood glucose fluctuates all the time. Sometimes it may be above the renal threshold, sometimes below.

For all these reasons, urine testing may alert a doctor to the possible presence of diabetes, but it is not diagnostic. A negative urine test does not exclude diabetes.

GLUCOSE IN THE BLOOD

Having a blood test

Many people are frightened of having a blood test. Occasionally, the anxiety builds up out of all proportion to the very brief test. There is no need at all to be worried – the discomfort is akin to nicking yourself shaving or catching yourself on a rose thorn gardening. When you go to the surgery or hospital you will be asked to roll up your sleeve, and to sit down with your arm resting on a table. A band will be placed temporarily around your upper arm to make the veins stand up. Some people clean the skin with alcohol, some do not. The person taking the sample will hold your skin taut and slip the needle through the skin. It feels sharp or stings very briefly as it goes through the skin but in most cases that is all you will notice and within seconds the blood sample will be taken. You will be given a piece of cotton wool to press on the vein. Keep your arm straight and press firmly for one minute. (Bending the arm kinks the vein and can cause bruises.) And that is that. A few tips: keep really warm until just before the sample is taken (it makes your veins easier to find); relax as you sit down and do some deep breathing if you are nervous; concentrate on your summer holiday (if you relax it hurts less). If you are an experienced blood testee and have an especially good vein, show it to the person taking the sample.

What happens to your blood?

The sample will be put into a little bottle containing a chemical to preserve the glucose. The bottle is carefully labelled with your name, number (if in hospital) and the date. It is then sent to the laboratory with the accompanying request form from your doctor. (Do check the form when your doctor gives it to you. Make sure your name and other details are correct.) In the laboratory a receptionist checks in the sample and the request card and allocates it a laboratory test number. Then a technician puts the bottle into a centrifuge and spins it down to separate the blood cells from the fluid in which they float (plasma). The plasma is then put into the analyser (usually as part of an automatic line of samples) which measures the plasma glucose concentration. The result is then

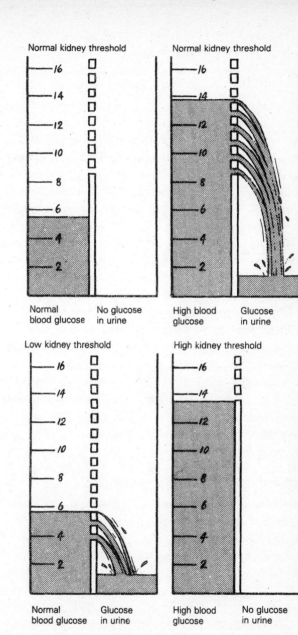

Normal kidney threshold

Normal blood glucose — No glucose in urine

Normal kidney threshold

High blood glucose — Glucose in urine

Low kidney threshold

Normal blood glucose — Glucose in urine

High kidney threshold

High blood glucose — No glucose in urine

Differences in renal thresholds

checked and printed or written onto a report form. The form will be sent to your doctor or his secretary. He must then extract your form from the heap of such forms he receives every day (in my own department this may be over a hundred forms a day) and match it with your records.

The plasma glucose concentration

Previously I have loosely referred to this as the blood glucose level. There are small differences between whole blood glucose concentrations and venous plasma glucose concentrations. There are also differences between glucose concentrations in a finger prick sample and one taken simultaneously from a vein.

Blood full of glucose and oxygen and other nutrients is delivered to parts of the body by arteries which divide into ever smaller branches. These branches eventually become capillaries, which actually deliver the nutrients to the tissues. Waste substances are then drained from the tissues by small vessels which link up to form veins. Finger pricks obtain blood from capillaries. The tissues have used up some of the glucose by the time the blood reaches the vein.

Most laboratories measure venous plasma glucose and it is to this that I will be referring throughout this book when I talk about glucose levels taken from a vein and sent to the laboratory. Finger-prick testing measures capillary blood glucose.

There are four categories of plasma venous glucose concentration: normality, impaired fasting glucose, impaired glucose tolerance and diabetes. Obviously if you have had something to eat you will be absorbing glucose from digested food and your plasma glucose is likely to be higher than if you are starving. So it is important to know whether you are fasting (i.e. have had nothing to eat or drink except water for 14 hours) or whether it is a random blood sample.

Normal

- Fasting venous plasma glucose concentration below 6.1 mmol/l (110 mg/dl).
- Random venous plasma glucose concentration below 6.1 mmol/l (110 mg/dl).

Impaired fasting glucose

• Fasting venous plasma glucose concentration 6.1–6.9 mmol/l (110–124 mg/dl).

Impaired glucose tolerance

• Fasting venous plasma glucose concentration below 7.0 mmol/l (126 mg/dl).
• Random venous plasma glucose concentration between 7.8 and 11.1 mmol/l (140–200 mg/dl).

Diabetes

• Fasting venous plasma glucose concentration above 7.0 mmol/l or more (126 mg/dl).
• Random venous plasma glucose concentration above 11.0 mmol/l (200 mg/dl).

In the presence of symptoms of diabetes, one fasting or one random blood test is sufficient to confirm the diagnosis. In the absence of symptoms, the diagnosis of diabetes can only be made on the basis of at least two separate confirmatory blood tests.

More people are having detailed tests of glucose tolerance because it is possible to treat more subtle glucose abnormalities. An oral glucose tolerance test (OGTT) is done if your fasting glucose is 6.1–6.9 mmol/l (110–124 mg/dl) (impaired fasting glucose). You will be asked to eat your usual diet (ie with no restrictions on sugary or starchy foods) the day before, fast for 8–14 hours before the test (you may drink plain water) and sit still during the test and not smoke. You will have a venous blood glucose test at the start and then be given 75 g glucose in a drink. Two hours later another venous blood glucose test will be taken.

Two hour glucose 11.1 mmol/l or more (200 mg/dl) – diabetes.
Two hour glucose 7.8–11.0 mmol/l (140–199 mg/dl) – impaired glucose tolerance.

Impaired fasting glucose

This condition has recently been defined as a fasting glucose of 6.1–6.9 mmol/l (110–124 mg/dl). You have a greater risk of having impaired glucose tolerance than other people and may develop diabetes. You should eat healthily, keep to the right weight for your height, and exercise regularly. Ensure that you have a fasting venous glucose blood test once a year.

Impaired glucose tolerance

This is defined as a fasting venous plasma glucose below 7.0 mmol/l (126 mg/dl) and a glucose two hours after a 75 g glucose load of 7.8–11.0 mmol/l (140–199 mg/dl). As many as ten per cent of people with impaired glucose tolerance will develop diabetes each year. People with impaired glucose tolerance also have a greater risk than the normal population of developing furring of the arteries (atherosclerosis) and hence heart attacks, strokes and other circulatory problems. A recent American study of 3234 people with impaired glucose tolerance, yet to be published, was called Diabetes Prevention Program (DPP). This showed that those who exercised for half an hour a day and dieted to lose weight reduced the risk of developing diabetes by 71 per cent. Metformin, a drug used to reduce glucose levels in people with diabetes (see pages 76–7) also reduced the development of diabetes, but exercise and weight reduction did better. Metformin is not yet licensed for this use in the UK although it may be. You should also stop smoking and have your cholesterol level checked.

WHAT NOW?

If you have been told that you have diabetes you should now possess the following information:
- A careful record of your diabetes symptoms (if any);
- One (symptoms present) or two (symptoms absent) venous plasma glucose concentrations written down in your own health record.

The next step is to find out who is going to assess you and your diabetes in general and who is going to care for you and your diabetes.

Every person with diabetes has the right to see a doctor with specialist training in diabetes. This doctor may be your own GP or one of his colleagues, but is more likely to be a hospital-based diabetes consultant working in a diabetic clinic. Unfortunately there are still some parts of Britain where such a specialist service is not readily accessible.

Either way, your GP will remain central in your health care, and it is very important that you discuss everything with him and keep him informed. Nowadays, most hospital diabetes clinics share diabetes supervision with the patient's GP – usually a very fruitful coalition for the patient.

SUMMARY

- There are many paths to the discovery of diabetes.
- Diabetes may be suspected when glucose is found in the urine, but this alone is not diagnostic. Some people without diabetes pass glucose in their urine. Some people with diabetes do not.
- The WHO criteria for diabetes are a fasting venous plasma glucose concentration above 7.0 mmol/l, or a random venous plasma glucose concentration above 11.0 mmol/l. Two such values are required to diagnose diabetes in someone with no symptoms of the condition.

3

ASSESSING A PERSON WITH DIABETES

Your doctor will want to listen to your story, ask some questions of his own and to examine you generally.

YOUR STORY

Tell the doctor exactly what you have noticed is wrong. Try to be specific about symptoms if you can. It is often helpful to give the 'headlines' first and then elaborate on them if necessary. Can you remember for how long the symptoms have troubled you? How bad are they? Are they interfering with your life? Have you had them before?

For example:

'Over the past two months I've been thirsty, drinking a lot of water and I keep passing urine. I've lost about a stone in weight.'

If your doctor asks for details you could say:

'I've got more and more thirsty over the past two months. Now I'm drinking about three big jugs of water a day and lots of tea. I get thirsty at night too. I'm going to the toilet every hour or two and I pass a lot of urine each time. I'm not sleeping very well because I have to get up to go to the toilet. Six months ago I used to weigh 11 stone and last night I only weighed 10 stone.'

But do not feel you have to have symptoms. Not everyone with diabetes does. It is also important to tell the doctor about any other symptoms you have, even if you do not think they are related to your diabetes. You might not think that easy bruising and thin skin could be related to diabetes, but they could if you were taking steroid tablets. These can cause diabetes and easy bruising.

Who are you and what do you do? It helps your doctor to know what sort of person you are and what job you do. He may ask what the job involves – is it heavy work, or is your timetable very variable? Are you a shift or night worker? Do you have responsibility for other people's lives? Are you self-employed? Is your diabetes interfering with any aspect of your life?

Previous medical history

It is important that you tell any new doctor about your medical past. This includes major illnesses and any operation. Doctors usually ask about tuberculosis, rheumatic fever, epilepsy, kidney disease, heart trouble and high blood pressure. In someone with newly diagnosed diabetes it is also helpful to know about thyroid disorders and pernicious anaemia, other autoimmune disorders (see pages 32–3), pancreatitis (see pages 35–6) or pancreatic surgery.

Obstetric history

How many pregnancies have you had and how many babies? How much did your babies weigh? Diabetic women often have a history of big babies. Did you have diabetes or glucose intolerance in pregnancy?

Family history

Does anyone in your family have diabetes now, or did anyone that you know of in the past? Diabetes runs in families.

Drugs and allergies

By drugs I mean any medicine or remedy in any form – injections, pills, capsules, tablets, mixtures, elixirs, herbal extracts, vitamins, ointments, potions. It is very dangerous not to tell your doctor what you are taking as it may react adversely with something he gives you. Some drugs can cause diabetes or worsen it. These include steroids (e.g. prednisolone) and thiazide diuretics (such as bendrofluazide or Moduretic) which are used to treat high blood pressure or ankle swelling.

Some people, especially those from Asia, have a traditional doctor and a NHS doctor. Some traditional remedies may lower the blood glucose slightly – karela, for example. The problem with many herbal remedies is that they may contain toxic impurities and that the dose of any active ingredient is variable. Other people see homeopathic doctors or other alternative practitioners. Tell each practitioner you are seeing the other. Never stop your medication without consulting your doctor – you could become seriously ill.

If you have ever had an adverse reaction to any drug or medication it is vital that you tell every doctor you see about it. Such adverse reactions or allergies might include coming out in spots on taking penicillin, skin irritation caused by using sticking plaster or something more serious.

Eating and drinking

Your doctor may ask you about the sort of foods you usually eat, although he will probably leave detailed questioning to the dietitian. Do you have religious or moral rules which preclude certain foods? It is also useful to know if you have to eat at unusual hours or cannot predict when you will eat or not.

Do you drink alcohol and if so, how much? Do you drink a lot of alcohol or have you ever drunk heavily in the past? It is important to be honest – large amounts of alcohol can damage the pancreas and cause diabetes as well as other conditions for which it is important to be checked (see page 140).

Smoking

As smoking causes many different illnesses, any doctor will ask whether you smoke.

Your overall health

People who have a full medical examination for the first time are often mystified by the lists of questions that the doctor asks them. If you have gone to the doctor because you are passing a lot of urine, questions about chest pain and cough may appear to be straying from the point. But you may have symptoms which you have forgotten or which seem unimportant to you, but which can help the doctor to come to a diagnosis. However most people say 'No' to most of these 'screening' questions.

EXAMINATION

Most doctors will ask you to undress fully. Leave your underpants on unless asked specifically to remove these. Tell the doctor if your religion prevents you from revealing your legs or imposes other restrictions. Most surgeries and hospitals have women doctors who could examine you if you prefer, but you may have to wait for one to be found. Similarly, if you would prefer to see a male doctor, ask. Ask, too, if you wish a relative or friend to chaperone you. Doctors are trained to examine patients while standing on your right hand side and they will usually ask you to lie down on a couch so that they can examine you more readily. Do not be afraid to ask for help in undressing or getting on or off the couch – there will always be someone to help you. It is easier for the doctor to examine you if you are relaxed – although all doctors understand that you may not be feeling at all relaxed! Try taking calm, deep breaths and letting your muscles relax.

Signs of diabetes

General behaviour and appearance You may look outwardly normal and there may be no sign that you have diabetes. Other people with diabetes may be rather tired and perhaps irritable or listless. With very high blood glucose levels and severe chemical imbalance, you may be confused, semi-conscious or unconscious – but this is an uncommon finding in newly-diagnosed diabetes.

If you have lost a lot of fluid you will be dehydrated. This can make your tongue dry and your skin may lose its usual elasticity. Many people with untreated diabetes lose weight and this may be obvious. A previously fit teenager can become very thin in a matter of weeks. This will all return to normal once your diabetes is treated. Some people may have white patches of pigment lack – vitiligo – a condition associated with autoimmune disorders, of which diabetes is one (see pages 32–3). People who have an infection may be flushed or feverish and have a raised temperature.

You may have spots or boils on your face or elsewhere. Some people may notice fatty lumps on their upper eyelids by the nose (called xanthelasmata) or may have a white fatty ring around the coloured iris of the eye (called a corneal arcus). These may be signs that your cholesterol level is raised (see pages 160–1). Some people have other skin problems with diabetes, which are discussed on pages 130–131.

Heart and circulation Your pulse rate will probably be normal (about 60–90 beats per minute), although if you are anxious, infected, very dehydrated or in a state of severe chemical imbalance it may be fast. Your arteries (the blood vessels which carry oxygen and nutrient-rich blood from the heart to the tissues) may feel tortuous and wiggly if you have atherosclerosis or furring-up of the arteries (see pages 138, 152). Smoking is the commonest cause of this, but diabetes can cause it too. if the arteries are very furred-up the doctor will not be able to feel the pulses in your feet and legs. Sometimes it is possible to hear turbulent blood flow over areas of atherosclerosis by listening with a stethoscope in the neck or the groin, for example. This noise is called a bruit.

Your blood pressure may be normal, low or high. If you are dehydrated you may have a low blood pressure, which may fall further when you stand up. This is called postural hypotension. High blood pressure (hypertension) is more common in people with diabetes than in other people and may need treatment (see pages 149–51). Some people with long-standing diabetes may have normal or high blood pressure sitting or lying down, which falls on standing (postural hypotension) because the nerves which control the blood vessels response to gravity have been damaged (see page 152).

Your heart will probably be of normal size and your heart sounds will probably be normal. If you have had untreated blood pressure for some time the heart may be enlarged because it has to pump more strongly to overcome the higher pressures in the arteries. Occasionally there may be murmurs (turbulent blood flow across the valves in the heart). These are usually of no major significance but may indicate that your largest artery, the aorta, has some atherosclerosis.

Your ankles may be puffy if your heart has been weakened – by a previous heart attack, for example. But there are many causes of swollen ankles, the most common being standing up all day in hot weather.

Your lungs Your doctor will probably check that your breathing is normal. In people who are severely ill with newly-diagnosed diabetes, there may be a very deep, sighing breathing, called Kussmaul breathing. This is to blow off acid from the body and is a sign that the person is very ill. The person's breath smells of acetone (pear drops or rotten apples). This is uncommon.

Most people with diabetes have normal chest expansion and normally resonant lungs (checked by tapping the chest with a finger), and their breath sounds are normal. if you have a chest infection, there may be signs of this on examination, including a cough with green phlegm. Doctors call phlegm 'sputum'.

Abdomen This is the area between the ribs and the groins. Most people call it their tummy or stomach, but strictly speaking the stomach is the bag inside on the left into which all your food is delivered when you swallow it. The abdomen can only be examined when you are lying flat and with your hands relaxed by your sides. If you tense your muscles the doctor will be unable to examine you. Occasionally the liver may be enlarged; this often settles with treatment. There may be tenderness over the bladder (in the lower abdomen) or kidneys (in your sides or loins) if you have a urinary tract or kidney infection.

If you have noticed itching, burning or discharge from the penis or the vagina, the doctor will examine these areas too and may take swabs to send to the laboratory. The swabs nearly always show *Candida albicans* – the thrush fungus – which is easily treated.

The nervous system and senses This means the brain and the nerves which lead, like electric cables, to and from it. Most people with newly diagnosed diabetes will have no abnormal neurological (to do with the nervous system) signs. The detail in which the nervous system is assessed will depend, to some extent, on your age and symptoms.

The eyes can be affected by diabetes in several ways (see pages 131–5). The blurring of vision due to the changes in blood glucose concentration can reduce your visual acuity (i.e. the ease with which you can focus on the letters on the eye chart). This is usually temporary. Changes can occur in the back of the eye and the doctor will look at this with a magnifying torch called an ophthalmoscope.

He may put drops in your eyes to make it easier to see the back of the eye.

The nerves which carry signals from the hands and feet to the brain can be affected by diabetes and this may mean that you have numb areas, especially on your feet, or have other changes in sensation (see pages 153–6). Sometimes nerves which tell muscles what to do may be affected too.

After checking sensation and movement in face, arms and legs, your doctor will check your reflexes. These are found on both arms and legs, and your doctor may tap your elbows, wrists, knees and ankles with the tendon hammer to see if the muscles jerk reflexively. This shows that the nervous pathways are intact.

Feet Your feet are particularly vulnerable if you have diabetes. Your doctor will look at the shape of your feet and toes and at deformities or unusual pressure areas. The skin is checked for injuries, ulcers, infection and general texture. He will feel the pulses on the top of the foot and behind the ankle. I have already discussed the need to check the sensation in the feet. Your doctor will notice your shoes as well.

Joints and ligaments These can be affected by diabetes long-term, but it is unusual to see problems in a newly diagnosed diabetic.

All these findings will be noted down. Then the doctor summarises your problems. Here is an example of a case history as a doctor might write it down.

JOAN HOPKINS, AGE 42, HAIRDRESSER

Patient complains of:
- thirst
- polyuria
- 1 stone weight loss
- vaginal discharge

History of presenting complaint:
Well until two months ago

Gradual onset thirst (water by bed, carries drinks shopping)
Passes large volumes day/night = 10–12/2–3 times
11 stone in May 1989, now 10 stone
One week white vaginal discharge, severe itching and soreness

Previous medical history
No major illness
Varicose vein surgery 1984
Fractured right arm 1987

Obstetric history
Two pregnancies
Two children (Sarah 1978 birthweight 7 lb; John 1980, 9 lb)

Family history
Married, husband electrical fitter
Mother diabetic (on tablets), father died stroke aged 69

Drugs
None

Allergies
None known

Diet
Vegetarian, but eats milk, cheese. Alcohol, 4–6 units a week.

Smoking
Stopped four years ago

DIRECT QUESTIONS

Cardiovascular/respiratory systems
Dry cough following cold at present. Usually no symptoms

Gastrointestinal system
Weight falling
Appetite good, craves sugary foods
Slight constipation
No other symptoms

Genitourinary system
Urinary symptoms as above
Some burning on passing urine, no blood
Discharge and pruritus vulvae as above
Periods regular, LMP 10.2.92

Nervous system
Slight blurring of vision (one month)
No other symptoms

Endocrine system
No thyroid or adrenal symptoms

ON EXAMINATION
Tired, unwell
No anaemia, cyanosis (blueness), jaundice (yellowness)
No xanthelasmata or arcus
No lymph node enlargement
Normal breasts

Cardiovascular system
Pulse 84 beats/mm, regular. Blood pressure 170/95 (lying and standing)
Carotid (neck artery) pulses normal, no bruits
Heart not enlarged
Heart sounds normal, no added sounds
No evidence cardiac failure
Peripheral pulses present, equal

Respiratory system
Respiratory rate 14/min
Expansion normal, equal
Percussion note resonant, equal
Breath sounds normal, no added sounds

Abdomen
Non-tender, no scars or masses
No enlargement liver, kidneys, spleen

Vaginal examination
Curd-like white discharge (swab sent), perineal redness, otherwise
examination normal

Nervous system
Eyes – visual acuity left 6/9, right 6/9
Lens normal
Fundi (the back of the eye) normal
Power and sensation normal, upper and lower limbs
Normal reflexes

Feet/legs
Blister right little toe (new shoes!)
Varicose vein surgery
Ingrowing toenail left great toe
Sensation and circulation normal

Diagnosis
Diabetes mellitus
Hypertension
Candida albicans
Blister and ingrowing toenail

The next stage would be some investigations.

TESTS

Blood glucose concentration

If the diagnosis has not been confirmed with a laboratory venous
glucose sample, then it must be (see pages 10–14).

 If the diagnosis is known, the doctor may still want to check
today's glucose level. Nowadays, many doctors do this with a
desktop meter.

Glycosylated haemoglobin

This is a measure of long-term glucose balance. Haemoglobin is the
chemical which makes your red blood cells red. When the haemoglobin is being incorporated into the red cells, glucose can bind with
it. This process is called glycosylation. The more glucose there is in

the circulation, the greater the proportion of haemoglobin that is glycosylated. This form of haemoglobin is called haemoglobin A$_{1C}$ and usually forms less than 7 per cent of the total haemoglobin (some laboratories have different normal ranges).

Other tests

A full blood count will check whether you are anaemic or have a raised white blood cell count which may indicate infection. Measurement of blood electrolyte level (see page 245) will indicate your body salt levels. Urea and creatinine assess state of hydration and kidney function (pages 143–5). Cholesterol and triglyceride are blood fats which may be raised in untreated diabetes (pages 160–1). A chest X-ray is done to exclude chest infections and look at the heart size. An electrocardiogram (pages 138–9) checks the heart function. Microbiological examination of a midstream urine sample can show a urine infection.

SUMMARY

- Tell your doctor what (if anything) you have noticed wrong.
- Tell him your previous medical history, obstetric history and family history.
- Tell him what medication you take and whether you suffer from any allergies.
- Describe your eating habits and be honest about smoking and drinking alcohol.
- Your doctor will usually examine you carefully to check your general health and the effect (if any) that the diabetes has had upon it. The detail of the examination may vary.
- Then he may do some tests including blood glucose level and haemoglobin Al$_c$.

4

WHAT IS DIABETES? WHY ME?

So now you know that you have diabetes and have had a careful initial assessment. But what is diabetes and why have you got it?

WHAT IS DIABETES?

Diabetes is a condition in which the blood glucose is above normal because your body can no longer use the glucose you absorb from digested food. The name was coined by Aretaeos the Cappedocian in the second to third century AD from a Greek word *diabetes* meaning 'siphon'. 'Diabetes is a mysterious illness ... being a melting down of the flesh and limbs into urine.' Centuries later it was found that in some forms of diabetes the urine tasted sweet like honey (mellitus) and in others it was tasteless (insipidus). You have diabetes mellitus. Diabetes insipidus is due to lack of the water-concentrating hormone, anti-diuretic hormone, and is nothing to do with diabetes mellitus.

But it is very important to understand that the problem is not just one of blood glucose balance. Diabetes can affect many of the chemical processes and tissues in the body. It is a multi-system disorder. This is why your doctor and diabetes team check you over so carefully. Many people, even those who have had diabetes for years, do not realise that diabetes care is not simply a matter of eating the proper diet and taking the diabetic tablets to correct the high blood glucose. For example, they do not connect their foot ulcer with having diabetes. But it is all part of the same condition.

You and your doctors must care for your whole body not just your blood glucose.

So the true definition must be: diabetes mellitus is a chronic multi-system disorder defined by an abnormally high blood glucose concentration.

BODY GLUCOSE BALANCE

Food

We obtain glucose by digesting the carbohydrate foods we eat. These starchy or sugary foods (e.g. bread, potato, beans, rice, pasta, sugar, sweets, candy, biscuits) are first prepared by processing or cooking in an infinite variety of ways (for example, boiled potatoes, mashed potatoes, fried potatoes, chips, crisps etc.) Then we eat them. They are broken down into a lumpy mush by chewing and then swallowed. Already digestive enzymes (breakdown chemicals) in the saliva are starting to work on the food. The chewed mush passes down the gullet or oesophagus into the stomach (see diagram on page 29). There it is churned around and mixed with stomach juices which contain acid. This kills off most bacteria and helps to further break down the food. The stomach pushes the food out into the first part of the gut, the duodenum, where the digestive juices from the pancreas and the gall bladder (bile) are mixed in with the food. As it passes on through the duodenum into the jejunum and then the ileum, the food is being broken down into a thin soup containing simpler and simpler substances. As the soup of food and digestive juices passes through the small bowel (duodenum, jejunum and ileum) the simple particles into which the food has been digested are absorbed through the bowel wall into the bloodstream. This includes glucose, which is the simple sugar into which most carbohydrate foods are broken down. Other simple sugars include lactose (from milk) and fructose (from fruit, although fruit sugar is also broken down into glucose). Undigested food, e.g. fibre, and other wastes are passed from the small bowel into the large bowel or colon and are eventually passed as faeces.

Glucose is the body's main fuel. As the glucose absorbed from the small bowel travels along in the bloodstream it first passes through the liver. The liver acts as a storage depot for glucose. Much of the glucose will stay in the liver until it is needed. But, without help, glucose cannot leave the bloodstream and enter the body cells (the tiny units from which all body tissues are made).

The chemical which allows glucose to enter liver cells and those of other tissues is called insulin. It is made in the pancreas in clusters of cells called the islets of Langerhans. These islets are dotted about the pancreas amongst the rest of the cells which are busy making digestive juices. Within the islets of Langerhans are the beta cells whose main job is to make insulin. You cannot see

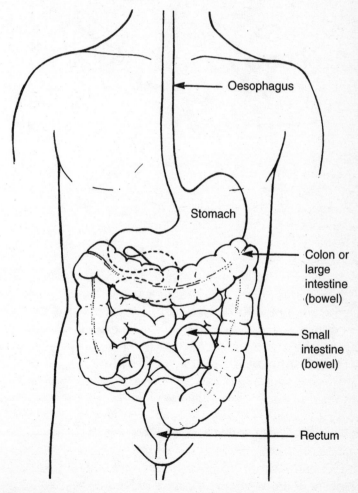

Oesophagus

Stomach

Colon or large intestine (bowel)

Small intestine (bowel)

Rectum

The digestive system

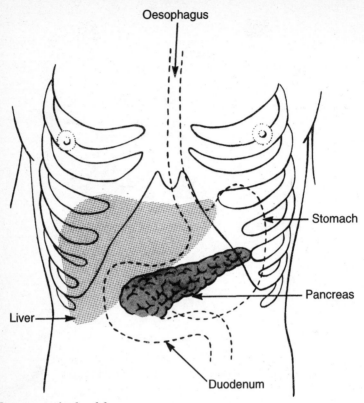

The pancreas in the abdomen

your pancreas, or feel it, for it lies hidden behind the stomach and in front of the backbone, deep in your abdomen.

Insulin is a hormone, a chemical made in one group of cells and released into the bloodstream to influence processes elsewhere in the body. It is made inside the beta cell and stored as granules until it is needed. In a non-diabetic, a rise in glucose triggers special nervous and chemical signals in the pancreas which stimulate the beta cells to release their stored insulin into the bloodstream. A fall in glucose 'switches off' insulin release.

The way in which insulin links with the body's cells and enables glucose to enter has been discovered in considerable detail through years of painstaking research all over the world. On the surface of many cells are specially shaped areas called insulin receptors. They are shaped to be an exact fit for insulin, rather like a keyhole waiting

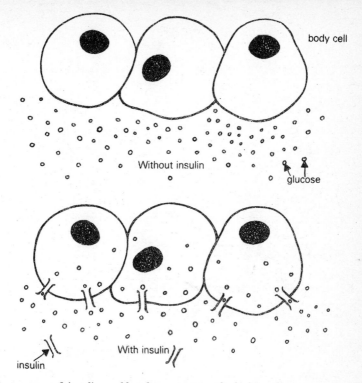

The presence of insulin enables glucose to enter the body's cells.

for a particular key. The insulin acts as the key. When the insulin key fits into the keyhole, a chain of chemical changes occurs in the wall of that cell and glucose is passed through the cell wall, rather like a key opening a door.

So glucose cannot enter the body's cells without insulin, and insulin cannot work without insulin receptors.

Cells are like little factories – they have a considerable variety of functions. Once inside the cell, glucose is either burned up as a fuel or stored for future use. It is stored in big clumps called glycogen. When the blood glucose levels fall, as in vigorous exercise for example, the beta cells stop releasing insulin and the lack of insulin allows breakdown of glycogen back into glucose. This is either used up there and then or released into the bloodstream for other cells to use. The cells which use most glucose are muscles. It is glucose which fuels your press-ups or your walk to work. It is glucose which keeps your heart muscle pumping. But muscles can also use other fuels derived from fats. One part of the body is wholly dependent on glucose – the brain. It is glucose which keeps your brain ticking over and fuels those brilliant (and for that matter, not-so-brilliant) ideas.

Normally the body keeps all its body systems in balance and if any of its processes are upset it reacts to return them to normal (homeostasis – see page 8). Through its complex systems of insulin release and the storage of glucose or the breakdown of glycogen, the body maintains the blood glucose levels at about 4–8 mmol/l no matter what you do. A huge chocolate pudding or a 10-mile run cause no major fluctuation in blood glucose level. But if you have diabetes this finely tuned system fails. Two main factors appear to be involved – insulin manufacture and release, and insulin receptors.

TYPES OF DIABETES

There are two main types of diabetes – Type 1 and Type 2

Type 1 Diabetes Mellitus
(Insulin-Dependent Diabetes Mellitus)

This is the form of diabetes which predominantly affects children and young people. It is also called juvenile onset diabetes. This form of diabetes is due to a complete failure of insulin production. Type 1 diabetes occurs in about 0.5% of the population (all ages).

People with Type 1 diabetes appear to inherit a lack of protection from diabetes. Our genetic material is handed down to us in chromosomes which are double strands of a special protein called deoxyribonucleic acid or DNA for short. DNA is made of tiny particles called amino acids which are arranged in sequences. One of these amino acids (on Chromosome 6) is replaced with others in people with diabetes. One theory is that the person is then vulnerable to an upset, such as a viral infection, which can trigger the body to destroy its own beta cells. This process is called an autoimmune reaction (*auto* = self, *immune* = defence mechanism). It is really a natural example of chemical warfare, going on inside you. Foreign substances, called antigens, for example chemicals carried by bacteria, are detected by the body's defence cells – the white blood cells. They react by making antibodies which destroy the antigens. In diabetes, the white cells perceive substances on the wall of the beta cells as antigens and make antibodies which destroy them.

As the beta cells die, less and less insulin is made and released and the blood glucose rises rapidly. In Type 1 diabetes, islet cell antibodies can be detected months or years before the development of diabetes, but when the major destructive process begins, it is rapid and most of the beta cells are destroyed within weeks. So other processes must be at work too.

People with newly-diagnosed Type 1 diabetes are usually under 40 years of age, sometimes children, who are slim (or even thin) and have had severe thirst, polyuria and weight loss for a few weeks. They usually feel ill. If they do not receive insulin quickly they will become extremely ill. Before the discovery of insulin in 1922, children with Type 1 diabetes did not survive. But with insulin people feel better within days.

Without insulin you will break down body fat into chemicals called ketones. High ketone levels make the blood acid – ketoacidosis. This causes deep breathing, vomiting and coma. Get medical help urgently (see pages 208-9).

Type 2 Diabetes Mellitus
(Non Insulin-Dependent Diabetes Mellitus)

This form of diabetes is much more common than Type 1 and tends to occur in the over 40s. Overall, one in 70 adults has Type 2 diabetes and knows it, another one in 70 has it without realising – a total incidence of about 3%. Again, the incidence is increasing. However, the incidence of Type 2 diabetes varies among different communities. Known diabetes is about four times more common in the Asian community than in the rest of the population. Within the Asian community Type 2 diabetes starts in a younger age group (being most often diagnosed in those in their 30s or 40s) and the incidence increases with age so nearly one in five Asian people over 60 is known to have diabetes. This is an underestimate – the true incidence in some sections of the Asian community can be as high as 25 per cent. Diabetes is also more common in people whose ancestors came from Africa or the Caribbean Islands.

There is some debate as to the exact cause of the problem. Once again the vulnerability to diabetes is inherited – more strongly than in Type 1 diabetes. Indeed, it has been estimated that as many as 25 per cent of the first-degree relatives (that is parents, brothers, sisters) of someone with Type 2 diabetes had, have or will develop diabetes.

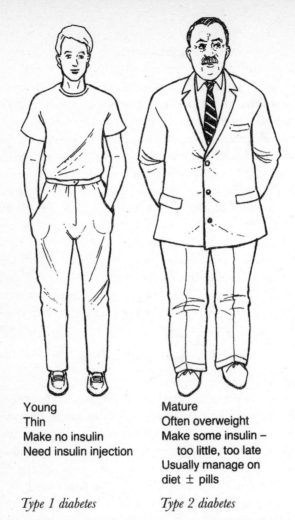

Young
Thin
Make no insulin
Need insulin injection

Type 1 diabetes

Mature
Often overweight
Make some insulin –
    too little, too late
Usually manage on
diet ± pills

Type 2 diabetes

People with Type 2 diabetes are capable of making insulin – indeed for years it was thought that they might even make more than non-diabetic people. However, recent work has shown that older ways of measuring insulin measure insulin-related chemicals as well as insulin, producing falsely high 'insulin' levels.

There are several theories. One is that Type 2 diabetes is due to a lack of insulin receptors or to abnormalities within the receptor. Overweight people have been shown to have fewer insulin receptors and it was thought that such people would have to make more insulin to try to overcome this problem. Eventually, the exhausted beta cells 'wear themselves out'. High plasma insulin levels have been found in overweight people with Type 2 diabetes. Another theory is that the beta cells are making some insulin, but not enough and they are not releasing it at the right time. This can be demonstrated by giving people a glucose meal or injecting sterile glucose into a vein and measuring the insulin response.

There has been much excitement at the discovery that in people with Type 2 diabetes the beta cells are replaced with a solid, stranded material called amyloid. An apparent amyloid precursor has been found in beta cells and in the bloodstream. But, as yet, there is no proof that this is the cause of diabetes rather than the end result of a destructive process.

It seems likely that several factors may combine to produce the same end result – an inability to cope with glucose. Overweight people do usually need more insulin per unit body weight (e.g. a unit of insulin per kilogram of body weight per 24 hours) to return their glucose to normal than a slim person (e.g. a third of a unit of insulin per kilogram per 24 hours). This is probably a cause of diabetes in some instances.

Other causes of diabetes

Pregnancy Diabetes or glucose intolerance can occur during pregnancy because of the dramatic rises in sex hormones at that time. This is called gestational diabetes. It may disappear completely after the baby is born, but can continue permanently. If you have had gestational diabetes in one pregnancy you are likely to have it again in later pregnancies. And you are more likely than other women to become diabetic later on so you should maintain a normal weight, exercise regularly and have an annual check on your blood glucose.

Pancreatic damage or surgery If you have had inflammation of the pancreas, the most common cause of which is long-term alcohol excess, or an operation on the pancreas, the beta cells may be removed or damaged and you may develop diabetes. In addition, the cells which make pancreatic digestive juices may also be damaged and you may not digest your food properly. Weight loss and fatty, pale faeces, should alert you and your doctor to the need to add pancreatic extracts to your food or to swallow them as capsules. People who have drunk sufficient alcohol to cause this condition may also have heart damage, brain damage and nerve damage. There are other causes of pancreatic inflammation too.

Drugs – steroids, other hormones, and thiazides Steroids are the hormones (see page 30) made by the adrenal glands, which sit on top of the kidneys. In the small quantities usually produced in the body, they are essential for our survival. They are also useful in treating allergic conditions, like asthma, severe inflammation, some forms of muscle problem and artery inflammation. In these big doses, they can cause diabetes. The more steroids you have to take, the higher will be your blood glucose. When the dose falls, so will your glucose levels, but you may remain diabetic.

The sex hormones in the contraceptive pill can cause glucose intolerance or worsen existing diabetes.

Thiazide diuretics are pills given to increase urine production in conditions like high blood pressure and heart failure with swollen ankles. If you have any tendency to diabetes, thiazides may bring it out. However, they do not seem to cause problems with glucose balance if used to treat high blood pressure in people with existing diabetes.

Other hormone conditions Thyroid hormone overactivity (thyrotoxicosis) or growth hormone overactivity (acromegaly) can be associated with diabetes. Overproduction of steroid hormones by the body can also cause diabetes.

Iron deposition in the pancreas can cause diabetes. This occurs in people on treatment for thalassaemia (an inherited blood condition) and in haemochromatosis.

Tropical diabetes This does not occur in Britain. It is seen in tropical countries and is thought to be related to starvation or perhaps to contaminants in food.

WHY ME?

Some of you will have been able to identify the type of diabetes you have, but many may still be unsure. Do not worry, it is not essential to label your diabetes as the treatment will simply be tailored to you and your needs.

Some of you may be teetotal men or women on no medication with no family history of diabetes. You may not be able to find anything to blame for your diabetes – in your case it has just happened. Although it is human nature to look for an event or person to blame when we become ill, it is not always a good idea to do this as it can lead to frustration and retrospection when one should be looking ahead to feeling better and getting on with life. Your diabetes is not your fault.

SUMMARY

- The two main types of diabetes are Type 1 and Type 2 diabetes.
- Type 1 diabetes occurs mainly in thin under 40s, with rapid onset of severe symptoms. It requires insulin treatment. It is caused by insulin deficiency.
- Type 2 diabetes occurs mainly in overweight over 40s, with more gradual onset of variable symptoms. It is treated by diet alone, or diet and pills or insulin. It is caused by a combination of inadequate insulin release and insulin resistance.
- Both Type 1 and Type 2 diabetes can occur at any age, in men or women, whatever their weight.
- Other causes of diabetes include pregnancy, pancreatic damage, steroids, thiazides and other drugs.
- Whatever its cause, diabetes can always be treated.

5

GETTING STARTED

The doctor has told you that you definitely have diabetes. You may have been expecting it, or it may have come as a shock. Until they are told that the diagnosis is certain most people have been hoping that it is all a mistake. 'This can't be happening to me.' It can be especially startling for people who have had no symptoms of diabetes. 'How can I be ill if I don't feel ill?'

COMING TO TERMS WITH DIABETES

All of us think that our bodies should work perfectly. Illness is what happens to other people. When people become ill, especially when they develop a long-term illness, they react in different ways. Some people think it must be someone's fault. They look for someone, or something to blame. 'If my wife hadn't left me I would never have got diabetes.' 'It's all because that man drove into my car. It was the shock that did it. He gave me diabetes.' But as the previous chapter shows, most people who have diabetes are born with the potential to develop the condition.

Other people think it is all their own fault. 'I must have done something wrong.' 'I ate too much sugar.' They perhaps feel that they are being punished. 'God is punishing me because I have done something wrong. He is trying me.' But it is not their fault that they have diabetes. Nor is it anyone else's fault.

For some, the discovery of diabetes is a numbing blow and they feel as if their world has come to an end. Everything seems impossible, their plans are shattered, and there is no hope. Some people favour the ostrich approach. 'If I don't think about it, it will go away.' 'It isn't really happening. It is all a dream.' But if you bury your diabetes in the sand, you will get sandy too.

There are people who are very matter-of-fact about their diabetes. They betray little emotion about it all and carry on at work and at home as if nothing has happened. Some people are good at coping with new problems in this way. Others find themselves reacting with anger or sorrow later.

Most people with newly diagnosed diabetes have a mixture of emotions. Shock, some anger at fate for giving you this, some tears that you are not as well as you thought you were, some pretending it is not happening. But most people cope.

No one comes to terms with diabetes overnight. But, gradually, you need to try to accept that you have a condition which will, in the majority of cases, be with you for ever. It will need some attention from you every day. This may just be in terms of watching what you eat and checking your blood glucose occasionally, or it may be managing your insulin injection treatment. You will need regular medical check-ups – at least once a year. Your diabetes can make you unwell in years to come, but this is less likely if you look after yourself now and continue to do so.

Do not be too tough on yourself. There is no right or wrong way to come to terms with having diabetes. It is not wrong to shout or cry or bottle it up. Learn about your condition and its management step by step. No one is ever a perfect diabetic. After all, no one is ever a perfect human being.

Fears and worries

Most people know very little about diabetes until it happens to them or to one of their family. They just hear about the dramatic aspects and the old wives' tales. So let me put some of these stories right straightaway.

Diabetes rarely makes people collapse dramatically, as portrayed in television dramas. Diabetes does not make people go mad. Diabetes will not stop you from having a family. Diabetes will not stop you from being a good mother, father, wife, husband. Diabetes rarely interferes with people's jobs. Diabetes will not make you go blind, if you look after yourself. Diabetes will not stop you from enjoying your food. Diabetes will not stop you from having fun.

Think positively

Some people feel that becoming diabetic, despite its demands on their body and their time, actually enriches their life. A young woman who had recently developed diabetes said 'Being diabetic has made me a stronger person.' Another, who had changed from an overweight, inactive person eating junk food to a slim man who ate healthy food and exercised regularly said 'I'm fitter now than I've ever been.'

THE FIRST FEW DAYS

information you need from your doctor

The diagnosis You need to know that you definitely have diabetes. Ask your doctor to tell you the diagnostic blood glucose values.

The cause Has the diabetes arisen because of an inherited tendency to diabetes? Is it secondary to another condition or being worsened by another condition which needs separate treatment? If so, what is it and what treatment does it require?

If you are taking medication which has precipitated your diabetes (e.g. steroid pills) or which is worsening it (e.g. thiazides – water or blood pressure pills) you need to know this. Should you stop this medication, reduce the dose or change it to something else? It can be dangerous to stop steroid pills suddenly.

Chemical imbalance Is your problem mainly the glucose imbalance of your new diabetes or are other body chemicals awry? Does any of the chemical imbalance need urgent treatment? If so, what?

Tissue damage Has your diabetes damaged any of your body tissues? If yes, which tissue and what treatment is needed? Is the treatment urgent?

Diet

The foundation of diabetes treatment is sensible eating – the right foods in the right quantities at the right times. But don't panic. If you eat the wrong thing occasionally nothing terrible will happen. Eventually you will be able to tailor the rest of your diabetes treatment to the healthy eating pattern that suits you best.

What to eat and drink If you eat or drink a glass of cola or some boiled sweets, the glucose they contain enters the bloodstream rapidly and your blood glucose rises fast. But your body cannot cope with glucose as well as other people's, so you will not clear all this glucose. Your blood glucose will remain high for some time. If, on the other hand, you eat starchy, high-fibre carbohydrate foods like beans or wholemeal bread, they will be digested slowly and the glucose that they contain will arrive in the bloodstream slowly so that your body has a chance to deal with it. So cut down on sugar and sugary foods.

Your body is not very good at coping with fat, either. Your blood fats may be high (see pages 160–1). So it is sensible to eat less fat. Cut the fat off your meat and be sparing with butter and greasy foods.

Quench your thirst with a variety of drinks – water, tea, coffee or sugar-free 'diet' drinks. Do not drink colas and other fizzy drinks that contain glucose or sugar (sucrose). Avoid alcohol at present – you can drink alcohol in moderation when your diabetes is sorted out.

How much to eat If you are thin obey your appetite. If you feel hungry eat. If you are overweight you must watch the amounts you eat. Cutting out sugar and reducing fat will help you to lose weight but you should also watch the total quantities that you eat. Try to take smaller helpings. You may need to eat less than your appetite demands. Fill the gaps with salad and vegetables – lettuce, cabbage, celery, tomato etc.

When to eat Eat three meals a day, spaced out evenly. If you are on insulin treatment, eat three snacks a day as well – mid-morning, mid-afternoon and before bed.

Diet alone An adjustment to your diet may be all you need to control your diabetes. In this case it is very important that you stick to it. After all, no one wants to take tablets or injections unless they are strictly necessary.

Pills

Your doctor may prescribe pills (see Chapter 8) to help your pancreas to release more insulin and to help the insulin to work more efficiently in the body tissues. These pills are called oral hypoglycaemic drugs (*oral* – taken by mouth, *hypo* – low, *glycaemic* blood glucose). Ask the name of your pills. Write it down. Make sure you know exactly what dose to take and at which times of day.

Most glucose-lowering drugs carry the risk of lowering the blood glucose below normal – that is, below 4 mmol/l. If this happens you may notice unusual feelings or become unwell (see pages 109–110). It is called hypoglycaemia. The symptoms include confusion, slow thinking, sweating, shaking and palpitations (a fast heartbeat). If you feel like this, eat some glucose or sugar and contact your doctor or diabetic sister (diabetes specialist nurse) when you feel better.

Insulin

If you are not making any insulin you will need insulin injections to replace the missing insulin. This is nothing to be frightened about. The injections are given through special, very fine needles which sting no more than a gnat bite when they go into the skin. Soon, you will learn how to give the injections yourself and it will become as routine as styling your hair or shaving. Chapter 9 describes insulin treatment in detail.

Today you need to know the name of your insulin, the dose your doctor advises and when to take it – usually about 20 minutes before breakfast and 20 minutes before your main evening meal. Write this information down.

The doctor, diabetes specialist nurse or other diabetes team member will show you how to draw up your insulin (or set your insulin pen) and how to inject. Often people give their own first injection and continue to give their own insulin. It is not nearly such a big hurdle as most people imagine. You just pinch up a fold of skin and fat, put the needle in, push the plunger down, pull the needle out and press on the injection site briefly. It can take less time to do than reading the last sentence aloud.

Insulin can cause hypoglycaemia. If you feel muddled, slow thinking, sweaty, shaky or have palpitations, eat some glucose or sugar and then call your diabetes adviser or GP.

Diabetes card

Your diabetes adviser will give you a card to carry with you all the time. It is important that you carry it. If you have an accident or become ill and have to go to hospital, the doctors need to know that you have diabetes.

Carry glucose

If you are on glucose-lowering pills or insulin injections, you must carry glucose tablets (e.g. Dextrosol, Lucozade, Boots etc.) or sugar with you all the time just in case you become hypoglycaemic. Hypoglycaemia is usually easy to cope with, but it is important to be prepared.

Checking your own blood glucose

You need some means of monitoring your own condition so that you can see if your diet and any other diabetes treatment is working. At one time everyone with diabetes tested their urine for glucose either by dropping urine and water onto fizzy tablets, or by dipping a strip into the urine. Nowadays, people with all types of diabetes are monitoring their own blood glucose directly. You do not have to do this at the beginning but most people find that self-monitoring of blood glucose gives them a lot more confidence in looking after their diabetes.

Your diabetes adviser will help you to learn how to monitor your own blood glucose (see also Chapter 6). It is well worth it.

Work

In most instances, you will not need time off work. However, if you are feeling unwell or if you are starting insulin treatment, it is sensible to take a few days off work until your diabetes is sorted out and you are feeling better.

A few people taking insulin (and sometimes glucose-lowering pills) will need to review their job. Airline pilots, drivers of passenger-carrying vehicles or large goods vehicles, divers and those in some other high-risk occupations will probably not be allowed to continue in their current post. Discuss this with your doctor and your employer, as the situation is changing (see pages 167–70).

Driving

The British Driving Licence which many of you will be carrying states 'You are required to tell the Drivers Medical Branch, DVLC, Swansea, 5A99 ITU at once if you have any disability (includes any physical or mental condition which affects (or may in future affect) your fitness as a driver if you expect it to last more than 3 months).' Diabetes is such a condition and you are compelled by law to inform the DVLC (now called DVLA) as soon as diabetes has been diagnosed. The new licence mentions diabetes specifically. There are similar requirements in other countries. (See pages 170–2).

Motor insurance companies regard diabetes as a 'material fact'. In other words you are strongly advised to tell your car insurance company that you have diabetes.

Do not drive a car, or ride a bicycle or motor bike for a week after starting glucose-lowering pills or insulin injections – discuss the exact length of time with your diabetes adviser.

Back-up

All over the world there are groups of people with diabetes who are willing to befriend new diabetics and help them to learn how to manage their condition. Diabetes UK is one of the oldest of these organisations and there are local Diabetes UK groups throughout the country. Ask your diabetes adviser for the name and address of your nearest Diabetes UK group. Join your local diabetes association – it will provide information and support.

Help

Very important Before you leave the clinic, surgery or hospital, make certain that you have written down the name(s) and telephone numbers of the people to contact if you are in difficulty with your diabetes. This includes an out-of-hours contact number. If things do go wrong you can almost guarantee that it will be at 3 am on a Bank Holiday.

If you need help, telephone sooner rather than later. The father of one of my patients with diabetes always taught his son that 'No question is ever stupid if it has to be a question'. All health care professionals would rather answer a simple question now than have to give you emergency treatment later. Many people are worried about troubling their GP and even more worried about troubling hospital staff. Diabetes is a condition in which there is constant personal contact between patients and staff at all levels. Much of the day-to-day contact is by telephone. So you need never be afraid to bother the doctor or the rest of the diabetes team – that is what we are there for.

SUMMARY

- Learn to live with your diabetes.
- Make sure you write down the information you need to keep you going for the first few days – what is going on, what tests or changes in existing treatment are needed, what to eat, what pills or insulin to take, how to check your glucose, what to do about work.
- Carry a diabetic card and emergency glucose or sugar.
- Tell the DVLA and your motor insurance company you have diabetes.
- Join Diabetes UK and get in touch with your local support group.
- Make sure you know who to call for help. Write down their telephone number. Find out who your diabetes adviser is (diabetes specialist nurse). They will provide specialist diabetes advice.
- Do not be afraid to ask for help. That is what we are here for.

6

BLOOD OR URINE GLUCOSE TESTING

This is the key to freedom. If you can know, with certainty, what your blood glucose is at any time, anywhere, then you can adjust your own treatment.

Technology is moving very fast. By the time this book is published there will be new testing techniques. Most tests rely on obtaining a drop of blood from a finger tip or ear lobe and placing it on a strip which either changes colour or transmits signals directly to a meter. The colour changes can be read by eye or by a meter.

THE LABORATORY IN YOUR HAND

We believe laboratory results because we know that tests are done carefully, with trained precision and quality assurance on well-maintained equipment. If you are to produce similarly accurate results, you too must perform the test carefully, with trained precision on well-maintained equipment. If you do not follow the instructions exactly, literally down to the last second, the results you obtain will be at best meaningless, at worst disastrous.

But these tests are simple and, with practice, you will have no difficulty in obtaining results comparable with those of a big laboratory.

Preparing your fingers

Most people use their fingers, although a few use their ear lobe while looking in a mirror. Your hands should be clean – wash them

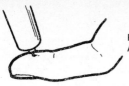

Prick clean warm finger to obtain a big drop of blood. A finger-pricking device is better than a lancet alone.

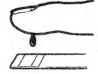

Drop blood on to a stick, covering test pad completely. Do not rub or smudge.

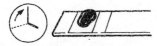

Leave drop on test pad for specified time (check manufacturer's instructions).

Clean blood from test pad and wait extra time (check manufacturer's instuctions).

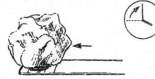

Wipe, e.g. BM-test 1–44   Blot e.g. Glucostix.

Insert into meter according to instructions or

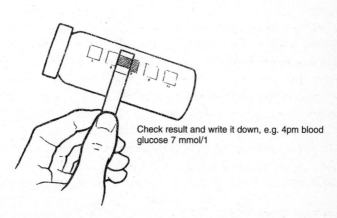

Check result and write it down, e.g. 4pm blood glucose 7 mmol/1

Measuring blood glucose

in warm water, rinse all soap off and dry them on a clean towel. There is no need to use antiseptic swabs – in any case, they make your result inaccurate. If your hand is warm nothing else need be done. If you have difficulty getting blood out or it is cold, try to warm your hand up. Also hold it downwards towards your legs and shake the hand vigorously. You will see the fingertips go pink with blood.

Pricking your fingers

You can simply use a sterile lancet (they are manufactured for single use only). Most people find an automatic finger-pricker helpful. These devices include Autolancet, B-D Lancer 5, Glucoject, Glucolet, Hypolance, Microlet, Autolet, Monojector, Penlet, Soft-touch and others. Load the lancet into the device and then press a platform onto the side of your finger. To start with you may find it easier to rest your hand on a table. Then trigger the device. If you are the only person using the finger-pricker you can reuse platforms if they are clean. If someone else uses the device they must have a new platform as well as a new lancet – and so must you when you next use it. There are usually several different platforms for different pricking depths so find the one that suits your fingers.

If your finger is warm the blood will ooze out on its own. If not, milk it up from the base of the finger. Do not squeeze the finger-tip tightly as this dilutes the blood with fluid and gives you sore fingers.

MEASURING THE BLOOD GLUCOSE CONCENTRATION

Colour-change strips

The first testing system was Dextrostix from which the blood had to be washed before reading. These are rarely used today. The two commonest visually read colour change strips are BM glycemie strips 1–44 (Chemstrips bG in USA) and Glucostix. There are others including Hypoguard.

Before starting you should check that the strips are in date. Hold the strip with the reagent pad upwards and drop the blood onto the pad, covering it, just enough – not too much and not too little – with no smears. Instantly start timing with a watch with a second hand.

The glucose in the blood is reacting with the glucose oxidase in the pad to produce a colour change in the dyes with which the pad is impregnated. As soon as the time indicated in the instructions is up,

Finger Prickers and Compatible Lancets

Compatible Lancets	Auto Lancet	Autolet	Autolet Lite	Autolet Mini	B-D Lancer 5	Glucoject	Glucolet	Hypolance	Microlet	Monojector	Penlet II	Soft Touch	Softclix II
Ames		•	•				•						
Baylet	•	•	•	•	•		•	•	•	•	•	•	
BID Microfine +	•			•	•	•	•		•	•	•	•	
Finepoint	•		•	•			•		•		•		
GlucoTip		•	•	•	•	•			•			•	
Microlet	•	•	•	•	•		•	•	•	•	•	•	
Milward Steri-let	•	•	•	•	•		•	•	•	•	•	•	
Milward Steri-let Ultra -Fine	•	•	•	•	•		•	•	•	•	•	•	
Monolet	•	•	•	•	•		•	•	•	•	•	•	
Monolet -Extra		•	•	•									
Softclix 11													•
Unilet GP	•			•	•	•			•	•	•	•	
Unilet Superlite		•	•				•						
Unilet GP Superlite	•			•		•			•		•	•	
Unilet Universal Comfort Touch	•	•	•	•	•	•	•		•	•	•	•	
Vitrex	•	•	•	•	•		•	•	•	•	•	•	

*N.B.: Finger pricking devices are not prescribable at NHS expense.

C/I = Contraindications. S/P = Special precautions. INT = Drug interactions. ADR = Adverse drug reactions.
Prices – Normal type = NHS price, P = private prescription price, R = recommended retail price inc. VAT.

Blood Glucose Testing Strips and Meters

Meter	Sensitivity Range (mmol/l)	Manufacturer	Retail Price (exc. VAT)	Advantage II	BM Accutest	BM Test 1–44	Glucometer Esprit Sensors	ExacTech	GlucoMenTest Sensors	Glucostix	Glucolide	Glucotrend Plus	Hypoguard Supreme	Hypoguard Supreme spectrum	MediSense G2	MediSense Optium	Medi-Test Glycaemic C	Pocketscan	Prestige Smart System
AccuChek Advantage	0·6-33·3	Roche Diag.	£25·00	•															
Accutrend	1·1-33·3	Roche Diag.	£34·00		•														
Accutrend GC*	1·1-33·3	Roche Diag.	£199·00		•														
Exec Tech	2·2-25	Medi Sense	£59·00					•											
GlucoMen Glyco	1·1-33·3	Menarini Diag.	£35·00						•										
Glucometer 2!	1-44	Bayer	–							•									
Glucometer 4!	0·6-33·3	Bayer	–								•								
Glucometr Esprit	0·6-33·3	Bayer	£24·99				•												
Glucometer GX!	1-44	Bayer	–							•									
Glucotrend 2	0·6-33·3	Roche Diag.	£25·00									•							
Glucotrend Premium	0·56-33·3	Roche Diag.	£49·00									•							
Glycotronic C	1·1-33·3	BHR	£31·00															•	
Hypoguard Supreme Plus	2·22·0	Hypoguard (UK)	£35·00										•						
Hypoguard Supreme Extra	2·2-22·2	Hypoguard (UK)	£40·00											•					
MediSense Card	1·1-33·3	Medi Sense	£35·00												•				
MediSense Optium	1·1-33·3	Medi Sense	£45·00													•			
MediSense Pen	1·1-33·3	Medi Sense	£35·00												•				
Medisense Precision QID	1·1-33·3	Medi Sense	£35·00												•				
Pocketscan	1·1-33·3	Lifescan	£17·50															•	
Prestige Smart System	1·4-33·3	DiagnoSys Medical	£29·00																•

● Meters are not available at NHS expense.   * Combined Glucose/CholesterolMeter   ! Meter no longer marketed

© *Reproduced courtesy of August MIMS 2001. This information is updated monthly so for the latest advice consult the current edition.*

wipe the blood off firmly with cotton wool (BM strips) or blot it off firmly (Glucostix). Wait the remaining time and match the colour with the range on the bottle from which you took the strip. Use a good light, and keep out of the rain or wind while doing the test.

Blood glucose meters

Although meters are not available on the NHS, if properly used they make it much easier and more accurate to monitor your finger-prick blood glucose. Often, your local diabetes clinic or centre will be able to give you one – ask.

Meters use a variety of electronic techniques to read the colour change in the blood-testing strip. They are very accurate if used strictly according to instructions. This includes calibrating each new batch of strips (which must, of course, be the right ones for that particular meter). With some meters if you do not put enough blood on, or smear it, the result will be inaccurate. You must also follow any timing instructions carefully. Some meters will download into a computer to give you graphs and charts of your results. Examples of various meters are: AccuChek Advantage, Accutrend, ExacTech, Glucometers, Glucotrends, Hypoguards, Medisenses, One Touch Profile, Pocket Scan and Prestige Smart System. New devices appear often.

Devices are now being produced which measure glucose via skin pads (Glucowatch) or fine needle sensors. They still have to be calibrated with finger-prick glucose tests. Their place in diabetes care is still being evaluated and there are still some problems with their use (skin soreness with Glucowatch for example). They are not available on the NHS. Glucowatch may help those who are troubled by frequent hypoglycaemia without warning.

How do you get blood testing equipment?

All these devices should be obtained via your diabetes adviser. You can buy one from a pharmacist or medical shop. However, if possible get an expert to show you how to use it. In Britain, lancets and test strips are available on GP prescription. Meters are provided in various ways, depending on your diabetes service. Prescriptions are free if you take diabetic pills or insulin.

When to test

Whenever you want to or need to. If you are worried about your glucose, check it. Routinely you should check at least once a day. If you are a new diabetic, have changed your treatment, are pregnant or feel unwell, check your glucose four times a day. The standard times are before each meal and before bed. Pregnant women may be asked to check some after-meal (post-prandial) levels as well. If you are taking glucose-lowering pills, it is usually sufficient just to test before breakfast, fasting. On any treatment, if your blood glucose is above 19 mmol/l (342 mg/dl) and you feel ill, check every 2–4 hours and check urine ketones (page 31, 209).

Recording the result

Some meters have memories which will record a specific number of glucose tests. There are also systems in which the meter can download directly into a computer. However, most patients still write down their results in diaries. These results are your record, not the clinic's, although it helps if your doctor and/or diabetes adviser go through the results with you. There is no point in writing down imaginary results. Who are you fooling? Yourself. Most doctors can spot an invented record, even if they say nothing. If you have done no tests, say so.

It is important to be able to spot trends, so write the results in columns with the time of day at the top. The figure on page 52 shows a page from a particularly careful young woman's record. Scattered numbers in your appointment diary are helpful at the time but hard to evaluate later.

PROBLEMS

Poor vision

If you cannot see at all, there are talking meters – ask your diabetes adviser or your diabetic association. If you can see a little but not well enough to match colours, some meters have a large number display – ask to see one. If you have diabetic eye disease your colour vision may not be optimal. Use a meter. People who know they are colour blind should do this.

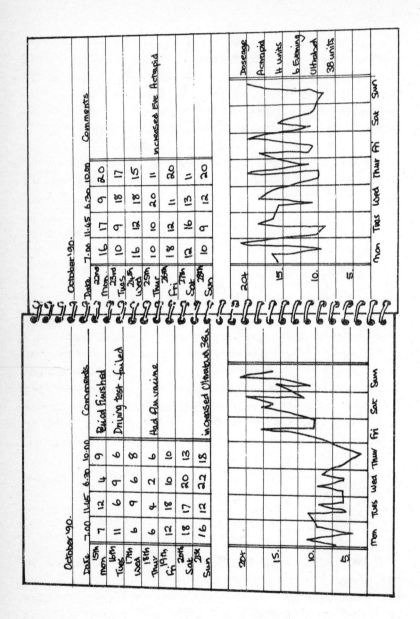

Blood glucose diary

Carelessness

Most problems are due to failure to follow the instructions for the strips or meter. Overfamiliarity breeds contempt. If you do not time the reaction properly you will get nonsense results. If you wipe the blood off on your trousers (I have seen it done) you will get very dirty trousers, and a dubious result. Get a proper sample and do not smear the blood. Keep the strips dry and in date.

Sticky finger

If you have anything sweet on your fingers all the test strip will measure is your finger candy level. This is a common trap in people with hypoglycaemia who have been eating glucose tablets. They get a high reading, think they are better, then become hypoglycaemic again.

The aim

You are aiming for a blood glucose concentration between 4 and 7 mmol/l (72 and 126 mg/dl). Below 4 mmol/l is heading for hypoglycaemia. Above 10 mmol/l (180 mg/dl) is too high and, if such high levels persist, may make you feel unwell, in addition to putting you at risk of tissue damage. It takes time and hard work to keep the blood glucose between 4 and 7 mmol/l, so do not get upset by the occasional value over 10 mmol/l. If you are taking glucose-lowering pills or insulin, you should go to bed with a blood glucose of 6 mmol/l or more (108 mg/dl) to protect you from night-time hypoglycaemia. Before breakfast you should aim for a fasting blood glucose between 4 and 6 mmol/l (72 and 108 mg/dl) Discuss your target with your diabetic adviser.

URINE GLUCOSE TESTING

This is an indirect method of estimating the blood glucose. Its limitations are discussed on page 10. However, many people still use it and some doctors advise urine testing for some non-insulin-treated patients. Ensure that your strips are in date and dry. Hold the strip into the stream of urine, tap off the excess liquid and start timing it. Glucose oxidase in the pad reacts with glucose and the dye in the pad to produce a colour change. When the time is up, match the colour against the chart on the bottle. If you prefer, pass urine into a completely clean container and dip the strip in. Then proceed as above.

It helps if you and your diabetes adviser check your renal threshold (page 9) before you use urine testing. You can do this by collecting urine for known time periods and matching urine glucose with simultaneous blood glucose samples. If you lose glucose into the urine very easily, or with difficulty, urine testing is not helpful in monitoring your diabetes.

Do the urine tests at the same intervals as blood tests, but remember that the urine reflects an average of the ups and downs of blood glucose over the time it has been filtered through the kidneys and collected in the bladder. Blood glucose testing is more accurate and gives you the glucose level at the time of the test.

The aim

You are aiming to have no glucose in the urine. The old counsel of keeping a touch of sugar in the urine may lead to persistently high blood glucose levels, as most people have a renal threshold around 10 mmol/l (180 mg/dl).

SUMMARY

- Blood glucose testing is the key to freedom for people with diabetes.
- Aim for a finger-prick glucose between 4 and 8 mmol/l (72–144 mg/dl).
- Choose the method which suits you and use it carefully.
- Test regularly to keep a check on your diabetes, and at other times when you are worried or ill, or when you are doing something unusual.
- Write the results down in a way that is easy to read.
- Act on abnormal results as advised by your diabetes team.
- Use urine testing if you prefer or if you cannot do blood tests, but be aware of its limitations.
- Aim to have no glucose in the urine.

7

HEALTHY EATING

The dictionary defines a diet as 'a mode of living, now only with especial reference to food'. This emphasises the integral part that eating plays in our lifestyle. Food is our means of staying alive, our comfort, a way of sharing or giving, our responsibility to our families and a great pleasure. The diet you need for your diabetes is still all of these things. In fact, it is the normal, healthy diet we should all be eating. In general, people with diabetes eat a much healthier diet than the rest of the population.

There are two parts to your diet. What you eat and drink and how much you eat and drink. It does not need to be complicated. You do not need to weigh out every morsel of food. You do not have to calculate complex exchanges, although some people on insulin injection treatment find these helpful. Nothing terrible will happen if you make the occasional mistake.

WHAT YOU EAT

Food is made up of carbohydrates, proteins, fats, fibre, minerals, vitamins and water. Carbohydrates, proteins and fats are be used by the body as fuels, for growth or for storage. Their fuel potential is measured in calories or kilojoules (one calorie = 4.2 kilojoules). Fats contain twice as many calories, weight for weight, as carbohydrates and proteins. If you take in more calories than you need, you will get fat. Fibre, minerals, vitamins and water do not contain calories and are neede to keep healthy.

Carbohydrates

These are starchy or sugary foods. Examples are bread, oats, potato, Chapati's, yam, plantain, pasta, rice, beans, root vegetables, sugar, glucose, sweets, cakes and candies. Some dietitians abbreviate carbohydrate to CHO. This can be confusing, as Bill and Myra (whom I described in *Diabetes Beyond 40*) found out.

Bill and Myra were in their mid-seventies when Bill developed diabetes. They both listened carefully to the enthusiastic young dietitian as she explained about Bill's diet. She wrote it all down for them and they took the diet sheet home to study carefully. They puzzled and puzzled over it. For every meal Bill was supposed to eat a strange food called CHO. Neither of them could remember what the dietitian had said about CHO but it was obviously important. So Myra set out with her shopping bag to buy some. She tried two supermarkets and in each a helpful assistant searched along the shelves – no CHOs. She tried a delicatessen and two pharmacies. Finally a pharmacist explained that CHO was simply an abbreviation for carbohydrate!

Complex carbohydrates

These are also known as unrefined or starchy carbohydrates. The starch in bread, potato, pasta, rice, beans, cereals and other similar foods is broken down by digestion into more simple carbohydrates such as glucose. As I explained in Chapter 5, these starchy carbohydrate foods are better for people with diabetes than are sugary foods, because starches take a long time to be digested and so release their glucose slowly.

Complex carbohydrates are often mixed with fibre in food. Fibre is the substance that stiffens plants and makes up their cell walls. It is not digested and remains in the bowel to act as roughage. There are two sorts of fibre – insoluble fibre and soluble fibre. Insoluble fibre is found in vegetables, bran, wholemeal bread and brown rice. It forms a tangle in which the starchy carbohydrate is embedded. Soluble fibre is that found in kidney beans, lentils, oats, baked beans and other legumes. It forms a glue-like solution containing the starchy carbohydrate. Soluble fibre is especially good at improving glucose balance in people with diabetes.

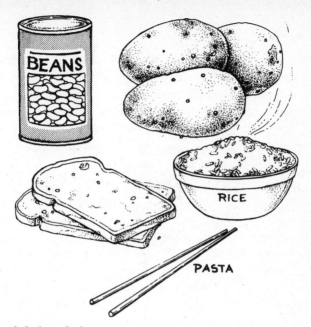

Some carbohydrate foods

Work in Oxford and elsewhere showed that in people with diabetes a diet in which 50–60 per cent of all calories are eaten as starchy carbohydrate high in fibre produced better glucose control than the old low carbohydrate diet. Base your meals and snacks on starchy carbohydrate, high in fibre.

Simple carbohydrates

These are also known as refined or sugary carbohydrates. The word 'sugar' is confusing. The granulated sugar we buy from the supermarket to put in our tea or cook with is sucrose, but the word sugar is also used more loosely in conversation to mean anything that tastes sweet. People talk about their blood sugar when they mean their blood glucose.

Simple carbohydrates include sucrose (which is made up of two glucoses), glucose itself, fructose or fruit sugar, and foods containing these – sweets; candies; sweet drinks such as pop, soda and cola; fruit; jelly (jello in America) and jams (jellies).

Simple carbohydrates are digested and absorbed rapidly, producing a sudden peak of glucose in the bloodstream. However, if they are associated with large amounts of fibre (for example as part of a wholemeal bread and jam sandwich, or in an apple or pear) the glucose will be absorbed more slowly. For many years people with diabetes were told that they must never eat sucrose but they were allowed fruit freely. This was illogical as some fruits contain sucrose. Studies have shown that the blood glucose rises no more after meals containing small amounts of sucrose with large amounts of starchy, high-fibre carbohydrate than after a meal containing the same number of calories eaten as complex carbohydrates alone. So eat an occasional treat such as cake, biscuit or dessert if you want

You can buy 'diabetic' foods in which the sucrose has been replaced by fructose. There is little evidence that long-term use of fructose is better than sucrose and it may, in fact, be worse. Fructose is broken down to compounds which may raise the blood glucose in people whose blood glucose is not optimally controlled. Furthermore, it may encourage a rise in one of the blood fats,

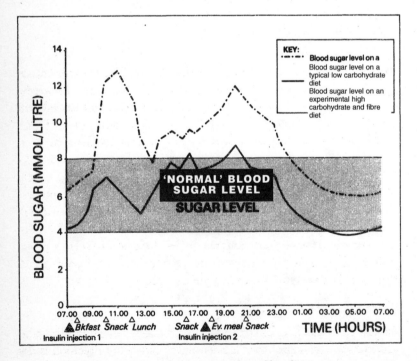

Improved diabetic control on a high carbohydrate fibre diet

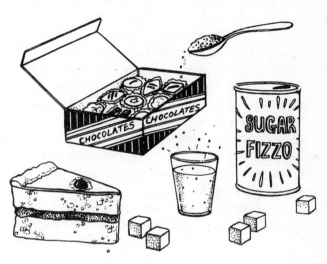

Foods containing simple sugars

triglyceride, which could be harmful long-term. The sensible course is to count fructose as a simple sugar like sucrose. Eat a moderate amount of natural fructose, as fruit for example, but do not eat extra fructose – there is no need to do so. You should eat lots of fruit and vegetables, both raw and cooked, at least 5 portions a day.

Avoid sugar in tea or coffee. Try to do without, or if you cannot, use an artificial sweetener in moderation – tiny quantities go a long way. (See Diabetes UK's leaflets on sweetners.) Use the smallest possible amount and try to do without if possible. Do not drink sweet drinks such as lemonade, colas, pop and other canned drinks. Use the 'diet' versions in moderation. Try mineral waters or dilute real fruit juice with mineral water or carbonated water. Small amounts of undiluted fruit juice are all right.

Carbohydrate exchanges

In the past much emphasis was placed upon weighing food and calculating exchanges exactly. Such time-consuming precision is not necessary. However, at first, weighing and reading the contents may help you to learn about different foods. Some people find it helpful to know how much carbohydrate there is in different foods so that they can eat similar amounts at each meal time or snack time. The standard exchange is 10 grammes of glucose. Thus a medium-sized apple is considered to contain the equivalent carbohydrate to 10 grammes of glucose. However, the way in which the food is prepared (e.g. boiled potato, mashed potato, crisps, potato soup) and the state of your insides determine how rapidly each form of that particular food is digested and its carbohydrate content absorbed.

Research workers in Oxford, Canada and elsewhere have used a measure called the glycaemic index to attempt to produce a more accurate comparison between carbohydrate foods. This compares the blood glucose rise, under standard conditions, after a particular carbohydrate food, with a standard carbohydrate load, has been eaten. The glycaemic index of the same food may vary depending on how it is prepared. For example, the blood glucose will rise more after apple juice than after cooked apple. It will rise least after eating a raw apple. This is why elaborate calculations of carbohydrate exchanges are misleading and unnecessary, and the diet for diabetes is not carbohydrate-restricted.

Proteins

These are found in meat, fish, milk, cheese, quorn, beans and pulses, soya, nuts and cereal foods. They are rarely found on their own and often have fat with them. We need protein for growth and repair. It is especially important that children have enough protein to develop their muscles and grow up. About 10–20 per cent of dietary calories should come from protein.

In the old days, people with diabetes were encouraged to eat lots of protein because it did not make the blood glucose rise straightaway. (In times of insulin lack, however, the body breaks down its own protein stores to make glucose – this process is called gluconeogenesis.) Cheese, was 'free', in other words, they could eat as much as they wanted. Sadly, cheese is laden with fat and we now know that too much fat is bad for your heart and blood vessels (see pages 160–1).

Eat some protein-containing foods each day. Vegetarians can find protein in plants such as soya, beans, peas and lentils as well as animals. Quorn is a useful meat substitute.

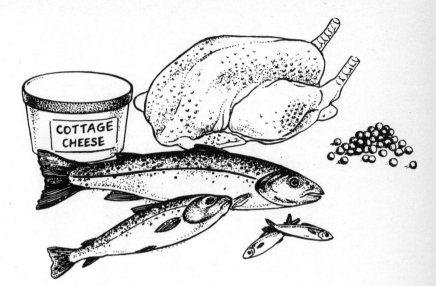

Protein foods

Fats

Fats are greasy or oily foods such as full cream milk, cream, butter, cheese, margarine, olive oil, sunflower oils, lard, dripping and meat fat. Nuts contain a lot of fat. There are also hidden fats in many foods – meat, cakes, biscuits, pastry and made-up meat dishes such as sausages and pork pies. Fats are very calorific – a small amount of fat gives you a lot of energy – or puts a lot of weight on.

People with diabetes need to be wary of fats for several reasons. Firstly, because many people with diabetes are trying to lose weight. People with diabetes are at risk of heart disease and often have high blood-fat concentrations. You should try to reduce your fat intake until 30 to 35 per cent of your daily calories comes from fat.

Buy low fat spreads rather than butter, use low fat yoghurt, eat lower fat cheeses (such as cottage cheese or Edam), and drink skimmed milk. Grill rather than fry, and drain the fat off oven-cooked meat. Reduce the amount of fat you use in cooking – do not add fat to stews or casseroles, and do not use it as a garnish on vegetables. Avoid rich puddings and gateaux. Scrape the spread onto your bread – any extra is excess calories. Cut off visible fat on

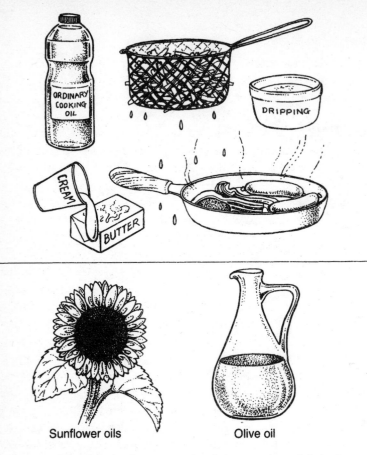

Sunflower oils   Olive oil

Some saturated fats (abve) polyunsaturated and monounsaturated (below)

your meat. Do not have bread and butter and cheese – just have the bread and cheese.

Polyunsaturated and monounsaturated fats

Your most important aim is to reduce your total fat content. However, you should also look at the type of fats you are eating. Saturated fats, such as those found in butter, cream, cheese and the fat on meat, are particularly likely to fur up your arteries. Some nuts also contain saturated fats. Polyunsaturated fats (such as sunflower spread) or monounsaturated fats (such as olive oil) are better for you. You should also include oily fish (e.g. herring, mackerel, sardines, salmon) in your diet.

Minerals and vitamins

If you eat a varied diet as described above, you will not need to add vitamin or mineral pills to your diet.

We all tend to eat too much salt or sodium chloride. There is no need to add extra salt at table. Many doctors believe that excessive salt intake elevates the blood pressure. It is sensible to restrict added salt to the minimum – there is plenty in our food. Avoid salt substitutes as they are high in potassium. Try herbs and spices to add flavour.

There is one situation in which you may need extra salt and that is if you are dehydrated or salt and water deficient. Dehydration can be caused by excess sweating (e.g. by exercising very vigorously for a long time or in hot weather), diarrhoea or vomiting, or by severe insulin lack causing polyuria. In this situation it is better to drink slightly salty water or salt-replacement solutions such as Diorylate than plain water. Ask your doctor about this. If the drink is unpalatable it is too salty.

Potassium is another mineral which we need in moderate amounts but which is harmful in excess. Most people do not need to worry about this – your body will keep you in perfect balance. However, if you are taking water pills (diuretics) for swollen ankles or shortness of breath, or as a treatment for high blood pressure, it is sensible to eat plenty of potassium-containing foods. These are citrus fruits, bananas, dried fruit such as apricots and tomatoes.

The majority of people obtain the vitamins they need from their food. If you are a very strict vegetarian or vegan you may become deficient in vitamin B_{12}. You will need to supplement this. There are now non-animal sources of B_{12} supplements. Ask your doctor.

Drinks

If you add up the number of drinks of all kinds that you take in each day you may be surprised at the total. Most people drink a minimum of six glasses or cups of fluid a day. Doctors usually assume that an average-sized adult needs three litres of fluid a day. Someone who is eating and drinking normally will have some of this as separate drinks and the rest mixed in with food – apples, soup and vegetables, for example. You can tell if you are taking in enough fluid by looking at your urine. It should be a pale straw colour. If it is very yellow or dark (what most of us would call concentrated) you need to drink more.

But which drink? You can have as much water as you want. Tea and coffee are fine in moderation, but too much caffeine will make you jittery. Recent research suggests that there is no need to change to caffeine-free coffee to protect your heart, but some people like it as an alternative to ordinary coffee. Fruit juice is good in small amounts but watch the sugar content. Check the labels of canned drinks – some of them have added sucrose or glucose. 'Diet' drinks are best in moderation. Some people like beef extract drinks or vegetable juices – watch the salt content. Milk shakes and yoghurt drinks are often rather fatty and sugary.

Alcohol

Having diabetes does not stop you drinking alcohol, but stick to the common sense limits. These are 14 units a week for women and 21 units a week for men. A unit of alcohol is a half-pint of beer or lager, a standard measure of spirit or a wine-glass full of wine. Be careful about low-sugar lagers. They have been brewed on to convert more of the sugar to alcohol. On the other hand, low-alcohol lagers and wines may contain a lot of sugar. Choose ordinary wine or lager. Never drink on an empty stomach.

> Monty had clinched a highly successful deal. He had a drink in the hotel bar with his boss before walking home. Because he has insulin-treated diabetes he had a pint of low-sugar lager. Half-an-hour later a policeman found him staggering across a road. Because Monty's breath smelled of alcohol the officer thought that he was drunk and took him to a police station. He became more and more confused and they put him in a cell to 'sober up'. Fortunately, the custody sergeant searched his pockets and found his diabetic card and some glucose tablets. When they had cured his hypoglycaemia they took him home.

Hypoglycaemia or a low blood glucose is described on pages 108–9. Alcohol prevents the liver from releasing glucose from its stores and can cause hypoglycaemia in non-diabetics as well.

There is now a wide range of non-alcoholic drinks. Many people space out alcoholic drinks with these. Check the label, as some of these are quite sugary.

If you drink very heavily for a long time you can damage your pancreas so badly that diabetes is caused.

'Diabetic' foods and other special foods or additives

'Diabetic' foods There is no need to buy expensive 'diabetic' foods. Diabetes UK's does not reccomend 'Diabetic' foods. 'Diabetic' foods are made with fructose or sorbitol rather than glucose or sucrose. As discussed above, there is no evidence that fructose is better for diabetics than glucose, and it contains the same number of calories so it cannot be used as part of a weight-reducing diet. Sorbitol causes bowel upsets if large amounts (i.e. more than 30 g) are eaten. If you want some chocolate, have a little bit of ordinary chocolate after a mixed meal.

Artificial sweeteners These can make soft drinks and puddings more palatable. You need only tiny amounts. Use a variety of different sweeteners sparingly. It is better to learn how to enjoy less sweet tastes. Artificial sweeteners are not suitable for cooking

'Health' foods, pills and additives I once met a man who was taking 40 different doses of 'health pills' a day. I had to tell him that he might well be overdosing on some compounds. Others were probably harmless but unnecessary.

Most of us get all we need to keep fit from a balanced diet. We do not need additives. If you are tempted to buy from a health food shop, check the labels carefully. A herbal remedy may not have undergone the stringent tests and manufacturing controls demanded of the pharmaceutical industry. Consult your doctor and do not stop your usual diabetes medication. One herbal remedy used in diabetes care was Goats Rue. The active component of this is metformin – now manufactured as a glucose-lowering drug (see pages 76–7).

The diabetic diet has changed

Those of you who have had diabetes for many years, or who have had relatives with diabetes, may have found this section confusing. Ideas about diabetic diets have changed considerably over the years. In the 18th century Rollo advocated a low calorie diet containing rancid meat! In the first part of the 20th century the only treatment for diabetes was starvation with severe carbohydrate restriction. This idea that diabetics could not eat carbohydrate persisted for some years after the discovery of insulin. Unless people were overweight they were allowed unlimited fats and proteins. Nowadays we know that too much fat is harmful and that people need lots of complex carbohydrate mixed with fibre for a healthy diet.

HOW MUCH YOU EAT

When you eat food it is either used as fuel straightaway, or stored for future use in one of the body's fuel depots. One of these is the liver – another is fat. So if you eat more than your body needs you will put on weight. To paraphrase Mr Micawber:

- Daily intake 2000 calories, daily expenditure 2000 calories, result happy balance;

- Daily intake 2500 calories, daily expenditure 2000 calories, result obesity.

So, it should be simple to lose weight. Eat less than you need each day and you will lose weight. But we all know that it is not as easy as that. Food is nice. Food is friendly. It is comforting. It fills our tummies. Eating less can make you feel hungry. Feeling hungry is not nice. It can be very hard to cut down.

A further problem is that everyone is different in their fuel needs. We all know some really slim person who eats like a horse and never puts weight on. We also know people (perhaps us) who have difficulty losing weight even if they eat very small helpings. So how does one lose weight?

The first step is to be honest with yourself. Write down every single thing you eat and drink for a week. And write down how much (e.g. how many spoonfuls of cereal or pudding, how many slices of bread). Sit down and look at that list.

1. Avoid unnecessary calories Are you eating anything that you don't actually like? If yes, then stop – why eat food you do not enjoy? Are you eating other people's leftovers – the children's for example? If yes, stop. You are not a rubbish bin.

2. Avoid mechanical eating Do you sit in front of the television dipping into a bag of crisps? Or eat a packet of biscuits while you are typing? Are you actually enjoying each mouthful? If you must chew while you are doing things, try sugar-free chewing gum, or celery.

3. Regain control Is most of your eating out or in your home? If you are eating out, you often have less control over your food. Could you take a packed lunch rather than eat greasy canteen chips? Is there a greengrocer's you could choose rather than the burger bar? If you are eating in, can you control what you eat? Does someone else cook for you? Involve them in your need to lose weight. All of us like to see someone enjoying our cooking, and there is a natural tendency to encourage second helpings. Explain that you are not rejecting them or their cooking, but following doctor's advice to lose weight. (One study showed that the wives of diabetic men are much more likely to change their own eating to help their husbands stick to their diet than are the husbands of diabetic women.)

4. Say no This may be the hardest part. Start saying no. No to fatty foods. No to sugary foods. No to second helpings. But don't be too hard on yourself.

5. Say yes Go through your diet sheet with the dietitian and focus on foods you like. Look at less fattening ways of cooking other favourite foods.

6. Eat less Have smaller portions. Use a smaller plate so that the helpings look bigger. Put a teaspoonful back each time.

7. Fill up on non-fattening vegetables – these include artichokes, asparagus, green beans, broccoli, Brussels sprouts, carrots, pumpkin, radish, spinach, swede, watercress, marrow, lettuce, cabbage, cucumber, celery, tomato, courgette, marrow, and onions.

8. Stay busy Occupy your mind so that you are not thinking of food all the time. Learn new hobbies. Try to avoid situations where you will feel pressure to over eat.

9. Exercise Burn off some of the fat. See chapter 17.

10. Be honest with yourself and your dietitian or doctor. Many people swear that they are eating tiny amounts of food 'barely enough to keep a bird alive'. But studies have shown that people who say this and cannot lose weight are actually eating more than they need – often nibbling continuously. You may not even realise you are doing it.

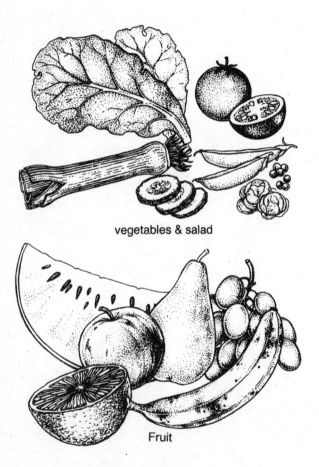

vegetables & salad

Fruit

Eat five helpings of fruit and vegetables a day

Doreen is 32 and weighs 18 stone (252 pounds). She is trying to lose weight. <u>This is what Doreen thought she had eaten on Monday.</u>

Breakfast half a grapefruit, black coffee, one slice toast with low fat spread and one teaspoon marmalade.

Lunch chicken sandwich (2 slices bread, low fat spread), tomato, lettuce, cucumber, apple.

Cup of tea.

Dinner Weight Watcher's frozen meal 240 calories, Perrier water, lemon water ice (made with artificial sweetener), coffee.

<u>This is what Doreen actually ate:</u>

Made mother's early morning tea – ate broken biscuit.

Got children's breakfast – ate piece of toast while making theirs.

Breakfast half a grapefruit, black coffee, one slice toast with low fat spread and one teaspoon marmalade (licked marmalade spoon).

Out shopping tasted cheeses at display in supermarket – five mouthfuls. Met friend and had cup of coffee with cream in department store.

Lunch chicken sandwich (2 slices bread, low fat spread), tomato, lettuce, cucumber, large spoonful of mayonnaise, apple.

Afternoon job in office Julie's birthday. Ate most of a slice of birthday cake, cup of tea.

Prepared children's tea. Ate several peanuts and the sausage that burst in the frying pan.

Dinner Weight Watcher's frozen meal 240 calories, Perrier water, half a glass of husband's wine, lemon water ice (made with artificial sweetener), coffee.

Grapes.

Midnight Very hungry. Went downstairs and ate two biscuits.

---

11. Don't give up If you have a set-back, just keep trying. Everyone is human. Remember, every ounce lost is a step towards becoming slim.

Diabetes treatment and weight loss

If you are overweight, weight loss is an important part of your diabetes treatment. However, it is important to adjust the dose of glucose-lowering pills or insulin if you start eating less and losing weight. If you do not reduce your insulin as your weight falls, you are likely to become hypoglycaemic. Careful blood glucose monitoring can help you here. A benefit of weight loss is often better blood-glucose control.

ASIAN FOODS

If you enjoy sharing traditional food with family and friends in the community, or have to obey religious rules about food and drink, you can still eat a diet that suits your diabetes. You do not have to give up your favourite or everyday foods. Traditional Asian diets usually contain healthy amounts of vegetables, fruit, and carbohydrate such as rice (use brown rice), pulses such as lentils (e.g. dal), beans (e.g. rajam) and chickpeas (e.g. cholas, cabuli chanas), breads (chapatti – use wholemeal flour). Reduce sweet foods such as jelabi, kulfi and gur. Some dishes (e.g. halva) could be sweetened with aspartame or saccharine. Pay attention to the cooking of your food. It is important not to use too much fat such as ghee or the various cooking oils. What oil you do use should be carefully measured and high in polyunsaturated fats (e.g. sunflower oil) or monounsaturated fats (e.g. olive oil). Some meat dishes and vegetable preparations (e.g. aubergines) are cooked in fat, and fat is often used to prepare carbohydrate foods such as nan, poppadums, poorata and pooris. Some dishes such as samosas are fried. Consider different ways of cooking, such as stir-frying using very little oil. Milk, yoghurt and butter (ghee) are saturated fat, so use skimmed milk and low fat yoghurt, and avoid butter. When making tea use sweeteners such as canderal after heating if you need a sweet flavour. Avoid yoghurt drinks such as lassi (unless made with low fat yoghurt). Nuts contain fat too. You can eat whatever spices you wish. Certain foods, and also herbal remedies, may contain medicines which interact with your treatment from the hospital, so be careful. Karela lowers the blood glucose, so tell your doctor if you are eating this vegetable or any herbal preparation.

	METRIC					
Height without shoes (m)	Men Weight without clothes (kg)			Women Weight without clothes (kg)		
	Acceptable average	Acceptable weight range	Obese	Acceptable average	Acceptable weight range	Obese
1.45				46.0	42–53	64
1.48				46.5	42–54	65
1.50				47.0	43–55	66
1.52				48.5	44–57	68
1.54				49.5	44–58	70
1.56				50,4	45–58	70
1.58	55.8	51–64	77	51.3	46–59	71
1.60	57.6	52–65	78	52.6	48–61	73
1.62	58.6	53–66	79	54.0	49–62	74
1.64	59.6	54–67	80	55.4	50–64	77
1.66	60.6	55–69	83	56.8	51–65	78
1.68	61.7	56–71	85	58.1	52–66	79
1.70	63.5	58–73	88	60.0	53–67	80
1.72	65.0	59–74	89	61.3	55–69	83
1.74	66.5	60–75	90	62.6	56–70	84
1.76	68.0	62–77	92	64.0	58–72	86
1.78	69.4	64–79	95	65.3	59–74	89
1.80	71.0	65–80	96			
1.82	72.6	66–82	98			
1.84	74.2	67–84	101			
1.86	75.8	69–86	103			
1.88	77.6	71–88	106			
1.90	79.3	73–90	108			
1.92	81.0	75–93	112			

	NON-METRIC					
Height without shoes (ft.in)	Men Weight without clothes (lb)			Women Weight without clothes (lb)		
	Acceptable average	Acceptable weight range	Obese	Acceptable average	Acceptable weight range	Obese
4 10				102	92–119	143
4 11				104	94–122	146
5 0				107	96–125	150
5 1				110	99–128	154
5 2	123	112–141	169	113	102–131	152
5 3	127	115–144	173	116	195–134	161
5 4	130	118–148	178	120	108–138	166
5 5	133	121–152	182	123	111–142	170
5 6	136	124–156	187	128	114–146	175
5 7	140	128–161	193	132	118–150	180
5 8.	145	132–166	199	136	122–154	185
5 9	149	136–170	204	140	126–158	190
5 10	153	140–174	209	144	130–163	196
5 11	158	144–179	215	148	134–168	202
6 0	162	148–184	221	152	138–173	208
6 1	166	152–189	227			
6 2	171	156–194	233			
6 3	176	160–199	239			
6 4	181	164–204	245			

Guidelines for body weight

Fasting

Many religions have fast days or periods of restrained eating. Ramadan and other fasting periods can be observed safely if you wish although your religioun may grant you exemption on the grounds of your condition. Discuss fasting with your diabetes adviser before you begin. You may need to reduce your pills or insulin, or take them only during the hours of darkness when food is permitted, for example. It is important to work out exactly what to do about your treatment during periods of fasting in order to avoid hypoglycaemia (see page 104).

SUMMARY

- A diet is what you eat.
- Your body cannot cope with sugary foods, whose carbohydrate is quickly absorbed.
- Eat plenty of starchy, fibrous carbohydrate, which is digested slowly. Your body can cope with that.
- Eat as little fat as possible.
- Eat a small amount of protein.
- Avoid manufactured 'diabetic' foods.
- Drink alcohol only in moderation.
- Do not eat excess salt.
- Eat less of everything if you are overweight.
- Enjoy what you eat.

8

GLUCOSE-LOWERING PILLS

If dietary measures do not return your blood glucose to normal your doctor will probably prescribe glucose-lowering pills (also called oral hypoglycaemic agents). The indications for insulin treatment are listed in Chapter 9. Glucose-lowering pills will only work if your pancreas is still making some insulin. You still need to eat a healthy diet, and exercise regularly.

Glucose lowering pills include: insulin-production boosters called sulphonylureas (e.g. gliclazide); glucose absorption and uptake/release modifiers called biguanides (e.g. metformin); insulin sensitizers called thiazolidinediones (e.g. rosiglitazone); meal-time glucose regulators (e.g. repaglinide); a sucrose-digestion blocker called acarbose; and a high-fibre product called guar gum.

SULPHONYLUREAS

There are several drugs in this class with different duration of action. Some are taken once a day, others more often. Take them before meals.

Chlorpropamide was the first. It is still used although now largely replaced by newer sulphonylureas. It is extremely long-acting – over 24 hours – so should be taken once daily at the same time each day.

Glibenclamide is the most commonly used worldwide although less so in Britain nowadays. It enters the islet cells and stays there for many hours.

Gliclazide is often used. There is a twice a day, or a very long-acting version. It produces a more natural insulin response to glucose than earlier sulphonylureas. It may also reduce blood stickiness, which could help the circulation. Glipizide has a similar duration of action.

Tolbutamide is shorter-acting. The pills are quite large.

Glimepiride is a newer very long-acting agent which can be taken once a day. You should have regular haematology and liver tests when taking it.

SULPHONYLURGA PILLS

Name of pill (Drug Co. names in brackets)	Dosage range (per 24 hours)	Dosage frequency
chlorpropamide	50–500 mg	once a day
glibenclamide (Daonil, Semi-daonil, Euglucon)	2.5–15 mg	once/twice a day
gliclazide (Diamicron)	40–320 mg	once/twice a day
gliclazide (Diamicron 30 MR)	30–120 mg	once a day
Glimepride (Amaryl)	1–6 mg	once a day
glipizide (Glibenese, Minodiab)	2.5–20 mg	once/twice a day
gliquidone (Glurenorm)	15–180 mg	one to three times a day
tolbutamide	500–2000 mg	one to three times a day

This is a general guide. Note that the safe dose for you may be lower than this.

How do they work?

The sulphonylureas work in several ways. They boost insulin release by the pancreas in response to a glucose load. They also have effects in the liver and tissues, helping the insulin to work more effectively at receptor level and perhaps in the cells (see pages 30–1).

When not to use sulphonylureas

Not at all in insulin-requiring diabetes, in pregnancy, for breast-feeding mothers.

With caution in liver disease, kidney disease, adrenal insufficiency, thyroid disease, and in older people.

Drugs which interfere with sulphonylureas or vice versa

There are many, including sulphonamide antibiotics (e.g. Septrin) and chloramphenicol, phenylbutazone, ibuprofen and similar drugs, aspirin, warfarin, other anticoagulants, beta blockers, monoamine oxidase inhibitors, sulphinpyrazone and barbiturates. Thiazides and steroids may increase the blood glucose.

Side-effects

The most obvious side-effect is hypoglycaemia. Others include allergic reactions like skin rashes, and gastrointestinal upsets – nausea or bowel symptoms, for example. Alcohol causes flushing with some glucose-lowering pills, especially chlorpropamide. Rarely, they cause liver damage or abnormalities of blood cells. In most instances the side-effects disappear once the drug is stopped. In the early 1960s the American University Group Diabetes Program suggested that tolbutamide use was associated with an increased risk of heart disease. However, this study has since been criticised. Sulphonylureas are now used extensively. Glibenclamide was shown to be safe in a large study called UKPDS (see page 159) They rarely upset people and are taken by millions world-wide.

Hypoglycaemia on sulphonylureas

Obviously, sulphonylureas are meant to lower your blood glucose. However, if you take more pills than you need, eat too little or exercise unexpectedly your glucose may fall lower than you want. You may become hypoglycaemic. The symptoms and signs of hypoglycaemia are detailed in Chapter 10. If you suspect that you are hypoglycaemic you must test your blood glucose. If this is at all difficult or you feel very unwell, eat some glucose immediately. It is extremely important to follow this up with a good meal containing long-acting carbohydrate. Then contact your diabetes adviser. Because you still have the sulphonylurea in your bloodstream, it will encourage your pancreas to keep releasing insulin every time your blood glucose rises. So you may keep becoming hypoglycaemic. With chlorpropamide, severely hypoglycaemic people can have recurrent glucose falls for a day or more, until the drug has worn off.

Glibenclamide is the commonest cause of hypoglycaemia in during sulphonylurea treatment – probably because it is prescribed often and can last for 20 hours. One in three people taking glibenclamide report hypoglycaemic episodes, so you must be alert for this. The high frequency of hypoglycaemia on glibenclamide is why some doctors prefer alternative sulphonylureas nowadays.

METFORMIN

This is the only drug of its class still in use. It is prescribed in a dose of 500–3000 mg daily in divided doses. It does not boost pancreatic insulin production and so is unlikely to cause hypoglycaemia unless taken in overdose. It helps insulin to work in the tissues, reduces glucose absorption from the bowel and reduces liver glucose release.

Metformin is particularly useful in overweight people as it helps them to lose weight (if they stick to their weight-reducing diet). It can cause a loss of appetite as well as reducing glucose absorption.

When not to use metformin

Not at all in pregnant and breast feeding women, people who drink too much alcohol and those with severe disease of kidneys, liver, heart or lungs

With caution in elderly people

Drugs which interact with metformin Cimetidine, Anticoagulants

Side-effects

These are more common than with sulphonylureas but can usually be avoided by starting treatment with very small doses so that the body gets used to the metformin. Side-effects may include lack of appetite, nausea, vomiting and diarrhoea, an odd taste in the mouth, wind and indigestion. Rarely, anaemia due to vitamin B_{12} or folate malabsorption may occur. The most dangerous side effect is lactic acidosis – a severe acid derangement of the blood chemistry. This is very uncommon and usually occurs in people who have kidney failure, very low blood pressure, low blood oxygen levels, or very severe illness from any cause. Stop your metformin temporarily if you have an x-ray in which you are given an intravenous injection of contrast 'dye'. Discuss this with your doctor.

MEAL-TIME GLUCOSE REGULATORS

Repaglinide (Novonorm) is taken in doses of 0.5–4 mg before each meal with a maximum dose of 16 mg in each 24 hours. Nateglinide (Starlix) is taken 1 to 30 minutes before each meal starting with a dose of 60 mg for each meal. This can be increased to a maximum of 180 mg three times a day.

How do they work?

Meal-time (prandial) glucose regulators are designed to control the peaks of glucose you get after you have eaten. They increase the release of insulin at meal times. Because they act fast and clear quickly they can be taken to match meal-times but are unlikely to persist in the blood stream, so less likely to cause low glucose levels.

When not to use meal-time glucose regulators

Not at all in children under 18 years old, insulin-dependent diabetics, pregnant or breast-feeding women and those with severe kidney or liver disease.

With caution in older people and those with moderate kidney or liver disease, steroid insufficiency or malnourishment.

Drugs which may interfere with meal-time glucose regulators or vice versa

Monoamine oxidase inhibitors, beta blockers, ACE inhibitors (drugs ending in -pril such as ramipril), aspirin, non-steroidal anti-inflammatory drugs such as ibuprofen/Nurofen, octreotide, alcohol, steroids, oral contraceptives, thiazide diuretics (water pills), danazol, thyroid hormones, sympathomimetics (drugs such as ephedrine), rifampicin and simvastatin (cholesterol-lowering).

Side-effects

These are relatively new drugs and currently doctors are asked to report all side-effects to the regulatory bodies. Like sulphonylureas they can cause hypoglycaemia. Rashes, visual disturbances, elevation of liver enzymes (blood tests) and gastro-intestinal upsets have been reported.

THIAZOLIDINEDIONES

Thiazolidinedione is the name of a completely new class of glucose-lowering drugs designed to make your own insulin work better. At present these drugs are only licensed to be used in combination with metformin in overweight people, or with sulphonylureas in people who are unable to use metformin. The aim is to improve glucose control. They should only be started by a doctor experienced in the treatment of Type 2 diabetes. Rosiglitazone (Avandia) is taken in doses of 4 mg daily, increasing (in people on metformin, but not in those on sulphonylurea) to a total of 8 mg a day (as a single or divided dose). Pioglitazone (Actos) is taken as 15–30 mg daily with either metformin or sulphonylurea. At present you must not take both metformin *and* a sulphonylurea *and* rosiglitazone or pioglitazone. Neither drug can be taken as the only glucose-lowering medication, although this situation may change following further studies.

How do they work?

Thiazolidinediones work by increasing sensitivity to your own insulin. This means that your insulin works better and allows more glucose to get into body tissues, especially muscle. These drugs also reduce the amount of glucose released by the liver. Type 2 diabetes can be difficult to treat as people who have it are often resistant to the action of their own insulin. Thus, this new class of drugs may be particularly helpful.

When not to use thiazolidinediones

Not at all in pregnant or breast-feeding women; children under 18 years old; those with liver failure, severe kidney disease or heart failure; people on kidney dialysis treatment; and insulin-dependent diabetics.

Drugs which cause problems with a thiazolidinedione or vice versa

Insulin (these drugs can cause heart failure in insulin-treated patients), nonsteroidal anti-inflammatory drugs such as aspirin or ibuprofen (Nurofen) and pacitaxel (Taxol – a cancer drug).

Side-effects

Like other glucose-lowering drugs thiazolidinediones may cause hypoglycaemia. The first thiazolidinedione, troglitazone, was withdrawn because of deaths from liver failure. All drugs in this class can cause liver problems, and liver blood tests should be monitored. Other side-effects which have been reported include anaemia, fluid retention, weight gain, headache, gastrointestinal upsets, tiredness, visual disturbance, joint aching, blood in urine, impotence, dizziness.

ACARBOSE

Acarbose (Glucobay) is taken with meals, either chewed with the first mouthful or swallowed whole with liquid immediately before eating. Start with 50 mg a day with the main meal. This is increased according to glucose control by 50 mg doses every fortnight to 50 mg three times a day. After 6–8 weeks gradually increase to 100 mg three times a day. Increasing it faster than this runs the risk of abdominal side-effects. The maximum dose is 200 mg three times a day.

How does it work?

Acarbose works in the gut where you are digesting your meal. It blocks the enzyme (chemical) that converts sugar – sucrose – into glucose. This means that starch and sucrose may pass through the bowel and out with the faeces without being absorbed. If you eat a sugary meal this sugar will 'ferment' in your bowel and may give you wind, abdominal griping and diarrhoea.

Important warning: Because acarbose prevents the conversion of sucrose to glucose you must carry *glucose* tablets with you to eat if you have a low sugar reaction as sugar would not help.

When not to use acarbose

Not at all in bowel disorders such as colitis or Crohn's disease, ulcerated bowels, intestinal blockage, chronic disorders of digestion or absorption; pregnancy and breast-feeding; and liver or kidney failure (it is suggested that liver tests should be done during the first year of treatment).

Drugs which interfere with acarbose or vice versa

Drugs which absorb gut compounds, pancreatic enzymes (such as Creon), neomycin, cholestyramine (cholesterol-lowering granules) and digoxin. If acarbose is used in combination with other glucose-lowering treatment, blood glucose levels should be checked carefully as acarbose may increase the risk of hypoglycaemia, necessitating reduction of treatment.

Side-effects

Gastro-intestinal side-effects are common and include wind, bloating, fullness after meals, abdominal pain or discomfort and diarrhoea. Such effects can be reduced by a low-sugar diet and by avoiding rapid increase of acarbose doses. Rarely jaundice, liver inflammation and rashes are a problem.

GUAR GUM

Guar gum (Guarem) is rarely used nowadays. It comes as sachets which are dispersed in 200 mls of water. One sachet is drunk before each meal. The sachet can be sprinkled onto food.

Guar gum is a fibrous bulking agent which slows absorption of glucose by adding to the fibre content of your diet. It should not be given to children or those with gullet problems or bowel blockage. If used in combination with other glucose-lowering medication it can cause hypoglycaemia and the dose of your other medication may need to be reduced. It can cause wind, abdominal bloating and diarrhoea.

COMBINATION TREATMENTS

Some glucose-lowering pills can be used in combination to improve glucose control. This should only be done in full consultation with your doctor. The following combinations are in regular use:

Sulphonylurea and metformin
Sulphonylurea and thiazolidinedione
Sulphonylurea and acarbose
Metformin and thiazolidinedione
Metformin and repaglinide

PROBLEMS WITH PILLS

Failure to control the blood glucose

If combination treatment and a healthy diet and exercise do not maintain good blood glucose balance you need insulin. Although no one likes injecting themselves with insulin, it is much better not to delay starting treatment – you will feel very much better within days and it is not as awful as you imagine (see Chapter 9).

Vomiting and other illness

If you cannot keep your tablets down or have diarrhoea (which may mean that you do not absorb them), call your doctor. In the meantime check your blood glucose at least 6-hourly, and preferably more often. If you are too ill to measure your own glucose you need to be in hospital. Infections and other illness push the blood glucose up – you may need insulin to help to control it at this time. Vomiting is a danger signal in diabetes – it may reflect an illness that causes your blood glucose to rise or it may be due to a high glucose and major chemical imbalance. Like diarrhoea, it will prevent you from absorbing your treatment. Call for help early.

Failure to control the blood glucose

You may simply need more pills (assuming you are sticking to a healthy diet). Ask your doctor or diabetes adviser for guidelines so that you can increase you pills (within the safe dosage range) if your blood glucose levels rise.

The blood glucose may rise temporarily because of an illness or operation. A few days or weeks of insulin treatment will solve this. However, as the years go by, the pancreas produces less and less insulin until finally pills will work no longer. When this happens, no amount of adjustment of the type of pills or their dose will help and you need insulin injections. This is not a major problem. If you wait – 'just one more try with the pills', 'I'll try really hard with the diet' – you may find yourself suffering all the symptoms of untreated diabetes and feeling ill. If you need insulin, have it so that you will start feeling better quickly.

What should you know about your pills?

1. Their name: the proper (generic) name (e.g. glibenclamide) and any trade name (e.g. Daonil).

2. What they are for: lowering the blood glucose.

3. When to take them: before or with the meal for sulphonylureas and with or after the meal for metformin. Make sure you know the correct times.

4. How much to take: be careful – some drugs are marketed in different strengths, so you need to know the size of your pills and your dose in milligrammes (mgs) or grammes (gs). (One g = 1000 mg). 40 mg gliclazide is half an 80 mg pill; 160 mg gliclazide is two 80 mg pills. You may need to take a different dose morning and evening. (You may be offended that I am spelling this out but mistakes often occur.)

5. What unwanted effects may occur: hypoglycaemia with many; see above for other effects.

6. Possible interactions with other pills

7. How long to take them for: indefinitely unless you are told otherwise. This means making sure you get some more before your current supply runs out. Show the doctor the original bottle. Compare the pills the pharmacist gives you with the ones in your original bottle – they should be the same.

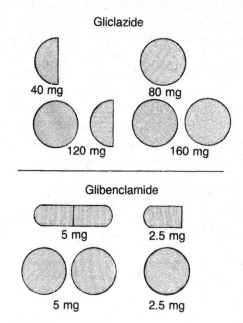

What are you taking? How much?

8. Cost: People on glucose-lowering pills are exempt from prescription charges in Britain.

9. Is your 'diabetic card' correct? Carry it always.

10. If you are taking a glucose-lowering pill, carry glucose with you always.

SUMMARY

*   Glucose-lowering pills only work if you are still making some insulin of your own.
*   Glucose-lowering pills can cause hypoglycaemia.
*   Metformin helps lower the blood glucose effectively. It may help overweight people lose weight.
*   Make sure you know what you are taking, when, how much and what for.

- Carry a 'diabetic card' or other identity card.
- Carry glucose if taking glucose-lowering pills.
- Monitor your blood glucose concentration.
- Seek help early with vomiting illness, or other illness in which your blood glucose is rising.

9

INSULIN TREATMENT

If your body can no longer make enough insulin to keep your blood glucose normal, you need insulin treatment. Many people are frightened about this, but nowadays, you need not be worried. The injection itself hurts no more than a gnat bite and even small children can learn how to draw up and inject insulin. Furthermore, if you have a modern insulin pen, you do not even have to use a needle and syringe – just select the dose on your pen and slip the fine needle into a fold of skin and fat.

WHO NEEDS INSULIN?

People who have Type 1 diabetes need insulin. This includes the majority of people whose diabetes comes on before the age of 30 years. If you make no insulin then no other treatment will work.

People who cannot control their blood glucose with diet, exercise and glucose-lowering pills also need insulin. This treatment has failed because you are no longer making enough insulin for the pills to work. Note that I have said that the *treatment* has failed – not you. It is not your fault that your pancreas is failing to produce enough insulin. You will feel much better on insulin treatment, so do not put it off.

If your diabetes is usually controlled by diet alone or by diet and pills, you may need insulin treatment temporarily when you are ill. Examples are during infections, heart attacks or operations or after accidents. In most cases you can return to your usual treatment once you have recovered.

Pregnant women who have diabetes which they cannot control by diet alone, or who usually take glucose-lowering tablets, must have insulin treatment until the baby has been born.

WHAT YOU NEED TO KNOW ABOUT INSULIN TREATMENT

Essential information

Write this down and carry it with you at all times. It is essential for your survival.

- The name of the insulin(s) your doctor has prescribed;
- The dose(s);
- When to inject it;
- Where to inject it;
- How to keep your insulin in good condition;
- Where to get your insulin from;
- The name of your insulin-injection system (i.e. which syringe and needle, or which pen);
- How to look after your insulin-injection system;
- Where to get your insulin-injection system from;
- How to use your insulin and your injection system;
- What to do if you feel odd or ill, including hypoglycaemia;
- Who to contact if you need help (day or night).

Desirable information

The 'essential information' is minimal. It will not allow you to adjust your treatment yourself. Nor will it allow you to sort out many emergencies yourself. Further information will help you to understand how your treatment works and may well save you inconvenience or illness. As Dr Lawrence said, 'It is not enough that your doctor should put you on the proper lines of treatment. You must learn to follow it and carry it out yourself in your own home'. Learning as much as you can about your insulin and the way in which you use it and your body responds will make the difference between having to adapt your life to your treatment and adapting your treatment to suit your life. Information that it is desirable for you to have, therefore, covers the following:

- What type of insulin?
- How does it work?
- What effects does it have on the body?
- How can you adjust the dose and timing?
- What to do in emergencies?
- What other insulins and injection systems are there?

Because I believe that all of you will want to control your treatment, rather than have it control you, I will combine the essential and desirable information in the following sections.

INSULIN

Types of insulin

Rapid-acting The insulin that your body used to make was a clear colourless substance. This type of insulin is produced as a water-like liquid. It used to be called soluble insulin (regular insulin in America). Hypurin soluble is one example. Nowadays most clear insulins are called neutral and some are analogues – modified insulin. Some trade names are Actrapid, Humalog, Humulin S (Humulin R in America), Novorapid and Velosulin. These insulins are clear and work fast.
NB. A new *slow*-acting insulin called glargine is clear – so be careful.)

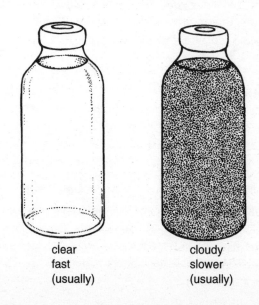

Insulin

clear
fast
(usually)

cloudy
slower
(usually)

Rapid-acting insulin can be injected directly into the bloodstream (this is only done in hospital). There it starts to work within minutes. Injected under the skin it starts to work within half an hour and most brands have their greatest effect between two and six hours. Ultrafast analogue insulins such as Humalog (Insulin Lispro) and Novorapid (Insulin Aspart) peak in half an hour and clear after 2 hours.

Rapidly acting insulins will deal with one meal eaten within minutes of injection. Some people may have an injection of rapid-acting insulin before each meal.

Slow-acting These insulins have all been treated to delay their onset of action after injection. Cloudy insulin is always slower-acting. Some of these insulins are slowed down by using crystalline forms, others by adding protamine and others by incorporating zinc. One of the problems with the slow-acting insulins, is that their duration of action may vary from person to person. An insulin that lasts 24 hours in one person may need to be given twice daily in someone else. In general the following insulins are usually medium-acting and are therefore given twice a day: Humulin I, Isophane, Insulatard, Protaphane and Semitard. Monotard comes somewhere in between. These insulins are usually considered longer-acting and are often given once daily: Lentard, Lente and Humulin Zn. These insulins are usually considered very long-acting and are only given once daily: Hypurin Protamine Zinc and Ultratard. Insulin glargine is a long-acting insulin designed to give a smooth background profile for boosts of faster-acting insulin. It is clear.

Fixed-proportion mixtures These are mixtures of rapid-acting and isophane insulins provided by the manufacturer. They include Humalog Mix 25 or Mix 50, Humulin M2, M3, M5 and Mixtard 10 to 50. If you increase the dose of one of these insulins the dose of both the short and medium-acting components will increase.

How is insulin made? Human, pig and beef insulin

Originally the only source of insulin was animal pancreas – either beef or pig. The need for good supplies of pig pancreas meant that much insulin was made in Denmark. Beef insulin is rarely used today. It is less like human insulin than the porcine variety, which differs in only one tiny detail.

Preparation		Manufacturer	Species	Form	Onset, peak activity and duration of action in hours (approx)
Neutral Insulin Injection	Humalog (insulin lispro)	Lilly	🧍	V, P, C₂ C₃, C₄	
	Human Actrapid (pyr)	Novo Nordisk	🧍	V, P, C₁ C₆	
	Human Velosulin (emp)	Nova Nordisk	🧍	V	
	Humulin S (prb)	Lilly	🧍	V, P, C₂ C₃, C₄	
	Hypurin Bovine Neutral	CP Pharm	🐄	V, C₂, C₃	
	Hypurin Porcine Neutral	CP Pharm	🐖	V, C₂, C₃	
	Insuman Rapid (prb)	Hoechst	🧍	V, C₅, P	
	NovoRapid	Novo Nordisk	🧍	V, P, C₁ C₆	
	Pork Actrapid	Novo Nordisk	🐖	V	
Biphasic Insulin Injection*	Humalog Mix25	Lilly	🧍	P, C₂, C₃ C₄	
	Humalog Mix50	Lilly	🧍	P	
	Human Mixtard 10 (pyr)	Novo Nordisk	🧍	P, C₁, C₃ C₆	
	Human Mixtard 20 (pyr)	Novo Nordisk	🧍	P, C₁, C₃ C₆	
	Human Mixtard 30 (pyr)	Nova Nordisk	🧍	V, P, C₁ C₃, C₆	
	Human Mixtard 40 (pyr)	Novo Nordisk	🧍	P, C₁, C₃ C₆	
	Human Mixtard 50 (pyr)	Novo Nordisk	🧍	V, P, C₁ C₃, C₆	
	Humulin M2 (pd)	Lilly	🧍	C₂, C₃, C₈	
	Humulin M3 (prb)	Lilly	🧍	V, P, C₂ C₃, C₄	
	Humulin M5 (prb)	Lilly	🧍	V	
	Hypurin Porcine 30/70	CP Pharm	🐖	V, C₂, C₃	
	Insuman Comb 15 (prb)	Hoechst	🧍	V, C₅, P	
	Insuman Comb 25 (Pd))	Hoechst	🧍	V, C₅, P	
	Insuman Comb 50 (prb)	Hoechst	🧍	V, V₅, P	
	Pork Mixtard 30	Nova Nordisk	🐖	V	
Isophane Insulin Injection	Human Insulatard (pyr)	Nova Nordisk	🧍	V, P, C₁ C₆	
	Humulin I (pit)	Lilly	🧍	V, P, C₂ C₃, C₄	
	Hypurin Bovine Isophane	CP Pharm	🐄	V, C₂, C₃	
	Hypurin Porcine Isophane	CP Pharm	🐖	V, C₂, C₃	
	Insuman Basal (prb)	Hoechst	🧍	V, C₅, P	
	Pork Insulatard	Nova Nordisk	🐖	V	
Insulin Zinc Suspension (Mixed)	Human Monotani (pyr)	Nova Nordisk	🧍	V	
	Humulin Lente (prb)	Lilly	🧍	V	
	Hypurin Bovine Lente	CP Pharm	🐄	V	
Insulin Zinc Suspension (Crystalline)	Human Utratard (pyr)	Nova Nordisk	🧍	V	
	Humulin Zn (prb)	Lilly	🧍	V	
Protamine Zinc Insulin Injection	Hypurin Bovine PZI	CPPharm	🐄	V	

(prb)-produced from proinsulin synthesised by bacteria using recombinant DNA technology   (emp)-produced by enzymatic modification of porcine insulin
(pyr)-produced from a precursor synthesised by yeast using recombinant DNA technology   (insulin lispro)-human insulin analogue, rDNA origin
*Speed of onset is proportional to amount of soluble insulin **Key:** V = vial. P = pre-filled pen. C = cartridge. (C₁= compatible with NovoPen3;
C₂ = compatible with BD Pen Ultra; C₃ = compatible with Autopen; C₄ = compatible with HumaPen; C₅ = compatible with OptiPen Pro1; C₆ = compatible with Innovo.) **Pen needles:** Micro-Fine + and NovoFine are compatible with all pre-filled and reusable pens.

Reproduced courtesy of August MIMS 2001. The information is updated monthly, so for the latest advice consult the current edition.

About 15 years ago, insulin became the first drug to be manufactured using genetic engineering. By altering their genetic material, harmless bacteria were made to produce human insulin. The bacteria were then killed and the insulin purified. This meant that people with diabetes were no longer dependent upon animals for their insulin supply. It also meant that they could, at last, have the insulin that their bodies would have been making were they not diabetic. Because animal insulins are 'foreign' to the body, antibodies (pages 32–3) to the insulin are produced, which may necessitate increasingly larger doses of insulin to achieve the same glucose-lowering effect. Antibody formation may also cause variability in response to insulin. It has been suggested that these antibodies may be implicated in tissue damage. High antibody levels have been linked with the formation of big dents at injection sites (see page 101). (Antibodies can be made to human insulin too, but this happens much less often.) Modern highly purified insulins (from whatever origin) are less likely to cause antibody formation than were older insulins. Genetically engineered insulin made by bacteria is denoted by 'crb' or 'prb' on the label. Yeasts can be used – 'pyr' on the label. It has also proved possible to modify porcine insulin using enzymes – 'emp' on the label. Most insulin-dependent diabetics in Britain now use human insulin and use of animal insulins is declining.

Strength All insulin in Britain is provided in a concentration of 100 units per millilitre. It is called U100 insulin. Other countries may have different strengths so beware if you try to obtain insulin abroad. You must use U100 syringes to give 100 insulin.

Preservative All insulin contains preservative to keep it sterile until the expiry date. This is why it smells slightly antiseptic and why you can keep sticking your needle into the bottle without infecting the insulin.

How is insulin packaged

Insulin usually comes in vials or cartridges with a self-sealing rubber bung. Every bottle is labelled with the name and expiry date, among other information. Every time you obtain a new bottle of insulin and every time you use it, check that it is the right sort of insulin for you (if you are taking Humulin S and Humulin I, make sure you have not been given Humulin M2, for example), and check that it has not expired.

Increasingly, insulin is provided in cartridges. These are about the same size as ink cartridges and have a self-sealing rubber bung at one end (which will be penetrated by the double-ended pen-needle) and a plug which will be depressed by the pen plunger at the other end. It is possible to get insulin out of a cartridge using an ordinary syringe and needle but this should only be done in an emergency (e.g. broken pen and no back-up insulin) and is not to be recommended. As with insulin bottles make sure that you have the correct insulin and it is within its expiry date.

Because insulin is a protein it is digested if swallowed. Researchers are trying to put insulin into capsules which release their insulin only in the large bowel, beyond the reach of digestive enzymes. However, there are still many problems to be overcome, including that of ensuring good absorption and accurate dosage. These problems also arise with intranasal insulin – insulin which is sniffed up the nose. Both these ways of administering insulin are experimental and seem unlikely to replace insulin injections. Insulin-producing islet cells can also be implanted into the liver and other tissues – this means that they can produce insulin in the body. Several people with diabetes have received islet cell transplants but this remains a research technique. There is currently a large project studying this in the UK. It is difficult to obtain enough pure islets and they have to be protected from rejection by your body. So for the time being if you need insulin, it must be received by injection.

How to look after your insulin

Insulin is a protein. This means that, like an egg, it is permanently altered by freezing or heating. But while you can still eat a previously frozen or cooked egg, insulin which has been altered in this way is useless.

Some researchers were testing a new type of insulin. A large batch was produced abroad and flown in specially. The cargo handlers unloaded the plane and left the containers on the tarmac to be collected later. It snowed and all the insulin froze. The entire consignment was worthless.

Bill is a sales representative and travels a lot. One day he nearly forgot his insulin. His wife ran after him and handed the bottles through the car window. He put them on the dashboard. He left the car parked in the sun all day. It was one of the hottest days of the year. The business trip lasted several days and although Bill stuck to his diet and his usual doses of insulin, his blood glucose went up and up and he started to feel thirsty. It was not until he returned home and started a fresh supply of insulin that he began to feel better. Eventually he realised that the insulin he took on his trip must have been damaged by the heat of the sun.

You can carry your current bottle(s) around with you – most insulin-pen users carry their pen in their pocket for up to 28 days under 25°C. However, you must protect your insulin from freezing or cooking when you travel. Keep all your spare insulin in the fridge between 20 and 10°C. It is usually safest to keep it well away from the freezing compartment. Always, always have at least one spare bottle or cartridge in your house, or baggage if travelling. If you use a pen you should also have a bottle of insulin and a syringe and needle just in case of pen loss, damage or malfunction. Remember that if your bag is stolen you could lose your insulin. Consider keeping it in a safe pocket when travelling. (See Chapter 18)

Although your insulin is self-sterilising, it is sensible to keep it clean. This means cleaning the bung before inserting the needle. Some people use alcohol-impregnated swabs but there are sprays or bottles of alcohol or other antiseptics. Ask your doctor or nurse which they advise.

INSULIN-INJECTION SYSTEMS

Syringes

When I first became interested in diabetes, most insulin-treated patients were using glass syringes, many with re-usable needles. It was hard to keep the syringe clean, it was breakable and injections could be painful. Disposable syringes and fine disposable needles were used in hospital but were not available on outside prescription. Many clinics gave them out to patients when they could. Then, primarily as a result of efforts by the British Diabetic Association, now Diabetes UK, supported by many individual patients and other concerned people, disposable syringes, pens and needles became available on prescription. No one needs to use a glass syringe nowadays.

Syringes are made by several companies. They are marketed with fixed or detachable needles. Those with a fixed needle are probably the most practical for the majority of patients. People who are injecting insulins which should not be mixed should have a separate needle and syringe. That way they can draw up each insulin separately and inject them through the same needle left in the skin. Few people will be giving insulin like this.

Syringes range from 0.3 ml (30 units), to 0.5 ml (50 units), to 1 ml (100 units) and are marked in units of insulin. They are designed for single use only. Keep the syringe packet intact and dry until you use it or it will not be sterile.

It is your responsibility to keep your syringes and needles secure and to inform the police should they be lost or stolen. Similarly, be careful about disposal. Your GP can prescribe needle clippers which will hold about a thousand needle ends and can then be thrown away safely. You can also obtain sharps boxes from the surgery or hospital depending on the system locally. Never throw a syringe and needle away in your domestic rubbish without first ensuring that no one else could possibly prick themselves or (a sad reflection on our society) use it.

Insulin pens

Several insulin pens are available, (see your diabetes nurse for the latest models). They use an insulin cartridge with a self-sealing bung at one end and a rubber plug at the other. The disposable needle is double-ended – one end goes into the bung and the other, finer, needle goes into you. The insulin dose can be selected simply by depressing the plunger the right number of times (one press can give half to two units of insulin so check on your own pen), or by dialling up the correct dose and twisting or depressing the cap to inject the insulin. The pen is easy to carry and easy to use, and more and more people with diabetes are replacing their syringe and needle with one of these devices.

As there are several on the market and more on the way, it is important to chose a pen which suits your needs. Some older pens are simply covers for a syringe with a replacement plunger. There are easier pens to use but this is the only system in which you can

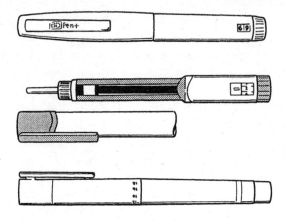

Three types of insulin pen syringes (there are many more)

use any type of insulin. Otherwise, most pens and insulins are not interchangeable. So, unless you are prepared to change your insulin, you may find that the decision has been made for you. However, if you do have a choice, insist on actually handling several pens. Does it fit your hand? Can you dial up a dose and expel the insulin easily? Does the pen show you how much insulin you have used and how much is left? Can you correct mistakes before injection? Does the pen have a 'locking device' so that insulin is not expressed until you wish it? Also find out what the back-up is like. What happens if you have a problem with the pen? Will the company give you another straightaway? Ideally you should have two pens – one for use and one spare but this may not be possible while pen numbers are limited.

Other devices

Several cannulae are available which can be left under the skin for a day or more. The insulin is injected into a self-sealing port. Most people find that injections are so trouble-free anyway that an indwelling device which could catch on clothes or become infected is not necessary. A few find it preferable.

Insulin jets use technology developed for mass immunisation to drive insulin through the skin under high pressure. This does not require an injection as such. Some people find these devices very helpful but others find that they get bruising at jet sites and that insulin oozes out again. They are more popular in America than in Britain.

Other aids include magnifiers to place over the markings on the syringe to aid vision when drawing up and guides to hide the needle. The advent of insulin pens has made insulin injections much easier and fewer people seem to have the problems with insulin administration which necessitated concealing devices.

Insulin pumps

Normally the pancreas releases insulin all the time – in tiny bursts every few seconds. Larger amounts are released when the blood glucose rises. Thus it is simplistic to believe that even four injections of insulin a day can accurately mimic normal pancreatic function.

This has led to the development of continuous subcutaneous insulin infusion (CSII) by pumps which are worn all the time. Pumps were very popular several years ago but became less so, although there has been a recent resurgence of interest. Some of the reasons for their decline in popularity are the need for very intensive supervision, the high frequency of problems (including ketoacidosis and, less commonly, severe hypoglycaemia), the discomfort, inconvenience and embarrassment of a box attached to a tube attached to a needle *in situ* for 24 hours a day, every day, and the demonstration that they provide no better glucose balance than very carefully monitored conventional insulin therapy. CSII is still an option for patients who, despite frequent monitoring and appropriate insulin treatment and adjustment, cannot maintain good glucose balance. However, it is not an easy option and should be chosen carefully after thorough discussion with your diabetes adviser.

There are other, implantable, insulin pumps, for example intra-peritoneal (implanted into the abdominal cavity). Despite media excitement these are still at the experimental stage and are used only as a last resort. There are rare patients whose life has been saved by one of these devices but there are probably only a few such people in Britain with diabetes so severe as to need this drastic measure.

INSULIN TREATMENT PATTERNS

There are as many versions of insulin treatment as there are diabetologists (doctors specialising in diabetes). Some patterns are
more common than others. In general, once daily insulin is not an
effective way of achieving good glucose balance and is reserved for
elderly patients who have problems managing their condition or for
very small children. Occasionally once-daily insulin is used in
people who have some residual pancreatic insulin production but
not quite enough to keep their blood glucose normal. Many people
use twice daily insulin and increasingly people are using pens before
each meal.

In general, you need insulin for two types of glucose balance –
coping with meals and helping with body housekeeping (dealing
with the glucose produced by the body itself). Fast-acting insulin
copes with meals. Cloudy, longer-acting insulin copes with body
housekeeping. Most people need about two-thirds of their total
daily insulin in the morning and one-third in the early evening.
About a third of your insulin will probably be fast-acting and about
two-thirds longer-acting. The type of insulin pattern you need must
be tailored for you personally and no one else. There is no right or
wrong insulin pattern. Your final insulin pattern may be completely
different from anything described in this book – if it gives you good
glucose balance and you can manage it then that is the right insulin
pattern for you.

Twice-daily insulin

This is usually a combination of clear, fast-acting insulin mixed with
cloudy medium-acting insulin given before breakfast and before the
evening meal:

- Morning fast works until lunchtime;
- Morning medium works from lunch to evening meal;
- Evening fast works until bedtime;
- Evening medium works overnight until next morning.

Multiple pen injections with background insulin

This uses a cloudy, long-acting insulin, (e.g. Insulatard, Ultratard)

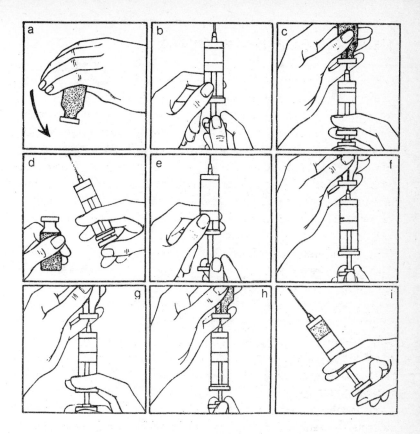

Drawing up and mixing insulin

a) Gently rotate bottle to mix insulin
b) Draw up air
c) Inject air into cloudy insulin bottle
d) Put cloudy insulin down
e) Draw up air
f) Inject air into clear insulin bottle. Draw up clear insulin
g) Express air bubbles and check you have drawn up correct dose of clear insulin
h) Draw up correct dose of cloudy insulin
i) Ready for injection

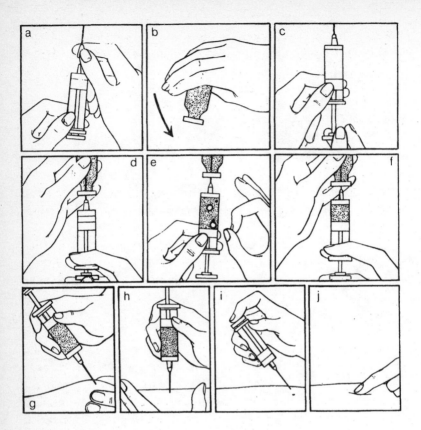

Injecting insulin

a) Attach needle to syringe or pen if necessary
b) Gently rotate vial or pen to mix insulin
c) Draw up air and inject into the insulin bottle
d) Draw up insulin or dial dose on pen
e) Clear air bubbles, or do a 2 unit 'air shot' with pen
f) Check syringe contains correct insulin dose
g+h) Inject insulin into fatty layer under skin. Wait 10 seconds
i) Withdraw needle
j) Press on the hole

taken before bed as background to several pen injections of fast-acting clear insulin taken before each meal, whenever it is eaten:

- Pre-breakfast fast works until lunchtime;
- Pre-lunch fast works until evening meal;
- Pre-evening meal fast works until bedtime;
- Bedtime medium or long works overnight and into the next day.

Insulin should be injected about 20 minutes before eating, to allow time for the insulin to be absorbed. You need to find your own best injection time.

Increasingly, people are finding that the new ultra-fast analogue insulins, Humalog and Novorapid, allow a more flexible lifestyle. Because they are absorbed so rapidly they can be given immediately before each meal, or even immediately afterwards. They work for that particular meal. This means that meal times can be more flexible. Also, if you do not know when the food will be served, or how much carbohydrate it will include, you can give your insulin after you have finished eating. You cannot do this with other insulins. Once you have injected an ultra-fast insulin you must eat or you will quickly become hypoglycaemic. The ultra-fast insulins can also be useful if your glucose is unexpectedly high as they will reduce it quickly. Insulin Glargine, which will soon be available in the UK, was designed to provide a smooth long-acting background to this sort of regimen.

DRAWING UP INSULIN

This is shown in the illustrations on pages 97–8. Obviously, if you do not draw up the correct dose your insulin will not have the desired effect on your blood glucose. Insulin is very concentrated and mistakes are easy. One study demonstrated that a large proportion of insulin doses drawn up by people with diabetes, nurses and doctors were inaccurate. This is another reason for using an insulin pen. If you are doubtful about the accuracy of a particular dose, discard it and start again. A small air bubble can cause a major inaccuracy, especially with small insulin doses.

It helps gently to rotate cloudy insulin bottles or pens between your hands. But do not shake the bottle – the resultant froth takes a long time to settle. Cloudy insulin straight from the fridge may seem a little 'sticky'. New syringe plungers should be depressed fully before attempting to draw up insulin. Working the syringe plunger up and down vigorously is not necessary and can cause tiny fragments of rubber to come off.

Most problems seem to arise with mixing insulins. Now that so many fixed proportion insulins are available there is less need to mix. If you are mixing your own remember that you must *never* get cloudy insulin into your clear bottle. If you make an error discard that insulin and try again. Also remember that the only stable mixtures are those between soluble or ultrafast insulin and cloudy isophane insulins. Other longer-acting insulins will start to convert your clear insulin to cloudy in the syringe and this will obviously alter its onset and duration of action. Always inject such a mixture immediately.

INJECTING YOUR INSULIN

Where

Inject insulin under the skin (subcutaneously). If you inject it into the skin surface you will get painful, white, firm blisters which leave red spots. If you inject it too deeply, the needle enters the muscles, which may be painful, and the insulin will be absorbed too quickly. Most of your subcutaneous tissue is fat with little blood vessels running through it. They will carry the insulin away gradually. Take a good pinch of skin and subcutaneous tissue and slide the needle in at an angle. Your diabetes nurse will advise you.

> Ali is a young athlete who trains hard every day. When he developed diabetes he found it very difficult to inject his insulin because he had so little subcutaneous tissue. His glucose level kept falling precipitously within an hour of his injection because he had injected the insulin into the muscle. Eventually he devised a technique whereby he pinched up the skin firmly and put the needle in virtually horizontally.

The best places to inject insulin are the top of the thighs, upper buttocks, abdomen, and upper arms. You can also use your 'spare tyre' if you have one. A few people use their calves, but I would not advise this. It requires careful technique to avoid intramuscular injection and should not be done if you have poor circulation or varicose veins. Use as much of your chosen area as possible. Do not overuse any part of an injection site.

> Augustus was 75 and had had insulin-treated diabetes for 20 years. He rarely came to diabetic clinic and usually refused examination when he did come. One winter he was admitted to hospital with pneumonia. The doctor who admitted him was horrified to discover a black hole on the front of each thigh. 'That's where I puts me insulin,' said Augustus.

A less dramatic consequence of overusing a particular site is lumps or dents. The lumps are called insulin hypertrophy and the dents insulin atrophy. Insulin absorption from these sites will be erratic. If you have an area like this, change your injection site.

Many factors can affect the rate and amount of insulin absorption. Insulin is absorbed fastest from the arms, then the abdomen, then the legs, then the buttocks. However, if you increase the circulation to the injection site by warming it (by sunbathing or sitting in a hot bath, for example) or by exercising the muscle underneath (by running, for example), your insulin will be absorbed faster than usual and your blood glucose may fall unexpectedly. If the injection site gets cold (outside in winter, for example) the insulin will be absorbed very slowly – until you warm up – and then it may be absorbed quickly and when you are not expecting it. Cigarette smoking causes erratic insulin absorption because of the adverse effect of nicotine on the circulation. All of this means that the same dose of insulin in the same site may be absorbed at a different rate on Monday (football), Tuesday (sauna), Wednesday (sitting watching television) and Thursday (stopped smoking).

How

There is no need to clean your skin unless it is very dirty – and you should have daily all-over washes if you have diabetes. Spirit or alcohol hardens the skin and causes stinging injections. However, if possible, you should wash your hands before drawing up and injecting. Pinch up the skin and subcutaneous tissue with one hand, hold your pen or syringe with the other and quickly put the needle through the skin. When you are sure that the needle tip is in the

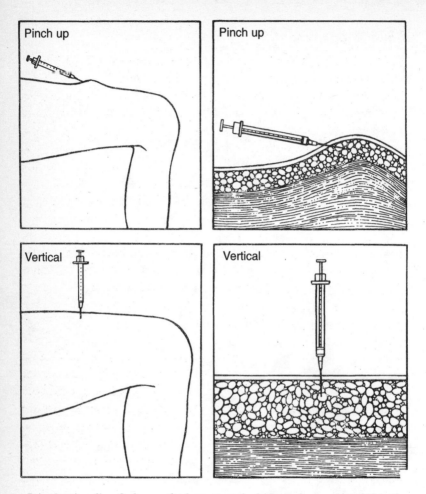

Pinch up

Pinch up

Vertical

Vertical

Injecting insulin. Only use the bottom method if you have a lot of fat; the top method is safest.

subcutaneous layer push down the plunger or twist the pen top to inject your insulin steadily, count to ten, and quickly withdraw the needle. Put your finger firmly over the hole. Do not worry if you see a little blood, it is from a tiny vessel and will soon stop. Quick firm injections are less likely to sting than a slow tentative approach. Practise on an orange first, using a spare syringe and needle with some water.

What happens now?

You eat. Once you have injected the insulin you cannot get it back. It will be absorbed and will lower your blood glucose. It is therefore important that you eat after injecting all insulins unless told otherwise. However, you should not fall into the old trap of adapting your meals to suit your insulin. This limits you and there is no reason why you should not adjust your insulin to suit your meal plans. Ask your diabetes adviser how to do this. If your meals are very erratic, a pre-meal pen insulin pattern may suit you best.

ADJUSTING YOUR INSULIN

Once you are confident about insulin injections and understand how each of your insulins affects you, you can learn to adjust your own treatment. There are several common sense rules. At first, decide what you think you should do and then telephone your diabetes adviser to check that you have got it right. Follow their advice. Gradually you will be able to sort it out yourself. Alter only one insulin in any one day unless your blood glucose level is very high or very low. Alter your insulin by only one or two units at first, until you become more confident. Remember that if you increase your insulin there is a small risk of hypoglycaemia, so be especially alert for this. Each change in your cloudy insulin dose will take about three days to settle down. It is therefore not a good idea to alter cloudy insulins more often than once every three days. You can alter your clear insulin each day if necessary. Never stop your insulin.

Some practical problems and what to do

Cracked or broken insulin vial or cartridge Throw it away – keep at least one spare vial or cartridge of each sort of insulin.

Bent needles You are not keeping the needle in a straight line with the bottle while drawing up or injecting. Try to keep your hands steady.

The syringe jams Throw it away. Syringes may jam if you work the plunger vigorously – there is no need to do this. They sometimes jam with Ultratard insulin, especially if it is cold. Wait until the insulin is at room temperature. If you still have problems contact your diabetes adviser.

Painful injection You may be injecting too deeply or too shallowly, or too jerkily, or at the wrong angle with needle pulling on skin. Wet alcohol or other cleansers can sting – either let them dry or do not use them. You may have a tender area, in which case try somewhere else.

Spots at injection sites Either you are injecting too shallowly or your skin is being irritated by a cleanser. If your skin is very red, tender, swollen and spotty, you may have an infection (this is very rare). If you think you have an infection, see your doctor that day.

ESSENTIAL EMERGENCY INFORMATION

Low blood glucose or hypoglycaemia

If you have too much insulin for your current needs, your blood glucose will fall below normal (i.e. less than 4 mmol/1, or 72 mg/dl). You will become hypoglycaemic. This is rarely dramatic or severe and in the vast majority of episodes you will realise that your glucose is falling long before you feel more than slightly off-colour. However, you must be prepared for this – which means that from your first insulin injection and as long as you continue on insulin you must carry glucose or some other sugar on your person at all times and have it by you at night. You must also carry a 'diabetic card' so that others can help you in the very unlikely event of your needing assistance.

Read about hypoglycaemia in Chapter 10. For practical purposes, if you feel odd or unwell in any way check your glucose. If you find checking your glucose at all difficult, stop and eat some glucose immediately.

Because it takes a few days or weeks to establish a pattern of insulin treatment to suit you, you are at increased risk of hypoglycaemia during this time. *Do not* drive a car, operate machinery, work at heights, or take responsibility for other people's lives (e.g. carry a small baby, work as a nurse) for a week after starting insulin or beginning a new pattern of insulin treatment or a new type of insulin. Discuss the exact safety period with your diabetes adviser.

High blood glucose or hyperglycaemia

Few people with diabetes have normal blood glucose levels all the time. Each person should discuss high blood glucose levels with his or her diabetes adviser before it becomes a problem. These are very general guidelines and there is more detail in Chapter 11. Blood glucose levels always in double figures – i.e. 10 mmol/l or more (180 mg/dl or more) – are unacceptable and you should work to reduce them. This is not always easy, so do not demand too much of yourself. If your blood glucose is over 19 mmol/l, you must do something about it now.

One high glucose level If you know this is due to overeating, take 1–4 units of extra rapid-acting insulin to cover that meal and plan better next time (i.e. don't eat so much or have more insulin before the meal). Check your glucose again in two to four hours. If you feel well and the repeat glucose is under 19 mmol/l, do not worry.

A rising glucose level but feeling well If the glucose is persistently high it means that your insulin dose is not covering what you are eating and your body housekeeping. If you are overweight consider eating less. If not, increase your insulin according to blood glucose; try 1–4 units of whichever insulin acts at that time of day. Check your urine for ketones. Contact your diabetes adviser within 48 hours. If more than a trace of ketones (i.e. more than one plus) are present, contact your diabetes adviser that day.

A rising glucose level and feeling ill This is an emergency. Continue your usual insulin and if your glucose is 19 mmol/l or more (342 mg/dl or more), give yourself 4–8 extra units of insulin (or the dose your diabetes adviser has advised in teaching sessions) and contact your doctor immediately. He should see you within hours. Continue to measure your glucose every two to four hours and write the results down. Check your urine for ketones. If there is more than one plus of ketones you are markedly insulin deficient. You need medical help. While these urine ketones persist, give yourself 2–8 extra units of insulin (preferably fast-acting) every four hours if your glucose remains above 19 mmol/l. Do not forget to have your usual insulin as well. If you feel worse or medical help is delayed you should be seen in hospital. Call an ambulance if necessary.

If you become too ill to check your own blood glucose you need to be in hospital now. Call an ambulance by dialling 999 in the UK or the emergency number of the country you are in.

If your breathing becomes deep and sighing and you have urinary ketones, you must be in hospital whatever your blood glucose. You have ketoacidosis. Call an ambulance.

If you are vomiting (with or without raised blood glucose levels) you need to see a doctor within the next few hours – call one. If you have any problems contacting a doctor, go to hospital.

NEVER STOP YOUR INSULIN

You need insulin to survive. If you stop taking it you will become acutely insulin deficient. Ketones will build up in your blood and you may become comatose. Even if you have a hypoglycaemic episode you should not stop your insulin. Eat glucose and more food, and, if necessary, reduce the dose. Contact your diabetes adviser for help. But do not stop your insulin.

If you stop your insulin because you are vomiting from gastro-enteritis or some other infectious illness you will be cutting off your insulin at a time when your blood glucose levels are rising in response to the infection. This is a recipe for disaster. You will become very ill, very quickly. Occasionally people with diabetes encounter doctors not familiar with insulin-treated diabetes who try to stop their insulin. This situation can be difficult to handle. Explain politely that you have been told never to stop your insulin – and why. Show them this book. Suggest they contact your diabetes adviser.

Most people do not have dramatic problems with a minor bout of gastroenteritis. However, it can be hard to handle if you are newly insulin-treated, which is why you need immediate advice. Often you will get better at home with fluids and more insulin. Otherwise fluids and insulin into a vein in hospital will soon solve the problem. Do not be afraid to ask the hospital for help. But in most instances you will be able to manage at home.

SUMMARY

- If your body cannot make insulin you must give it by injection.
- Find the insulin injection method and pattern which suits you.
- Learn how to adjust your insulin according to your blood glucose measurements.
- Look after your insulin and equipment.
- Know who to contact for help.
- Always keep a back-up supply of insulin and needles and syringes or cartridges.
- Pay attention to detail when drawing up your dose of insulin and injecting it. Get it right.
- Remember the variability of insulin absorption from different injection sites.
- Always carry your 'diabetic card'.
- Always carry glucose.
- Beware of hypoglycaemia.
- Plan what to do if your glucose rises or you become ill.
- Vomiting is a danger sign. Heed it.
- Remember, tailor your insulin treatment to suit your needs.
- Never stop your insulin.
- If you feel ill seek medical help sooner rather than later. Do not delay.

10

HYPOGLYCAEMIA OR LOW BLOOD GLUCOSE

If you are taking pills or insulin to lower your blood glucose you must read this chapter carefully. Hypoglycaemia is rarely a major problem but it is common and you must learn to recognise its earliest symptoms and act on them promptly.

HYPOGLYCAEMIA: BACKGROUND INFORMATION

How common is hypoglycaemia?

People with insulin-treated diabetes average about 10 hypo-glycaemic episodes each year. About one in three people on insulin will need treatment for hypoglycaemia from someone else each year. In other words, each year you have a one in three chance that you will have an episode that you have difficulty treating on your own. Learning how to recognise your early warning signs and taking prompt action will reduce this risk. People with diabetes taking glucose-lowering pills are less likely to become hypoglycaemic but it can occur and you too must be able to recognise the symptoms. It may take you longer to get your glucose back to normal should you become hypoglycaemic.

How can you prevent problems with hypoglycaemia?

Firstly, by keeping a close eye on your blood glucose and planning ahead – more of this later in the chapter. Secondly, by learning to recognise all of your own hypoglycaemia symptoms, however minor, so that you can treat them immediately. I believe that people with diabetes are better at recognising their own hypoglycaemia than they realise. Hypoglycaemia may actually make you forget what happened, but you can sometimes write symptoms down at the time – once you have eaten your glucose, of course. Have a high index of suspicion; if you are new to insulin ask yourself if every unusual feeling may be due to a low glucose. As I write this I can almost hear diabetes advisers who read this saying 'She'll turn them all into terrified neurotics, thinking every itch and sniff is a hypo and afraid to do anything in case they go hypo.' Oh no, I won't! My readers have more common sense than that. You must control your diabetes if you are to get on with enjoying life as you want it. To control your diabetes you must have the power to rule it. In knowledge lies power. Once you have learned your early warning signs you can treat an early hypoglycaemic attack with a quick mouthful of glucose tablets and carry on. You will not have to wait until it gets so bad that you have difficulty in managing it yourself.

What is hypoglycaemia?

There is no generally accepted definition of hypoglycaemia, although most would accept a laboratory venous blood glucose below 2.5 mmol/l as indisputably hypoglycaemic. For practical purposes, in a person with diabetes on glucose-lowering treatment, it is a finger-prick blood glucose level below 4 mmol/l (72 mg/dl), with or without symptoms; or symptoms or signs substantially and rapidly improved by giving glucose, sucrose or glucagon (see pages 115–6).

SYMPTOMS OF HYPOGLYCAEMIA

These are usually divided into two sorts. Firstly, there are those due to the brain being deprived of its main fuel, glucose. Medspeak for these is 'neuroglycopaenic symptoms'. Secondly, there are those due to the body's emergency response. Medspeak for these is 'adrenergic symptoms'. In practice, the symptoms of hypoglycaemia for any one person do not necessarily fit the classical pattern. Each person must learn to recognise his or her own symptoms as early as possible.

Problems with thinking and awareness

These may be very early signs. Lack of concentration should lead you to suspect that you are hypoglycaemic. You may find yourself taking a very long time to do a simple sum or unable to understand a newspaper article. You may be unable to make decisions – simple ones like 'Shall I have tea or coffee?'. You may start to become muddled or find that your thoughts or what people say does not make sense. You may not be able to find the right words, or you may start to talk and talk. You may become very confused and get lost, or be unable to finish a task. Your eyes may feel heavier and heavier until you fall asleep.

Not wanting to eat

One part of your brain may tell you that you need food while another says 'Yeucch!' and refuses. Hopefully the first part will win.

'I've started so I'll finish'

One common feeling is that you must complete the task you were engaged in as your glucose started to fall. If you are driving a car this inner voice telling you to drive on must be resisted at all costs. Stop immediately you suspect you may be hypoglycaemic. I once watched a hypoglycaemic man trying to get an apple from a polythene bag. Despite my holding glucose tablets out to him he insisted on opening the bag. It kept slipping in his sweaty fingers. In the end I stuffed the glucose into his mouth and as he came to he allowed me to open the bag and hand him an apple.

Emotions

Quiet people may feel like being noisy and vice versa. You may feel extraordinarily happy or giggly – everything is a huge joke. Or you may feel very sad – everything is low and miserable. Quite often people who are hypoglycaemic get cross. You may become irritable because you cannot calculate your change in a shop, or shout at your wife because she asks what you want for dinner and you cannot decide. Or you may become furious with everyone for no particular reason. You may feel that everyone is against you – and this feeling may be worsened by people's attempts to help you to get better. (Carers should, however, remember that people with diabetes have the same emotions as everyone else. Nothing is more infuriating than people saying, 'There, there, you're not really cross, you're hypo, have some glucose, dear' when the person is genuinely angry and not in the least hypoglycaemic.)

Problems with movement and co-ordination

Co-ordination skills are often reduced early in hypoglycaemia. You may feel very clumsy – buttons won't do up and you cannot open your packet of glucose tablets. You drop things. You may start staggering and eventually be unable to walk. Your arms and legs may not work properly and, rarely, you may be unable to move part of your body.

Weakness or superhuman strength

You might expect that lack of fuel would make your whole body weak and this is often the case. You may feel as if you are wading through porridge. However, occasionally people briefly become extremely strong and can run or fight. You may feel invincible.

Altered vision

Blurring of vision sometimes occurs. Or you may see the world with abnormal clarity – as if it is new and wonderful. One of my friends said that the sky always turned pink when he became hypoglycaemic.

Palpitations

This means increased awareness of unusually rapid heart beats. It can occur as the glucose level is falling.

Sweating

Torrential sweating which soaks your clothes is a clear sign of hypoglycaemia. However, it may be quite a late sign and occur only as the glucose is rising again.

Trembling

This is a fine shaking of your hands. It may add to the problems of inco-ordination, making it difficult for you to take glucose.

Anything else

There is a huge variety of symptoms of hypoglycaemia; some seem unique to one person. Any unusual sensation should be assumed to be due to hypoglycaemia until proved otherwise.

SIGNS OF HYPOGLYCAEMIA

These are for friends and family to note – although some may be apparent to the hypoglycaemic person.

Not himself or herself

The early signs may be very subtle and apparent only to someone who knows the person well. Very small changes that you cannot pinpoint but which make you vaguely uneasy or look twice may indicate hypoglycaemia. Look three times.

Problems with thinking or alertness

The lack of concentration may be more apparent to you than to sufferers themselves. Their thoughts and movements may be painfully slow. I have learnt that when a patient in the diabetic clinic is taking an inordinately long time to understand or answer what seem to be simple questions he or she is nearly always hypoglycaemic. It may be hard to keep such patients to the point and they may not appear able to obey simple instructions. Undue sleepiness in the day or difficulty waking someone in the morning is another sign.

Emotions

This is probably one of the factors in the 'not himself' sign. But more obvious emotional changes often appear – undue quietness in the 'life-and-soul of the party', extrovert behaviour from an introvert. Irritability and a desire to be left alone is common. 'I don't want help. I'm not hypo. Go away.' People with diabetes will be annoyed to read the next bit but it is something I have learned the hard way. If someone on insulin says that they are definitely not hypoglycaemic, especially if they are very cross or fed up when they say it, their glucose is often falling fast (but see page 110).

Teresa McLean in her book *Metal Jam* says: 'Although a part of my brain often knows that I am feeling hypo, the state itself stops me being able to do anything about it. Nor am I able to admit my problem to anyone I am with. If asked, I always deny that anything is wrong. It is this inability to explain to others that I need sugar once a hypo has started which baffles everyone around me.'

Marion was returning from a long mountain walk. She was stumbling and seemed likely to fall. We asked if she thought she might be hypoglycaemic. 'I'm not hypo. Of course I'm not hypo. How could anyone who was hypo do this?' And before we could stop her she had climbed a rock and was balancing on one leg, other leg outstretched with toe pointed balletically. When we retrieved her, Marion's finger prick blood glucose was 2 mmol/l.

Sometimes people with hypoglycaemia may think that people trying to help them are attacking them and resist with all their force – I was hurt by a hypoglycaemic 80-year-old. She also injured two ambulancemen, a nurse and a large, rugby-playing medical student.

Problems with movement and co-ordination

Clumsiness or stumbling combined with lack of co-ordination, slurred speech and confusion can make a markedly hypoglycaemic person appear drunk. However, such gross problems are uncommon and you must watch for smaller difficulties – dropping a cup while washing up or stubbing a toe on a paving stone perhaps. I have noticed that hypoglycaemic people may bump into you while walking beside you. Rarely, it can seem as if someone with hypoglycaemia is having a stroke, but in this case glucose will restore completely normal function within minutes.

Inappropriate or unusual behaviour

Rarely, severe hypoglycaemia can make people do odd things – sunbathe on a windowsill in the evening, attack people with a brush, unpack something they have just packed. They may talk nonsense or run up a hill they have just walked down. They may simply stand and smile without moving. Don't laugh. Treat the hypoglycaemia.

Fast pulse, pallor, trembling and sweating

The shakiness and sweating will be obvious. Feel the pulse – it is usually fast (say 100 beats per minute rather than 70). The skin may become very pale, or occasionally flushed, sometimes patchily.

Coma and fits

Although first aid books may give the impression that all hypogly-caemia is coma this is not true. Coma or lack of consciousness is rare in hypoglycaeniia. Sometimes people who are unconscious from hypoglycaemia have a convulsive fit. This may appear frightening but both the coma and the fits are immediately relieved by glucose.

DON'T PANIC

By now both those of you with diabetes and your carers and family may be worried. No one has all these features and most people never have dramatic changes with hypoglycaemia. Coma is rare. I have collected these signs and symptoms from thousands of people with diabetes seen over many years. Furthermore, hypoglycaemia is one of the most wonderful medical conditions to treat – give glucose and the patient recovers in minutes and is soon his or her usual self again.

TREATMENT OF HYPOGLYCAEMIA

Test your glucose if you can

If the symptoms are minimal and you are in a safe situation, test your blood glucose and confirm that you are indeed hypoglycaemic. If you are, eat some glucose. If you find any aspect of blood testing difficult, abandon it and eat glucose.

Eat glucose or sucrose

The best emergency treatment for a low blood glucose is glucose. It will be absorbed most quickly in liquid form – for example as a glucose drink such as Lucozade. However, this may not be convenient to carry around. Glucose tablets (Boots, Dextrosol, Lucozade and others) are simplest. Try to wash them down with water or another drink if possible. There are also sweets which contain glucose. Sucrose, as sugar lumps or in sweets or candies, also works quickly, but the sucrose has to be digested to glucose before absorption.

For water sports, Hypostop glucose gel is easier. It is in a leakproof plastic bottle which you can put in a pocket in a swimming costume or boating gear.

If you are unable to feed yourself, your friends or relatives may have to post glucose tablets into your mouth. Firm, direct command

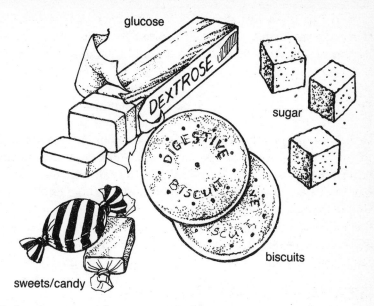

Foods to be consumed for treatment of hypoglycaernia

is best. 'Eat this now. No, don't spit it out. Eat it *now.*' Again, a glucose drink may be quicker. Some people insist on a particular food to cure their hypoglycaemia – like an elderly lady who became hypoglycaemic in the diabetic clinic, a strawberry jam sandwich. Balance what you eat to the severity of the hypoglycaemia.

Eat food

The elderly lady was partly right. Once you have eaten or drunk your glucose, have something more substantial to keep your blood glucose up. A sandwich, a couple of digestive biscuits, a bowl of muesli or a muesli bar. If you do not eat something solid and you still have too much insulin in your circulation, it will use up all the glucose you have just eaten and you will become hypoglycaemic again.

Glucagon

Partners and relatives of insulin-treated diabetics should always have glucagon in the house. This is rarely necessary if you are taking glucose-lowering pills. Take glucagon with you when you are travelling. It is a hormone which works in the opposite way to insulin – it raises the blood glucose by releasing it from the liver stores. Unlike insulin, it is not stable in solution and comes in a pack containing a bottle of dry powder, water and a syringe and needle. The pack must be in date.

Use glucagon if the hypoglycaemic person will not or cannot swallow – for example, if the person is so confused that you cannot persuade him to eat glucose, or if he is unconscious. If you have to use glucagon (either for yourself or for another person), do not rush. First put an unconscious person in the recovery position (pages 116–7). Get the box out, hold it and take a deep breath in and out (to calm yourself). Then open the box carefully. Draw up the water into the syringe (some syringes are pre-filled with water) and squirt it into the bottle containing the powder. Mix gently. Then draw back all the solution into the syringe and hold it needle up. If there are air bubbles tap up to the top and squirt them out. Then inject the glucagon deep into the big muscles in the side of the thigh. It does not matter if some goes subcutaneously, nor if it enters a vein, provided there are no air bubbles. If the person is fighting you or you cannot undress him, inject through the trousers. This technique is only to be used in dire emergencies. Injections through clothes, even tights, carry the risk of introducing bits of fibre under the skin, which can act as a focus for infection.

Glucagon has a temporary effect only. Once the person is awake and rational you must feed him. This may be difficult because glucagon makes some people feel sick and 'hungover'.

Coma and fits

The main danger is not that of the low blood glucose itself but of the unconsciousness. You must protect the airway before you do anything else. Check that there is nothing in the unconscious person's mouth. Then roll the person onto his side, being careful to keep the mouth away from the floor. The illustration on page 117 shows the recovery position, in which it is safe to leave the patient while you get the glucagon or call for help. Otherwise you must not leave him unattended until he has woken up. If he is having a fit, move all the furniture away so that he cannot injure himself and keep him on his side. Do not attempt to force anything into his mouth. The tongue is bitten in the first instant of the fit and you will only cause further injury – to the patient and, perhaps, to yourself.

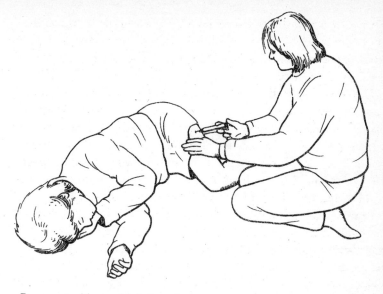

Recovery position and injecting glucagon

Once you have injected the glucagon, keep the person on his side and wait. He will wake up within a quarter of an hour. If he does not, immediately phone an ambulance. Phone your doctor or an ambulance in any case if you are at all worried. The doctor can always wake the person up by injecting concentrated glucose into a vein.

While it is dangerous to give anything by mouth to someone who is unconscious in case they inhale it, years of experience, especially with children, has shown that small amounts of glucose rubbed inside the cheek or gums, may help to rouse them. Small amounts of Hypostop can be used in this way. Always lie the patient on his side with his airway clear and watch that you do not get bitten fingers.

WHY WERE YOU HYPOGLYCAEMIC?

As soon as you feel better work out why you became hypoglycaemic. The main causes are:

* Too much insulin or too many glucose-lowering pills;
* Not enough food;
* Unexpected or strenuous exercise.

Too much insulin or too many glucose-lowering pills

Everyone is capable of making mistakes – did you take more insulin or pills than you intended? Did you inject the insulin more deeply than usual so that it entered the muscle? Check your needle length. Is your insulin dose too big – look back over your previous blood glucose tests to see whether you often have lower readings at this time. Is your pill dosage too high? Check the label on the bottle.

Not enough food

This is a common reason for hypoglycaemia. Did you miss a meal because you were in a hurry or did not like it? Were the portions smaller than expected? The wise person with diabetes has a muesli bar or biscuits in a bag, briefcase or pocket to ensure that she has something to eat at any time. Dieting to lose weight without first reducing your dose of insulin or glucose-lowering pills is another reason for frequent hypoglycaemia (especially in weight-conscious young women).

Unexpected or strenuous exercise

Running for a bus, playing an expected game of tennis, finding a tough job in the garden, unloading a lorry that you were not expecting – exertion like this can lower your blood glucose fast. Eat extra glucose while you are exercising. Note that I said unexpected exercise – if you know you are going to exercise you should plan ahead (see Chapter 17).

HYPOGLYCAEMIC UNAWARENESS

After many years of diabetes, about one in five people lose awareness of some or all their symptoms of hypoglycaemia. About one in 15 have no warning symptoms at all. This appears to be related to long duration of diabetes, and, in some cases, to diabetic autonomic nerve damage (see pages 140–1). You may regain awareness if you take great care to avoid hypoglycaemia altogether. Ask your diabetes adviser for help. Beta blocker pills used to treat high blood pressure or angina (see pages 151 and 136) can diminish your warning of hypoglycaemia. Never stop these pills without first consulting your doctor.

Human insulin

There has been some anxiety that human insulins are more likely to cause problems with hypoglycaemia than are animal insulins. Human insulin was introduced at a time when there was also increasing encouragement to keep blood glucose concentrations as close to normal as possible. This strategy is to protect people from long-term tissue damage but it does mean that there is more risk of hypoglycaemia and less warning. It usually takes less time for the glucose to fall from 5 to 2 mmol/l (90–36 mg/dl), than to fall from 12 to 2 mmol/l (216–36 mg/dl). Insulin-treated diabetics with persistently normal blood glucose levels have less emergency hormone response to hypoglycaemia than those who usually have high blood glucose levels. One survey (around the time of some media publicity against human insulin) asked people to remember what their hypoglycaemia was like before and after starting human insulin. One in twelve of those who had warning of hypoglycaemia before the changeover said they had less warning since but one in 24 had more warning – and, of course, all of them had had another few years of diabetes.

If you have had diabetes for long enough to remember taking animal insulin you may have diabetic tissue damage which, among other effects, can reduce your warning of hypoglycaemia. A study in Switzerland showed that people requiring hospital treatment for severe hypoglycaemia were more likely to be taking human insulin than patients with diabetes admitted for other reasons. However, those admitted for hypoglycaemia also had better blood glucose control than the others. Another Swiss study compared human with pork insulin in 44 people. Each person took both, but neither patients nor doctors knew which insulin was being taken. A blood glucose below 2.8 mmol/l was recorded more often when subjects were taking the pork insulin. While taking human insulin, hypoglycaemic people were more likely to report restlessness and lack of concentration and less likely to report hunger than during hypoglycaemia on pork insulin.

A British survey of about 6000 insulin-treated people found just 19 who reported loss of warning of hypoglycaemia for which the only reason seemed to be taking human insulin, and who regained their warning symptoms on restarting animal insulin. Seven of them agreed to be made hypoglycaemic with either pork or human insulin under identical conditions without knowing which insulin they were receiving. There was no difference in their feelings, their blood glucose, or their emergency hormone response to either insulin. Further studies have confirmed that there is no difference in frequency or recognition of hypoglycaemia between those taking human and those taking animal insulin.

If I had diabetes I personally would want human insulin treatment. However, if you feel that you had better warning of hypoglycaemia on animal insulin, or you have any other concerns about human insulin, discuss it with your doctor and, if you are still unhappy, ask to change to animal insulin. You may not be able to have insulin with exactly the same duration and pattern of action as your human one(s).

Watch your blood glucose

I am always a little surprised when people show me their blood glucose diaries with 2s (36 mg/dl) dotted about and then say that they have had no hypos since I last saw them. When I point to the 2s they say that they did not feel hypo then. Whether or not you feel hypoglycaemic, a blood glucose level of 2 mmol/l (36 mg/dl) is hypoglycaemic and requires immediate treatment and then review as to why it happened. So if the result is 2, *stop*, eat.

Some people are fine during the day, but their blood glucose dips at night. You may detect this by waking feeling hungover or with a headache. If you are on insulin make sure you always have a bedtime snack and do not go to bed with a glucose below 6 mmol/l (108 mg/ dl). It is sensible to set an alarm clock for 2 or 3 am from time to time to check your blood glucose level.

Tracey was 17. She wanted to learn to drive. I asked how her diabetes was. 'Good,' she said, 'I've been really careful.' I asked to see her diabetic diary. All the blood glucose levels were 4 or below. At least half were 2 mmol/l or less. I was horrified. She admitted she did feel low quite often. She was very upset when I said that she was not safe to drive. After she had calmed down and we discussed it all, it emerged that she thought a previous doctor had told her to keep her blood glucose levels as low as possible to avoid tissue damage. She had been doing exactly as she was told. We reduced her insulin dose and her blood glucose concentrations became normal. She passed her driving test a year later.

HONEYMOON PERIOD

In the weeks or months after startlng insulin treatment your few remaining islet cells, which had been 'stunned' by high glucose levels, may start making insulin again. You may become hypoglycaemic and your insulin requirements may plummet. This is called the honeymoon period. Eventually these cells will succumb to the autoimmune process and die. You will need bigger insulin doses again.

SEEK HELP

If you are experiencing problems with hypoglycaemia always ask you diabetes adviser for help.

SUMMARY

*   Hypoglycaemia is a low blood glucose – below 4 mmol/l for practical purposes, official definition below 2.5 mmol/l.
*   It is common in insulin-treated diabetics (about 10 episodes a year) and occurs in one in three people who are taking glibenclamide.
*   Hypoglycaemia is rarely serious.
*   Learn to recognise when your blood glucose is falling.
*   Teach your friends and family what to look for.
*   Always carry glucose if you take insulin or sulphonylurea pills.
*   Eat glucose immediately you become hypoglycaemic, followed by some starchy food.
*   When you are better, work out why you were hypoglycaemic. Was it too much insulin or too many pills, too little food, or unexpected exercise?
*   Bad hypos are rare. If you are on insulin keep glucagon in the house just in case.
*   Good observation and early treatment of hypoglycaemia can prevent trouble.
*   Seek advice early.

11

HYPERGLYCAEMIA OR HIGH BLOOD GLUCOSE

In theory, any blood glucose over 8 mmol/l (144 mg/dl) is high, i.e. hyperglycaemic. However, while everyone would like to have their blood glucose levels between 4 and 8 mmol/l (72 and 144 mg/dl), (4–7 mmol/l premeal), in real life it is very hard to achieve this all the time over years of diabetes. That does not mean that you should stop trying.

For practical purposes, this chapter is about blood glucose levels in double figures (i.e. 11 mmol/l or more – 200 mg/dl USA). Many of you will see blood glucose levels in this range from time to time; the occasional level between 11 and 20 mmol/l is rarely a disaster although it may make you feel below par and thirsty, and you may pass a lot of urine.

One of the difficulties in advising people with diabetes about how to respond to changes in blood glucose is that everyone responds differently to a given blood glucose. Some people who do not look after their diabetes walk around with blood glucose levels of 30 mmol/l (540 mg/dl) and claim to feel fine. Others feel awful if their glucose rises about 11 mmol/l (200 mg/dl). Part of this is due to the body getting used to the prevailing glucose level, but we all perceive things differently. In addition, other factors, such as the state of other body chemistry, will affect how you feel and how seriously to take a particular glucose level. This makes it hard to use particular blood glucose levels to indicate particular courses of action. Each of you must get to know your own body. Discuss with your diabetes adviser what you are going to do if your glucose rises – what follows is general guidance only.

PERSISTENTLY HIGH BLOOD GLUCOSE LEVELS

11–19 mmol/l (200–342 mg/dl)

Sadly, many people with diabetes have levels like this most of the time. Part of this may be a legacy of the days when you were told, 'Always keep a little sugar in your urine to stop you going hypo.' If there is glucose in the urine your blood glucose is likely to be over 11 mmol/l. This is over the threshold for the development of diabetic tissue damage. This means that if your average blood glucose is above this for long periods of time, you may develop diabetic tissue damage (see Chapter 12).

Thus, while for most people these blood glucose levels are not acutely dangerous, they may be slowly harming your body and should be reduced.

Over 19 mmol/1 (over 342 mg/dl)

Most people with insulin-treated diabetes will have one-off levels like this at some time. However, if most of your blood glucose levels are this high you are in danger. Although you may not feel very ill, a small upset – a row at work or a cold, for example – could push your blood glucose up fast. Then you could feel very ill. Levels like this require immediate action.

SOME CAUSES OF HIGH BLOOD GLUCOSE LEVELS

- Too little insulin or glucose-lowering pills;
- Too much food;
- Too little exercise;
- Monthly periods;
- Pregnancy;
- Infection;
- Injury or operation;
- Heart attack;
- Stress;
- Drugs and medicines.

Too little insulin or too few glucose-lowering pills

If you forget your insulin, run out or stop taking it, your glucose level will rise. If you forget your diabetic pills, run out or stop taking them, your glucose will rise. Glucose-lowering treatments are your lifeline – by all means reduce your treatment if your blood glucose is persistently low (see Chapter 10), but do not stop it. There is no excuse for running out of pills, and to run out of insulin is unforgivable. The occasional forgotten dose is human, but if you keep forgetting develop a system for remembering – an alarm clock beside the insulin if necessary. Do not stop your insulin during a vomiting illness.

Too much food

Lucy was an in-patient on the diabetic ward. She had been admitted with pneumonia which upset her blood glucose balance. Although the pneumonia soon improved her blood glucose levels went up and up. Eventually we discovered that she was having two breakfasts – one on the ward and a second one in the staff canteen. 'I do like a cooked breakfast,' she said, 'and I can't be bothered at home.' She liked the canteen's afternoon teas too.

If you eat more than the insulin in your body can cope with (whether your own insulin or that boosted by pills or injected insulin) then your blood glucose will rise. A few people need to put on weight if newly-diagnosed diabetes has made them thin. In most cases extra weight is the last thing you need. As you get fat, your insulin needs rise, your insulin dose or pills must be increased, this makes you hungry, you eat more, and so on.

A few people try to starve their glucose down. This is not a good idea. It causes fat breakdown which makes ketones.

Too little exercise

Damian was in the sixth month of his first job. The job was going well but his diabetes wasn't. His blood glucose levels had started to rise soon after he began the job and he seemed to need more insulin these days. He could not understand it because he was sticking to his diet. He discussed it with Mrs Baxter, the Diabetes Specialist Nurse. 'How much exercise do you get these days?' she asked. 'Not much,' replied Damian, ruefully. 'I really enjoy all the planning work I do in the office, but I miss the school football team. No one here seems interested in sport.' This was why his glucose levels had risen. He had been exercising less since he left school. He was not burning off the glucose as he used to. When Mrs Baxter checked his weight it had increased a little. She suggested eating a little less and using the factory swimming pool several times a week to keep fit. There he met several sportsmen and was soon playing squash regularly.

Regular exercise increases your sensitivity to insulin and improves the way in which you use glucose. It keeps you fit generally (see Chapter 17).

Monthly periods

The hormone changes which occur during a woman's menstrual cycle can have profound effects on blood glucose. Most diabetic women find that their blood glucose rises just before or as they lose blood. A few notice a tendency to hypoglycaemia then a rise in glucose. The changes last only a few days in most people and are often not severe enough to alter the insulin dose. However, some women adjust their insulin with every period. Find out what happens to your own glucose levels. Glucose levels may fall after the menopause.

Pregnancy

As the pregnancy progresses, your insulin needs will increase. Some women may be taking twice as much insulin by the end of pregnancy as they were at the start (see Chapter 16).

Infection

Any infection can upset your diabetes: a cold, 'flu, viral sore throat, cystitis (urine infection), chest infection, gastroenteritis, thrush, an abscess and so on. The degree to which your blood glucose rises during an infection is not always in proportion to the severity of the infection. However, the glucose can rise very fast – for example overnight it may go from 8 to 22 mmol/l (144 to 396 mg/dl). The reason for the rise in glucose (sometimes despite vomiting or eating less) is the release of emergency hormones (e.g. steroids and adrenaline) to help your body fight the infection. They release glucose from the liver into the bloodstream. So you need more insulin when you have an infection. As the infection settles you will need to reduce your insulin dose again. People on diet treatment alone may find that they need extra help – glucose-lowering pills or insulin injections while the infection resolves. Those on pills may find that they need insulin temporarily. Your body cannot fight the infection if your blood glucose level is high. This prevents your 'soldiers' – the white blood cells – from moving in to attack and engulf the bacteria. So a vicious circle may ensue – infection, glucose rises, defence slows, infection worsens, glucose rises more and so on. Get help early on to treat the infection and do not allow your blood glucose to rise. This means injecting your usual dose of insulin even if you are unable to eat and giving extra insulin if your blood glucose levels are high. You need energy to get better so if you cannot eat try drinking Lucozade, Coke, Pepsi, fruit juice, milk or soup. Ice cream or yoghurt may be easy to eat. But *on no account* stop your insulin.

Injury or operation

The body responds to injury – a broken leg, for example, as it does to infection. As far as the body is concerned, an operation is a form of injury. Stress hormones are released to help you recover and these release glucose into the bloodstream. You may need to increase your insulin while recovering from major injury. If you have an operation and cannot eat for a while you will usually be given insulin and glucose into a vein. The doses will be adjusted according to blood glucose levels until you are eating again. Then your usual insulin or pills can be restarted. With a major injury or operation people on diet alone may sometimes need insulin temporarily.

Heart attack

See pages 137–9. A heart attack is another form of stress and injury, and again emergency hormones are released pushing the blood glucose up. Your blood glucose level should be returned towards normal, making sure that you cannot become hypoglycaemic at a time when your heart may be irritable.

Stress

I have used the word 'stress' to mean a situation which evokes an emergency response in the body. The stress of everyday life can cause adrenaline release which may push the blood glucose up.

Mike was the shop steward in a glass factory. There had been increasing friction between a particular manager and the workers in the plate glass plant. This came to a head one Friday when the manager accused a man of sloppy work. Mike had a fierce argument with the manager and both sides eventually retired angry with the dispute unsettled. Mike drove home in a temper. When he checked his blood glucose it had risen from 9 mmol/l (162 mg/dl) at lunchtime to 19 mmol/l (342 mg/dl) – the highest evening level he had seen for years. He took three extra units of fast-acting insulin and by bedtime the glucose was down to 11 mmol/l (200 mg/dl).

Drugs and medicines

I do not mean street drugs, although these can upset your blood glucose (among other things) and are dangerous. Medical drugs are a common cause of hyperglycaemia. Steroids produce the greatest rise in glucose and the dose of insulin or glucose-lowering pills can double during a course of steroid treatment. If the steroids are stopped abruptly, the glucose will fall suddenly. This is important for diabetic asthmatics who may need short courses of steroids. Other drugs which may increase the blood glucose concentration are thiazide diuretics (see page 150), oral contraceptive pills and sometimes tricyclic antidepressants (e.g. amitriptylline). Thiazides can usually be changed to another medication to control high blood pressure or alleviate ankle swelling. Steroids are essential treatment for most of the conditions in which they are used, so you will have to adjust your diabetes treatment to follow the glucose rise (and its fall when the steroid treatment finishes).

WHAT DO YOU DO ABOUT HIGH BLOOD GLUCOSE LEVELS?

If the high value comes as a complete surprise, wash your hands and repeat the test carefully. You may have had sticky fingers.

Emergency advice for high blood glucose levels is given on pages 105–6. To adjust your insulin you need to know which insulin is acting (or rather, should be acting) at the times when the blood glucose is high, and how long it acts for. As cloudy insulins take a long time to clear from the body, it is best to wait three days between each dosage adjustment. Over-rapid changes in medium or long-acting insulin may lead to exaggerated glucose fluctuations and hypoglycaemia. It is also easiest (at least to start with) to adjust only one insulin dose (i.e. morning only or evening only) at a time, to avoid confusion. If you are nervous about increasing your insulin do it in one-unit steps. Check with your diabetes adviser. But do not simply sit and look at high blood glucose levels and do nothing.

People taking glucose-lowering pills can also adjust their medication if blood glucose levels are persistently high. But you must check with your diabetes adviser first. Each pill has a maximum dose which must not be exceeded (unlike insulin where you can have as much as your body needs). The maximum doses are shown on page 74 – but these may be lower in people with some medical problems, such as kidney impairment. Again leave three days in between each dosage adjustment.

SUMMARY

- If your blood glucose is in double figures, i.e. 11 mmol (200 mg/dl) or more, you are at risk of thirst and polyuria now.
- If your blood glucose remains in double figures you are at risk of tissue damage later.
- If you feel well but your blood glucose is rising, take extra insulin and adjust your diet or treatment to prevent future high glucose levels.
- If you feel ill and your blood glucose is rising, especially if you have urinary ketones, take extra insulin and get help urgently.
- Vomiting is a danger sign in people with diabetes. Get help.
- Causes of high blood glucose include too little insulin or too few glucose-lowering pills, too much food, too little exercise, monthly periods, pregnancy, infection, injury, heart attack, stress, drugs.

12

DIABETIC TISSUE DAMAGE

Diabetes is a multi-system disorder. In other words, it affects many parts or systems of the body. So far, I have concentrated on blood glucose balance, but other blood chemicals are also disturbed in diabetes. And more problems arise from damage to body tissues than are caused by ups and downs of blood glucose. Many people do not link their heart attack or poor vision to their diabetes, but they are connected. They are also potentially preventable if you take care of yourself from the beginning.

Diabetes tissue damage is traditionally divided into small blood vessel damage, such as that which occurs in eyes or kidneys; and large blood vessel damage, occurring in vessels supplying the heart and legs. But problems may be a combination of these and other factors. Also, classifications which seem obvious to doctors do not always reflect what people actually notice in themselves. I will therefore discuss the effects of diabetes as you may discover them and how your doctor may assess and treat you. This approach means that common and uncommon complications are mixed up. Don't panic. No one will have all of them! And if you do find a problem, your diabetes team can help you. In Chapter 13 I will review possible causes of these effects and what you can do to prevent them.

I have described potential problems according to parts of the body where you may find them, or the doctor examining you may find them.

SKIN

Infections

Minor skin infections These are common in diabetes, especially if the blood glucose is not well controlled. There may be boils or spots which will settle as the blood glucose settles. Occasionally boils develop into abscesses or carbuncles. These may need surgical incision and drainage, sometimes under a general anaesthetic. Rarely, a rash of purple-red spots up the legs or a generalised redness and heat indicates a spreading bacterial infection needing antibiotic therapy. More often purple or red marks on the legs are scars due to old knocks and scrapes.

Thrush This may develop in cracks and crevices of the skin – under breasts or in the groins – if you are overweight. This will respond to antifungal cream, control of high blood glucose and weight loss.

Diabetic dermopathy

Many people with long-standing diabetes develop red/brown or brown marks on the skin. These may occur at the site of minor injury or spontaneously. They may fade a little but can last many years. No treatment is needed and they are not serious.

Necrobiosis lipoidica diabeticorum

Necrobiosis lipoidica diabeticorum is a rare complication of diabetes, usually found in people whose blood glucose has been too high for a long time. It is a red-purple shiny dent in the skin, usually over the lower leg. It may settle slowly on its own. If not, steroid treatment is sometimes helpful, and some doctors use nicotinic acid tablets. The condition itself is not dangerous but it is occasionally sore and women may want to hide it with tights or make-up.

Eruptive xanthomata

These are little fatty lumps which are found in people with very high levels of the blood fat triglyceride. Such people may have fatty streaks in the creases of their hands too. Eruptive xanthomata are quite rare and are most often found on the upper limbs. People with these need to lower their triglyceride fast (see pages 160–1).

HEAD AND NECK:

General appearance

Facial appearance While not strictly a complication of diabetes, the following changes may alert you to the existence of a hormonal cause for your diabetes which was perhaps not obvious initially. A very round moon-face, with rosy red cheeks and (in women) excess hair on the chin, upper lip and sides may indicate steroid hormone excess (whether taken as tablets or due to overproduction in the body). Coarsening of the skin, heavy brows, a large protruding jaw and increased spacing of the teeth may indicate growth hormone excess (acromegaly – a rare condition). A slim face with an anxious expression and staring eyes may indicate thryoid overactivity.

Pimples and boils Facial pimples and boils on the back of the neck can cause much distress especially if you are young. They usually improve with good blood glucose balance. Acne can be treated with good skin care and sometimes tetracycline or related antibiotics.

Muscle weakness Facial muscle weakness can be due to a stroke (usually including cheek and side of the mouth) or to damage to one of the nerves supplying the face, in which case it may be more localised. If the facial nerves are not working (either due to a stroke or to nerve damage), you may not be able to control your mouth and saliva or food may dribble out of that side (rather like the effects of a dental local anaesthetic). Nerve damage may prevent the eyelid from opening fully. Facial weakness usually improves gradually.

Gustatory sweating This describes the flushing and sweating on the face precipitated by eating in someone with diabetic autonomic nerve damage (see page 147). It is best to avoid highly spiced foods if you have this problem.

Eyes

Squint with double vision This is another sign of weak muscles because of nerve damage. It may come on quite suddenly with pain or aching around the eye. Again this can resolve with time, improvement usually starting within weeks, although full recovery may take many months. An eye patch or glasses with a prism may help.

Cataract Cataract is common in people with diabetes. Even young children can have cataracts. In children this may be due to poor glucose balance. However, most people do not develop cataracts until they are much older. A cataract is a collection of debris inside the lens of the eye. The lens of the eye resembles that of a camera. If your camera lens is dirty you cannot see through it and the same applies in the eye. Cataracts can cause blurred vision. Sometimes the blurring is patchy.

Your doctor will check your visual acuity by asking you to read letters off an eye chart – 6/6 or 6/5 is good – and then looking at your eyes in a darkened room, usually after putting drops in to dilate (widen) the pupil. The drops (usually tropicamide) will wear off gradually or can be reversed, but do not drive until you can see normally. You should not be driving if your vision has deteriorated badly. Can you still fulfil the visual requirements for a driving license? When the cataract is 'ripe' an eye surgeon (ophthalmologist) will remove the lens under local or general anaesthetic. Usually an artificial lens will be inserted in its place.

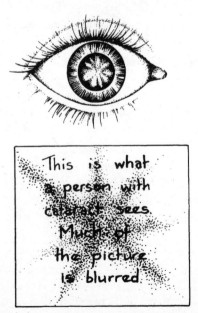

Cataracts

Diabetic retinopathy Retinopathy is one of the major complications of diabetes. It means disorders due to diabetes affecting the back of the eye. The retina is the part we see with (like the film in a camera). Diabetes is the most common cause of blindness in people of working age in Britain, but this situation is gradually improving. The development of diabetic retinopathy can be delayed or even avoided by keeping your blood glucose normal, and even if it does develop it can be treated successfully. After 15 years of diabetes virtually anyone with Type 1 diabetics will have some evidence of diabetic retinopathy. After 15 years of Type 2 diabetes, about 65 per cent will have some evidence of retinopathy. However, in many people this will simply be tiny red dots which do not affect vision.

Eye checks People with diabetes must have their eyes checked at least once a year. They can be checked in several ways, but the essential is for someone to look at the retina either with a special torch called an ophthalmoscope and/or by taking a photograph. In most instances this has to be done in a dark room after eye drops have been put in to dilate your pupil. To use the ophthalmoscope the observer (who may be a doctor, optometrist, ophthalmic optician or specially trained nurse) must come close to you and look through the black pupil in the centre of your eye. He will ask you to look straight ahead, and it makes it much easier if you can fix on a point ahead and keep looking in that direction even if his head is in the way. You can blink, and do not forget to breathe! Another way of checking is to take a photograph of the eye with a camera which focuses on the retina using infra-red light. This is called non-mydriatic retinal photography because it is usually done without needing to put eye drops in.

Background retinopathy This is the commonest form of diabetic retinopathy. At first all that can be seen are swollen veins. As the condition progresses, microaneurysms (tiny red dots near blood vessels) and haemorrhages (red smudges or blots) are found, alone or with fatty yellow exudates. Background retinopathy does not usually cause any loss of vision – you are unlikely to know you have it. However, it can progress to more severe problems, so it must be detected and watched carefully. If the exudates are over the macula (the area of best vision) they can reduce vision (see below).

The treatment of background retinopathy is a gentle return of your blood glucose and blood pressure to normal. Once this has been achieved, then keep it there.

Macular disease The macula is a tiny area of the retina where the central vision is concentrated. It can become swollen (macular oedema) or exudates can block the path of light or encircle it. If the macula is affected, visual acuity will be reduced and you will notice a problem. An ophthalmologist (eye doctor) may be able to improve matters with laser treatment. Again, you must gently return your blood glucose and blood pressure to normal.

Pre-proliferative and proliferative retinopathy This is the most serious form of diabetic eye disease. Pre-proliferative retinopathy is shown by irregular veins and soft white blobs on the retina – soft exudates or cotton-wool spots. One in two people with these changes develop proliferative retinopathy in two years. In proliferative retinopathy new blood vessels grow across the retina or out forwards into the clear jelly or vitreous through which we see. These new vessels are fragile and bleed easily, filling the vitreous with blood, through which you cannot see. The new vessels can also cause fibrous tissue which drags the retina off its supporting tissue

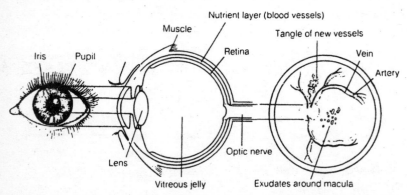

In the centre is a vertical section through a normal eye, while on the right is what the doctor sees when he looks through the pupil of someone with severe diabetic retinopathy

– retinal detachment. Up to one in four people with new vessels will lose vision in that eye in the next two years. Urgent laser treatment – within weeks – can greatly reduce the risk of blindness from proliferative retinopathy.

Unfortunately you may have no symptoms of pre-proliferative retinopathy or proliferative retinopathy until it is too late. Once a bleed has occurred you will either see a black film across your vision or black floaters across it. If you see anything like this you must see your doctor that day or go to the emergency department of an eye hospital. Urgent treatment may save your vision. If the retina is being pulled off its supports it may be possible to remove the vitreous and stop any further traction on the sensitive retina. This operation is called a vitrectomy.

Laser treatment is usually done as an out-patient procedure, with some local anaesthetic in the eye. The dilating drops needed can blur your vision for a while. The laser treatment does not hurt but it may make your eye ache or give you a headache.

Other eye problems Clots in the arteries or veins in the retina are more common in people with diabetes than in others, as is glaucoma. Glaucoma is an increase of pressure in the vitreous fluid bathing the inside of the eye. If you have a painful, tense, red eye you must go to your doctor immediately. Less dramatic signs of glaucoma are halos around lights, blurred vision and eye ache. Glaucoma is diagnosed by dropping local anaesthetic onto the eye and putting a measuring device called a tonometer onto the numbed cornea. It is readily treatable.

WARNING

Doctors need to use eye drops to dilate (widen) the pupil of the eye to see the retina. This may be dangerous in people who have:

*   Glaucoma;
*   A previous eye operation;
*   An artificial lens implanted during a cataract operation.

If you have any of these make sure you warn anyone about to put drops in your eyes – before they put the drops in!

Ears

Deafness Deafness is not always recognised as being linked with diabetes, but the auditory nerves can be damaged by diabetes, which causes hearing impairment. A hearing test will determine the type of problem and, if necessary, a hearing aid can be fitted.

Neck

The back of the neck is a classical site for carbuncles or boils. At the front, the thyroid gland may swell, indicating possible thyroid overactivity.

CHEST

The chest contains the heart and lungs, confined within the ribs, which are linked to the breastbone or sternum with springy cartilage. The underside of the chest cavity is formed by the muscular diaphragm. The oesophagus or gullet runs behind the heart and in front of the backbone or spine, carrying food from the mouth to the stomach.

Heart

Chest pain Most pains in the chest are not due to heart disease. The problem with describing symptoms in detail is that we all start feeling them as soon as we read about them – it is an occupational hazard for doctors and nurses. So don't start imagining things. Classically, heart pain is a tight, crushing pain in the centre of the chest, radiating across the chest and sometimes up the neck to the jaw or down the arms, usually the left. Because diabetes can affect the nerves, heart pain may not be classical in diabetics.

Angina Angina means tightness or narrowness – thus angina pectoris is tightness of the chest. This is a sign that part of your heart is not getting enough blood. Symptoms can be chest tightness, radiating to the neck or arms, which occurs with exercise, agitation, excitement or emotion – anything which makes your heart pound. Angina can be relieved by glyceryl trinitrate tablets or spray under the tongue. Pills such as nitrates, beta blockers (e.g. atenolol) and calcium channel antagonists (e.g. nifedipine) may prevent angina attacks.

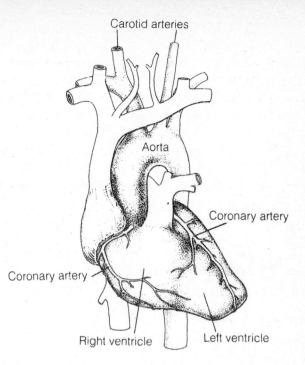

Carotid arteries

Aorta

Coronary artery

Coronary artery

Right ventricle

Left ventricle

The heart, showing the major arteries leaving it and the coronary arteries which supply the heart itself

Heart attack This is a non-specific name for the acute condition in which a clot in an artery supplying part of the heart muscle (coronary thrombosis) causes the muscle that artery supplies to die (myocardial infarction). This causes the same sort of pain that occurs in angina, but often it is more severe and prolonged. Angina is a temporary condition. A myocardial infarct is permanent. Other symptoms of myocardial infarction are being very frightened, sweating, nausea or vomiting, burping and shortness of breath. Some people have minor symptoms only. If you think you are having a heart attack call an ambulance. Then take one aspirin (unless you know that aspirin upsets you, or you have been told not to take it).

Nowadays, there is a specific treatment for coronary thrombosis – thrombolysis or 'clot-busting' drugs, e.g. streptokinase. People with untreated retinal new vessels should avoid thrombolysis in case they bleed (page 134). The sooner thrombolytic treatment is injected into a vein, the more likely it is to prevent myocardial infarction – permanent heart muscle damage. It works best within six hours of the onset of the symptoms, so call an ambulance immediately if you have symptoms of a heart attack. Electrocardiograms (FCGs) will confirm the diagnosis, as will later blood tests for enzymes leaking out of damaged heart cells. You will be kept under observation on a coronary care unit for a day or so, and will usually be given aspirin and beta blocker drugs (unless you are sensitive to them). You will gradually get up and about, and

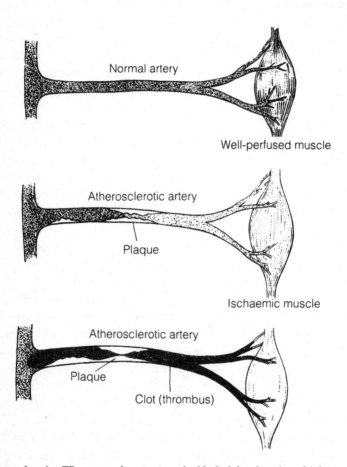

Atherosclerosis. The artery becomes partly blocked by deposits of plaque, on which clots may develop, blocking the artery completely. The muscle first becomes damaged and then dies completely

most people leave hospital in about a week. Most hospitals have a coronary rehabilitation programme. Many doctors will check how your heart responds to exercise with an exercise ECG to see if you need further treatment.

Coronary angiography is a common further investigation of angina or myocardial infarction. Dye is injected into your coronary arteries through a fine tube threaded up a groin artery to the heart. This is done under local anaesthetic with X-ray screening. You may feel hot when the dye is injected and may be left with a temporary bruise on your leg. People taking metformin should stop it beforehand. If particular types of coronary artery narrowing are seen, angioplasty (stretching the narrowing with a balloon) or coronary artery bypass surgery may be recommended. Make sure you understand exactly what the cardiologist or cardiac surgeon plans to do and what any risks are.

Coronary thrombosis is a common condition from which the majority of people recover to continue working and enjoying their hobbies. It takes about two to three months to get back to normal and you should not drive for the first month, or until your doctor says you can. If you have angina or coronary thrombosis you must not smoke, must watch your weight and blood pressure and should eat a low fat diet. When your doctor agrees, you should take regular exercise.

Lungs

Chest infection If you have a chest pain on one side of your chest or in the back of your chest which hurts when you take a breath in, especially if you are coughing up green phlegm or are breathless, you may have an infection in your lung. Call your doctor. People with diabetes are prone to infection. Antibiotics will soon resolve it.

Breathlessness may simply be due to general lack of fitness or being overweight. It can be a sign of many chest problems, including asthma, bronchitis and infection. If you have sustained heart damage, it can be due to water collecting in the lungs because the heart is not pumping vigorously enough to clear it. This is called pulmonary oedema or left ventricular failure and usually responds to diuretic pills. Diuretics make you pass urine and clear water (and sometimes potassium) from the body. They include frusemide and bumetanide. You may also be given angiotensin-converting enzyme inhibitors (ACE inhibitors), which ease the heart's work.

ABDOMEN

This lies between the lower ribs and the groins and is commonly called the tummy or (inaccurately) the stomach (see page 29). In fact the stomach lies inside the left abdominal cavity and delivers food to the duodenum and thence to the small intestine and the large intestine or colon. Faeces leave the body via the rectum. Behind the stomach lies the pancreas, which drains its digestive juices into the duodenum. The liver lies under the ribs on the right. The gall bladder hangs below the liver, from which it collects bile. The bile then drains into the duodenum to mix with the digestive enzymes from the pancreas. The kidneys are at the back of the abdominal cavity – one on each side. Urine drains from the kidneys down the ureters to the bladder, which is at the bottom of the abdominal cavity, just inside the pubic bone. In a woman, the ovaries and uterus lie behind the bladder. The urine passes out through the urethra. The urethra is short in a woman and passes in front of the vagina, which is in front of the rectum. In men the urethra is longer because it travels through the penis. The testes hang in the scrotum to keep them cool. The blood supply for the abdominal organs, and the legs, spurts down from the heart through the aorta which runs in front of the backbone. Used blood travels back up the vena cava, the great vein beside the aorta.

Gastrointestinal problems

Pancreatitis Pancreatitis is one cause of diabetes. It means inflammation of the pancreas and can cause very severe pain in the epigastrium – the part of the central abdomen just below the ribs. The pain may radiate to the back and be eased by sitting up. It is usually associated with vomiting. Chronic recurring pancreatitis may occur with several conditions including alcohol excess. Gall stones can cause pancreatitis too. A very high blood amylase level may support the diagnosis. Treatment is pain killers and fluid replacement through a vein.

Diabetic gastroparesis This is a partial paralysis of stomach emptying found in people with diabetes whose autonomic nerves are not working. The nerves are the cables which carry electronic signals to all parts of the body from the brain and which send messages back to the brain. The autonomic nerves are responsible for body functioning. If the stomach cannot empty you feel overfull after eating and may vomit often. This can be associated with indigestion pains. The treatment is good glucose balance and drugs such as metoclopramide, which encourage stomach emptying.

Diabetic diarrhoea This is another manifestation of autonomic neuropathy. It can wake you suddenly early in the morning and you may need to rush to the toilet several times. The treatment is good glucose balance and drugs like codeine which slow the bowel down. Antibiotics sometimes help.

Constipation Constipation can be due to dehydration, as in uncontrolled diabetes, or to failure of the nerves which tell the

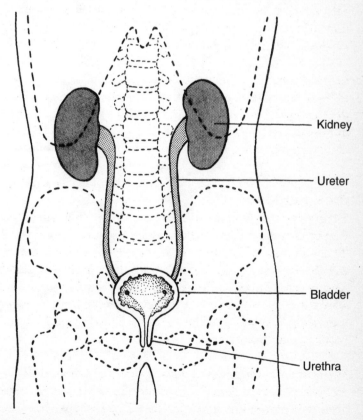

Kidney

Ureter

Bladder

Urethra

The urinary tract and kidneys

bowel muscles to move faeces along. Dehydration-induced constipation responds to fluid replacement. Laxatives or enemas can help the other kind of constipation.

Kidney and bladder problems

Infections Infections of the urinary tract and kidneys are more common in women than in men. This may be because a woman's short urethra can easily become contaminated with faecal organisms. However, diabetic men may also have urinary tract infections. Cystitis or bladder infection causes burning pain on passing urine, a sense of incomplete urination and the need to try to pass urine very frequently. The urine may be cloudy, or pink with blood, and smell horribly fishy.

Kidney infections or pyelonephritis may occur with or without symptoms of cystitis. You may have a high fever, vomiting and loin pain on the side of the affected kidney.

Antibiotics cure these infections. Cystitis rarely leads to hospital admission, but pyelonephritis can make you ill enough to warrant this. The blood glucose may rise and you may need more insulin or glucose-lowering tablets. You must drink plenty of clear fluids. Potassium citrate sometimes relieves the symptoms. If you have recurrent urinary tract infections be especially careful about perineal hygiene – women should wipe or wash from urethra to anus and not the other way round. Do not use strong soap in this sensitive area. Men should be careful to clean gently under the foreskin.

Nephropathy Nephropathy means kidney disease. The kidneys act as filters for water, salts and waste products. Blood is delivered in tiny tangles of blood vessels called glomeruli. Wastes, salt and water filter out of the blood vessels into collecting chambers and thence through concentrating tubules to the main drainage system to the kidneys. This urine then passes through the ureters to the bladder. In diabetes the walls of the blood vessels or capillaries thicken or become irregular. Wastes can no longer filter out to make urine. In other instances proteins leak out – in very small amounts – to produce microalbuminuria, and then in larger amounts to produce frank proteinuria. Dipstick urine tests can detect this protein leak. If you are losing a lot of protein, your blood albumin level will fall and you will be unable to keep water inside the bloodstream. You will develop swelling of the ankles, legs, face and elsewhere. This is called nephrotic syndrome.

You have millions of glomeruli in each of two kidneys so it may be many years (if ever) before you notice any ill effects of diabetic nephropathy. If the glomeruli are all damaged the wastes will build up in your blood. You may become tired and nauseated, with itchy skin and a lack of energy. You may develop shortness of breath, either because of fluid build-up or because the accumulation of wastes makes your blood acid. In particular, blood urea and creatinine concentrations will rise, as may blood potassium level. Your doctor will ask you to save all your urine for 24 hours and have a simultaneous blood sample taken to calculate the kidney clearance of creatinine from the blood into the urine.

As all these changes occur, the kidney damage may cause your blood pressure to rise, which can cause further kidney damage. In order to stop this vicious circle it is vital to keep your blood pressure normal (see pages 149–50).

There are many causes of kidney disease and your doctor will want to be sure that yours is due to diabetes and not a condition requiring different treatment. Diabetic nephropathy is virtually always linked with diabetic retinopathy (see pages 133–5). You will

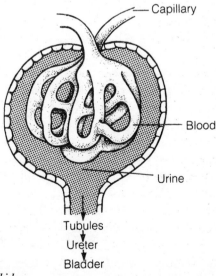

A glomerulus in the kidney

probably have an ultrasound scan, and perhaps an intravenous urogram to check kidney size, drainage and function.

Treatment depends on exactly what your problem is. Is it mainly protein loss and hence fluid build-up? Or is it accumulation of wastes? Initially good control of blood glucose and blood pressure, a diet, correct fluid balance, and instant treatment of urinary tract and other infections may be all that is needed to manage diabetic nephropathy. Diuretics can help in some cases. If the condition progresses you may eventually need peritoneal dialysis or haemodialysis. Renal transplant is successful in treating renal failure in people with diabetes. Nowadays, pancreas transplant may be done at the same time.

Bladder problems Such problems may include urinary incontinence and difficulty in emptying the bladder. In someone who has difficulty preventing urine leaks, a high blood glucose can cause increased urine flow and, especially in children or elderly people, urinary incontinence. Leaks can also occur if bladder sensation is lost through diabetic nerve damage. Nerve damage, autonomic neuropathy, can make it difficult to squeeze all the urine out of the bladder. If this is a problem, try pressing down behind the pubic bone to complete bladder emptying.

SEXUAL PROBLEMS AND PERIODS

Libido

Sex drive or libido can be diminished in anyone who is ill (for example with uncontrolled diabetes) and usually returns as you recover. If this problem persists, your doctor can check your sex hormone levels.

Menstruation

Periods (menstruation) can become irregular or stop altogether in someone with undiagnosed or uncontrolled diabetes. They usually return to normal as the diabetes comes under control. Periods and the menopause can affect glucose balance (see page 125).

Pregnancy

Pregnancy is not a complication of diabetes – but diabetes and pregnancy can complicate each other – see Chapter 16.

Impotence (Erectile dysfunction)

Impotence has many causes, and can affect most men at some time in their lives. In many instances a temporary inability to achieve an erection is due to emotional factors or the circumstances in which you are trying to have intercourse. Patience and an understanding partner can often resolve this sort of impotence. General ill-health, whether diabetes-related or not, can cause temporary impotence.

If you have no erections at all, whether with masturbation, spontaneously during the night, on waking, or when with a partner, it is more likely that you have a hormonal or mechanical sexual problem. If you are short of the male sex hormone, testosterone, this can be replaced to restore your sex life in most cases. Testosterone is useless in other cases – it increases the desire but not the performance. In diabetes, the problem may be inadequate blood supply to the penis due to furring up of the arteries, or to lack of the nerve signals which tell the penis to become erect. Arterial problems can sometimes be treated by vascular surgery. Occasionally, nerve problems improve with improved blood glucose balance. However, in some instances, the nerve damage is permanent.

Treatment for erectile dysfunction has changed over recent years and many men can now find a treatment to help them. It is important to have a full medical examination and blood tests before starting any treatment.

Sildenafil (Viagra) can be used in diabetic men. It increases blood flow to the penis during sexual stimulation. It only works if the penis has a functioning nerve supply and blood supply. The tablet is taken approximately one hour before sexual activity. Sexual stimulation is needed for an erection to occur. The initial dose is usually 50 mg. Lower doses are used in older men or those with kidney or liver problems. The dose can be increased to 100 mg. Viagra opens up the circulation and should not be used in people with low blood pressure, or in those taking nitrate medication. It should not be used in men who have had a recent stroke or heart attack, or have severe liver disease. It may cause a painfully, long-lasting erection (priapism). This is more likely if there are deformities of the penis, or in people with blood problems such as sickle cell anaemia or leukaemia. Viagra should not be used in men in whom the physical exertion of sexual intercourse might be dangerous (for example, in someone with severe heart disease). It may cause flushing and headache.

Alprostadil can be inserted into the urethra (Muse) or injected into the penis (Caverject) to stimulate an erection. This can be helpful in men who have a degree of diabetic nerve damage causing impotence. Muse comes as a medication stick which is inserted into the urethra with a special applicator after training by a nurse or doctor. Urinating beforehand makes it easier to insert. It may cause a burning feeling inside the penis, which usually settles. Men should sit or stand for the next 10 minutes, during which an erection usually develops, lasting about 30 to 60 minutes.

Caverject comes as a powder which has to be mixed with the fluid in a prefilled syringe. It is then injected into the corpus cavernosum (the part of the penis that fills with blood during erection). An erection usually occurs during the next hour. The first injection must be given by a trained nurse or doctor and the patient must be properly taught how to use Caverject. The injections can be painful and may cause bruising.

There is a risk of priapism with either form of alprostadil. Caverject must not be used in men with penile deformities or penile implants, nor in those with blood problems such as sickle cell disease or leukaemia.

There are vacuum devices which slip over the penis and can be used to draw blood into the penis to produce an erection. They are used less often nowadays. Very rarely, a surgeon may advise a penile implant to stiffen the penis. This involves major penile surgery and there is a risk of serious complications.

With any treatment for impotence if the penis does not go down after four hours, you must go immediately to a doctor or an Accident and Emergency department where they can remove the excess blood from the penis through a small needle to allow it to relax.

Impotence is an emotive subject. Often men do not want to talk it over with their wives or partners, but it is nearly always best to be open with each other. Your wife may be greatly relieved to know that you do still love her but have avoided sex only because you have a physical problem. Some couples find renewed pleasure in non-penetrative sexual activities. Others enjoy non-sexual pastimes together.

It is also sensible to tell your doctor about your worries. He will not be embarrassed and can always help. Many hospitals have a counselling service. Some have impotence clinics.

Infections

Thrush This can cause perineal itching and burning in diabetic men and women and can be passed on during sexual contact. It can make your skin red and sore, and causes a creamy curd-like discharge. It is easily treated by antifungal creams, which should be given to both partners for a full course of treatment. Women should ensure that the cream is also put into the vagina. A single pessary or tablet of antifungal medication can also help. The thrush fungus is common and seems to like a sugary, moist environment.

ARMS AND LEGS

Joints and tendons

Cheiroarthropathy This means stiff hand joints. It can also occur in the toes. It rarely limits what you can do. It is due to a tightening of the ligaments in the fingers. The same process can cause claw toes. Try finger exercises in the warm to keep your fingers supple.

Dupuytren's contracture This is a similar process causing tightening of the tendons in the palm. It occurs in non-diabetics as an inherited problem and sometimes with other conditions.

Problems with nerves

Peripheral neuropathy Peripheral neuropathy is nerve damage occurring in the nerves supplying the extremities or periphery of the body. The whole body is served by nerves. Some carry instructions from the brain to the body. These are called motor nerves. Other nerves carry information to the brain from body and skin sensors. They are called sensory nerves. The autonomic nerves carry signals to the heart, blood vessels, gut and bladder, for example. In diabetes, sorbitol and other abnormal substances can be deposited inside the nerve. The nerve sheath can be damaged, and its blood supply may become erratic. All this impairs transmission of the electronic signals running up or down the nerves. This may mean that no signals get through or that they are scrambled and send misleading messages to your brain.

Sensory neuropathy is the commonest form. It can affect any

sensory modality – touch, temperature, pain, vibration or position. The feet are more often affected than the hands. Classically, people with diabetes develop a 'glove or stocking neuropathy'. You may feel tingling or pins and needles in your feet or hands. Occasionally this can be painful. You may develop numbness, sometimes so marked that you can injure your foot and not notice. You may not to able to tell if your bath is too hot. I have seen someone with a serious burn on his numb foot from overhot bath water. Some people do not know exactly where their feet are in relation to the ground – rather like walking on cotton-wool. Your doctor may test sensation with sterile pins, wisps of cotton wool or the vibration from a tuning fork. Nowadays, many doctors use a bendy filament to gently test sensation. Absence of ankle reflexes may also indicate neuropathy.

Motor neuropathy is less frequent. It can affect one muscle or a group of muscles. If their nerve supply is interrupted they become atrophied and weak or paralysed. In diabetic amyotrophy, the thigh muscles are affected in this way.

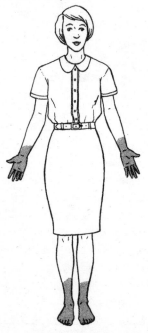

The extent of numbness in someone with glove and stocking peripheral neuropathy

There are many causes of neuropathy other than diabetes (including vitamins B$_{12}$ deficiency and alcohol) so these must be excluded. Good glucose balance is essential and may relieve tingling. Many drugs have been tried. Antidepressants like amitriptylline are effective – not because you are depressed but because of a specific effect on the nerves and receptors. Other agents like carbamazepine can relieve neuralgic pain. If you have loss of sensation you must protect the numb area(s) from injury and inspect them regularly.

Carpal tunnel syndrome This describes the trapping of the median nerve as it runs through a fibrous tunnel at the wrist. This entrapment causes pain or tingling in the thumb and next one and a half fingers. Symptoms are often worse at night. It can also cause finger weakness. A simple operation can release the trapped nerve.

Circulatory problems

High blood pressure (Hypertension) High blood pressure is included in this section because it is usually measured by a cuff around the upper arm (see page 20). Of course, your blood pressure exerts effects all around your circulation. You may be completely unaware that your blood pressure is high until it has exerted considerable damage on your heart and kidneys.

Your blood pressure is recorded as systolic (the upper, pumping pressure) over diastolic (the resting pressure). For example, 120/70. A doctor or nurse should check your blood pressure regularly. If your blood pressure is raised it should be rechecked later that visit, and again in one to four weeks depending on how high it is. The British Hypertension Society (BHS) guidelines say that in people with diabetes, the blood pressure should be below 140/80. However, some studies suggest that the blood pressure should be below 130/80 to gain optimal protection for people with diabetes. As blood pressure is a very important risk factor for the development of diabetic complications (see pages 161–2), it is essential to control it as well as possible providing the treatment does not make you feel light-headed or dizzy.

Most of us feel anxious when we visit the doctor and this can send blood pressure up. People for whom this 'white coat hypertension' is a major problem can measure their own blood pressure quietly at home. Blood pressure can also be measured over 24 hours with a little recorder than you wear as you go about your daily life (24-hour blood pressure monitoring). If you have hypertension you should consider buying a home blood pressure machine. These have to be used exactly according to instructions. The BHS has a list of devices which have been checked for accuracy.

Treatment for hypertension starts with weight reduction, trying to relax and reduce stress, and a low salt diet. Medication is nearly always needed too.

Bendrofluazide is a water tablet (diuretic). 2.5 mg is taken in the morning each day. Bigger doses are unnecessary. It may make you pass more urine. It should be avoided in severe kidney or liver failure, blood salt (electrolyte) abnormalities, pregnancy and breast-feeding, and in those allergic to sulphonamide drugs. Bendrofluazide has been in use for many years and has been shown in a large study to be helpful and safe in reducing high blood pressure in diabetes.

ACE inhibitors (ramipril, lisinopril, enalapril, captopril and others ending in -pril) have been shown in many studies to be helpful in people with diabetes in reducing blood pressure and protecting the kidneys. The doses vary. Most are long-acting and can be taken once daily. These drugs work by blocking the enzyme (chemical) which sets in train the process which constricts blood vessels and raises the blood pressure (angiotensin = blood vessel tightening). They are very effective in lowering blood pressure and can also increase the blood flow to the kidneys and reduce the workload of the heart. Most people with diabetes who have hypertension take them nowadays.

ACE inhibitors usually improve kidney function but rarely, especially if the arteries to the kidneys are furred up, they can cause kidney failure. It is therefore important that your urea, blood salts (electrolytes) and creatinine (see page 143) are checked before and dunng ACE inhibitor treatment. If you have severe arterial disease or severe kidney disease these drugs should be used with caution. ACE inhibitors should not be used in pregnancy (women of child-bearing age who need ACE inhibitors should be using good contraception) or breast-feeding. ACE inhibitors are well-tolerated but side-effects can include dizziness (from excessive blood pressure lowering), cough, swelling, tiredness, headache, nausea, diarrhoea or palpitations.

ACE II blockers (candesartan, valsartan and others ending in -sartan) can be used instead of ACE inhibitors as they are less likely to cause chronic cough. They have been shown to be effective in diabetic patients.

Beta blockers (atenolol and other drugs ending in -olol) are one of the first-line treatments for hypertension. Atenolol was shown in a large study to be safe and effective in people with type 2 diabetes. These drugs block receptors in arteries and elsewhere that lead to an increase in blood pressure. They also slow the heart rate. They can cause asthma and should be avoided in people with chest problems. Beta blockers should also be avoided in people with a tendency to unduly slow heart rate, or in those with very poor circulation in their legs. These drugs can cause tiredness, difficulty with sleeping, heart failure, hair loss and stomach upsets. If you have dry eyes or a skin rash see your doctor straightaway.

Calcium channel blockers (nifedipine modified release, felodipine and other drugs ending in -ipine) are also widely used to lower blood pressure in diabetes. Some smaller studies suggested that in general they could cause heart problems, but the two named have been shown in large studies to be safe in diabetic patients. They reduce muscle contractions in blood vessel walls, relaxing them and reducing blood pressure. They should not be given to pregnant or breast-feeding women, nor to those with some unstable heart conditions. Calcium channel antagonists can cause ankle swelling, headache, flushing, dizziness, tiredness, palpitations, rash and worsening of angina. Most of these drugs are taken once daily.

Doxazosin may be given to people with diabetes whose blood pressure is hard to control. This is an alpha blocker which works by relaxing blood vessels. It should be avoided in pregnancy or breast-feeding, and in liver disease. It can cause dizziness, headache, tiredness, weakness, swelling, nasal symptoms and nausea. It is usually taken at night, once daily.

There are over one hundred blood pressure-lowering drugs, so it should be possible to find the treatment that suits you and your blood pressure. The notes above briefly discuss the commonly used ones. Please read the packet insert with your tablets for full details or talk with your doctor. Many people need more than one type of tablet for good blood pressure control. It is important that you understand how and when to take your tablets and that you report any side-effects to your doctor. It is also important to take the tablets! If you don't take them they won't work. Most people will need lifelong blood pressure medication to gain most benefit from treatment. Furthermore, it can be dangerous to stop some tablets suddenly.

Postural hypotension If you have autonomic nerve damage your blood pressure may fall when you stand up. This can cause dizziness or fainting.

Peripheral vascular disease This problem is not confined to diabetics. It also troubles smokers and people with high blood fats. If the arteries supplying the legs become atherosclerotic (furred up) blood flow to the legs and feet is reduced. This may cause pain in the calves on walking – intermittent claudication (intermittent limping). The pain comes on sooner going upstairs or uphill and is eased by rest. If the blood flow is severely restricted you may develop sluggish circulation in your feet – they become very white if you raise them and take a long time to regain their colour on

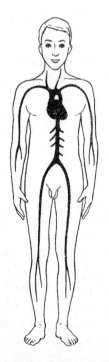

The major arteries

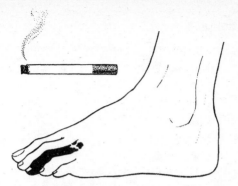

A gangrenous toe in a smoker with diabetes

lowering. Eventually they take on a reddish tinge and may start to hurt at night so that you have to hang them over the bedside. If you have this type of rest pain you must call your doctor urgently. If the circulation is completely blocked you will develop gangrene. Signs of this are bluish purple discoloration followed by blackening. Fortunately, this is rare. As with rest pain, this is a medical emergency. Call your doctor now.

Stopping smoking is essential – indeed some vascular surgeons may not treat people who continue to smoke. A low fat diet is sensible. Continued exercise may encourage collateral vessels to develop and the intermittent claudication may improve, so keep walking if you can (don't forget to protect your feet). Your doctor will examine your pulses and may listen to them with an ultrasound probe resting lightly on the skin. X-rays recording the flow of dye injected into a groin artery under local anaesthetic may show a narrowing, which can be relieved by stretching with a balloon (angioplasty) or by a bypass operation. People on metformin should stop taking it beforehand. If there is a clot it can sometimes be dissolved (see pages 137–8). If you have developed gangrene it is virtually impossible to rescue that toe or foot and it will probably have to be amputated. Because your circulation is very poor, a local amputation may not heal and your surgeon may advise a below knee amputation. However, advances in surgical techniques to improve the circulation may reduce the risk of major amputation. With good healing, expert rehabilitation advice and vigorous physiotherapy you can learn to walk (with an artificial limb if necessary) and could be expected to return to most jobs within a few months.

Diabetic foot problems

As can be seen from the descriptions above, your feet are very vulnerable. These are some potential problems:

- Claw toes;
- Numbness;
- Insensitivity to temperature;
- Clumsiness because of poor position sense;
- Abnormal gait because of the above;
- Abnormal weight distribution causing rubbing or callus;
- Poor circulation;
- Poor healing.

These can lead to small rubs and wounds which you may not notice and which soon become infected. It is therefore vital that you learn to look after your feet.

Examine your feet every day. Sit comfortably. Take your shoes, socks or tights off and look at the top and bottom of your feet very carefully in a good light. Do not forget to look at the tips of each toe and in between the toes. If you cannot see your feet properly or cannot get close enough, ask someone to help you. Sometimes a mirror can help. Is the skin red? Is it broken anywhere? Are there blisters? Is there skin thickening on the sole or elsewhere? Is there any swelling? Do you have athlete's foot? Touch your feet – can you feel touch? Are they cold? Are there local areas of hotness?

Wash your feet every day in lukewarm water and dry them very carefully, especially between the toes. Cut your toenails regularly, being very careful to cut them straight across without sharp points or edges which could dig into the sides of that toe or other toes. Put on clean socks or tights each day. Socks should be made of wool or cotton. Never wear nylon socks – they can rub and they do not absorb sweat, so the feet can get soggy. Ensure that your socks or tights are loose enough for all your toes to wriggle freely and that socks do not cause a tight ring around your ankle. (Women should never use garters to hold up stockings.) Buy shoes which feel comfortable in the shoe shop and that cannot rub you or pinch you anywhere. Very high-heeled or pointed-toe shoes are not suitable for diabetics. Be careful with sandals – they increase the risk of

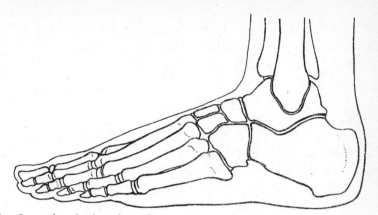

Your foot – these intricate bones bear your weight every day

small injuries. Use a shop which has a professional shoe fitter. If you work in the construction industry or on sites or in factories where there is a risk of foot injury, wear comfortable professional protective footwear (e.g. steel toe-caps). Ask your chiropodist for advice. Never use a hot water bottle in bed – use an electric blanket with a thermostat and turn it off before you get in. Never get into a hot bath unless you have checked the temperature with a bath thermometer. You should see a chiropodist regularly – this means at least once a year, and more often for those who cannot care for their own feet or who have 'at risk feet' – i.e. who have any of the problems listed above or who have ever had a foot ulcer or injury.

If you notice any change in your feet, discuss it with your chiropodist. Any breaks in the skin, however small, should be cleaned, covered by a non-adherent dressing (e.g. N-A) and checked daily. If injuries do not heal rapidly, start oozing pus or become surrounded by redness, you need to see a doctor straightaway because you probably need antibiotics. If in doubt contact your doctor. Wound care in diabetes requires expertise and experience. Some hospitals have wound care sisters or dressing clinics. Some chiropodists have a special interest in diabetes. Once the wound has been dressed, keep off it. This can mean resting for weeks, but if you walk on an ulcer it rarely heals. Total contact plaster casts can be used to redistribute the weight but must be applied only by experts. When you are resting your foot, put it up on a stool or sofa. Make sure that you do not rest the weight of your leg on your heel – you may get a pressure ulcer there. Support your whole calf (e.g. with a plastic foam trough or wedge) and leave the heel free from the bed or stool.

In someone with diabetes a tiny foot ulcer can cause trouble out of all proportion to its size. It may lead to severe skin and tissue infection, bone infection (osteomyelitis), blood poisoning and amputation. Look after your feet well and seek early advice about all problems, however minor.

Charcot joints Charcot joints are a bone problem which can occur in anyone with severe lower limb neuropathy. People with neuropathy sometimes ignore minor injuries because they do not feel pain properly. The neuropathy alters the circulation within the bone and makes it weaker. Walking on a minor injury causes damage to the thin bones and fractures can develop. The joints may gradually be destroyed. The joint becomes red and swollen and may eventually become misshapen. If you have diabetic neuropathy in your feet and have persistent problems after a minor injury, or an unexpected injury to your feet or ankles, insist on an x-ray. The management of Charcot joints usually requires a combination of orthopaedic surgeon and diabetes team.

SUMMARY

- Diabetes is a multi-system disorder.
- It can affect all the major body systems.
- These effects include problems with skin, eyes, heart, kidneys, stomach, bowels, sexual functions, blood vessels, blood pressure, muscles, nerves, ligaments and joints.
- Feet and eyes are especially vulnerable.
- The longer you have had diabetes, the more likely you are to have diabetic tissue damage.
- Most people are *not* seriously troubled by tissue damage, but many require treatment for some of its forms.
- Learn to check your body and report problems early.
- Attend your medical checks, even if you feel perfectly well.
- Diabetic tissue damage is not inevitable, you can greatly reduce the likelihood of being affected. The next chapter will tell you how.

13

PREVENTING DIABETIC TISSUE DAMAGE

We still have a lot to learn about diabetic tissue damage – thousands of people in many countries are researching in this area. However, some factors have been identified as being definitely or probably related to the development and progression of tissue damage in people with diabetes. You can do something about them. Do not wait until it is too late. All diabetic tissue damage becomes more likely with time. The longer you have had your diabetes, the more likely you are to have tissue damage. Virtually every person with diabetes will have some evidence of diabetic tissue damage eventually. What you do now will affect your health and well-being in years to come. The choice is yours.

STOP SMOKING

There is no doubt about the harmful effects of smoking. One in five of all deaths in the United Kingdom is due to cigarette smoking. Cigarettes kill one in two of those who smoke. Cigarettes also maim people. They cause cancers, for example in the lung, from which many people die a painful and lingering death. They fur up your arteries, causing strokes, intermittent claudication (pain in the legs on walking), and gangrene requiring amputation.

But if you have diabetes the risk is even greater. Your diabetes increases the likelihood of atherosclerosis causing coronary thrombosis and circulatory problems. If you smoke as well, your risks of dying from a coronary thrombosis are enormously increased. In addition to increasing your risk of death or disability, cigarettes can upset your blood glucose balance because the nicotine and other substances cause acute circulatory effects. For example, smoking a cigarette may upset your insulin absorption. Smoking can increase your blood fats. And smoking also poisons anyone who breathes in your smoke: if your wife does not smoke, she is more likely to die of lung cancer than if she had married a non-smoker. The same applies to your children.

If you retain only one piece of advice from this book it should be this: PEOPLE WITH DIABETES SHOULD NOT SMOKE. If you smoke, stop now, as you read this. You will improve both your health and that of those around you.

LOSE WEIGHT

Take all your clothes off and stand in front of a mirror. Be completely honest with yourself. Are you fat? If you are, then your fatness is not only increasing your risk of having a coronary thrombosis or high blood pressure, but is also making your diabetes harder to control. Seek your dietitian's help in losing weight. Once you have reached the right weight for your height, stay there.

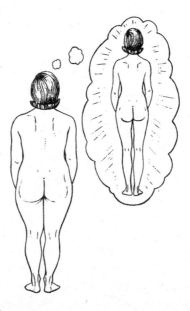

Be honest with yourself

KEEP YOUR BLOOD GLUCOSE CONCENTRATION NORMAL

People with high blood glucose levels are much more likely to develop diabetic retinopathy, diabetic nephropathy and diabetic neuropathy than those with normal blood glucose levels. The higher the glucose and the longer it is high, the more likely you are to have one of these forms of tissue damage. If you have been running blood glucose levels persistently over 7 mmol/l (126mg/dl) before meals, gradually reduce your blood glucose by decreasing your food intake (if you are overweight), increasing the amount of exercise you take and increasing your dose of insulin or glucose-lowering pills. See Chapters 8 and 9, and ask your diabetes adviser for help. Do not reduce your blood glucose abruptly – ease it down gradually over a few weeks.

There is now good evidence that keeping your blood glucose as near to normal as possible both reduces the risk of developing diabetic tissue damage and also slows the progression of existing tissue damage. The Diabetes Control and Complications Trial (DCCT) studied intensive glucose control versus usual glucose control in people with Type 1 diabetes. The intensively treated group were on very carefully controlled insulin treatment patterns with frequent dose adjustment to obtain near normal blood glucose levels. Those with intensive control had a mean blood glucose of 8.6 mmol/l (155 mg/dl) compared with 12.8 mmol/l (230 mg/dl) in the conventionally treated group. There were huge reductions in the risk of tissue damage in the intensively treated group – new retinopathy was reduced by 76%, obvious neuropathy by 54%, urinary protein by 54%. In those with existing retinopathy, the progression was slowed by 54%.

The UK Prospective Diabetes Study (UKPDS) studied people with Type 2 diabetes. Overweight people intensively treated with metformin had an average HbAlc of 7.4% whereas those on usual treatment had an HbAlc of 8.0%. This intensive treatment reduced diabetes-related complications by 32%. Patients on sulphonylurea or insulin had an HbAlc of 7.0% in the intensive group compared with 7.9% in the usual treatment group. In these patients intensive treatment reduced diabetes-related complications by 12%.

It should be noted that intensive glucose lowering does increase the risk of hypoglycaemia. This was particularly obvious in DCCT to start with, and great care had to be taken to avoid unduly low glucose levels.

LOWER YOUR BLOOD FATS

Another word for blood fats is lipids. Your blood fats are cholesterol (mostly made up of the 'good' high-density lipoprotein cholesterol or HDL, and the 'bad' low-density lipoprotein cholesterol LDL) and triglyceride. If your total cholesterol is high, with a low HDL and a high LDL; or if your triglyceride is high (especially in the presence of a low HDL), you are at risk of having a coronary thrombosis. The risk increases as the levels move away from the desirable range:-

Total cholesterol below 5 mmol/l (192 mg/dl)
HDL cholesterol above 0.9 mmol/l (35 mg/dl)
LDL cholesterol below 3 mmol/l (115 mg/dl)

Triglyceride below 2.3 mmol/l (203 mg/dl)

You can improve your blood fat levels by keeping your weight normal, and by eating much less fat. The fat that you do eat should be high in polyunsaturates and monosaturates, and low in saturated fat (see pages 61–3). Eat a high fibre diet. Reducing your sugar and alcohol intake helps to reduce your triglyceride level. Exercise will help too, and *you must stop smoking*.

Recently, the Heart Protection Study of 20,000 people, many of them diabetic, showed that people with diabetes who took the cholesterol-lowering drug simvastin, dramatically reduced their risk of having a heart attack or stroke. Also, people with peripheral vascular disease (see pages 152–3) lessened their risk of amputation or arterial surgery. *Everyone* with diabetes, whatever their cholesterol level, should now consider taking statin treatment.

Statins were specifically designed to block the manufacture of cholesterol in the body and help clear it from the circulation. The most commonly used ones are simvastatin, pravastatin and atorvastatin. They should be avoided in pregnant and breast-feeding women and in those with liver disease. Rarely, they may cause muscle inflammation, especially in people with kidney disease or under-active thyroid, or if used in combination with fibrates. Liver tests should be checked before prescribing and monitored during treatment. Stop your statin and see your doctor if you get muscle aches and pains. Statins can also cause tiredness, headache, gastrointestinal upsets and rashes. However, most people have no problems with them. Atorvastatin reduces both cholesterol and triglyceride; the others have little effect on triglyceride unless given at very high dose.

Fibrates are better at reducing triglyceride levels than cholesterol levels. Bezafibrate, fenofibrate and gemfibrozil have all been shown to be useful in people with diabetes. Again, liver function should be checked before prescribing and during treatment. They should not be given to people with liver or gall bladder disease, nor to pregnant or breast-feeding women. They can also cause muscle inflammation (see as for statins). They have a higher risk of gastrointestinal side-effects than statins, and may cause a rash or impotence.

Bile acid sequestrants – cholestyramine and colestipol – bind to bile acids from the bile after they have been excreted into the gut. This prevents them from being reabsorbed later, so the body has to make more and this uses up cholesterol. They come as granules in sachets and can be drunk dispersed in fluid or sprinkled on food. They tend to cause gastrointestinal symptoms.

Fybozest – soluble fibre – increases dietary fibre and can be used to achieve a small reduction blood fats.

Marine triglycerides – concentrated fish oils – are used to help reduce triglyceride when other methods are not succeeding. They are taken as capsules with meals.

KEEP YOUR BLOOD PRESSURE NORMAL

High blood pressure is as dangerous for people with diabetes as high blood glucose. There is mounting evidence that it is closely involved in the development and progression of diabetic tissue damage. UKPDS studied blood pressure lowering in 1148 people with Type 2 diabetes and hypertension with an average blood pressure of 160/94. They used captopril or atenolol to lower blood pressure to an average of 144/82 in a tight control group, compared with a less tight control group (154/87). Over the eight year follow up period there was a 32% reduction in deaths related to diabetes, a 44% reduction in strokes and a 34% reduction in progression of diabetic retinopathy in the tight control group as compared with the conventionally treated group. Other studies have shown similar results. Also studies of people with diabetic kidney disease have shown that deterioration of kidney function is considerably slowed in people with good blood pressure control.

EXERCISE REGULARLY

Regular, vigorous exercise helps to reduce the likelihood of having a coronary thrombosis. It also improves sensitivity to insulin, helps you to lose weight and helps to reduce your blood fats (see pages 61 and 194). Never start an exercise programme without first consulting your doctor. You should exercise at least three times a week for it to see benefit.

NOTICE WHAT IS HAPPENING TO YOU – AND ACT

Darren was a bricklayer. He led a busy life. At work all day, out every evening with his girlfriend. He injected his insulin twice a day and did the occasional blood test. These were usually high but he felt OK. One day while he was changing to go out he felt something wet on his sock. It was blood. When he looked at his foot his big toe was all red and there was a hole underneath, with pus and blood coming out of it. He washed it and covered it with elastoplast, finished dressing and rushed out to the party. His toe did not seem to hurt much, and it did not stop him dancing. Two days later he started to feel ill. He felt hot and sweaty and shivery. His glucose was over 22 mm.ol/l (396 mg/dl). His mother called the doctor. When the doctor looked at his foot, it was red up to the ankle and there was pus oozing out of the toe. Darren spent the next six weeks in hospital. He had to have an operation to drain the pus and intravenous drips with antibiotics, and insulin. After he got home he looked at his working boots and found a nail sticking up through the insole. His toes had become numb from neuropathy and he had not noticed the nail digging in.

If Darren had checked his feet daily, he would have seen the early signs of injury in time to act. Had he taken more care of his blood glucose he may not have developed neuropathy.

This sort of story, sadly, is not uncommon. Every day people with diabetes are being admitted to hospitals in Britain with problems due to self-neglect. No one expects you to do everything perfectly – and there will be days when you forget things. But try to develop a routine for checking your body over and learn to notice what your skin looks like and what you feel like. If something is wrong you will often be able to sort it out yourself, but the diabetes team are always there to help – and they like to be asked. The aim is not to turn you into a hypochondriac, but to have an observant, common sense approach to what is going on in your body. If you discover a problem, be prepared to admit to yourself and your advisers that all is not well, then seek help if needed and act on it.

SUMMARY

- Keep fit. Prevent diabetic tissue damage.
- If you smoke, *stop*. If you don't smoke, don't start.
- Keep your weight normal for your height.
- Keep your blood glucose concentration normal.
- Keep your blood fats down.
- Keep your blood pressure normal.
- Keep exercising.
- Keep an eye on yourself.
- Be realistic.
- Be kind to yourself.

14

LIVING WITH DIABETES

A DAILY ROUTINE

Once you have got over the surprise of discovering that you have
diabetes and have learned the basics of looking after yourself, you
need to get back to enjoying life. But you must give your diabetes
a little attention each day.

Establish a daily routine. Keep all your diabetes things together
in a box, case or bag. Insulin-treated people should keep their spare
insulin in a small box in the fridge (away from the freezing
compartment).

A diabetes kit

At home your diabetes kit should include:

* Your diabetes record book and a pen;
* Your insulin, pen or syringe and needles;
* Alcohol swabs (or industrial methylated spirit) to clean insulin
  bottle bung;
* A needle clipper (B-D Safe Clip);
* Your pills;
* Your finger pricker, platforms (if needed) and lancets;
* Your blood glucose test strips, bottle, meter;
* Cotton wool (if needed);
* A container for sharps;
* Urine testing kit for ketones (and glucose);
* A spare diabetic card;

- Your help telephone numbers;
- Some spare glucose tablets;
- Your glucagon.(Check your partner knows where to find it and how to use it.

Keep your diabetes kit out of reach of children – lock it away if there are children in your house. If the person with diabetes is a child, make sure his/her brothers and sisters cannot access the items. It is always sensible to have two of everything in case of breakages or loss (keep your reserve items in a separate place). If you are using an insulin-injection device, keep a syringe and needle in case of problems. You can draw insulin out of a cartridge if you have to.

Around town your diabetes kit should include:

- Your diabetes record book and pen;
- Insulin kit or that day's pills;
- Blood testing kit;
- Diabetic card;
- Glucose tablets;
- Your help telephone numbers;
- A fibre crunch bar or biscuits.

If you are often out and about you will probably find an insulin pen and a blood glucose meter easier to carry around than bottles of insulin, needles, syringes and a bottle of strips. See Chapter 18 for guidance on extended trips.

Tests and treatment

When you know what tests and treatment you need and when, decide how best to fit them into your daily routine. Most people test their blood (or urine) at least once a day, usually before a meal or before bed, sometimes two hours after the largest meal of the day. At first allow 5 to 10 minutes for each test and treatment time – you may soon be able to do blood tests in less than one minute and an insulin injection can take only a minute with a pen. Now and then, it is worth spending a little time thinking whether you could make your testing and treatment easier for yourself or more efficient in any way. Where do you keep your diabetes things? Are they easy to reach and can you find what you want simply? Would another method of insulin injection suit you better? Are there problems with glucose testing? It is often the small things that can make a task a prolonged nuisance or a quick job.

Body maintenance

Choose a convenient time each day (e.g. before bed or after your shower) to look at your feet carefully. Learn to listen all the time to what your body is telling you – notice if you have problems seeing or feeling, notice if you have bowel or bladder problems and so on. But notice in a common sense way. You do not need to become a hypochondriac:

> 'Do not distress yourself with imaginings. Many fears are born of fatigue and loneliness. Beyond a wholesome discipline, be gentle with yourself.'
> *Desiderata*, 1692

Medical checks

From the outset you must accept that you will need to have routine checks with health care professionals. It is important to attend these sessions. Take time off work if necessary – your diabetes clinic will give you a letter if you need one for work. If you cannot attend, make certain you are given another date within a few weeks.

At least once a year:

- See a diabetes doctor;
- See a diabetes specialist nurse;
- See a dietitian;
- See an optometrist or ophthalmic optician;
- See a chiropodist.

You may need to see some of these people more often at some points in your diabetic career, e.g. to plan pregnancy.

> Arthur was a self-employed decorator. He worked hard. He became diabetic seven years ago and was treated with a diabetic diet and glibenclamide tablets. He last attended the diabetic

clinic four years ago. He was too busy to waste time sitting around in clinic. 'Time is money,' he told his wife. He obtained his pills on repeat prescriptions and was always 'in a hurry – can't stop now, doc' when his GP suggested a check-up. Eventually the GP insisted. He was worried to discover that Arthur had diabetic retinopathy in both eyes. He asked him to have some blood taken and arranged a hospital visit. Arthur put the hospital appointment letter behind the clock and forgot it. He was sent another appointment – to no avail. His GP was told of his non-attendance and the hospital notes were returned to file.

One afternoon, Arthur arrived at the hospital in an ambulance. He had fallen off his ladder, knocked himself out and broken his leg in three places. When the casualty doctor tried to look in his eyes she couldn't see into the left one – it was full of blood. His blood glucose was 17 mmol/l (306 mg/dl) and his glycosylated haemoglobin was very high at 16 per cent. After Arthur regained consciousness he told staff what had happened. He had been unsteady on ladders for some time because 'my feet don't seem to feel where they are'. He had been painting the side of a house when he suddenly lost the vision in his left eye and as rapidly lost his balance. The vitreous haemorrhage (page 133) cleared and Arthur's fractures healed but he could no longer manage ladders and had to stop work.

Arthur's eye problems were treatable, he need never have had the haemorrhage into his eye. Had he followed his GP's advice and attended the clinic, he would probably still be working.

WORK

Applying for jobs

People with diabetes can do most jobs. Unless you have diabetic tissue damage (e.g. visual impairment or amputation) diet-treated diabetes should not affect your employment. People with diabetes treated with glucose-lowering pills or insulin injections cannot join the police, the armed forces or the fire service, or fly aircraft. Pill-treated diabetics may be allowed to drive trains, large goods vehicle (LCV) and passenger carrying vehicles (PCV) if they can show that they are caring for their diabetes properly, their glucose is well-balanced and they have no disabling tissue damage. If you are a vocational driver it is better to control your diabetes with metformin (pages 76–7) if possible. People with diabetes who are taking insulin are not usually allowed to hold LGV or PCV licences, drive a Post Office vehicle, drive a taxi or cab, drive trains, fly aircraft or work as cabin crew, work offshore (e.g. in the merchant navy, or on a liner), work as a diver or join the armed forces. The risk, albeit small, of hypoglycaemia may also prevent your working at heights (e.g. circus acts, steeplejacks) or in jobs in which a lapse of attention could be dangerous, either to you or to others (e.g. working with hazardous machinery, or as a lighthouse keeper or signalman).

Diabetes is a registrable disability for employment, but it may not be to your advantage to register – discuss this with your diabetes team, social worker or Diabetes UK. Even if you are not registered as disabled the Disability Discrimination Act 1995 would still apply to you if you were treated simply unfavourably at work simply because of your diabetes.

Existing jobs

In most cases, no one at work will realise that you now have diabetes, unless you tell them. If you are on glucose-lowering pills or insulin injections it is sensible to tell people with whom you spend a lot of time at work. In the unlikely event of your having a hypoglycaemic episode at work, they would then know what to do. If you are responsible for other people's safety and your diabetes is treated with insulin or sulphonylurea pills you must tell them about your diabetes. It is also sensible to tell your employer, so that you can have any time off that you need for medical reasons, and so that you can keep to your diet at work without difficulty.

> Brian is a lively 20-year-old. He rarely had problems ith his diabetes and saw no need to mention it at work. One morning he woke up late and missed his breakfast. He had his insulin and decided to have a snack at the travel agents where he works. There was a rush of customers and he forgot. Rita, his manageress, found him staggering around the office, sweating profusely and mumbling. He was trying to say 'sugar, give me sugar' but she did not understand. She panicked. Eventually a customer called an ambulance. The ambulance men found Brian's diabetic card and soon revived him with some glucose tablets.

Brian awoke to discover Rita in tears, 'I thought you were dying,' she sobbed. 'It was only a hypo, Rita,' he said as he comforted her. When Rita had calmed down he told her about diabetes and hypos. He took her out to lunch to apologise.

If you are a vocational driver you must tell your employer, and the motor insurance company that you have diabetes. If you are already working in other jobs normally barred to diabetics you have a moral obligation, and often a contractual one, to report your diabetes to your employer. In many instances employers will be helpful and will allow you to continue working in a safer role. You can appeal against dismissal made on medical grounds – and such appeals can be successful. It is up to you to demonstrate that your diabetes is safely under control and that you can look after it responsibly. Diabetes UK can often help with employment-related matters.

Some people run into problems with company pension schemes or life insurance. There is a huge variation in the attitude of different insurance companies to people with diabetes. If you have problems, Diabetes UK can usually help.

Studies of the work record of people with diabetes have produced varying results – one study in the early 1960s showed that about one in two men and one in three women with diabetes had no sick leave at all in a year. Another study showed that people with diabetes took less sick leave than the non-diabetics in their company. Employers are sometimes ignorant about diabetes – in the vast majority of cases they need have no worries about employing a person who has diabetes.

Diabetes UK can provide more information about employment. They can also help if you feel you have been subjected to discrimination.

Circumstances at work

There may be small changes you can make to improve your circumstances at work. If the canteen food does not correspond to a healthy diet, take your own meals. Keep some emergency rations – biscuits, fibre-crunch bars, for example – in your desk or work box if food is permitted in your workplace. Find somewhere clean to check your blood glucose or give your insulin. If your work involves uneven ground or heavy goods, consider protective footwear. If you have poor circulation, make sure that your feet are warm – there are regulations about the temperature of workplaces. If you are a non-smoker (and all diabetics should be) ask people not to smoke in your working area.

Shift work

There is no problem with this for solely diet-treated diabetics. If you are taking glucose-lowering pills, take them with your meals. It may be more difficult for people with insulin-treated diabetes to work shifts, so try to avoid these if you can. However, if you do work shifts you can adjust your treatment to cover this. Most people find it easiest to take a very long-acting insulin once a day and use an insulin pen with fast-acting insulin before each meal. Then it is not so critical when you eat your meals. It is sensible to have snacks in between and to use frequent blood-glucose monitoring.

OTHER ASPECTS OF DAILY LIFE

Driving

This has already been discussed on pages 44 and 168–9. You must be especially careful not to endanger your life or that of others by driving when your blood glucose is too low, or by driving when you can no longer see properly, cannot feel the pedals or steering wheel, or have other diabetic tissue damage which interferes with driving. It is illegal (and selfish) to continue to drive when you are no longer a safe driver.

If you are on glucose-lowering pills or insulin, never drive on an empty stomach and, after any change in treatment, check your blood glucose before driving, and at hourly intervals during long journeys. Always carry glucose, food and a can or box of non-alcoholic drink in the car.

The instant you suspect you are hypoglycaemic, pull into the kerb or hard shoulder *immediately* it is safe to do so, turn off the engine and remove the keys from the ignition. Eat some glucose. Turn on the hazard warning lights. Slide into the passenger seat if you can. Eat some food. Do not resume your journey until your blood glucose is at least 6 mmol/l (108 mg/dl) and you are fully in control of yourself. If you are involved in an accident whilst hypoglycaemic you can be charged with driving whilst under the influence of a drug, i.e. insulin.

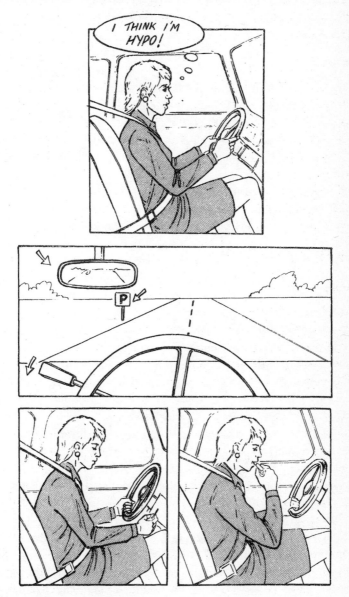

Hypoglycaemia and driving

The old advice was for a hypoglycaemic person to get out of the car so that you are no longer 'in control' of it. However, with today's busy traffic, it is dangerous to advise someone who may be confused or unco-ordinated to leave the relative safety of their car and stagger into the traffic.

Social life

Eating out need not be a problem for people with diabetes. You can avoid sugary puddings by having fruit, and it is usually possible to choose a relatively low fat meal – you do not have to eat the cream sauce! Most places will grill fish or steak, or provide a salad. And nowadays most restaurants and hotels serve wholemeal bread, and other high-fibre options. If you are invited out for a meal, go and enjoy yourself – or you can explain your needs to your host if you wish. There are so many religious, personal and medical food preferences nowadays, that a wise hostess will ask guests if they have any specific dietary requirements. Diabetes is no barrier to an active social life. Nowadays there is no need to drink a lot of alcohol to be sociable. Space out your alcoholic drinks with nonalcoholic ones, and always have something to eat when you drink alcohol because alcohol inhibits the release of glucose from the liver and can make you hypoglycaemic.

Teenagers with diabetes can become angry and frustrated if their parents insist that they are home for meals and at injection times. If you make sure that you carry something to eat and you use an insulin pen you do not need to rush home for meals and insulin and your social life can become a lot freer. Keep up to date with practical advances in diabetes care – they can make life much easier. This is one of many good reasons for joining a diabetic association such as Diabetes UK or your local diabetes centre youth group.

People are sometimes shy about discussing their diabetes with friends. Most people will be genuinely interested in your diabetes and how you look after it, if you wish to tell them. But remember that your friends may be shy of broaching the topic with you because they will not be sure whether you want to discuss it or not.

LIVING WITH DIABETES

During this century there have been many attitudes to diabetes by professionals and those who have it. Before the 1920s juvenile-onset diabetes was a death sentence. Once insulin was discovered there was a mood of great optimism – diabetes was no longer a problem. Joslin, a famous diabetes doctor, voiced a word of caution and predicted that diabetic tissue damage would gradually become more important. For people on insulin, early methods of treatment were painful and cumbersome – glass syringes and thick needles, complex methods of calculating the insulin dose, reliance on urine testing with all its inaccuracies. Then, with standardisation of insulin concentrations, easy self-monitoring of blood glucose and the advent of insulin pens, people with diabetes were again told that diabetes was no longer a problem, that they could do anything. People with diabetes who found the restrictions of insulin injections, self-testing and regular check-ups frustrating, or who could not achieve the smooth blood glucose balance promised by books and professionals, were made to feel as if they had failed in some way. They felt that it was wrong not to see life with diabetes through rose-tinted spectacles.

When glucose-lowering pills were discovered in the 1950s, people whose diabetes could be controlled on these, and those whose diabetes could be controlled by diet alone, were given the impression that their diabetes was only mild and not likely to cause them trouble. I had angry letters from people on pills when I wrote an article which said that there is no such thing as mild diabetes. Many of these people still have difficulty accepting that their foot or eye problems are due to diabetes. Others feel cheated – if it is a mild condition why are they in difficulty now? Now many people with non-insulin-requiring diabetes want to have the same access to blood glucose monitoring and health care that insulin-treated people have, but there may still be resistance to this within the health care professions, especially in a budget-conscious world.

Nowadays a balance is being struck between the reality of the need to give up some time and effort to looking after diabetes and the risk of tissue damage, and the possibility, in the majority of cases, of getting on with doing what you want in life and enjoying yourself to the full. There have been at least five diabetic presidents and innumerable diabetic sportsmen, company directors, singers, artists, musicians, builders, professors, doctors, nurses – the list is endless.

When I started writing books for people with diabetes it was not considered 'kind' to talk about tissue damage in detail. But to fail to do so seems to me to insult my readers' intelligence and to take away their opportunity for working towards reducing the risk of their diabetes causing long-term problems. The down side of giving such detailed information is that it provokes anxiety. However, a small trace of anxiety is what keeps one following health rules – I like eating, but I am stopped from stuffing myself every day by anxiety that I 'will get very fat and that will make me look horrible and I might die from a heart attack'. I am not so anxious that I starve myself – it just keeps a small rein on my appetite. On the other hand, because my grandfather smoked and died of lung cancer, I am so afraid that I might get cancer that 1 have never smoked. That is useful anxiety.

But too much worry and anxiety can be destructive.

Delia is 30 and has had diabetes for 15 years. She has always been a worrier, but in recent years she has been so frightened that she is going to develop kidney failure that she has been measuring her blood glucose six or more times a day and is always changing her insulin dose and omitting meals to lower her glucose. She is often severely hypoglycaemic because she tries to keep her glucose at 4 mmol/l (72 mg/dl) all the time. She had a car accident when she was hypoglycaemic and lost her driving licence. This meant that she became trapped in the village in which she lives, as public transport is poor. Gradually she stopped going out. She missed some of her diabetic clinic appointments and the diabetes nurse came out to her house to see how she was. Delia at first denied that there was a problem but eventually told the diabetes nurse all her worries. She agreed to come to clinic where careful tests proved that her kidneys were working well. She was offered some sessions with a psychologist. She was terrified – 'You all think I'm mad,' she wept. But once she understood that these sessions were simply to help her to come to understand a little more about herself and her diabetes she agreed. The diabetes team helped her to reduce her hypoglycaemia through regular meals and appropriate insulin changes. She saw the psychologist regularly. Now, four years later, her blood glucose levels are normal much of the time, she has regained her driving licence and is working part-time. She still worries sometimes, but is able to cope with this and no longer allows anxiety to overcome her.

Norman is 20 and has also had diabetes for 15 years. His aunt was diabetic and on insulin. He used to be taken to visit her when he was little. She was blind and walked with a white stick. She always walked with a limp and one day he fell against her leg and discovered that it was artificial. Despite all that the diabetes team taught him about the preventibilty of diabetic tissue damage, his childhood impressions were so strong that he always equated diabetes with inevitable blindness and amputation. He decided that if this was the future he would rather not know. He would have a short life and a merry one. He stopped attending diabetic clinic, never tested his blood glucose and gave himself some insulin once a day or so. As a result he had several episodes of ketoacidosis. During one of them he nearly died. He usually discharges himself from hospital as soon as he feels well enough to walk. On one occasion he ran out of the building when he was told that he needed to see the eye clinic urgently to treat his retinopathy. He rejected all offers of help. He moved house and was lost to follow-up. The diabetes team felt that they had failed because they had been unable to help him. On this occasion the psychologist working with the team helped the staff to accept that they could not help everyone. They needed to learn not to be too hard on themselves.

Every large diabetic clinic has two or three Delias and a few Normans (so I have combined many stories to protect individuals). Most people with diabetes are not so dramatically affected by their feelings. I have told these stories to show that feelings about diabetes can overwhelm a few people. Help is available. Not everyone needs a psychologist, and not every diabetes team is lucky enough to work with one. The first step is to find someone who understands about diabetes to share your worries with. If your worries have become so enormous that they have swamped you, professional help can rescue you, so do not be afraid to admit to yourself and the diabetes team that you could do with help. We all need help from time to time. We are all human and none of us is perfect.

Two Canadians, Heather Maclean and Barbara Oram, collected people's comments about their diabetes and discussed them in a book called *Living with Diabetes*. Not everyone they asked about diabetes viewed it as negative experience.

Lydia: 'I have a sense of having come to peace with my diabetes. I feel some sort of contentment. I think that has added to my sense of self-confidence. I feel now that I can do anything that I wish to put my hands on. There's a contentment about not having to think about diabetes any more, because it's a part of my life.'

Tim: 'I can say that diabetes has made me a better person. It's weird. I almost feel like I contradict myself when I say that, because I hate diabetes, yet diabetes has made me a stronger person ... Since I got my diabetes things have really picked up for me. Diabetes has done so many things to me. I used to be on the shy side and now I'm not. I feel more confident in myself. It has strengthened me.'

Sarah: 'I know I'm better organised as a result of my diabetes, because I have to be – not only better organised to deal with diabetes but all around. There're certain things I have to do and that spills over into the rest of my life. I tend to think ahead a lot more than a lot of people, because I can't get caught in situations I can't handle. In a way, when I look at my life, there's positive things that balance out – like the organisation, the diet – you have an extra incentive to eat well; also tuning into your own body. So I don't see it all as negative ... If I were given a chance to change one thing in my life and only one thing, I can tell you right now that I wouldn't waste that chance on diabetes. I've never said that before but, in saying it now, I know absolutely that it's true.'

SUMMARY

- Establish a daily routine for your diabetes care.
- Keep your diabetes kit well-organised and safe.
- Make life easier for yourself – tailor your treatment and your monitoring to your personal needs.

- Take advantage of new advances.
- Have regular medical checks.
- People with diabetes can do most jobs.
- Tell close colleagues that you have diabetes.
- Tell your employer if the diabetes may affect your safety or that of others. It is best to tell employer anyway.
- Tell the DVLA that you have diabetes. Avoid hypoglycaemia particularly while driving.
- Don't hide your feelings about your diabetes. Share them with people who understand. Accept help if you need it.
- Diabetes has some positive aspects.

15

THE DIABETES TEAM AND THE DIABETES SERVICE

Every clinic, surgery or health care service has a system. Learning how your particular care system works can help you to make full use of facilities which may help you. It can also help you to understand why things happen as they do, and enable you to make suggestions for improvements if necessary.

Diabetes is a common condition which requires long-term care. This means that a hospital diabetic service can care for 1000 to 4000 patients depending on its catchment area and the availability of other clinics. A GP may have 10 to 100 diabetic patients, depending on his list type and size and whether he also cares for his partners' diabetic patients, for example. The potential size of diabetic clinics means that they have to be well-organised and that many staff are involved.

THE DIABETES TEAM

Nowadays people with diabetes are cared for by a team of people, all of whom have particular skills. Different diabetes services have different teams, but most include a doctor with specialist training in diabetes, a diabetes specialist nurse, a dietitian and a chiropodist. Some larger teams include people with skills in psychology, eye care and wound care, among others. Some team members may spend their whole time working with people with diabetes, others have additional responsibilities.

The most important team member

The most important team member is *you*.

The traditional view of health care is that you, the patient, seek help from your doctor, who tells you what is wrong with you and gives you treatment. 'I have a sore throat, doctor.' 'You have tonsillitis. Take one of these tablets four times a day for a week.' This approach is effective and perhaps sufficient in many conditions, but diabetes is a condition in which you, the person who has it, have a major influence on your own outcome. By eating healthily, exercising, checking your condition regularly and adjusting your treatment according to your blood glucose levels, you can keep yourself well. You live with your diabetes all the time, so *you* can be the most knowledgeable person in the world about *your* diabetes. You are the most important member of the team.

Doctors

Nowadays, in Britain, no doctor aspiring to a hospital consultant post can be accredited in diabetes without stringent training. This occurs in hospital and usually includes three years' training in various aspects of general medicine as a senior house officer, and five years as a registrar in general medicine and in diabetes. There may be additional years in diabetes research. Posts have to be approved by the Royal College of Physicians for higher medical training and must include broad general medicine and all aspects of diabetes care, both in-patient and out-patient. As a consultant, this doctor will then be a physician (everyone trained in general medicine is a physician and called 'Doctor' not 'Mister') with a special interest in diabetes, sometimes known as a diabetologist. Most diabetologists also practice general medicine. Those pursuing a career in academic medicine follow a similar pathway to start with but do more research. Some teaching hospitals have diabetologists at lecturer, senior lecturer or professorial level.

Not all hospitals have a consultant post specialising in diabetes. All general physicians will have some experience in diabetes care and sometimes the diabetic clinic is run by a general physician.

General practitioners undergo a broad training in several specialties at senior house officer level and then join a practice as a trainee, moving on to full partnership in a practice. Some GPs move into practice from registrar posts in medicine and some from specialised diabetes posts. Some work in hospital diabetic clinics as clinical assistants to a consultant diabetologist. There are courses in diabetes care for hospital doctors and GPs. There are also professional organisations (Diabetes UK, the European Association for the Study of Diabetes) which offer excellent opportunities for updating knowledge, and for revision and peer review.

I believe that everyone with diabetes has the right to see a doctor specialising in diabetes care.

Nurses

One of the greatest advances in diabetes care has been the increase in the number of posts for nurses with specialist training in diabetes care. There are now over 500 such posts in Britain. A diabetes specialist nurse (or sometimes a diabetes specialist health visitor) has usually attended courses in diabetes care and spends all of her time caring for people with diabetes. She will often have received special training in teaching and is usually your main source of diabetes education. She will also know about all the practicalities of blood glucose testing and insulin administration and be able to advise you about adjusting your treatment. Diabetes specialist nurses usually work closely with a consultant diabetologist. Many diabetes specialist nurses will see you on the ward in hospital, in the clinic, at your GP's or at your home. They may give you an emergency number on which you can contact them for advice.

Nowadays it is becoming increasingly unusual to admit people to hospital to start insulin therapy. The diabetes specialist nurse can visit you at home and help you to learn how to manage your insulin.

Many practice nurses attend training courses in diabetes care and then help with GP diabetic clinics. Community-based nurses such as district nurses may also have some diabetes training.

Dietitian

Healthy eating is the cornerstone of the treatment of diabetes. dietitians have detailed training in nutrition and its effects on the body. They will be able to assess your usual eating pattern and help you to adapt it to a healthy diet. The dietitian will not only advise you about the types of food to eat but also guide you about how best to cook them. If you have concerns about food safety or storage, she can help there too.

Chiropodist or podiatrist

A chiropodist has received training in keeping your feet healthy and in assessing and treating any problems which arise. He may measure the sensation in your feet and check your circulation. He will be able to perform minor surgical procedures if necessary. The chiropodist can also advise you about your shoes (if you run or practise a sport, do not forget to ask about your sports shoes as well). Some chiropodists like to see a pair of your older shoes when they assess you, so that they can look at the way in which your walking has worn or rubbed them. Diabetics have priority access to chiropody in some districts.

Wound care specialist nurse

At present, few diabetes teams have a wound care nurse. She has received specialist training in the causes and assessment of ulcers and other skin conditions and in their treatment. Some people with diabetes have foot or leg ulcers and it is a considerable help to them to be able to see a wound care nurse regularly. There is some overlap between the role of the wound care nurse and the chiropodist, and the latter will treat and dress foot ulcers too, if necessary.

Ophthalmologist, optometrist or ophthalmic optician

Some teams work with doctors who specialise in eye problems (ophthalmologists). Occasionally an optometrist or an ophthalmic optician will join the team. They are not doctors but have training in assessing your vision and the state of your eyes and in providing a prescription for glasses if necessary. All of these professionals will examine the backs of your eyes with a special magnifying torch called an ophthalmoscope, or they will photograph them. Diabetics are entitled to a free eye examination from an optometrist or ophthalmic optician once a year.

Psychologist

A few diabetes teams have regular contact with a clinical psychologist. Some people with diabetes have difficulty coming to terms with their condition, others may have pre-existing psychological difficulties which make it difficult to care for their diabetes. Many people have temporary ups and downs in their life with diabetes. If your problems are interfering with your life you may find some sessions with a psychologist helpful.

A psychologist is someone who studies and treats the variations of the way in which the normal human mind works and the way in which people behave. (A psychiatrist is a doctor who treats abnormalities or illnesses of the mind).

A DIABETES SERVICE

This can mean your GP and his practice nurse working closely together and providing your diabetes care (using the resources of the hospital laboratory and working with a local chiropodist and dietitian), or it can mean a hospital-based service. Or it often means both, working closely together.

This is an example of how one person was cared for:

John is 73 years old. Last year he saw his GP because of thirst and passing a lot of urine. Dr Jones tested his blood glucose and found that he had diabetes. Dr Jones runs a diabetic clinic at her surgery, and with the help of a dietitian who comes once a month and the practice nurse, John's diabetes was well controlled for a year. Dr Jones also arranged regular chiropody at the community clinic. One week the chiropodist found that John had rubbed his toe on a new pair of shoes. It was ulcerated and badly infected. He cleaned it and dressed it and sent John straight to see Dr Jones. Dr Jones was worried about the infected toe so she telephoned the consultant diabetologist at the local hospital. He suggested that John come to the diabetic clinic at the hospital that day.

The diabetic clinic list was already full but anyone with an urgent problem is always seen. The receptionist was expecting John and the records clerk had made a new set of notes ready for him. The chiropodist worked there too, so he brought John in to see the consultant diabetologist, Dr Smith. Together they examined John's foot very carefully. John had a bad infection which was spreading up the foot. There was evidence of diabetic nerve damage and the circulation was poor. The consultant explained to John that he needed urgent treatment in hospital including intravenous antibiotics and more detailed assessment of his foot.

John was admitted that day and interviewed and examined in detail by Dr Smith's house officer, and then by his registrar. His foot was x-rayed, swabbed, cleaned and dressed. He had blood tests and other investigations to check his general health. His blood glucose was very high because of the infection, so he was given insulin treatment as well as the antibiotics.

That evening the vascular surgeon came to see him to assess his circulation and arranged an x-ray of the arteries in his legs. That was done next day and showed a narrowed artery, which was improved there and then by a procedure called angioplasty. The circulation to the foot improved and slowly the infection cleared.

While in hospital John was seen by the diabetes nurse, had a revision session with the dietitian and was given physiotherapy to keep his muscles strong while he was resting his foot. The wound care sister advised the ward nurses about dressing his toe. He got to know the whole medical team – Dr Smith, his registrar, senior house officer and house officer – because they saw him often.

After three weeks the foot was much better and John was ready to go home. Dr Smith's house officer telephoned Dr Jones to explain all that had happened and what the plan was now. She also gave John a letter for Dr Jones. John was back on his diabetes tablets again and the diabetes nurse visited him at home to make sure that his blood glucose remained normal. He saw the wound care sister once a week to dress the healing ulcer on his toe and she liaised with the district nurse, who came in daily. Dr Jones checked John's progress regularly. A month after his discharge from hospital, John saw Dr Smith and the vascular surgeon in the out-patient clinic. The toe ulcer was now healed and the foot was back to normal. The chiropodist had ordered special shoes to protect John's feet in future and John found them very comfortable.

Now Dr Jones sees John at the diabetic clinic in the surgery every two months but shares his care with Dr Smith at the hospital. Other members of the diabetes team see him at intervals. To make sure that there is no confusion John carries a booklet in which all the health care professionals write their findings. He shows it to each of them when he sees them and keeps a close eye on his own progress.

Using your diabetes service

The keys to the service will be:

* Your doctor's name;

- His telephone number (day and emergency);
- Your doctor's timetable (and his receptionist's/secretary's);
- Your diabetes specialist nurse's name;
- Her telephone number (day and emergency);
- Your number (e.g. NHS number, hospital record number);
- The name of your diabetic clinic;
- The time and day on which it is held (it may not be weekly);
- The appointment system's rules (and arrangements for emergencies).

Hospital and surgery switchboards can be extremely busy. Make certain that you have dialled the right number and wait comfortably. They will answer eventually. Never be put off by switchboard operators or receptionists. Be polite but firm. If you need help, insist on getting it. (But if you feel really ill, call your GP to see you at home or dial 999.) Find out if there is a directly dialled telephone number rather than the main switchboard – it may be much quicker.

Remember that the operator will need to know exactly who you want. Also have your hospital number and consultant's name to hand – virtually all departments will ask for these. You will need your GP's name and any practice number when you telephone the surgery – large group practices deal with thousands of patients.

When you make contact, remind the person you are calling who you are. Do not be upset if he does not recollect all your details. It is not that he does not care, it is just that all health care professionals are very busy. 1 may see 60–100 patients a week, for example. The nurse or doctor will need to know who you are and to have a memory nudge about where and for what they see you, as well as a brief summary of why you are telephoning – for example:

'Hello, Sister Brown, it's Mrs Plunkett from Wimbledon. I come to the diabetic clinic. I saw you three weeks ago when I came for my routine check-up and everything was fine. But now my sugar is high even though I've increased my insulin. I take Mixtard twice a day. I don't feel ill. What should I do now?'

'Hello, Mrs Plunkett. I remember seeing you – you had just come back from Majorca, hadn't you. I'll pop in on my way home and we can look at your glucose levels together.'

Another practical point is to make sure that the details in your hospital and GP surgery records are correct. If your name or address are wrong you may be the subject of dangerous confusion or never receive letters or appointments. Make sure the computer has it right. Many hospitals use sticky labels for blood forms and other identification. If you move or discover an error, ask staff to check that all the details in your records are right.

Help your doctor

'How is your diabetes, Mrs Green?' 'Well, it's a bit up and down.' 'Do you mean your sugar levels are up and down?' 'Yes, I don't know why.' 'Please can I see your diabetes diary?' 'Sorry, I left it at home.' 'Well, can you remember any of your sugar values?' 'Oh, up and down, you know ...' 'Have you changed your insulin?' 'No, I wasn't sure what to do.' 'Well, what insulin are you taking?' 'I don't know.' 'You don't know the name?' 'No, its in a bottle ...'

This sort of exchange is not uncommon. Mrs Green's doctor is doing his best to help her but it is impossible without clearer information. Please help the health care professionals to help you.

SUMMARY

To gain the most from the health care professionals who help you to care for your diabetes:

- Learn who they are, what they do and how to contact them.
- Learn how the diabetes service in your area works.
- Make sure that registration information is accurate.
- If you need help be polite but firm; ensure that staff know who you are and what the problem is.
- Help the diabetes team to help you.

16

PREGNANCY

Women with diabetes can have healthy pregnancies and healthy babies. However, you will have to take a little more care of yourself than non-diabetic women, even before you become pregnant. Start planning now.

PLAN YOUR PREGNANCY

If you have diabetes it is important to ensure that you become pregnant only when you and your partner want to start a family. This is partly because unsuspected pregnancy could upset your glucose balance (see page 125), but more importantly because babies need a perfect environment in which to develop and grow in the womb. This means that the body chemicals to which the baby is exposed must be within normal limits. Unless the blood sugar is normal from the moment of conception, there is a risk of the baby's development being impaired or, rarely, of malformation.

But how can you tell the moment at which your baby is conceived? Most women do not realise they are pregnant until they have missed a period, and by then the baby has already been growing in the womb for several weeks. In order to be sure that your baby has the best start in life, decide with your partner when you want to become pregnant, and until then use contraception and work on ensuring that your blood glucose is normal. Then stop the contraception. Take folic acid tablets.

Diabetes UK provides a lot of information about diabetes and pregnancy. Send for it straightaway.

Contraception

As soon as a girl has her first period, she is capable of bearing children. This means that mothers of diabetic girls should make sure that their daughters fully understand the facts of life. Ask your diabetes sister or doctor to help you if you find it difficult to discuss sexual matters. As soon as a diabetic woman starts to have sexual intercourse she should use contraception every time, except when she wants to become pregnant. As you are capable of child-bearing for 30 or more years, the ideal method is one which does not expose your body to any risks, nor upsets your diabetes control. The simplest methods are therefore barriers to sperm and spermicides. However, it is important that each couple uses the method which suits them and follows the instructions exactly. Barrier methods are effective only if used by people who take care to use them properly. The Pill only works if you take it precisely according to instructions. The rhythm method is not reliable and is inappropriate for diabetic women.

Condoms Condoms (or French letters) should be used with spermicidal coating (cream or foam). They will not upset your diabetes, can be used easily any time. They will also protect you and your partner from sexually exchanged disorders (including AIDS and gonorrhoea). If you have thrush or other minor fungal infections they may be passed on through intercourse, although they can occur in anyone and may be unrelated to sexual intercourse. Condoms may also reduce the risk of cervical cancer. The other advantage is that they are widely available in shops in Britain and easy to carry. They are less reliable than oral contraceptives, but the difference is small when condoms and spermicide are used together properly.

Diaphragms Diaphragms or Dutch caps have to be individually fitted for your vagina and you need to learn how to use them. Spermicidal cream is used with them. Once in place over the cervix they can be forgotten (although more spermicide is needed if you have intercourse more than once). They need to be removed and cleaned 6 to 8 hours after intercourse, and some women find that they have more frequent urinary tract infections and vaginal discharge when using a diaphragm. A diaphragm will protect your cervix from sperm, but you and your partner are not protected from infection.

Intra-uterine contraceptive devices IUCDs, or coils, can be used in diabetic women but there is a small risk of pelvic infection, which may, rarely, cause infertility. A long-acting progesterone device (Mirena) is increasingly popular.

Progestogen-only pills Otherwise known as 'mini -pills', these are the oral contraceptive of choice in diabetic women who wish to use the Pill. They have only a small risk of upsetting the blood glucose or blood fat balance. They have to be taken continuously (i.e. there should be no break during the fourth week of your menstrual cycle) – take your Pill with your insulin every day. Progestogen-only pills may temporarily suppress the periods altogether or cause erratic bleeding. They are slightly tess effective than combined Pills.

Combined oral contraceptive pills with low-dose oestrogen These can be used in diabetic women who are unable to use barrier methods reliably or who dislike them. They carry a risk of blood clots, raised blood pressure, heart problems, stroke, and worsening of blood glucose balance and blood fats in any woman, but these side-effects are more likely in diabetic women, especially if you smoke or are overweight. Oral contraceptives are the most effective means of preventing pregnancy.

Morning after contraception Contraception in the form of a specific combined oral contraceptive can be given up to 72 hours after unprotected intercourse. See your doctor, a family-planning clinic or your pharmacist as soon as possible if you have had a split condom or other problems with your usual contraception, or have had intercourse with no protection and do not want to become pregnant.

Sterilisation This should be regarded as irreversible but may be an option for men or women once they have completed their family. In a few instances, women with extremely severe diabetic tissue damage may be offered sterilisation as pregnancy would put them at risk.

Do we want a baby?

The decision to have a family needs a little extra thought if either parent has diabetes. Your children are more likely to develop diabetes than those of a non-diabetic couple. The risk of diabetes developing in your children is hard to calculate exactly – it depends on your country of origin, where you live now, your family history and many other factors. About 0.4% of the population have insulin-dependent diabetes. If both parents have insulin-dependent diabetes 30% of their children may develop diabetes; if the father has diabetes the risk is 9%; and if the mother has diabetes the risk is 1%. 3% of the population have non-insulin-dependent diabetes. If both parents have diabetes 75% of their children will eventually develop diabetes. If one parent has diabetes 15% of their offspring will develop diabetes. Diabetes is increasing in frequency and these figures are changing.

Although most people with diabetes who are planning a family will not have significant diabetic tissue damage, if you do have – especially if it is the woman who has diabetic complications – you need to consider whether you will be fit enough to go through pregnancy and bring up a child. Pregnancy may worsen diabetic complications, especially eye and kidney disease. Discuss this with your doctor. Diabetic complications are not necessarily a bar to pregnancy, but you will need specialist advice and very intensive supervision.

What blood glucose level should I aim for?

Advice varies. Aim to acheive non-diabetic glucose levels throughout pregnancy (body chemistry changes in pregnancy). Some doctors suggest the following finger-prick glucose levels – fasting 4–5 mmol/l (72–90 mg/dl); before meals 4–6 mmol/l (72–108 mg/dl); two hours after a meal 4–7 mmol/l (72–126 mg/dl); Ideally, measure your blood glucose before and after each meal, and before bed. Discuss your testing and targets with your diabetes adviser. Adjust your insulin every few days to optimise glucose balance. Aim for an HbA_{1C} within the non-diabetic range.

Such tight blood glucose control means that you are at risk of hypoglycaemia. Be very careful driving. Have a bed-time snack to avoid night-time hypoglycaemia. Keep glucagon (see pages 115–6) by you and teach your partner how to administer it to you. Always carry your diabetES card and glucose.

DIABETES TREATMENT DURING PREGNANCY

Adhere carefully to your healthy diet (see the dietitian for advice). Before pregnancy lose weight if you need to, but once pregnant do not starve yourself – it is not good for your baby.

It is unusual for women of child-bearing age to be taking glucose-lowering pills for their diabetes. If you are taking glucose-lowering pills your doctor will change you to insulin – this is because it allows more flexible and better glucose control and because of a possible risk of fetal malformation on pills.

Your insulin needs may fluctuate in the early stages of pregnancy, but as the weeks pass you will need more and more insulin. Keep increasing the dose according to your blood glucose levels, in close liaison with your diabetes team. By the end of pregnancy you may be taking twice your pre-pregnant insulin dose.

Care in pregnancy

When planning pregnancy ask if your local diabetes centre has a women's diabetic clinic or a pre-pregnancy clinic. As soon as you suspect you are pregnant see your doctor. Pregnancy testing kits bought in chemists are usually very sensitive and accurate if used properly. However, remember that pregnancy tests may be negative in the very early stages of pregnancy – a blood test can confirm pregnancy. If in doubt assume you are pregnant.

Pregnant women with diabetes should be cared for by an obstetrician and a diabetologist working closely together. Find out if there is a special pregnancy diabetic clinic near you. Helping a diabetic woman through pregnancy is hard work for everyone – especially the mother-to-be and partner. You will need to test your blood glucose and adjust your insulin carefully. You need extra ultrasound scans to check your baby's progress (some centres do special fetal heart scans routinely). There will be frequent visits to the antenatal clinic or pregnancy diabetic clinic. The reason for all this care is that diabetic women and their babies are more prone to the complications of pregnancy than non-diabetic women. For example, your blood pressure may rise or you may develop excess fluid around your baby. Your baby's growth is monitored very carefully because he may grow too big or not fast enough. In addition to the pregnancy checks, you should have your eyes and kidney function checked at the beginning of pregnancy and regularly throughout.

Delivery

This is always in a hospital with a special care baby unit in case your baby needs monitoring after birth (most hospitals do this routinely). There are differences of opinion as to when and how to deliver babies of diabetic mothers. Some centres allow women to go the full forty weeks if the baby is developing normally and the mother is well. Vaginal delivery is best provided the mother's pelvis is the right size and there are no problems with mother or baby. However, many obstetricians prefer to deliver the baby at about 37 or 38 weeks and would have a low threshold for caesarean section to ensure that the baby has no problems during labour. Discuss the options with your obstetrician – your treatment must be tailored to you and your baby.

While you are in labour you will have an intravenous drip with glucose in it and insulin (if necessary) adjusted to your blood glucose level. This way you can have the energy and insulin you need finely tuned for you. As soon as the placenta is delivered your insulin requirements will fall to your pre-pregnant levels. It is very important that you remember this to avoid hypoglycaemia. You may stay in hospital a little longer than your non-diabetic friends.

Your baby may need extra glucose for the first day or so as he becomes used to life away from the diabetic womb. Previously, babies of diabetic mothers were often large red cherubs. This is less common with near-normal glucose balance in pregnancy. Occasionally the baby of a diabetic woman may have breathing problems. This is why it is important that there are facilities for special care of the newborn where your baby is born.

Home again

All the hard work in pregnancy is worthwhile when you take your new baby home. At this time you can relax your blood glucose control a little. You do not want to become hypoglycaemic while you are caring for a baby so aim for 6–8 mmol/l (108–144 mg/dl). Eat three meals and three snacks a day (you may find you need a midnight snack if your baby often gets you up at night). If you are breast-feeding you may need more carbohydrate and may also need to reduce your insulin. Make sure you drink plenty. Try not to put on weight.

But what about father?

With all this attention focused on your partner you may feel a little left out. But it is very important that you share in the pregnancy throughout as your partner will need a great deal of support. If you do not already know how to do blood glucose tests, learn so that you can help her. Learn how to give insulin so that you can help with injections if necessary. And, very important, learn your partner's early warning signs for hypoglycaemia so that you can encourage her to eat glucose if necessary. Make sure that you have some glucagon (pages 115–6) available in case she is unable to eat when hypo. Studies have shown that persistently high glucose levels are much more likely to harm the baby than hypoglycaemia, but it is still important to treat hypos promptly. Night-time hypoglycaemia seems particularly common during pregnancy – if your partner's breathing is unusual, she seems to be having a bad dream, is thrashing around or is sweating a lot, wake her and give glucose if appropriate. But you do not need to stay awake all night watching!

The frequent clinic visits can become tiring so try to help with transport if you can. Although diabetic women should not find pregnancy any more tiring than non-diabetics, the extra hassle may take its toll, so help at home with housework and any other children is always appreciated. Stress can upset diabetes so your partner needs a relaxing home environment at this time. You do too. It can be hard to strike the balance between helping your partner to keep an eye on her diabetes and general health and becoming over anxious. Discuss any concerns with the diabetes and antenatal team or your own doctor.

SUMMARY

- Women with diabetes are fertile and can have healthy pregnancies and healthy babies.
- Pregnancy should be planned.
- Use contraception if you do not want to become pregnant.
- Barrier is best (if used properly).
- Family Planning Association: www.fpa.org.uk
- Keep your HbA_{1C} normal from before pregnancy until delivery.
- Beware hypoglycaemia.
- Tell your doctor immediately you suspect you may be pregnant.
- Pregnancy is hard work for a diabetic woman, but the rewards are infinite.
- Don't forget dad!

17

SPORT AND EXERCISE

People with diabetes can enjoy most sports and other physical activities – and may excel in them.

EXERCISE IS GOOD FOR YOU

Exercise is good for everyone – it helps to keep your body trim and to keep your weight normal. It helps to strengthen your heart and lungs. It also improves your sensitivity to insulin and hence your glucose tolerance. Regular exercise – by which I mean 30 minutes, 5 times a week, within the training zone (see page 197) – reduces your risk of having a heart attack. Exercise is good relaxation and most people who exercise regularly will also tell you that it makes them feel good.

Even small increases in exercise, however mild, can be good for people with diabetes. This section includes help for people who want to do strenuous exercise or take up particular sports, but even a walk round the garden each day will help. Do not let the detailed suggestions for rock climbers or rowers put you off. Each of us enjoys different activities and has different daily timetables and pressures. There is no point in choosing a form of exercise which you hate. You will soon stop doing it. Your exercise programme also needs to be practical. Can you get to your chosen activity easily? Do the timings fit in with your job? Try to increase your physical exertion in ways that you can fit into your lifestyle. Use the stairs rather than the lift. Park a few spaces away from the supermarket entrance. Walk around the block in the sunshine.

FUEL FOR EXERCISE

Body movement is produced by muscles. Different muscle groups contract and relax to produce different movements. Muscles contract and relax as you exercise. They need fuel to contract. The body supplies this in the bloodstream as glucose and fatty acids (produced from fat). The glucose and the fatty acids have to enter the muscle cells to provide the energy for contraction. Muscles store some glucose as glycogen – so this is used up when you first start to exercise. Soon your muscles need more fuel. You need a small amount of insulin to allow glucose and fatty acids into the muscle cells.

In a person without diabetes, as glucose leaves the bloodstream and the blood glucose level falls, the pancreas shuts off insulin production. This allows the liver to release glucose from its stores. Similarly, fatty acids can now be released from fat stores. So the blood glucose level does not fall below normal unless someone runs a marathon, or participates in some other endurance event. Glucose also arrives in the bloodstream from digestion of carbohydrate food in the gut.

In someone with insulin-treated or sulphonylurea-treated diabetes, glucose and fatty acids can enter the muscle cells, because there is usually plenty of insulin around. However, insulin production cannot be turned off as the blood glucose levels fall. High insulin levels prevent the liver from releasing glucose from its stores, and fatty acids cannot be released from body fat. But the muscles keep taking more and more glucose from the bloodstream, and the blood glucose level falls lower and lower. Eventually, you will become hypoglycaemic – unless you have eaten some glucose, which is absorbed from the gut into the bloodstream. Other carbohydrate food will also eventually be absorbed as glucose – but more slowly because it has to be digested first (see page 196).

So how do you exercise if you have diabetes and have no internal control over insulin production? It is not as critical as it seems. If you are planning new or vigorous exercise, reduce the insulin (e.g. by 10–50% of your usual dose) or reduce your pills (e.g. by half a pill) which will be acting at that time. Eat more long-acting carbohydrate (i.e. high-fibre, starchy carbohydrate) at the meal before, and have some glucose immediately before exercising, and if necessary during exercise (e.g. at half-time). After exercising have some more long-acting carbohydrate. Check your blood glucose levels before and after (if necessary during) your exercise and use this information to work. out what to do next time. Your diabetes adviser will be able to help you.

A word of warning. Do not exercise vigorously with a high glucose level, especially if you have ketones in your urine. If you have no insulin in the circulation, exercise will push your blood glucose up further as the liver releases glucose but the muscles cannot use it. Fatty acids cannot be used either and the liver breaks them down into ketones. This makes your blood acid. You will eventually develop diabetic ketoacidosis (page 106). Give yourself some insulin to return the glucose towards normal (but not hypoglycaemic) and wait for it to work. It is better not to exercise vigorously that day if you can avoid it but to allow your diabetes control to improve. This can also happen if you overeat before or during exercise.

FIT TO EXERCISE?

Before starting an exercise programme discuss what you are planning to do with your doctor. Virtually everyone can exercise, but if you have heart problems or muscle or joint problems you may need to choose the form and vigour of your exercise carefully. If you have just had laser treatment for retinopathy or a vitreous haemorrhage you should not exercise until given the all-clear by your doctor. You must not do exercises which could knock, rub or put pressure on a foot or leg ulcer.

As a general rule, never exercise so energetically that you cannot hold a conversation with someone while exercising. Learn how to take your pulse at the wrist. The pulse rate should not exceed the maximum rate for your age. The pulse rate at rest is about 60 to 80 beats a minute. Your training rate should be 60–85% of your maximum. You can calculate this by subtracting your age in years from 220. Thus for a 50-year-old man the maximum heart rate is 220–50 = 170 beats per minute. His training rate is 120–144 beats per minute, which should be sustained for 20–30 minutes each week for maximum benefit. If you do not exercise regularly start at the 60% end (102 beats per minute in this case), and work up towards 85 per cent (144 beat/mm) over several weeks or months. People with diabetic nerve damage may not have a normal heart rate – talk to your doctor.

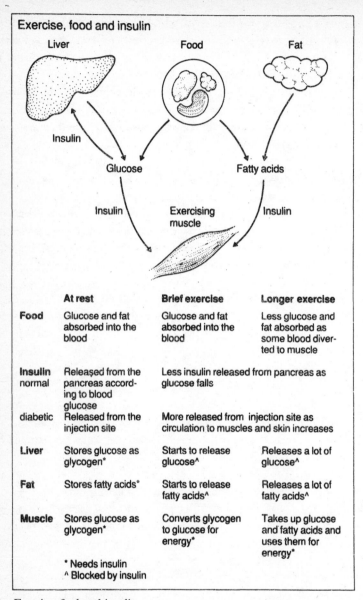

Exercise, food and insulin

	At rest	Brief exercise	Longer exercise
Food	Glucose and fat absorbed into the blood	Glucose and fat absorbed into the blood	Less glucose and fat absorbed as some blood diverted to muscle
Insulin normal	Released from the pancreas according to blood glucose	Less insulin released from pancreas as glucose falls	
diabetic	Released from the injection site	More released from injection site as circulation to muscles and skin increases	
Liver	Stores glucose as glycogen*	Starts to release glucose^	Releases a lot of glucose^
Fat	Stores fatty acids*	Starts to release fatty acids^	Releases a lot of fatty acids^
Muscle	Stores glucose as glycogen*	Converts glycogen to glucose for energy*	Takes up glucose and fatty acids and uses them for energy*

* Needs insulin
^ Blocked by insulin

Exercise, food and insulin

Work up to it gently. There is no point finishing your first exercise session drenched in sweat and gasping for air with an impression of imminent demise. Next morning your continued existence will be made only too plain by the discovery of muscles you didn't know you had, none of which now work and all of which ache abominably. The end result is usually a fervent determination never to exercise again! Warm up first with some gentle loosening-up exercises and then begin a graded programme which suits your own fitness level and needs. Stretch those stiff muscles and joints carefully. If it hurts don't do it. Wind down gently at the end.

Ask your doctor's advice on exercising safely *before* you start – not while he is treating your tennis elbow!

SPORT FOR ALL

There are hundreds of sporting activities to choose from, but you do not need to take up an organised sport. Walking in your favourite countryside or energetic gardening can both give you regular exercise. But if you decide to take up a particular sport, how do you decide whether you, as a person with diabetes, can do it? I wrote these guidelines for this book and modified them following very helpful discussions with co-members of the British Diabetes Association Sports and Exercise Working Party.

CAN I DO THIS ACTIVITY?

How fit am I?

- You should always discuss exercise with your doctor.
- Is your exercise tolerance good? (Can you walk upstairs easily, run for a bus, mow the lawn, for example?)

TRAINING ZONE FOR EXERCISE

Your age in years	Your heart rate in beats per minute	
	60% maximum	85% maximum
20	120	170
30	114	161
40	108	153
50	102	144
60	96	136
70	90	127

- Has your doctor told you to avoid any activities?
- Do you have diabetic eye disease, foot problems, heart disease or other diabetic tissue damage? If yes, discuss exercise with your doctor.
- If you have had a heart attack follow the hospital's cardiac rehabilitation programme or contact the British Association for Cardiac Rehabilitation.
- If you have active new vessel disease of the eye avoid excessive exertion until the eyes have been adequately treated. If you exercise too strenuously it can precipitate a bleed from these new vessels into the eye.
- If you have foot ulcers you should avoid weight-bearing altogether on the affected foot. If you have a poor nerve supply or poor blood supply to your feet you should, in addition, have your feet checked regularly by a state registered chiropodist.

Is my blood glucose balance safe?

- Is your blood glucose under control?
- Do you know how to adjust your diet and treatment for different exercise levels? If not, ask your diabetes adviser.
- Do you take insulin or pills which may cause hypoglycaemia? If so, can you recognise and treat hypoglycaemia?
- Do you have hypoglycaemia often or without warning? If yes, consult your diabetes adviser.

Can I do this particular exercise safely?

- Does it involve short bursts of activity or prolonged, endurance exertion?
- Can you eat, take your treatment (if necessary) and test your blood glucose during the exercise?
- Can you keep food and diabetes equipment with you and have you planned what to do if you become hypoglycaemic?
- How easy would it be for you to predict your energy expenditure and plan your eating and treatment before, during and after exercise?
- If the activity is done outdoors what would happen if you needed assistance? Are you alone or with others? Are you close to a telephone or transport?
- Does the activity involve heat or cold, heights or depths, water

or air? All of these can influence your blood glucose balance in addition to the exercise itself.

Is this sport or activity suitable for me?

There are regulations for some sports which relate to people with diabetes. Diabetes UK has a list of most of them.

This may seem a formidable list, but remember it is designed to include 70-year-olds as well as teenagers. Most of my readers will have no problem practising the majority of sports and will require this list only when contemplating unknown or potentially hazardous activities. Providing they learn from the experts and observe safety rules carefully, people with diabetes can take up sports such as rock-climbing or slalom canoeing. Tim, with newly-diagnosed diabetes, learned to climb on a Diabetics UK/Outward Bound mountain course, sought further training, put in a great deal of practice and, a year later, climbed the Old Man of Hoy – a 500-foot stack of rock towering above dangerous seas. But you do not have to opt for such dramatic activities. Choose one that interests you then talk with your health care team about any diabetes or other health issues which might affect your ability to do this activity safely.

Disabilities such as amputations or blindness are no barrier to most sports. I have met people who are wheelchair-bound who go canoeing and even abseiling. I also know a blind man who has scaled Mont Blanc and enjoys a range of sports including water-skiing and judo. And several people whose vision has been severely impaired have successfully completed Outward Bound mountain courses with me at Eskdale.

THE PERSON SUPERVISING THE ACTIVITY

If a sports instructor is unfamiliar with diabetes it may help to go through the following list with him. Suggest he asks himself the following questions.

Can a person with diabetes do it safely?

- Do you understand what diabetes is and what it means? Are you aware of the different types of diabetes and their treatment?
- Are there regulations about people with diabetes doing this activity – do they apply here?

- The main risks are hypoglycaemia and the effects of tissue damage (the latter are covered in the section for people with diabetes, pages 198–200). Do you understand what hypoglycaemia is and how you can recognise it? (See page 104 and Chapter 10). Hypoglycaemia, which sometimes causes confusion or coma, may affect not only the individual but also (indirectly) others involved in the activity, bystanders and those involved in rescue.
- If the person becomes hypoglycaemic will he be a danger to himself or to others? If yes, will he and you be able to recognise the warning symptoms and will he be able to eat and cure the hypoglycaemia? If he does become seriously hypoglycaemic can you safeguard him (and others) and treat/rescue him if required?
- Learn about high glucose (page 195).

Can this person with diabetes do it safely?

- Is he physically and mentally fit enough to start this activity?
- Have you gone through pages 197–9 with the person?
- Can he adjust his diabetic treatment and diet to enjoy this activity safely without losing control of his diabetes?

Can I supervise him?

- Do I, personally, feel competent to supervise him in this activity? Will I need additional help?
- It is natural to worry about looking after someone with a medical condition with which you are unfamiliar, but diabetes is no barrier to performing well in most activities – sometimes at national or international level. Some sporting bodies do have regulations banning people with diabetes who take insulin. However, many have no clear policy. Most national diabetes associations will advise people with diabetes and sporting organisations. Diabetes UK has information on a wide range of activities and the regulations, if any, and will be pleased to help both sports trainers and sportsmen and women.

COMMON PROBLEMS

Preventing hypoglycaemia

Reduce your insulin or sulphonylurea pills, eat enough fast and slow carbohydrate and test your glucose. It is as simple as that, but may be a little more difficult in practice.

Reduce your insulin or pills How much should you reduce your insulin? It is usually enough to reduce it by 2–4 units, but some people may need to halve the dose of the insulin which will be acting at the time of the activity. Thus for a morning activity, reduce your morning fast-acting insulin. For an afternoon activity reduce your lunch-time fast-acting or your morning medium-acting insulin. For an evening activity reduce your evening short-acting. You may also wish to reduce your evening medium or long-acting insulin a little to reduce the risk of nocturnal hypoglycaemia. For regular vigorous activity reduce your total insulin dose by at least 20%.

As an approximate guide, reduce the dose of pills taken before the exercise by a quarter to a third of your usual total daily dose.

Eat more (but not if you are not on glucose-lowering pills or injections). You need slow, starchy, high-fibre carbohydrate to last you through the exercise and to help you recover in the hours afterwards. You need glucose for rapid energy that will provide a boost when you want it. As a rough guide, double the carbohydrate in the last meal before vigorous exercise, have one and half times the normal amount before moderate exercise. Have a double snack before strenuous exercise, or replace the snack with a glucose sport drink. Many people use chocolate bars though they do have a high fat content which slows glucose absorption. Slip in some glucose as tablets or drink if you feel low during the exercise. Afterwards eat a mixture of fast and slow-acting carbohydrate and adjust your food to your blood glucose test and what you are doing next. Do not forget a bedtime snack.

'But I want to slim,' you wail! So, greatly reduce your insulin or sulphonylurea pills before exercise and keep a very close eye on your blood glucose levels. People on metformin alone do not need to eat extra before exercise; hypoglycaemia is most unlikely and most people on metformin alone usually have a weight problem so more food is not a good idea.

As you become familiar with a particular activity, you will be able to fine-tune your insulin and food. Most people who exercise regularly will not need large increases in their food.

Measure your blood glucose Do this often to start with and then as needed. It is the key to success. Blood glucose testing has freed people with diabetes from anxiety about the effects of exercise and other experiences upon their diabetes. Don't worry about your glucose – test it and establish the facts. Then you can learn from each training session. Remember that you may become hypoglycaemic up to 2 days after exercise. Keep testing.

TYPES OF EXERCISE

Sprinting

This uses the glycogen stored in your muscles. Some people eat plenty of carbohydrate in the days before an event to top-up muscle stores. You will probably not want a lot in your stomach immediately before racing, so make sure you eat a meal high in starchy fibrous carbohydrate earlier in the day. Some people may take some neat glucose as a non-fizzy drink, tablets or gel just before running to start topping-up their bloodstream and thus their muscles once the muscle glycogen has been used up by the sprint. It may be difficult to eat right away because intensive exercise can make you feel a little nauseous or cramped. Eat as soon as you comfortably can when you have finished sprinting. Again, train gradually and learn how much carbohydrate loading to do beforehand and how much insulin or tablets and food to take that day as you train.

Endurance exercise

This includes marathon running and walking. You will soon use up your muscle glycogen stores and start drawing glucose out of the bloodstream so you need to eat not only beforehand but also to keep topping up as you go along. Adjust your insulin so that there is not too much insulin around to allow your liver to release glucose when you need it. Reduce your insulin or sulphonylurea pills by 50 per cent when you start training if you have never walked or run a long way before. If you have trained you will be able gradually to work out how much to take. What you eat as you go along depends on the type of exercise and how competitive it is. Fluids and electrolytes are important, especially so if you are running and/or it is hot, and your glucose top-ups can be part of your drinks. Walkers can browse on fruit and nuts, biscuits and muesli bars with the occasional chocolate bar and glucose for emergency energy. For a day's strenuous walking with a heavy rucksack you need three big meals with plenty of starchy high-fibre carbohydrate, and six double snacks (i.e. the carbohydrate equivalent of twelve of your normal snacks). Once you get into training you may manage on less but start off with this. Whether walking or running you must have some glucose with you in a pocket or hip/bum bag.

ENVIRONMENTAL HAZARDS

Water

Look at the second-hand on your watch. Take a deep breath in and hold it. How long can you hold your breath for? That is the length of time you have to sort yourself out if you get into difficulties underwater. This is the most hazardous environment for the hypoglycaemia-prone diabetic. This is also why under-water diving is not a safe sport for some people taking insulin. If you are entirely confident in your knowledge of diabetes self-care and your freedom from hypoglycaemia you can dive with a buddy who has a good knowledge of diabetes safety. With any water sport it is essential that you do not become hypoglycaemic while on, in or under the water. It is rare for someone to become unconscious from hypoglycaemia (see pages 113–4) but if it did happen this could be disastrous while swimming or canoeing. Follow the rules for all exercise, but I would also suggest 2–4 glucose tablets just before setting off or entering the water. This means that you will be exercising on a rising glucose. Never go on/in water alone and always wear a life jacket or buoyancy aid or swim where there is a lifeguard. A wet suit alone is not enough – it will not always keep your head above water if you become unconscious. On boating or canoe trips keep snacks in a water-proof container tied into the boat. Rowing is one of the most strenuous sports there is and often requires both sprint and endurance effort. You must stoke up with enormous amounts of carbohydrate. In this sport the rest of the eight will not be pleased if you break stroke to eat half-way through a race! However, as Steve Redgrave has demonstrated, insulin-treated diabetes does not stop you from winning Olympic gold medals.

When I checked Josephine's blood glucose before she got into her kayak, it was 13 mmol/l (234 mg/dl). She was an accomplished canoeist. Fifteen minutes later she was going round and round in erratic and uncoordinated circles. Her blood glucose was now 2 mmol/l (36 mg/dl). A bottle of Hypostop glucose gel revived her and after a couple of biscuits, she continued the session.

Hypostop glucose gel is useful for water activities. It comes in a leakproof polythene bottle and can be tied onto your clothing or pinned into a pocket. It is easy to take in water. One diabetic acquaintance who dives carries and eats Mars bars underwater. If you need to eat in unusual places, practise first.

Large numbers of people with diabetes enjoy water sports safely and so can you if you wish. Learn from a recognised trainer and use some common sense to prevent hypoglycaemia.

Heights

Most activities involving heights are safety-roped, so they are often safer than water sports. Fear is a common factor for all of us at great heights and this causes adrenaline surges with racing heart, sweating and shaking – just like a hypo. If in doubt you must assume you are hypo and eat glucose. Rock climbing is a strenuous sport punctuated by periods of waiting.

Eat glucose just before you start climbing so that you are exercising on a rising glucose. If you are safeguarding someone else (e.g. on belay) you must be certain that you cannot become hypoglycaemic. As belaying takes two hands, eat a sugary carbohydrate and some dextrosol *before* you tell the climber he or she can start climbing. (It is, of course, essential to tell your climbing partner that you have diabetes and unforgiveable to become hypoglycaemic when you have someone else's life in your hands.) People can become hypoglycaemic abseiling too – although fear should increase the glucose as emergency hormones are released. Nevertheless, I have seen people become hypoglycaemic while in a state of fear. So, again eat glucose before you set off to ensure that your descent is as controlled as you would wish. People with diabetes go parachute-jumping and hang-gliding – seek expert advice before tackling such hazardous sports. For any of these sports you must have some means of keeping glucose on your person no matter what position you end up in.

Depths

Caving or pot-holing may include some climbing and some water. In addition to these dangers, one of its main features is that you are inaccessible once deep in the cave system. You must be certain that you have enough to eat and plenty to spare for unexpected delays. As with hang-gliding, think carefully before taking yourself and your diabetes down a pot-hole.

COMPETITIVE AND TEAM SPORTS

If you are simply pursuing a sport on your own for pleasure you need not be under pressure to compare your performance with that of others and you will not be a member of a team who are relying on you to pull your weight.

Joe and John were orienteering. They had to navigate and run a complex course competing against 10 other pairs and against the clock. There was a prize for the fastest team to find all the markers. Joe had diabetes. They jogged off and all was well to start with. They found the first two markers. Then they could not find the third. John started to get cross. 'We've slowed down, the others are catching up.' Then he noticed the landmark he had been looking for and raced towards it. Joe had been feeling slightly wobbly and was just getting some glucose tablets out of his bum bag. He tried to eat them as he ran after John and choked on the crumbs. Then he dropped the pack into some undergrowth. He stopped to look for it. John looked back. 'Come on, slow coach,' he shouted. 'Run, why are you stopping?' Joe was feeling rather dizzy by now but he did not want to let John down and so he stumbled on up the hill. When he reached the top, panting, John was already racing downhill to the next marker. Joe followed. He was sweating and shaky and everything seemed very hazy. When Joe did not appear at the next marker, John went back to look for him and found him semiconscious at the bottom of the hill where he had fallen. Fortunately, after he was revived with a can of glucose drink he just had a few bruises.

Hypoglycaemia can induce a state of mind in which people do not want to stop what they are doing (see page 110). Furthermore, it is natural to ignore minor symptoms so as to avoid letting a friend or team mates down, especially when an event is timed. It is best to ensure that the hypo does not happen in the first place. But if it does, it is faster (and safer) in the long run to stop and deal with it, as continued exercise will make it worse. John knew that Joe had diabetes and what to do to help him. Make sure your team mates know this. If you are playing professionally or in national competitions (as several people with diabetes do), you will have built up extensive experience of your exact treatment and food needs during training with the rest of the team. Use training to perfect your skills in the game and in diabetes management.

ACTIVITIES FOR ALL

Most people are not marathon runners or rock climbers although many take part in team sports. Physical activity is good for all of us. It will help you lose weight. Any increase in exercise, however small, helps. Do a little more each day. Try to walk a little further – do not use the car for short trips, use the stairs not the lift, walk around the house more. Even if you cannot get about much, moving the muscles you **can** use helps – for example, lift your arms up and down each hour. Ask your physiotherapist or nurse to advise you.

SUMMARY

- Exercise is good for people with diabetes.
- Consult your doctor before starting exercise or sport.
- Learn how to exercise and train safely.
- Learn how to adjust your diet and treatment for exercise.
- Gain a realistic understanding of the potential dangers in any new sport and how to safeguard yourself and others.
- Plan ahead.
- Tell your team mates and instructors that you have diabetes.
- Train for your diabetes care as well as the activity and physical fitness. Learn by experience.
- Have a go, with expert help.

18

TRAVEL

People with diabetes can and do travel all over the world. To ensure that your holiday or business trip is memorable for the right reasons put a little forethought into your travel arrangements. The following points are a general guide – choose those which are appropriate to your trip.

PLAN AHEAD

Where are you going?

Clearly a journey from Manchester to Birmingham is less complicated than an expedition to Tierra del Fuego. Are you going to a familiar place or breaking new ground? While there is no reason why someone with diabetes should not travel in remote mountains or in the depths of the rain forest, to do this you have to be very confident of your diabetes self-care if you are insulin-dependent. If diabetes is new to you consider spending your first holiday after diagnosis somewhere familiar or not too far off the beaten track. You are unlikely to have much choice in your destination with a business trip. A mystery tour (deliberate or unintentional) can be fun, but if you are taking glucose-lowering treatment with pills or insulin you may prefer to be able to plan to avoid unexpected delays or being stranded. It is always useful to learn how to read a map, if you do not already know how.

Is a visa required? Do you need immunisations? If yes, have all of them, including any non-compulsory ones advised by your doctor. Sarah (page 52) had a high glucose level for several days after her influenza immunisation – similar effects may occur with other immunisations so it is better to have them well before you travel. Always keep your tetanus shots up to date.

What language is spoken? Clearly it is easier visiting an English-speaking country. If you do not speak the language of the country you are visiting, it is wise to have a basic phrase book, or better to learn some words before you go. At the very least, learn the words for 'diabetes' 'insulin injection' (if necessary), 'help' and 'doctor'. Diabetes UK can often help with general information and translations of useful phrases. Ensure that you have some small denomination local currency with you to buy food or make telephone calls if necessary. If you can afford it, carry enough money, travellers cheques or credit cards to get yourself home if an emergency arises.

When are you going?

How far ahead is your journey? Tomorrow? Or do you have time to plan? If you are someone whose job or hobby often takes you away from home at short notice, keep a diabetes travel pack ready to go. At what time of year is your journey? You need to consider the weather in your country of departure and what the weather will be like when you get where you are going. Extremes of heat and cold, wet and dry, or high winds, can affect everyone's health, and may require special care with your diabetes equipment and insulin or tablets. (For example, insulin goes off if it overheats – see pages 92–3. It does not work if it has been frozen. Blood-glucose testing strips must be kept dry or they will not produce accurate results.) Always keep your insulin with you.

With whom are you travelling?

'I travel alone, sometimes I'm East, sometimes I'm West. No remembered love can ever find me.' Noel Coward enjoyed solitary travel. But if you have diabetes and get into difficulties – hypoglycaemia or gastroenteritis, for example – you may be very pleased to see your remembered love, or just a good friend. The choice is yours, but common sense suggests that, for prolonged trips or distant ones, people with diabetes are safer travelling with a companion. If you are travelling with other people you must tell them about your diabetes.

Patrick was on an initiative course with ten of his work-mates. They had been together for a week, trying a wide range of activities. The others noticed that Patrick did not look well, but he brushed their concern aside. 'I'm fine,' he said. 'Let's go and have a pint, I'm parched.' Patrick drank a lot – mostly beer. Next day the group set off on a two-day exercise, navigating over the moor to a hut to sleep, then walking back to base. Patrick was soon at the back of the group, puffing and panting. The others asked if he was all right. 'A bit of a hangover,' said Patrick, ruefully. It took them a long time to reach the hut. Patrick vomited several times in the night. 'Bad beer,' he gasped. Next morning he was drowsy and clearly could not walk. After much anxious discussion, two of his friends stayed with him while the rest went for help. When the group's tutor and a rescue party opened the door, the whole hut smelled of rotten apples. They searched his rucksack and found some insulin and a glucose-testing kit. Fortunately for Patrick, the tutor's wife was diabetic. He realised what was wrong, checked Patrick's glucose – which was 44 mmol/l (792 mg/dl) on the strip and gave him some insulin. Then they took him to hospital. Patrick could have died from this episode of ketoacidosis. Next time he told his companions about his diabetes.

It is also good to tell your companions about hypoglycaemia, if you are taking glucose-lowering medication. If you are prone to bad hypos, teach a close companion how to give glucagon (see pages 115–6). If your friends know that you have diabetes, they will not wonder why you have special dietary needs, and you need not hide your blood testing from them.

How long?

Consider the duration of the journey itself and the length of the whole trip. During a long journey you will need to eat, and may need to check your glucose. You may travel across time zones, in which case many people find it easier to stay on home time until you arrive, and then change to foreign time. On the return trip, stay in foreign time until you reach your home country and time zone (see pages 215–6).

Ensure that you have enough supplies of insulin and other medications to last the whole trip and to cover losses or breakages. Your doctor and chemist will need notice of your requirements, especially if you are going away for a long time.

How are you travelling?

This affects several aspects of your diabetes care. If you are travelling under your own steam – walking or cycling, for example, you need to fuel your exercise (see pages 194–5). If you are using your own car you must follow all the driving rules (see pages 170–2) and do not forget your Green Card, or other documentation if you are travelling abroad. With public transport you are completely dependent on others. A good general rule is to assume the worst – that the train will stop for no apparent reason in the middle of a featureless landscape for three hours and cause you to miss your connection; or that your Mediterranean holiday will terminate in a day and night at a small, hot airport clutching a straw donkey, two funny-shaped bottles of potent local spirit and a bag of olives (leaking) while your plane awaits a vital component available only from the other side of the world. Your planning (i.e. food, drink and treatment) should take such contingencies into account. Sufferers from motion sickness should, if possible, try to avoid the mode of travel most likely to precipitate this. People with diabetes can take motion sickness pills if they wish. Follow the dosage and precautions advised by your doctor or pharmacist.

Accommodation

Where will you be staying? In a hotel? A tent? Self-catering cottage? Bed and Breakfast? Youth hostels? Obviously if you have a room to yourself it will be easier to look after your diabetes in private. A fridge or FRIO pack will ensure that your insulin stays cool. if you are sharing with strangers, keep your diabetes kit secure – be particularly careful to lock up your insulin and syringes. (This is another reason why an insulin pen is simpler – you carry it with you – although you should still secure your back up supplies.)

Food

One of the joys of travelling is the opportunity to try exotic foods. Do your best to stick to healthy eating, but do not worry if you cannot follow it exactly. A good start is to find out about the country's staple carbohydrate foods before you go. These include bread (i.e. pumpernickel, chapati, rye-bread, unleavened bread, corn-bread, nan, crisp-bread, pitta), rice, potatoes, yams, pasta, sweet potato, cassava, maize, porridge, plantain, lentils and beans. Fruit provides carbohydrate too.

Wash it well or peel it. To fill up there will always be local vegetables. Most places will provide salad – but this must be well-washed. If in doubt, you are better with cooked vegetables (or wash the salad yourself). Choose grilled meat or fish if possible and avoid very fatty meat or meat dishes such as paté fois gras. Eat cheese sparingly. Avoid obviously sugary sweets and puddings.

Try local beverages if you wish, but do not overdo the alcohol. Use bottled mineral water on which you break the seal if you are unsure about the purity of tap water. Have some fruit juice if you wish, but remember that it is often sugary.

As soon as you arrive find out hotel or bed and breakfast meal times. Identify local restaurants and shops. Check opening hours of shops, holy days, religious festivals, early closing, etc. If you are on glucose-lowering drugs or insulin it is essential that you eat regularly, so do not be caught out. Always carry some energy rations (check first – some countries will not allow you to bring in certain types of food). Prepacked fibre crunch or muesli bars are easy to carry. Take some boxed or canned drink too.

Activity

What are you going to do while you are away? Lying on the beach uses less energy than tramping around ancient monuments. If your activity level is going to differ greatly from what you would do at home, adjust your diet and treatment to cope with this (see pages 194–5). Do not be tempted into hazardous activities 'because we're on holiday' without giving them the same thought that you would at home. Are they properly supervised? How can you prevent yourself becoming hypoglycaemic?

Getting around

Local transport may be excellent or non-existent. It is all part of the adventure – your rickshaw may deliver you promptly from door to door or you may fail to decipher the hieroglyphics on the bus and end up ten miles in the wrong direction (I've done this in London!). Carry your diabetes kit and some food with you so that you do not need to worry if you are late back for a meal.

Local hazards

Without wishing to put you off, exotic travel can have a wide range of hazards. Bears, crocodiles, spiders, scorpions and assorted snakes spring to mind. But there are smaller dangers which may catch you unawares – malaria and other parasitic diseases. Always take your antimalarial prophylaxis exactly as instructed. Do not paddle in rivers or lakes in tropical countries. Be careful on the beach. Any small injury – a blister, cut or bite – may become infected in hot countries so look after your skin very carefully and carry a first aid kit. Gastroenteritis is very common – avoid it (see page 217).

What happens if something goes wrong?

You must have full medical insurance. It should provide treatment while you are away and, if necessary, get you home with a medical escort if you become very ill abroad. The hospital in which I work serves Heathrow airport. I see people with diabetes who have become ill abroad and who have been unable to find proper medical advice. They hang on, getting iller and iller, until their booked flight home. They struggle onto the plane and have a terrible journey, often requiring help from other passengers. By the time they arrive they are dehydrated and collapsed and have to be rushed to hospital to be resuscitated.

Always check the small print very carefully as many insurance policies will not cover you for pre-existing illness. Be particularly careful with policies included in package holidays – you may need to ask your travel agent to show you the rules. Shop around, as with car insurance, there are wide variations.

When you return

Carry on with your antimalarials. Keep your diabetes diary safely so that you can use it to plan another trip.

STEP BY STEP

Diabetes UK Travel Guide

Diabetes UK has good information on most countries, with Travel Guides including useful phrases in the language of the country concerned. Other national diabetes organisations may provide similar support. Send for your Travel Guide as soon as you know you are going away.

Are you fit to go?

If you are in any doubt about your fitness ask your doctor before you book your ticket.

Booking

Tell the airline, hotel and travel company that you have diabetes. Some airlines will provide a diabetic diet if asked in advance but it is usually best just to eat the same as everyone else. Many hotels will help. Your package tour organiser should know too. If you are elderly or have a physical difficulty, wheelchairs can be provided at stations, ports and airports if you give advance warning.

Diabetes check-up

Before a long or very distant trip the following points should be checked.

- Glucose balance. What to do with treatment while travelling and while away, including emergencies.
- Tissue damage. Is there any and do you need to take any special precautions?
- Dietitian – for dietary advice.
- Chiropodist – for foot check and foot care advice.
- Doctor's letter to confirm that you have diabetes and the generic names of all medications. Note of allergies and other medical conditions.
- Supplies for your diabetes travel pack.

Diabetes travel pack

This should contain the following:

- Medic-alert or SOS medallion or bracelet (if you wish);
- Diabetic card;
- Letter from doctor confirming diabetes;
- Letter in language of country visited confirming diabetes;
- Treatment (take twice the amount you need)
  – insulin, syringes, needles, needle clipper
  – cool bag for insulin (4–25°C)
  – insulin pen, pen needles, insulin cartridges (plus a needle and syringe) or
  – glucose-lowering pills;

- Testing
  - blood testing strips (with meter if used), finger-pricker, lancets, platforms if needed
  - urine-testing strips for glucose and ketones
  - diabetic diary with pen;
- Hypoglycaemia treatment (if on glucose-lowering pills or insulin)
  - glucose tablets
  - hypostop
  - glucagon kit (if on insulin).

Medical kit

This should contain the following:

- Other medication;
- Antidiarrhoeal (e.g. codeine phosphate);
- Antibiotic (e.g. ampicillin or erythromycin if penicillin-allergic) if your doctor agrees;
- Motion sickness pills;
- Headache pills (e.g. paracetamol);
- Antiseptic wipes;
- Antiseptic cream;
- Assorted dressings;
- Roll of tape (e.g. Micropore);
- Foot care items from chiropodist;
- Non-adherent dressing (e.g. N-A dressing);
- Absorbent gauze;
- Triangular bandage;
- Open weave bandage;
- Eye pad;
- Safety pins (use nappy pins with protected ends);
- Round-ended tweezers;
- Round-ended scissors;
- Sunscreen cream;
- Thin foil space blanket;
- Torch;
- Paper tissues;
- Polythene bags.

NB Never use a safety pin next to the skin. Never put tape or bandages all the way around a toe or limb – it may constrict the circulation.

Out and about kit

- Diabetes travel pack;
- Plastic bottle of mineral water with screw top;
- Box(es) or can(s) of drink;
- Wholemeal biscuits or foil-wrapped fibre or muesli bars;
- Local money to put in pay phone;
- Selected items from your medical kit.

Packing

Take clothes to protect yourself from extremes of temperature, but do not pack so much that your suitcase is too heavy to carry.

Remember that in some forms of transport your suitcase will be taken away and stowed in the hold. Keep your diabetes kit with you in your hand luggage. A shoulder bag is useful for your out and about kit. Some people like a bum bag or ski bag worn around the waist. It is possible to fit all your diabetes kit and your out and about kit (except the water) into a large bum bag.

Setting off

People whose diabetes is controlled on diet alone and most of those on tablet treatment will not need to make any special treatment adjustments for the day of travel, although those on glucose-lowering pills may wish to reduce their morning dose for a very long or arduous journey.

Not flying

For all but short journeys, if you take insulin injections, you should reduce your morning dose by 10 per cent. It is better to have blood glucose levels above 6 mmol/l (108 mg/dl) while travelling to avoid hypoglycaemia. Test your blood glucose before each full meal and before bed, or 4–6 hourly.

Flying on insulin

You may cross time zones. For short flights and if the time difference is less than four hours this rarely requires much change in your insulin. Just make sure you cannot become hypoglycaemic. For longer journeys consider the day of travel as a special day and resume your normal insulin at breakfast-time in the country to which you are travelling (by breakfast I mean their first meal in the morning). On the day of travel you may be awake for longer than usual whether or not it is night or day on the ground below. Add up the insulin you usually have in each 24 hours and use common sense to make the suggested changes at an appropriate time of day. For example, on westward flights, take extra fast-acting at extra meals after checking your blood glucose. On eastward flights reduce your insulin.

Customs and security

You do not have to declare your diabetes at either of these points, but with the current concern about drug smuggling, syringes and needles are likely to be commented upon if found in a routine search. This is no problem, but a note in the language of the country you are visiting can make explanations easier. (Some countries have the death penalty for drug smuggling.)

WHILE AWAY

Many people travel to experience something different from everyday life. This can include temperatures, humidity, terrain, sleeping/waking patterns, food and many other facets of life. Some of these could change your glucose balance.

Heat

Protect your skin from the sun.

> Marie has diabetic neuropathy. She went on holiday to Italy. The sun blazed in a cloudless sky. Each morning she covered herself in sunscreen cream before going out. One day she paddled in the pool during the morning. By lunchtime her feet were scarlet. The blisters ruined her holiday and took a month to heal.

Hot weather also increases the circulation to your skin so your insulin may be absorbed more rapidly and may work earlier and more strongly than you expect.

Cold

This decreases the circulation to your skin as the body conserves its heat. Thus your insulin may be absorbed more slowly than you expect, only to appear later when you warm up. If your circulation is poor, especially in your feet, the circulation may be reduced to a critical level and you may lose the blood flow to your toes. Gangrene is a rare consequence. If you have poor circulation keep your feet well insulated from the cold.

Hypoglycaemia reduces your ability to shiver to keep warm. This means that if you become severely hypoglycaemic in cool weather your body temperature will fall. Once you have eaten and your blood glucose rises to normal you will start to shiver and warm up. This is a potentially dangerous problem in harsh environments. In this situation, anyone with diabetes who appears hypothermic must also be treated for hypoglycaemia, and anyone who is hypoglycaemic must also be treated for hypothermia.

Gastroenteritis

Sadly, many holidays include a day or so with Traveller's Tummy or Montezuma's Revenge. This is largely preventable by eating well-cooked food which has not been left standing, drinking bottled mineral or spring water, eating only well-washed salad and peeled fruit. If you do develop diarrhoea and/or vomiting, retire to bed near a toilet with some sealed bottles of water, some cans of Coca Cola or Pepsi Cola (they contain glucose and salts), some glucose tablets and a packet of plain biscuits. Make sure someone knows you are ill. Check your blood glucose every two hours – you will probably have to increase your insulin. Keep sipping fluids and sucking glucose tablets. Nibble biscuits if you can. Call expert help sooner rather than later.

Foot care

Every year diabetic clinics wave goodbye to their patients as they set off on holiday, then anxiously await their return. Every year, despite huge efforts to prevent this, people return with ulcers or infections on their feet. A few lose their legs. The story is always much the same.

'I bought these new sandals in the market, real leather and ever so cheap, too. Then we went to look at the castle. It was very hot and a bit further than I thought and the road was all pebbly. The blisters didn't look too bad. I put a plaster on them. I thought the swelling was the heat. I couldn't rest them not with all that sightseeing to do, could I? They didn't hurt so I thought it was all right. They do look a bit red, now I come to take the plaster off.'

Take your chiropodist's advice before you go away. Never wear new
shoes for the first time on holiday. Take your most comfortable
shoes and avoid sandals – sand and grit combine with sweaty feet
from the heat and walking to cause rubs and blisters, and you can
knock or cut your feet easily. Wear well-fitting training shoes with
socks that are neither too big nor too small and will absorb the
sweat. Make sure you take your foot care supplies with you. People
with peripheral vascular disease (see pages 152–3) and neuropathy
(see pages 147–9) are at special risk.

Have fun

By now you may be wondering if it is worth it. Obviously I have
had to include a very wide range of potential problems but
remember that most of them will not happen to you. Think ahead
and be prepared. Then go off and enjoy your trip.

Useful phrases

These are some translations of 'I am a diabetic on insulin. If I am
found ill, please give me two teaspoons of sugar in a small amount
of water or three of the glucose tablets* which I am carrying. If I
fail to recover in ten minutes, please call an ambulance.'

France Je suis un diabétique sur insuline. Si on me trouve malade,
donnez-moi s'il vois plait, deux cuillières à thé de sucres dans un
peu d'eau ou trois des comprimés de glucose que j'ai sur moi. Si au
bout de dix minutes je ne reviens pas à moi, appelez une
ambulance.

Germany Ich bin Diabetiker und brauche täglich Insulin. Finden
Sie mich krank, geben Sie mir bitte zwei Essköffel Zucker in Wasser
aufgelöst. Der Zucker befindet sich in meiner Tasche oder
Handtasche. Finden Sie mich ohmachtig, rufen Sie bitte einen Artz
oder einen Krankenwagen.

Italy Sono un diabetico e sono attualmente sottoposto a
trattamento con insulina. Se fossi colto da malore, per favore datemi
due cucchiai di zucchero in una piccola quantità di acqua o tre delle

---

*Make sure you *are* carrying glucose tablets!

pastiglie di glucosio che porto con me. Se non mi reprendo entro dieci minuti, per favore chiamate un'ambulanza.

Norway Jeg har sukkersyke og bruker daglig insulin. Hvis jeg blir funnet syk, vennligst gi meg to spiseskjeer sukker rørti vann. Det er sukker i mm lomme eller min veske. Hvis jeg er bevisstløs eller ikke våkner, vennlist tilkall lege eller sykebill.

Portugal Sou um doente Diabético usando diairamente insulina. Se me encontrar doente deem-me faz favor duas colheres de sopa de açùcar em agua. Encontraro açùcar no men bolso ou saco. Se me encontrar inconsciente sem recuperar, faz favor de chamar um medico ou uma ambulancia.

Spain Soy diabético(a) y tomo insulina. Si usted me encuentra enfermo(a) temga la bondad de darme dos cucharillas de azùcar en un poquito de agua o tres de los cornprimidos de glucosa que llevo encima. Si no me recupero dentro de diez minutos, tenga la bondad de llamar un ambulancia.

Sweden Jag är diabetiker med dagliga insulininjektioner. Om Ni finner mig omtöcknad, var snäll och ge mig två teskedar med socker, gärna upplost i vatten. Det skall finnas socker i min ficka eller väska. Om jag är medvetslos eller ej svarar på tilltal kallapå en doktor eller ambulans.

Yugoslavia Ja sam dijabeticar i dnevno uzimam insulin. Ako me nadjete bolesnog, molim vas dajte ml dvije supene kasike secera rastopljenog u vodi. Secer se nalazi u mom dzepu ili torbi. Ako sam u nesvijesti i ne osvijestim ne, molim vas zovite doktora ili prvu pomoc.

SUMMARY
* Plan your holiday. Do not forget your diabetes travel pack.
* Do not forget your medical kit.
* Do not forget your out and about kit.
* Eat clean.
* Look after your feet.
* Enjoy yourself.

19

SETTING GOALS

Goals for diabetes care in Europe were agreed internationally. Because the St Vincent Declaration is such an important document it is quoted in full.

DIABETES CARE AND RESEARCH IN EUROPE: ST VINCENT DECLARATION

'Representatives of Government Health Departments and patients' organisations from all European countries met with diabetes experts under the aegis of the Regional Offices of the World Health Organisation (WHO) and the International Diabetes Federation (IDE) in St Vincent, Italy on October 10–12, 1989. They unanimously agreed upon the following recommendations and urged that they should be presented in all countries throughout Europe for implementation.

Diabetes mellitus is a major and growing European health problem, a problem at all ages and in all countries. It causes prolonged ill-health and early death. It threatens at least ten million European citizens.

It is within the power of national Governments and Health Departments to create conditions in which a major reduction in this heavy burden of disease and death can be achieved. Countries should give formal recognition to the diabetes problem and deploy resources for its solution. Plans for the prevention, identification and treatment of diabetes and particularly its complications – blindness, renal failure, gangrene and amputation, aggravated coronary heart disease and stroke – should be formulated at local, national and European regional levels. Investment now will earn great dividends in reduction of human misery and in massive savings of human and material resources.

General goals and five-year targets listed below can be achieved by the organised activities of the medical services in active partnership with diabetic citizens, their families, friends and workmates and their organisations; in the management of their own diabetes and the education for it; in the planning, provision and quality audit of health care; in national, regional and international organisations for disseminating information about health maintenance; in promoting and applying research.

GENERAL GOALS FOR PEOPLE – CHILDREN AND ADULTS – WITH DIABETES

*   Sustained improvement in health experience and a life approaching normal in quality and quantity.
*   Prevention and cure of diabetes and of its complications by intensifying research effort.

FIVE-YEAR TARGETS

*   Elaborate, initiate and evaluate comprehensive programmes for detection and control of diabetes and of its complications with self-care and community support as major components.
*   Raise awareness in the population and among health care professionals of the present opportunities and the future needs for prevention of the complications of diabetes and of diabetes itself.
*   Organise training and teaching in diabetes management and care for people of all ages with diabetes, for their families, friends and working associates and for the health care team.
*   Ensure that care for children with diabetes is provided by individuals and teams specialised both in the management of diabetes and of children, and that families with a diabetic child get the necessary social, economic and emotional support.
*   Reinforce existing centres of excellence in diabetes care,

education and research. Create new centres where the need
and potential exist.

- Promote independence, equity and self-sufficiency for all
people with diabetes – children, adolescents, those in the
working years of life and the elderly.
- Remove hindrances to the fullest possible integration of the
diabetic citizen into society.
- Implement effective measures for the prevention of costly
complications:
    - reduce new blindness due to diabetes by one third or more;
    - reduce numbers of people entering end-stage diabetic renal
      failure by at least one third;
    - cut morbidity and mortality from coronary heart disease in
      the diabetic by vigorous programmes of risk factor
      reduction;
    - achieve pregnancy outcome in the diabetic woman that
      approximates that of the non-diabetic woman.
- Establish monitoring and control systems using state of the art
information technology for quality assurance of diabetes
health care provision and for laboratory and technical
procedures in diabetes diagnosis, treatment and self-
management.
- Promote European and international collaboration in
programmes of diabetes research and development through
national, regional and WHO agencies and in active
partnership with diabetes patients organisations.
- Take urgent action in the spirit of the WHO programme,
'Health for All: to establish joint machinery between WHO
and IDF, European Region, to initiate, accelerate and facilitate
the implementation of the recommendations'.

BUT WHAT ABOUT ME?

Dr R.D. Lawrence, himself diabetic, said

'In the successful treatment of diabetes the patient, the nurse,
the practitioner and the specialist are often partners working
together to establish the patient's health. In the long run the
most important part, the melody, is played by the patient.'

He wrote that over 60 years ago. This book aims to give you some of the notes and harmonies you need to compose your own tune. But I hope it will also help you to use all the players and instruments in the diabetes orchestra.

The British Diabetic Association (BDA) founded by Robin Lawrence and H.G. Wells formulated guidelines for people with diabetes. It is now called Diabetes UK. Again, the implications of these guidelines are so important that I am quoting them extensively, with permission from Diabetes UK.

WHAT DIABETES CARE TO EXPECT – ADULT

Introduction

To keep well and healthy, everyone with diabetes needs good and regular health care. The early detection, treatment and continued control of your diabetes is very important as this will reduce your chances of developing the serious health problems (complications) linked to diabetes, such as heart disease, kidney disease and blindness.

Diabetes UK has produced this booklet to set out your rights, your roles and the standards of care you should expect from the National Health Service (NHS). This booklet is for everyone with diabetes, whether on tablets, insulin injections or diet alone. It aims to give you the information you need to live with your diabetes on an everyday basis.

Included is a section for health care professionals, which you may also find useful.

What care you should expect from your diabetes care team

To achieve the best possible diabetes care, you need to work together with health care professionals as equal members of your diabetes care team. It is essential that you understand your diabetes as well as possible so that you are an effective member of this team.

You need to discuss with your consultant or GP the roles and responsibilities of those providing your diabetes care and to identify the key members of your own diabetes care team.

Members in your diabetes care team

- yourself
- consultant physician/diabetologist

- GP
- diabetes specialist nurse (DSN)
- practice nurse
- dietitian
- optometrist/ophthalmologist
- podiatrist/chiropodist
- psychologist
- medical specialists
- pharmacist

You may see some members of your diabetes care team more often than others.

When you have just been diagnosed, your diabetes care team should:

- give you a full medical examination
- work with you to make a programme of care which suits you and includes diabetes management goals (see the annual review check list on pages 229–31)
- arrange for you to talk with a diabetes specialist nurse (or practice nurse) who will explain what diabetes is and discuss your individual treatment and the equipment you will need to use
- arrange for you to talk with a state registered dietitian, who will want to know what you usually eat, and will give you advice on how to fit your usual diet in with your diabetes. A follow-up meeting should be arranged for more detailed advice
- tell you about your diabetes and the beneficial effects of a healthy diet, exercise and good diabetes control
- discuss the effects of diabetes on your job, driving, insurance, prescription charges and, if you are a driver, whether you need to inform the DVLA and your insurance company
- provide you with regular and appropriate information and education, on food and footcare for example
- give you information about Diabetes UK services and details of your local Diabetes UK voluntary group

Once your diabetes is reasonably controlled, you should:

- have access to your diabetes care team at least once a year. In this session, take the opportunity to discuss how your diabetes

affects you as well as your diabetes control
- be able to contact any member of your diabetes care team for specialist advice, in person or by phone
- have further education sessions when you are ready for them
- have a formal medical annual review (see pages 229–31) once a year with a doctor experienced in diabetes

On a regular basis, your diabetes care team should:

- provide continuity of care, ideally from the same doctors and nurses. If this is not possible, the doctors or nurses who you are seeing should be fully aware of your medical history and background
- work with you to continually review your programme of care, including your diabetes management goals (see the annual review check list on pages 229–31)
- let you share in decisions about your treatment or care
- let you manage your own diabetes in hospital after discussion with your doctor, if you are well enough to do so and that is what you wish
- organise pre- and post-pregnancy advice, together with an obstetric hospital team, if you are planning to become or already are pregnant
- encourage a carer to visit with you, to keep them up to date on diabetes to be able to make informed judgements about diabetes care
- encourage the support of friends, partners and/or relatives
- provide you with educational sessions and appointments if you wish
- give you advice on the effects of diabetes and its treatments when you are ill or taking other medication

Plus
If you are treated by insulin injections you should:

- have frequent visits showing you how to inject, look after your insulin and syringes and dispose of sharps (needles). Also how to test your blood glucose and test for ketones and what the results mean
- be given supplies of, or a prescription for the medication and equipment you need*

- discuss hypoglycaemia (hypos): when and why they may happen and how to deal with them

If you are treated by tablets you should:

- be given instruction on blood or urine testing and have explained what the results mean
- be given supplies of, or a prescription for the medication and equipment you need*
- discuss hypoglycaemia (hypos): when and why they may happen and how to deal with them

If you are treated by diet alone you should:

- be given instruction on blood or urine testing and what the results mean
- be given supplies of equipment you may need

YOUR RESPONSIBILITIES

Effective diabetes care is normally achieved by team work, between you and your diabetes care team. Looking after your diabetes and changing your lifestyle to fit in with the demands of diabetes is hard work, but you're worth it!

You will not always get your care right; none of us does, but your diabetes care team is there to support you. Ask questions and request more information especially if you are uncertain or worried about your diabetes and/or treatment. Remember the most important person in the team is you.

---

*Your hospital team will only give you your first prescription. Further prescriptions for medication, test strips, etc will be provided through your GP

People with Type 1 diabetes and tablet controlled Type 2 diabetes are entitled to free prescriptions for medication. Equipment such as blood glucose meters and finger pricking devices normally have to be purchased, but test strips, lancets, most insulin pens and pen needles are available on prescription. Discuss this with your GP

A prescription exemption certificate is available from your local health authority or equivalent in Scotland and Northern Ireland.

The following list of responsibilities is given to help you play your part in your own diabetes care.

It is your responsibility:

- to take as much control of your diabetes on a day-to-day basis as you can. The more you know about your own diabetes, the easier this will become
- to learn about and practice self-care, which should include dietary education, exercise and monitoring blood glucose levels
- to examine your feet regularly or have someone check them
- to know how to manage your diabetes and when to ask for help if you are ill, eg chest infection, flu or diarrhoea and vomiting
- to know when, where and how to contact your diabetes care team
- to build the diabetes advice discussed with you into your daily life
- to talk regularly with your diabetes care team and ask questions
- to make a list of points to raise at appointments, if you find it helpful
- to attend your scheduled appointments and inform the diabetes care team if you are unable to do so

WHAT CARE SHOULD YOU EXPECT IN HOSPITAL

You may be admitted to hospital for reasons related or unrelated to your diabetes. In hospital, responsibility for the management of diabetes should be shared between you and the health professionals. Good diabetes control is important for a speedy recovery and early discharge.

You should:

- receive a full explanation of your treatment during your stay in hospital and have the opportunity to discuss any particular worries. If you do not receive an explanation, ask for it
- inform the ward team of your usual diet, tablets or insulin treatment. Bring your own supplies with you. If they are

removed for safe keeping, make sure that they are returned to you at the end of your stay

- have access to the hospital diabetes care team doctor, nurse, state registered dietitian and chiropodist. Make sure they know you have been admitted

- be allowed to discuss your diabetes so you can manage some aspects of it yourself, such as blood/urine monitoring and injections, if you wish. However; the staff may need to check your technique and results and they may need to do additional tests of their own

- if you are treated by insulin, expect that it may be given via a glucose/insulin drip into a vein if for some reason you are not allowed to eat or drink. If you are having anaesthetic an anaesthetist will arrange care of your diabetes during and immediately following the operation

- if you are treated by tablets, be prepared that your treatment may need to be changed while in hospital, which may involve being transferred from tablets to insulin during your stay

- expect to be able to use your own emergency supplies of biscuits, sugary drinks, fruit or glucose tablets to treat hypoglycaemia if you are on insulin or sulphonylurea tablets. You should bring these supplies with you. If you do experience a hypo, inform your nurse or doctor

- expect to be informed and consulted about any changes in your treatment or diet which may be necessary during your stay in hospital. For example, if you have Type 2 diabetes you will sometimes be temporarily treated with injections of insulin while in hospital. This will be because your illness or operation has upset your diabetes control.

If you are unsure about the treatment or diet you are receiving in hospital, speak to your doctor, nurse or state registered dietitian.

Health care professionals should:

- find out the patient's normal routine with regard to insulin or tablets, blood glucose/urine monitoring and diet
- explain fully to the patient and, if appropriate, the carer what is going to happen throughout his/her stay in hospital, and how the diabetes will be managed until discharge

- discuss any necessary change of treatment with the patient
- inform the diabetes care team of the admission
- discuss with the patient whether they would like to manage aspects of their blood glucose/urine monitoring and treatment. If insulin, sugar or meters are taken away from patients for their benefit, this should only happen after discussion and with the patient's (or carer's) consent
- inform the patient of meal times and offer advice on how to order food and how to get hold of sugar if needed
- allow the patient to keep his/her own snacks and emergency hypo supplies with them in their locker and ensure that snacks are available
- ensure that you are up-to-date on all aspects of diabetes management and that there are written guidelines available on blood glucose monitoring, injection technique and treatment of hypoglycaemia
- ensure that only staff who have attended an appropriate training programme carry out blood glucose testing
- follow the blood glucose monitoring quality assurance programme that should be in place in your hospital. Poorly performed tests are dangerous and expensive
- ensure that the correct timing is entered on the drug chart for oral hypoglycaemic agents and insulins, taking into consideration the timing of medication with respect to meal times
- aim to return to the patient's usual treatment as soon as possible, especially if insulin is being given intravenously
- be aware that particular attention needs to be given to pressure area care for people with diabetes
- provide culturally appropriate diabetes care
- check that arrangements have been made for the patient to have regular check-ups following their stay in hospital

If English is not the patient's first language, bring in an interpreter and involve family members and friends where appropriate.

ANNUAL REVIEW CHECKLIST

It is important to remember that your annual review is to enable you to lead a normal and healthy life. It must be about what you want and need as well as what health care professionals recommend.

The following should be checked at least once a year.

Laboratory tests and investigations

- Blood glucose control: an HbA_{1C} blood test will measure your long-term blood glucose control. The range to aim for should be 7% or below.
- Kidney function: urine and blood tests to check for protein will show that your kidneys are working correctly. There should not be any protein in your urine.
- Blood fats (lipids, cholesterol and triglyceride levels): a blood test that measures your blood fat levels. A total cholesterol of 5.2 mmol/l or less and a fasting triglyceride of 2.0 mmol/l are accepted as national target ranges.*

Physical examinations

- Weight is often calculated as a Body Mass Index (BMI) which expresses adult weight in relation to height. From this you will be advised if you need to lose weight to better control your diabetes. Your GP will record your BMI in your notes.
- Legs and feet should be examined to check your skin, circulation and nerve supply. If necessary, you should be referred to a state registered chiropodist/podiatrist.
- Blood pressure should be taken. You should aim for your blood pressure to be at or less than 140/80. If it is at higher levels discuss this with your doctor to discuss why your blood pressure may be high. Keeping your blood pressure down has been proven to be beneficial for people with diabetes (UKPDS research trial).
- Eyes should be examined regularly through a 'fundoscopy' review, where your pupils are dilated to enable your optometrist/ophthalmologist to detect any early changes at the

---

Please note all normal and good ranges will vary from person to person – this is meant to be a guide so you know what to aim towards. If you have any questions, ask your diabetes care team.

back of the eye (retinopathy). Photographs may be taken to record the appearance at the back of your eyes.

- If you're on insulin, your injection sites should be examined.

Lifestyle issues:

The review should also provide enough time to discuss:

- your general well-being; how you are coping with your diabetes at home, work, school or college
- your current treatment
- your diabetes control, including your home monitoring results
- any problems you may be having

It should include discussion about smoking, alcohol consumption, stress, sexual problems, physical activity and healthy eating issues. You should feel free to raise any or all of these issues with your diabetes care team.

WHAT CARE TO EXPECT IF YOUR CHILD HAS DIABETES

Introduction

This leaflet is for parents of children with diabetes. It describes the sort of care your child needs to keep well and healthy. We use the term child/children to mean anyone who is seen in a paediatric setting, including teenagers.

The main aim of treatment for diabetes is to relieve the unpleasant symptoms of high and low blood glucose by maintaining 'near normal' blood glucose levels. Good diabetes control is not always easy to achieve. Most young people – and their parents – have difficulties with this at one time or another. But, with the support of your specialist children's (paediatric) diabetes care team, your child will be able to lead an active, healthy life with normal growth and development.

Meet your diabetes care team

As you know, it's hard to take in the news that your child has diabetes, let alone the mass of information about diabetes that you will be confronted with when he or she is diagnosed.

You will probably feel frightened and overwhelmed. The

232 DIABETES The Complete Guide

health care professionals you see will be aware of this. They should give you plenty of time to ask questions and should repeat information if needed. The important thing for you is not to be afraid to ask questions. In fact, keep asking until it makes sense.

Children with diabetes have special needs to do with the fact that they are children. This is why it is essential that your child is looked after by a specialist children's diabetes care team, and is seen at a special clinic just for children with diabetes. This way, you and your child can meet other parents and children who are in the same position as you – and meet all the members of the team at one visit.

You and your child are important members of the team too – after all, you will be living with diabetes day to day. Your own and your child's input and experience are just as important as your contact with the diabetes care team.

Your specialist children's diabetes care team should include:

Consultant paediatrician with a special interest in diabetes – has an overall responsibility for your child's diabetes care, hand in hand with the other members of the team. Their experience in childhood conditions and special knowledge of diabetes means that your child can have the best possible care and advice.

Paediatric diabetes specialist nurse – has special expertise in children and diabetes, and can give advice and support for managing diabetes in hospital, at home, at school, and in other settings.

Paediatric dietitian – food is an important part of a child's life, even more so when the child has diabetes. The paediatric dietitian can give advice and support on the subject of your family's food. This will help your child to have good diabetes control and healthy growth.

Children's clinical psychologist – diabetes affects many aspects of life for the child and the family, and this can lead to emotional stress. If needed, you should be able to contact a children's clinical psychologist with experience in diabetes.

Family GP – will still look after your child for non-diabetes matters. There should be good communication on your child's health between your GP and the diabetes care team.

Senior paediatric ward nurse with experience in diabetes – hopefully your child will not have much contact with the hospital ward after diagnosis, but the senior ward nurse can give advice if other members of the team are not available or if your child does need to go into hospital again.

We have described the ideal specialist children's diabetes care team. Resources vary throughout the country and the team in your health authority may differ from the one we have just described. If you are unhappy about the care your child is receiving, speak to your children's diabetes care team and contact Diabetes UK, your local Community Health Council (number in the phone book) or your GP, who should be able to tell you what is available in your area.

CARE AT DIAGNOSIS

At hospital or at home

These days with newly diagnosed diabetes, children may receive their initial care and treatment either at hospital, at home or a combination of both, depending on your child's health and the facilities available in your area.

If your child is going to be cared for in hospital and is under 16, s/he should be admitted to a paediatric ward staffed by health care professionals experienced in childhood diabetes. There should be facilities for you to stay with your child at the hospital, and the amount of time your child spends away from home should be kept to a minimum.

In some cases, your child may be treated at home by a children's diabetes care team if s/he does not have ketoacidosis (a complication of diabetes that needs to be treated in hospital). Your child may be able to spend the day at home and sleep at the hospital at night. Such 'home-based' diabetes services for children, though not widespread, are being developed in some areas.

What care to expect

Whether your child is to be at hospital or at home in the first few days after diagnosis, there are certain things that should happen:

- You should be given an explanation of diabetes from a senior member of the medical team, and appropriately written information on diabetes to back this up.
- You should be given time to absorb the fact that your child has diabetes, and a chance to talk over the emotional impact of diabetes on your child and the rest of the family.
- You should be able to talk over your concerns with senior staff while your child is in hospital or being looked after at home.
- One of the diabetes care team should inform your GP about your child's diabetes, and offer to get in contact with the school or nursery.
- You should have several sessions with a paediatric dietitian who can give you dietary advice and help you make any changes that are needed to your family's eating habits.
- You should be seen by a paediatric diabetes specialist nurse.
- You should be given information about Diabetes UK, family support groups in your area, and how to claim Disability Living Allowance to help cover the home supervision of your child now that s/he has diabetes.

Continuing care

At diagnosis and in the weeks and months following your child's diagnosis, members of the diabetes care team, (see pages 232–3), will give you and your child more detailed information on how to manage their diabetes. This should include:

- Information and advice on how and where to inject, injecting devices, and how to dispose of needles and finger pricking lancets.
- How and when to test for glucose and ketones, what the results of these tests mean, and when to seek advice.
- Information about how insulin, food, exercise, stress and excitement interact, and how they affect blood glucose levels.

- A discussion about hypoglycaemia (hypos), with clear information about its causes, symptoms and treatment. This should include the use of glucagon and/or Hypostop. You should be given information on convulsions (fits), which can occasionally be caused by hypos, and how to deal with them.
- An explanation of what is called the 'honeymoon' phase – the time shortly after diagnosis when your child may need less insulin.
- An explanation that your child may find it hard to adjust to early day-to-day life with diabetes.
- You should be given a telephone number to call for 24-hour advice from members of the diabetes care team or the paediatric ward.

As always, there should be time to ask questions and talk about your worries with your diabetes care team. Ask for more information if you need it, and find out how to contact members of the team if any problems arise.

Once your child's diabetes is reasonably controlled

After a time, you will become more confident in managing your child's diabetes. However, the diabetes care team should always be available when and if you need them. They will maintain contact to continue their education programme and to support you. Don't hesitate to ask for more help or information.

You can now expect the following:

- You and your child should see a paediatric diabetes specialist nurse, consultant and dietitian frequently in the weeks and months after diagnosis. Once you feel more confident in managing your child's diabetes, you will need to visit the clinic at least three or four times a year as part of your child's regular diabetes care.
- At these visits, your child's general health will be checked and their blood glucose levels will be reviewed by looking at your home records, and by some extra tests of long-term blood glucose control.
- You should have a chance to get further education about diabetes and discuss any other concerns you may have about diet, insulin, hypos or any other aspect of living with diabetes.

- As your child gets older there will be opportunities to discuss how s/he is coping with diabetes and life in general.

Clinic visits are an opportunity for you, your child and the diabetes care team to discuss any matters related to diabetes. This could be practical aspects such as difficulties with blood tests, or an emotional aspect such as your child's fear of being 'different' because of his/her diabetes. Members of the diabetes care team, such as the paediatric diabetes specialist nurse, may visit you at home for education and support.

Emotional support

Learning that your child has diabetes is a traumatic event for any family. Adapting to and managing diabetes upsets the normal routine at home and can place a strain on family relationships.

Diabetes can be fitted into an active and healthy life, and a settled home life, but you need help and support to do this. There may be some emotional or behavioural problems that you are finding difficult to manage on your own; perhaps your child is refusing to do blood tests, is worried about being bullied at school, or is anxious about changing to an adult diabetes care team.

This is why diabetes care should also include input from a psychologist and/or counsellor if needed. Don't be afraid to ask your diabetes care team for help in this area.

Diabetes at school – including pre-school facilities

It is important that there is good communication between your child's school staff and the diabetes care team. In most instances the diabetes specialist nurse will visit the school to talk to your child's teacher and other staff about diabetes. S/he can explain about hypos, your child's meal and snack times, exercise and who to contact in an emergency.

MEDICAL CHECKS

Children with diabetes should have a complete medical check by the diabetes care team. This may take the form of a yearly review or it may take place at each visit.

These checks will show how your child is managing with

injections, diet and diabetes control. They also allow the team to check for any signs of diabetes complications, which can affect the feet, eyes, kidneys and circulation.

Complications are rare in children, and we know that good diabetes control greatly reduces the risk. However, it is sensible for your child to have regular checks (at least once a year) so that any problems can be picked up early and treated.

The check

The check should include:

- blood test
- urine test
- blood pressure check
- injection sites check
- foot examination
- diet review
- weight and height check
- eye examination (from the age of 12 onwards)
- discussion of any worries you may have, and setting realistic targets for control and management for the coming year

The diabetes care team should note how many hypos, admissions to hospital and days missed from school due to diabetes your child has had.

Making the most of your appointment

Communicating with health care professionals is not always easy. Here are some points to help you make the most of your time.

Before

- decide what you want to get from the visit
- make a list of the points you want to raise
- inform yourself – if you know more about the things that are concerning you, you'll be in a better position to ask questions
- find out about how much time you will have

During

- confirm how much time you'll have – and ask for more if you need it

- use your list to check that you have covered all the points you wanted to raise
- make notes to refer to later
- ask for clarification if you're unsure about what is being said you could say 'Can I check that what you meant is ...'
- try to listen actively, asking questions and giving feedback
- ask for more time to think about an answer if you need to

After

- review what you think has been agreed and achieved
- make a note of anything you need to do before your next appointment
- make a date for the next appointment

Changing to an adult clinic

As your child gets older, the diabetes care team will be trying to encourage him/her to take on some more responsibility for doing his/her own injections and blood tests and keeping a record of his/her test results.

In this way, your child will start to understand how food, exercise and insulin affects their diabetes, and how to make adjustments to keep in control.

When your child reaches the mid-teenage years (generally 16 or over) s/he will probably come under the care of a new diabetes care team, specialising in adults with diabetes. Exactly when this happens depends on the individual child and the facilities available in your area.

Your child will have got used to their children's team and perhaps made friends with other children attending, but the children's team and the adult team should work together to make sure the transfer is as smooth as possible.

EUROPEAN PATIENTS' CHARTER

In 1991, the European Region of the International Diabetes Federation (IDF) and the St Vincent Declaration Steering Committee at the World Health Organisation Europe produced the first European Patients' Charter for people with diabetes. It has been circulated to all diabetes associations affiliated to IDF Europe. It is your charter – read it carefully.

YOUR GUIDE TO BETTER DIABETES CARE: RIGHTS AND ROLES

A person with diabetes can, in general, lead a normal, healthy and long life. Looking after yourself (self-care) by learning about your diabetes provides the best chance to do this. Your doctor and the other members of the health care team (made up of doctor(s), nurses, dietitian(s), chiropodist(s)) are there to advise you and to provide the information, support and technology so that you can look after yourself, and live your life in the way you choose.

It is important that you should know:

1. What should be available from your health care providers to help you reach these goals;
2. What *you* should do.

YOUR RIGHTS

The **health care team** (providers) should provide:

A **treatment plan** and **self-care targets**;
- **Regular checks** of blood sugar (glucose) levels and of your physical condition;
- Treatment for **special problems** and emergencies;
- **Continuing education for you and** your family;
  Information on available social and economic support.

Your role is:
- To build this advice into your daily life;
- To be in control of your diabetes on a day-to-day basis.

CONTINUING EDUCATION

The following are important items you should learn about:

1. Why to control blood glucose levels;

2. How to control your blood glucose levels through proper eating, physical activity, tablets and/or insulin;
3. How to monitor your control with blood or urine tests (self-monitoring), and how to act on the results;
4. The signs of low and high blood glucose levels and ketosis, how to treat them and how to prevent them;
5. What to do when you are ill;
6. The possible long-term complications – including possible damage to eyes, nerves, kidneys and feet, and hardening of the arteries; their prevention arid their treatment;
7. How to deal with life-style variations such as exercise, travelling, and social activities including drinking alcohol;
8. How to handle possible problems with employment, insurance, driving licences, etc.

TREATMENT PLAN AND SELF-CARE TARGETS

The following should be given to you:

1. Personalised advice on proper eating – types of food, amounts and timing;
2. Advice on physical activity;
3. Your dose and timing of tablets or insulin – and how to take them; advice on how to change doses based on your self-monitoring;
4. Your target values for blood glucose, blood fats, blood pressure and weight.

REGULAR CHECKS

The following should be done **at each** visit to your health care professionals.
NB These may vary according to your particular needs.

1. Review of your self-monitoring results and current treatment;
2. Talk about your targets and change where necessary;
3. Talk about any problems and questions you may have;
4. Continued education.

The **health care team** should check:

1.   Your blood glucose control by taking special blood tests, such as HbA_{1C} or fructosamine (or fasting blood glucose in non-insulin-treated people); this can be done two to four times per year if your diabetes is well controlled;
2.   Your weight;
3.   Your blood pressure and blood fats, if necessary.

The following should be checked at least **once per year:**

1.   Your eyes and vision;
2.   Your kidney function (blood and urine tests);
3.   Your feet;
4.   Your risk factors for heart disease, such as blood pressure, blood fats, and smoking habits;
5.   Your self-monitoring and injection techniques;
6.   Your eating habits.

SPECIAL SITUATIONS

1.   Advice and care should be available if you are planning to become or are pregnant.
2.   The needs of children and adolescents should be cared for.
3.   If you have problems with eyes, kidneys, feet, blood vessels or heart, then you should be able to see specialists quickly.
4.   In the elderly, strict treatment is often unnecessary. You may want to discuss this with your health care team.
5.   The first months after your diabetes has been discovered are often difficult. Remember you cannot learn everything during this period – learning will continue for the rest of your life.
6.   You should receive clear information on what to do in emergencies.

YOUR ROLE

To take control of your diabetes on a day-to-day basis. This will be easier the more you know about your diabetes.

Learn about the practice of self-care. This includes monitoring glucose levels and how to change your treatment according to the results. To examine your feet regularly.

Follow good life-style practices: these include choosing the right food, weight control, regular physical activity and not smoking

Know when to contact your health care team urgently, including for emergencies.

Regular talk with your health care team about questions and concerns you may have.

Ask questions – and repeat them if you are still unclear. Prepare your questions beforehand.

Speak to your health care team, other people with diabetes and your local or national Diabetes Association and read pamphlets and books about diabetes provided by your health care team or diabetes association. Make sure your family and friends know about the needs of your diabetes.

If you feel that adequate *facilities* and *care* are not available to help you look after your diabetes then contact your local or national Diabetes Association.

National Service Framework Diabetes

The Government has consulted widely about national guidance for the care of people with diabetes and is preparing a National Service Framework to be used by all health care professionals and those responsible for purchasing health care in districts and localities. It is hoped that it will be released in 2002.

NOW TAKE CONTROL OF YOUR DIABETES

This book and these guidelines will help you to look after your diabetes and to obtain the help that you need to do so. Gradually you will come to understand your diabetes. You will take command of it. But never be afraid to ask for help.

Remember: **you control your diabetes, your diabetes does not control you.**

Keep fit and enjoy life.

GLOSSARY

Acarbose A drug which prevents digestion of sugar into glucose in the gut.

ACE inhibitor Angiotensin-converting enzyme inhibitor – drug used to treat high blood pressure and heart problems. All the names end in –pril.

Acidosis Condition in which the blood is more acid than normal.

Adipose tissue Body fat.

Adrenal gland Gland found above the kidney which makes adrenaline and steroid hormones.

Adrenaline (American name Epinephrine) Flight, fright and fight hormone produced by the adrenal gland under stress.

Angina Chest pain caused by insufficient blood supply to heart muscle (a form of ischaemic heart disease). Also known as angina pectoris.

Angiogram X-ray examination of an artery.

Ankle oedema Swelling of the ankles.

Aorta The largest artery in the body running from the heart through the chest and abdomen. The aorta carries blood from the heart for distribution into other arteries around the body.

Arteriopathy Abnormality of artery.

Atherosclerosis Hardening and furring up of the arteries.

Artery Vessel which carries blood from the heart to other parts of the body.

Arthropathy Abnormality of joint.

Autonomic nervous system Nerves controlling body functions such as heart beat, blood pressure and bowel movement.

Autonomic neuropathy Abnormality of the nerves controlling body functions.

Background retinopathy The common form of diabetic retinopathy with microaneurysms, dot and blot haemorrhages and exudates.

Balanitis Inflammation of the penis.

Bed sores Ulcers in the skin and sometimes into deeper tissues over pressure points in someone lying or sitting in the same position for a long time.

Beta blocker Drugs which reduce high blood pressure, steady the heart and prevent angina. All the names end in -olol, e.g. atenolol.

Biguanide A type of blood glucose-lowering pill e.g. metformin.

Bladder Usually means urinary bladder. Bag in the pelvis where the urine collects before urination.

Blood pressure (BP) Pressure at which blood circulates in the arteries.

Candida albicans Another name for the thrush fungus

Carbohydrate (CHO) Sugary or starchy food which is digested in the gut to produce simple sugars like glucose. Carbohydrate foods include candy or sweets, cakes, biscuits, soda pop, bread, rice, pasta, oats, beans, lentils.

Cardiac To do with the heart

Cardiac enzymes Chemicals released by damaged heart muscle.

Cardiac failure Reduced functioning of the heart, causing shortness of breath or ankle swelling.

Carotid artery Artery which runs through the neck to supply the head and brain.

Carotid angiogram X-ray of dye passing up the carotid arteries into the brain arteries.

Cataract Lens opacity.

Cells The tiny building blocks from which the human body is made. Cell constituents are contained in a membrane.

Cerebral embolus Clot from another part of the body which lodges in an artery supplying the brain.

Cerebral haemorrhage Bleed into the brain.

Cerebral infarct Death of brain tissue due to insufficient blood supply.

Cerebral thrombosis Clot in an artery supplying the brain.

Cerebrovascular disease Disease of the arteries supplying the brain.

Charcot joints Damaged joints in areas of neuropathy (rare).

Cheiroarthropathy Stiffening of the hands.

Chiropodist Someone who prevents and treats foot disorders.

Chiropody Treatment and prevention of foot disorders.

Cholesterol A fat which circulates in the blood and is obtained from animal fats in food.

Computerised tomogram (CT) scan X-Ray which can take multiple, very detailed films from different angles. Commonly used to look at the brain, but whole body CT scanners are also available.

Congestive cardiac failure Impaired pumping of the right ventricle of the heart, causing ankle swelling.

Conjunctivitis Inflammation of the conjunctiva (white of the eye and inner eyelid).

Constipation Infrequent and/or hard bowel motions.

Continuous ambulatory peritoneal dialysis (CAPD) An out-patient system of filtering wastes from the body of someone in kidney failure. Clean fluid is run into the abdominal cavity, takes up the waste substances and is run out again.

Continuous subcutaneous insulin infusion (CSII) A system for the constant pumping of insulin through a fine needle left under the skin all the time. Also known as an insulin pump.

Coronary artery Artery which supplies the heart muscle.

Coronary thrombosis Clot in an artery supplying heart muscle.

Creatinine Chemical produced by breakdown of protein in the body and passed through the kidneys into the urine. A measure of kidney function.

Cystitis Inflammation of the urinary bladder.

Diabetes mellitus Condition in which the blood glucose concentration is above normal, causing passage of large amounts *(diabetes* a siphon) of sweet urine *(mellitus* = sweet like honey).

Diabetic amyotrophy A form of diabetic nerve damage which causes weak muscles, usually in the legs.

Dialysis Artificial filtration of fluid and waste products which would normally be excreted in the urine by the kidneys.

Diarrhoea Frequent and/or loose bowel motions.

Diastolic blood pressure Blood pressure between heart beats.

Diet What you eat.

Dietitian Someone who promotes a healthy diet and recommends dietary treatments.

Diuretic Pill which increases urinary fluid loss. Diuretics are used to treat cardiac failure and most are also effective blood pressure-lowering drugs.

Dot and blot haemorrhage Tiny bleeds into the retina in diabetic retinopathy.

Dupuytren's contracture Tightening of the ligaments in the palm of the hand or fingers.

Dysphasia Difficulty in talking.

Dysuria Pain or discomfort on passing urine.

Echocardiography Examination of the heart using ultrasound waves from a probe run over the skin of the chest.

Electrocardiogram (ECG or EKG) Recording of the electrical activity of the heart muscle as it contracts and relaxes.

Electrolytes Blood chemicals such as sodium and potassium.

Enzyme Body chemical which facilitates other chemical processes.

Epinephrine *see* adrenaline.

Erectile dysfunction *see* impotence.

Essential hypertension High blood pressure for which no specific cause can be found.

Exudate Fatty deposit on the retina in retinopathy.

Fat Greasy or oily substance. Fatty foods include butter, margarine, cheese, cooking oil, fried foods.

Femoral artery The main artery supplying a leg. The femoral pulse can be felt in the groin.

Femoral arteriogram X-ray of dye injected into a femoral artery.

Fibrate Drugs which reduce cholesterol e.g. bezafibrate

Fibre Roughage in food. Found in beans, lentils, peas, bran, whole-meal flour, potatoes, etc.

Fluoroscein angiogram X-ray of fluoroscein dye passing through the blood vessels in the eye.

Gastrointestinal To do with the stomach and intestines.

Gastroenteritis Inflammation or infection of the stomach and intestines.

Glaucoma Raised pressure inside the eye.

Glomeruli Tangles of tiny blood vessels in the kidneys from which urine filters into urinary drainage system.

Glucose A simple sugar obtained from carbohydrates in food. Glucose circulates in the blood stream and is one of the body's main energy sources.

Glycaemia Glucose in the blood.

Glycogen The form in which glucose is stored in liver and muscles.

Glycosuria Glucose in the urine.

Glycosylated haemoglobin *see* haemoglobin A_{1C}

Guar gum A substance which slows the absorption of carbohydrate from the gut.

Gustatory sweating Sweating while eating.

Haemodialysis Artificial filtration of blood in someone with kidney failure.

Haemoglobin A_{1C} Haemoglobin (the oxygen carrying chemical in the red blood cells) to which glucose has become attached. A long-term measure of blood glucose concentration.

Haemorrhage Bleed.

Heart Muscular organ which pumps blood around the body.

Heart attack General non-specific term for myocardial infarction or coronary thrombosis.

Hormone A chemical made in one part of the body and acting in another part of the body.

Hyper- High, above normal.

Hyperglycaemia High blood glucose concentration (i.e. above normal).

Hypertension High blood pressure.

Hypo- Low, below normal.

Hypoglycaemia Low blood glucose concentration (i.e. below normal)

Hypotension Low blood pressure

Hypothermia Low body temperature.

Impotence Difficulty in obtaining or maintaining a penile erection. Also called erectile dysfunction

Infarction Condition in which a body tissue dies from lack of blood supply – irreversible.

Insulin A hormone produced in cells of the islets of Langerhans in the pancreas. Essential for the entry of glucose into the body's cells.

Insulin dependent diabetes (IDD) Diabetes due to complete insulin deficiency, for which treatment with insulin is essential. Lack of insulin leads to rapid illness and ketone production. Juvenile onset diabetes. Insulin-dependent diabetes. *See* Type 1 diabetes.

Insulin receptor Site on the cell surface where insulin acts.

Intermittent claudication The intermittent limping caused by insufficient blood supply to the leg muscles.

Intravenous pyelogram X-ray of the kidneys showing the excretion of dye injected into a vein.

Ischaemia Condition in which a body tissue has insufficient blood supply – reversible.

Ischaemic heart disease An illness in which the blood supply to the heart muscle is insufficient.

Islet cells Cells which produce insulin.

Islets of Langerhans Clusters of cells in the pancreas. One form of islet cells produces insulin.

Juvenile onset diabetes Diabetes starting in youth. This term implies a need for insulin treatment. Type 1 diabetes.

Ketoacidosis A state of severe insulin deficiency causing fat breakdown, ketone formation and acidification of the blood.

Ketones Fat breakdown products which smell of acetone or pear drops and make the blood acid.

Kilocalories, cals or kcals. A measure of energy, for example in food or used up in exercise.

Kilojoules Another measure of energy. One kilocalorie = 4.2 kilojoules.

Left ventricle Chamber of the heart which pumps oxygenated blood into the aorta.

Left ventricular failure Reduced functioning of the left pumping chamber of the heart, causing fluid to build up in the lungs and shortness of breath.

Lens The part of the eye responsible for focusing (like the lens of a camera).

Lipid General name for fats found in the body.

Liver Large organ in upper right abdomen which acts as an energy store, chemical factory and detoxifying unit and produces bile.

Macroangiopathy Macrovascular disease.

Macrovascular disease Disease of large blood vessels such as those supplying the legs.

Macula Area of best vision in the eye.

Macular oedema Swelling of the macula.

Malaise Feeling vaguely unwell or uncomfortable.

Maturity onset diabetes Diabetes starting when a person is over the age of 30. This term usually implies that the person is not completely insulin deficient, at least initially. Non-insulin dependent diabetes. Type 2 diabetes.

Metabolism The chemical processing of substances in the body.

Microalbuminuria The presence of tiny quantities of protein in the urine.

Microaneurysm Tiny blow-out in the wall of a capillary in the retina of the eye.

Microangiopathy Microvascular disease.

Microvascular disease Disease of small blood vessels such as those supplying the eyes or kidney.

Moniliasis Thrush.

Myocardial infarction Death of heart muscle caused by lack of blood supply.

Myocardium Heart muscle.

Necrobiosis lipoidica diabeticorum Diabetic skin lesion (rare).

Nephropathy Abnormality of the kidney.

Nerve Cable carrying signals to or from the brain and spinal cord.

Neuroelectrophysiology Study of the way nerves work.

Neuropathy Abnormality of the nerves.

Nocturia Passing urine at night.

Non-insulin dependent diabetes (NIDD) Diabetes due to inefficiency of insulin action or relative insulin deficiency which can usually be managed without insulin injections, at least initially. Ketone formation is less likely. Maturity onset diabetes. Non-insulin dependent diabetes. *See* Type 2 diabetes.

Nutritionist Someone who studies diets. Nutritionists may be dietitians and vice versa.

Obese Overweight, fat.

Obesity Condition of being overweight or fat.

Oedema Swelling.

Ophthalmoscope Magnifying torch with which the doctor looks into your eyes.

Oral Taken by mouth.

-pathy Disease or abnormality, e.g. neuropathy, retinopathy.

Palpitations Irregular or abnormally fast heart beat.

Pancreas Abdominal gland producing digestive enzymes, insulin and other hormones.

Paraesthesiae Pins and needles or tingling.

Peripheral nervous system Nerves supplying the skeletal muscle and body sensation such as touch, pain, temperature.

Peripheral neuropathy Abnormality of peripheral nerves e.g. those supplying arms or legs.

Peripheral vascular disease Abnormality of blood vessels supplying arms or legs.

Photocoagulation Light treatment of retinopathy.

Podiatrist Someone who prevents and treats foot disorders.

Podiatry Treatment and prevention of foot disorders.

Polydipsia Drinking large volumes of fluid.

Polyunsaturated fats Fats containing vegetable oils such as sunflower seed oil.

Polyuria Passing large volumes of urine frequently.

Postural hypotension Fall in blood pressure on standing.

Potassium Essential blood chemical.

Pressure sores *See* Bedsores.

Protein Dietary constituent required for body growth and repair.

Proteinuria Protein in the urine.

Pyelonephritis Kidney infection.

Prandial glucose regulator Mealtime glucose regulator. Drug which reduces blood glucose peak after eating e.g. repaglinide

Pruritis vulvae Itching of the vulva or perineum.

Receptor Place on the cell wall with which a chemical or hormone links.

Renal To do with the kidney.

Renal glycosuria The presence of glucose in the urine because of an abnormally low renal threshold for glucose.

Renal threshold Blood glucose concentration above which glucose overflows into the urine.

Retina Light sensitive tissue at the back of the eye.

Retinopathy Abnormality of the retina.

Right ventricle Chamber of the heart which pumps the blood from the body into the lungs to be oxygenated.

Right ventricular failure
Reduced functioning of the right pumping chamber of the heart, causing fluid to build up in the legs and ankle swelling.

Saturated fats Animal fats such as those in dairy products, meat fat.

Sign Something you can see, touch, smell or hear.

Sodium Essential blood chemical.

Statin Drug which reduces cholesterol, e.g. simvastatin.

Steroid hormone A hormone produced by the adrenal gland.

Stroke Abnormality of brain function (e.g. weakness of arm or leg) due to disease of the arteries supplying the brain or damage to the brain.

Subcutaneous The fatty tissues under the skin.

Sulphonylurea A form of blood glucose-lowering pill.

Symptom Something a person experiences.

Systolic blood pressure Pumping pressure.

Testosterone Male sex hormone.

Thiazolidinediones Drugs which reduce insulin resistance and lower glucose, e.g. rosiglitazone.

Thrush Candidiasis or moniliasis. Fungal infection caused by candida albicans fungus. Produces white creamy patches and intense itching and soreness.

Thrombolysis Clot dissolving.

Thrombosis Clotting of blood.

Thrombus A blood clot.

Transient ischaemic attack (TIA) Short-lived stroke with full recovery within 24 hours.

Triglyceride Form of fat which circulates in the bloodstream.

Type 1 diabetes Insulin-dependant diabetes. No other form of treatment will control the blood glucose.

Type 2 diabetes Diabetes which can initially be treated by diet and/or glucose-lowering tablets. Insulin-treatment may eventually be needed. Previously called non-insulin-dependent diabetes.

Ulcer Open sore.

Ultrasound scan Scan of a part of the body using sound waves.

Uraemia High blood urea concentration.

Urea Blood chemical, waste substance excreted in urine.

Ureter Tube from the kidney to the urinary bladder.

Urethra Tube from the urinary bladder to the outside world.

Urinary incontinence Unintentional leakage of urine.

Urinary retention Retention of urine in the bladder because it cannot be passed.

Urinary tract infection (UTI) Infection in the urine drainage system.

Visual acuity Sharpness of vision.

Vitreous Clear jelly in the eye between the retina and the lens.

Vitreous haemorrhage Bleed into the vitreous.

USEFUL ADDRESSES

Diabetes UK
Diabetes UK (National office)
10 Queen Anne Street, London W1M 0BD
Telephone 020 7323 1531
Fax 020 7637 3644
e-mail www.diabetes.org.uk
Careline telephone 020 7636 6112 (language line available)
Fax 020 7462 2732
Minicom 020 7462 2757
e-mail careline@diabetes.org.uk

Diabetes UK Cymru
Quebec House, Castlebridge, Cowbridge Road East,
Cardiff CF11 9AB
Telephone 02920 668276
e-mail wales@diabetes.org.uk

Diabetes UK North West
65 Bewsey Street, Warrington WA2 7JQ
Telephone 01925 653281
e-mail n.west@diabetes.org.uk

Diabetes UK Northern and Yorkshire
Birch House, 80 Eastmount Road, Darlington DL1 1LE
Telephone 01325 488606
e-mail north&yorks@diabetes.org.uk

Diabetes UK Northern Ireland
John Gibson House, 257 Lisburn Road, Belfast BT9 7EN
Telephone 02890 666646
e-mail n.ireland@diabetes.org.uk

Diabetes UK Scotland
34 West George Street, Glasgow G2 I DA
Telephone 0141 332 2700
e-mail scotland@diabetes.org.uk

Diabetes UK West Midlands
I Eldon Court, Eldon Street, Walsall WSI 2JP
Telephone 01922 614500
e-mail w.midland@diabetes.org.uk

Other diabetes associations

European Association for the Study of Diabetes
Rheindorfer Weg 3
D-40591 Dusseldorf
Germany
Telephone +49 21175 84 690
Fax +49 21175 84 6929
e-mail www.easd.org

International Diabetes Federation
1 rue Defacqz
B-1000 Brussels
Belgium
Telephone +322 537 1889
Fax +322 537 1981
e-mail www.idf.org

The International Diabetes Federation website provides contacts and
addresses for diabetes associations throughout the world.

CONTACTS WHICH MAY BE HELPFUL

Children with diabetes
www.childrenwithdiabetes.com/index_cwd.htm

Diabetes Discrimination in Employment
www.users.globalnet.co.uk/%7Eifduk

Diabetes Insight
www.diabetic.org.uk

Diabetes Monitor
www.diabetesmonitor.com

Diabetes Network International
www.dni.org.uk

Diabetic Medicine On-line
www.blackwell-science.com/dme

European Association for the Study of Diabetic Eye Complications
www.diabeticretinopathy.org.uk

Foot care information
www.bigfoot.com/~diabeticfoot

Insulin Pumpers UK
www.insulin-pumpers.org.uk

These websites contain information about diabetes. The accuracy of this information has not been checked and Dr Hillson does not endorse or accept responsibility for websites or contacts shown in this book.

INDEX

Page numbers in *italic* refer to the illustrations

abdomen:
    examination, 21
    tissue damage, 140-4
abscesses, 130
abseiling, 204
acarbose, 73, 79-80, 81
ACE inhibitors, 139, 150-1
acetone, 21
acne, 131
acromegaly, 36, 131
Actrapid, 87
adolescents, 172
adrenal glands, 36
adrenaline, 125, 127, 204
air travel, 215-16
alcohol, 18, 35-6, 41, 64-5, 172, 211
allergies, 18, 36
alprostadil, 146
Amaryl, 74
amputation, 153
amyloid, 35
angina, 136
ankles, swollen, 20
antibodies, 32-3, 90
antidepressants, 127, 149
arms, tissue damage, 147-9
arteries, 20, *152*
Asians, 18, 33, 70
atherosclerosis, 14, 20, *138,* 152, 157
autoimmune reactions, 32
autonomic nervous system, 118, 131, 140-1, 147

babies, 186, 190-1
bed-wetting, 2
beef insulin, 88

beta blockers, 118, 151
beta cells, 29, 32, 35
biguanides, 73
bile acid sequestrants, 161
bladder, problems, 2, 142, 144
blindness, 51, 133, 199
blood:
    circulation, 20
    electrolytes, 26
    glucose levels, 8, 159
    monitoring glucose levels,
    10-14, 25, 43, 45, 46-51,
    52, 202
blood glucose meters, *49*, 50,
    51, 53
blood tests, 8, 10, 26, 165
blood pressure, 20, 143, 149-52,
    161-2, 230
blurred vision, 5, 21, 111, 132,
    132
boating, 203
Body Mass Index (BMI), 230
boils, 130, 131, 136
brain, fuel, 32
breast feeding, 191
breathing, 21
breathlessness, 139
British Diabetic Association
    (BDA), 92, 223

caffeine, 64
calcium channel blockers, 151
calories, 55
Candida albicans, 21
cannulae, 94
canoeing, 203-4
carbohydrate exchanges, 59-60
carbohydrates, 28, 55-60, *57-9,*
    201, 210
carbuncles, 130, 136
cards, diabetes, 43

carpal tunnel syndrome, 149
cars, driving, 44, 167-8, 169, 170-2,
    171, 210
cartridges, insulin, 91
case histories, 22-5
cataracts, 132, *132*
causes of diabetes, 32-6, 40
Caverject, 146
caving, 205
cells, insulin receptors, 30-1, *31*
Charcot joints, 156
cheiroarthropathy, 147
chemical imbalance, 40
chest infections, 139
chest pain, 136
childbirth, 190-1
children:
    care of, 231-8
    cataracts, 132
    inherited diabetes, 188-9
    Type 1 diabetes, 32-3
chiropodists, 181, 224
chlorpropamide, 73, 74, 75, 76
chocolate, 65
cholesterol, 20, 26, 160-1, 230
chromosomes, 32
circulatory problems, 149-53
clear (rapid-acting) insulin,
    87-8, *87*, 96-100
climbing, 204
clinics, 15, 166, 178-82, 190,
    232, 236
cloudy (slow-acting) insulin,
    87, 88, 96-100, 103
co-ordination problems, 111, 113
coffee, 64
cold weather, 216-17
colour-change strips, 48-50
comas, 106, 113-14, 116-17
complex carbohydrates, 56-7, *57*
computers, 50, 51
concentration, lack of, 109-10,
    112
condoms, 187
constipation, 3, 141-2
consultants, 223, 232
contraception, 187-8
contraceptive pills, 36, 127, 188

corneal arcus, 20
coronary arteries, 137-9
coronary thrombosis, 137, 139,
    157, 160, 162
creatinine, 26, 143
CSII pumps, 95
Customs and Excise, 216
cystitis, 142

daily life, 164-77
Daonil, 74
deafness, 136
dehydration, 19, 64, 141
dents, injection sites, 90, 101
dermopathy, diabetic, 130
diabetes care teams, 178-82,
    223-4, 239-41
    children's, 231-3, 236
diabetes insipidus, 27
diabetes kit, 164-5, 213-14, 215
diabetes mellitus, 27, 28
diabetes service, 182-5
Diabetes UK, 44, 92, 169, 172,
    180, 212, 223, 224, 233,
    234
    Travel Guides, 212
'diabetic' foods, 65
diabetologists, 179, 223
diagnosis, 7-15, 40
Diamicron, 74
diaphragms, contraceptive, 187
diaries, 51, *52*, 120
diarrhoea, 81, 141, 217
diet, 55-2, 226
    alcohol, 64-5
    Asian, 70
    carbohydrates, 55-60
    control of diabetes, 40-1
    drinks, 63-4
    and exercise, 201
    fasting, 72
    fats, 61-2
    on holiday, 210-11
    and hypoglycaemia, 115, 118
    minerals and vitamins, 63
    proteins, 60
    quantities to eat, 66-70
    as source of glucose, 28

special foods, 65
dietitians, 180, 224, 232
digestive system, 28-32, *29*
disability, registering, 168
diuretics, 17-18, 36, 63, 127,
    139, 150
diving, 203
DNA, 32
doctors, 7-8, 14-15, 16-26, 166, 178,
    179-80, 182, 183-5
doxazosin, 151
drinks, 41, 59, 63-4, 211
    see also alcohol
driving, 44, 167-8, 169, 170-2, *171*,
    210
drugs, 17-18
    causes of diabetes, 36, 40
    glucose-lowering pills, 42, 73-84
    and hyperglycaemia, 127
Dupuytren's contracture, 147

ears, deafness, 136
eating out, 172
electrocardiograms, 26, 138
electrolytes, 26
emotions, 110, 112-13
endurance exercise, 202-3
energy, loss of, 3
erectile dysfunction *see* impotence
eruptive xanthomata, 130
Euglucon, 74
European Association for the
    Study of Diabetes, 180
examination, 19-22, 230-1
exercise, 14, 118, 124-5, 162,
    193-206
eyes, 131-5
    blurred vision, *4*, 5, 21, 111, 132,
        132
    cataracts, 132
    checks, 133, 230-1
    macular disease, 134
    ophthalmologists, 133, 181
    retinopathy, 133, 134-5
    signs of diabetes, 20
    squints, 131
    testing blood glucose
    levels with poor vision, 51

facial appearance, 131
fasting, 72
fats:
    in blood, 160-1, 230
    in diet, 41, 55, 61-2, *62*
    see *also* overweight
fatty acids, 194, 195
feet, *155*, 230
    care of, 154-6, 162-3,
        166, 181, 217-18
    in cold weather, 217
    examination, 22
    numbness 148
    peripheral vascular disease,
        152-3
fibrates, 161
fibre, 55, 56, 58, 80, 160, 161
fingers:
    blood tests 46-8, *49*, 53
    cheiroarthropathy, 147
fish oils, 62, 161
fits, 113-14, 116-17
fixed-proportion insulins, 88
flying, 215-16
food *see* diet
fructose, 57, 58-9, 65
fruit, 57-8, 59, *68*, 210

gall bladder, 140
gangrene, 153, *153*, 217
gastroenteritis, 106, 212, 217
gastrointestinal problems, 140-2
gastroparesis, diabetic, 140-1
general practitioners (GPs),
    7-8, 14-15, 16-26, 167,
    178, 179-80, 182, 185,
    224, 233
genetics, 32, 33, 188-9
gestational diabetes, 35
Glargine Insulin, 87, 88, 99
glaucoma, 135
glibenclamide, 73, 74, 75, 76
Glibenese, 74
gliclazide, 73, 74
Glimepiride, 74
glipizide, 74
gliquidone, 74
glomeruli, kidneys, 142-3, *143*

glucagon, 115-16, *117*
gluconeogenesis, 60
glucose:
    in diet, 41
    digestion, 28-32
    during exercise, 194-5, *196*
    hyperglycaemia, 105-6, 122-8
    hypoglycaemia, 104, 108-21, *115*
    impaired glucose tolerance, 13,
    14
    levels in blood, 8, 159
    monitoring blood levels, 10-14,
    25, 43, 45, 46-51, *52*, 202
    in pregnancy, 189
    tolerance tests, 13
    in urine, 2, 7, 8-9, *11*, 53-4,
    123
glucose-lowering pills, 73-84,
    173, 226
    acarbose, 79-80
    dosage, 74, 128
    guar gum, 80
    hypoglycaemia, 42, 108
    meal-time, 77-8
    metformin, 76-7
    in pregnancy, 190
    problems with, 81-2
    sulphonylureas, 73-6
    thiazolidinediones, 78-9
    and weight loss, 70
glucose tablets, 43, 80, 144
Glucowatch, 50
Glurenorm, 74
glycaemic index, 60
glycogen, 31-2, 194
glycosylated haemoglobin, 25-6
growth hormone, 36, 131
guar gum, 73, 80

haemochromatosis, 36
haemoglobin, glycosylated, 25-6
hands, tissue damage, 147, 149
hang-gliding, 204
head, tissue damage, 131-6
health care teams *see* diabetes care
    teams
heart, 136
    examination, 20

    palpitations, 111, 113
    pulse rate, 20, 195
    tests, 26
    tissue damage, 136-9
heart attacks, 126, 137-9, 193
herbal remedies, 18, 6
high blood pressure, 20,
    149-52, 161
holidays, 207-19
homeostasis, 8, 32
'honeymoon period', 121
hormones:
    causes of diabetes, 36
    and hyperglycaemia, 125, 126
    sexual problems, 145
    steroids, 17, 36, 40, 125,
        127, 131
hospitals, 178, 179, 184, 227-9
    children in, 236-7
hot weather, 216
Humalog, 87, 88, 99
human insulin, 88, 119-20
Humulin 1, 88
Ilumulin M2, 88
Humulin M3, 88
Humulin M4, 88
Humulin R, 87
Humulin S, 87
Humulin Zn, 88
hygiene, 101
hyperglycaemia:
    causes, 105-6, 123-7
    treatment, 105-6, 127-8
hypoglycaemia, 104, 108-21
    alcohol and, 64
    causes, 117-18
    in cold weather, 217
    glucose tablets, 43
    in pregnancy, 189, 192
    and sport, 200-1
    and sulphonylureas, 75-6
    symptoms, 42, 109-14
    treatment, 114-17
    unawareness of, 118-20
    while driving, 170-2, *171*
Hypostop glucose gel, 114, 117, 204
hypothermia, 217
Hypurin Protamine Zinc, 88

Hypurin soluble insulin, 87

illness, glucose-lowering pills and,
    81
immunisation, 207-8
impaired fasting glucose, 12,
    13-14
impaired glucose tolerance,
    12, 13, 14
impotence, 145-6
incontinence, 144
infections, 3-5
    chest, 139
    and hyperglycaemia, 125-6
    skin, 130
    thrush, 147
    urinary tract, 142
injection sites, 101, 231
injections:
    glucagon, 115-16, *117*
    insulin, 42, 92-104, *98, 102,*
    225-6
injuries, and hyperglycaemia,
    126
Insulatard, 88, 96
insulin, 85-107
    care of, 91-2
    in digestive system, 29-32, *31*
    drawing up, *97-8,* 99-100
    and exercise, 194, *196,* 201
    history, 173
    hyperglycaemia, 105-6, 123-4,
    127-8
    hypoglycaemia, 104, 118, 119
    injections, 42, 92-100, *98, 102*
    packaging, 90-1
    in pregnancy, 189, 191
    stopping, 106
    sulphonylureas, 74-5
    treatment patterns, 96-9
    Type 1 diabetes (IDDM), 33
    Type 2 diabetes (NIDDM), 34-5
    types, 87-8
    ultra-fast, 99
    and weight loss, 70
insulin atrophy, 101
insulin-dependent diabetes,
    32-3

insulin hypertrophy, 101
insulin jets, 94-5
insulin pumps, 95
insurance, 44, 169, 212
intermittent claudication, 152
International Diabetes
    Federation (IDF), 220, 238
intra-uterine contraceptive   devices
    (IUDs), 188
intranasal insulin, 91
iron deposition, 36
islets of Langerhans, 29, 91, 121
Isophane, 88

joints, 22, 147, 156
juvenile onset diabetes, 32-3

ketoacidosis, 33, 106, 195,
    209, 233
ketones, 33, 51, 106, 124, 195
kidneys, 8-9, *11,* 140, *141,*
    142-4, *143*
    function tests, 230
Kussmaul breathing, 21

labour, 191
lactic acidosis, 77
lancets, 48, *49,* 50
languages, foreign, 218-19
Lawrence, Dr R.D., 223
legs, 25, 230
    tissue damage, 147-9
Lentard, 88
Lente, 88
libido, 144
lifestyle, 231
ligaments, 22
lipids, 160, 230
liver, 28-9, 140
lumps, insulin sites, 101
lungs, 21, 139

McLean, Teresa, 112
macular disease, 134
malaise, 3
marathon running, 202-3
meal-time glucose regulators,
    73, 77-8

medical checks, 166-7, 229-31,
   240-1
   annual reviews, 229-31
   children's, 236-7
medical history, 17-18
medical kit, 214
menstruation, 125, 144, 187
meters, 49, 50, 51, 53
metformin, 14, 65, 73, 76-7,
   78, 81, 82, 201
minerals, 63
Minodiab, 74
mixing insulin, 100
Mixtard, 88
Monotard, 88
monounsaturated fats, 62, 160
morning-after contraception,
   188
motion sickness, 210
mountaineering, 204
muscles:
   during exercise, 194
   facial, 131
   fuels, 31-2
   tissue damage, 148
Muse, 146

nails, care of, 154
nateglinide, 77
National Health Service, 223
National Service Framework, 242
neck, tissue damage, 136
necrobiosis lipoidica diabeticorum,
   130
needles, 92-3, 103, 216
nephropathy, 142-4, 143, 159
nerves:
   examination, 21-2
   muscle weakness, 131
   tingling, 3
   tissue damage, 147-9, 156,
   159, 162-3
neuropathy, 147-9, 156, 159, 162-3
Novorapid, 87, 88, 99
numbness, 22, 148, 148
nurses, 180, 182, 224, 232-3

oestrogen, contraceptive pills, 188

operations, and hyperglycaemia, 126
ophthalmologists, 134, 181, 224, 230
oral contraceptives, 36, 127, 188
oral hypoglycaemic agents see glucose-
   lowering pills
orienteering, 205
overweight, 34-5, 41, 158

palpitations, 111, 113.
pancreas, 36, 65, 140
   inflammation of, 35-6
   insulin production, 29-30
   iron deposition, 36
pancreatitis, 140
parachute jumping, 204
penis, impotence, 145-6
pens, 93-4, 94, 96-9
periods, 125, 144, 187
peripheral neuropathy, 147-9
peripheral vascular disease, 152-3
phlegm, 21
phrases, foreign language,
   218-19
pig insulin, 88, 90, 119
pimples, 131
pins and needles, 3
pioglitazone, 78
plasma glucose concentration,
   10, 12-13
podiatrist, 181, 224
polyunsaturated fats, 62, 160
polyuria, 2
pork (porcine) insulin, 88, 90, 119
postural hypotension, 20
pot-holing, 205
potassium, 63
pregnancy, 17, 144, 186-92
   cause of diabetes, 35
   checking glucose levels, 51
   insulin needs, 86, 125
prescriptions, 226
preservatives, insulin, 90
progestogen, contraceptive pills,
   188
Protaphane, 88
proteins:
   in diet, 55, 60, 61
   in urine, 142

psychologists, 181-2, 224, 232, 236
pulse rate, 20, 195
pumps, insulin, 95
pyelonephritis, 142

rapid-acting (clear) insulin, 87-8, *87*, 96-100
    ultra-fast insulin, 99
recovery position, 116, *117*
reflexes, 22
renal glycosuria, 9
renal threshold, 9, *11*, 54
repaglinide, 73, 77, 81
restaurants, 172, 211
retinopathy, 133, 143, 159, 162
    background retinopathy, 133-4
    pre-proliferative/proliferative retinopathy, 134-5
rock climbing, 204
rosiglitazone, 73, 78
rowing, 203
running, 202

St Vincent Declaration, 220-1, 238
salt, 63, 150
saturated fats, 62, 160
schools, 236
Semitard, 88
sex hormones, 35, 36
sexual problems, 144-6
shift work, 170
shivering, 217
shoes, 154-5, 181, 218
side-effects:
    acarbose, 80
    meal-time glucose regulators, 78
    metformin, 76-7
    sulphonylureas, 75
    thiazolidinediones, 79
sildenafil, 145
simple carbohydrates, 57-9, *59*
simvastin, 160
skin:
    problems, 20
    sunburn, 216
    tissue damage, 130

slow-acting (cloudy) insulin, *87*, 88, 96-100, 103
smoking, 14, 18, 20, 101, 152, 157-8
social life, 172
socks, 154, 218
sorbitol, 65, 147
spermicides, 187
sports, 197-206
sprinting, 202
sputum, 21
squints, 131-2
statins, 160-1
sterilisation, contraception, 188
steroids, 17, 36, 40, 125, 127, 131
stomach, 140
stress, 126-7, 192
stress hormones, 126
strokes, 131, 162
sucrose, 57-9, 79-80, 114
sugar, 57, 59
sulphonylureas, 73-6, 78, 81, 82, 201
sunburn, 216
support groups, 44
surgery, and hyperglycaemia, 126
sweating, 111, 113, 131
sweeteners, artificial, 59, 65
swimming, 203
symptoms:
    diabetes, 1-6, 4, 16-20
    hypoglycaemia, 109-14
syringes, 92-3, 103-4, 216

tablets, glucose, 43, 80, 114
teenagers, 172, 231, 238
tendons, 147
tests:
    annual reviews, 230
    blood, 8, 10, 26, 165, 230
    monitoring glucose levels, 43, 45, 46-51, *52*
thalassaemia, 36
thiazide diuretics, 17-18, 36, 127, 150
thiazolidinediones, 73, 78-9, 81
thirst, 1-2
thrush, 5, 21, 130, 147, 187

thyroid overactivity, 36, 131, 136
tingling hands and feet, 3
tiredness, 3
tissue damage, 6, 40, 119, 123,
    129-56, 173
    prevention, 157-63
tolbutamide, 74, 75
transplants, islet cells, 91
travel, 92, 108, 207-19
trembling, 111, 113
tricyclic antidepressants, 127
triglyceride, 26, 59, 130, 160-1, 230
tropical diabetes, 36
Type 1 diabetes, 32-3, *34*, 85, 159
Type 2 diabetes, 6, 33-5, *34*, 78,
    159

ulcers, 156, 181
Ultratard, 88, 96, 104
unconsciousness, 113-14, 116
urea, 26, 143
urethra, 140
urinary tract, *141*
    infections, 142
urine, 140
    glucose in, 2, 7, 8-9, *11*, 53-4, 123
    incontinence, 144
    infections, 142
    ketones, 106, 195
    polyuria, 2

protein in, 142
tests, 7, 26, 230

vegetables, 59, 67, *68*, 211
vegetarian diet, 60, 63
Velosulin, 87
Viagra, 145-6
vision, blurred, 5, 22, 111, 132, *132*
vitamins, 63
vitiligo, 19
vomiting, 81, 106, 124, 217

walking, 202-3
water sports, 114, 203-4
water tablets *see* diuretics
weather, 216-17
websites 252
weight, Body Mass Index (BMI), 230
weight loss, 2-3, 14, 66-70, 150,
    158
Wells, H.G., 223
work, 43, 167-70
World Health Organisation, 220,
    238
wound care nurses, 181
wounds, 155-6

x-rays, 26, 77, 139
xanthelasmata, 20
xanthomata, 130

Public Health

An action guide to improving health

Public Health
An action guide to improving health

SECOND EDITION

John Walley

Professor of International Public Health,
Nuffield Centre for International Health and Development,
Institute of Health Sciences, University of Leeds

John Wright

Consultant in Clinical Epidemiology and Public Health,
Bradford Teaching Hospitals NHS Trust,
Bradford, and
Professor of Clinical Epidemiology,
University of Bradford

OXFORD
UNIVERSITY PRESS

OXFORD

UNIVERSITY PRESS

Great Clarendon Street, Oxford ox2 6DP

Oxford University Press is a department of the University of Oxford.
It furthers the University's objective of excellence in research, scholarship,
and education by publishing worldwide in

Oxford New York

Auckland Cape Town Dar es Salaam Hong Kong Karachi
Kuala Lumpur Madrid Melbourne Mexico City Nairobi
New Delhi Shanghai Taipei Toronto

With offices in

Argentina Austria Brazil Chile Czech Republic France Greece
Guatemala Hungary Italy Japan Poland Portugal Singapore
South Korea Switzerland Thailand Turkey Ukraine Vietnam

Oxford is a registered trade mark of Oxford University Press
in the UK and in certain other countries

Published in the United States
by Oxford University Press Inc., New York

© Oxford University Press, 2010

The moral rights of the authors have been asserted
Database right Oxford University Press (maker)

First edition published 2001
Second edition published 2010

British Library Cataloguing in Publication Data

Data available

Library of Congress Cataloging in Publication Data

Data available

Typeset in Minion
by Cepha Imaging Private Ltd., Bangalore, India
Printed in Great Britain
on acid-free paper by the
MPG Books Group, Bodmin and King's Lynn

ISBN 978-0-19-923893-4

10 9 8 7 6 5 4 3 2 1

Dedicated to
Dr John Hubley, our esteemed colleague, friend
and
co-author of the first edition.

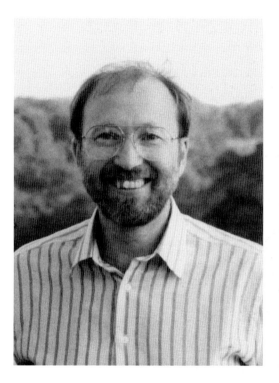

Preface

We face major challenges to health that threaten to reverse the advances in life expectancy achieved in the last century. New diseases such as AIDS, and the rise of chronic non-communicable diseases compete with traditional burdens of disease such as TB and malaria. Poverty remains the single most important cause of disease, acting through factors such as poor education, poor housing, and malnutrition but wider global threats of over-population, over-consumption, and climate change all contribute to uncertainty about our future health. Perhaps most worrying of all is the inexorable increase in health inequalities between high and low income countries.

Public health professionals have a crucial role to play in meeting these challenges and reducing the threats to global health. They can help to monitor disease and health needs, and plan effective and appropriate health care services to meet these health needs. They can act as advocates and change agents across health, education, housing, agricultural and water sectors to tackle the wider determinants of poverty and prevent ill-health.

Today's public health professionals need a broad focus and an armoury of skills including epidemiology, needs assessment, health planning, medicines management, design of interventions, planning, management, intersectoral working and involving communities. This book provides a foundation for doctors, community nurses and other public health professionals in training as well as those in practice. For this second edition we have had the chance to update our previous chapters, but more importantly to cover important new areas such health policy, non-communicable disease and quality and safety of care. We hope it can help, inform, and contribute to tackling today's health problems.

We would like to thank our contributors and reviewers, and those who have helped us edit this book, in particular Lynn Auty and Carolyn Clover, and to our families for helping us to complete this second edition.

John Wright and John Walley
Leeds/Bradford 2009

Contents

Contributors *xv*
Acknowledgements *xvii*

1 Public health and the burden of disease *1*
John Walley
    What is public health? *1*
    Who is involved in public health? *2*
    Health for all *3*
    Burden of diseases *4*
    Determinants of disease *5*
    The demographic and health transition *7*
    Conclusion *10*
    Further reading *10*

2 Public health interventions *11*
John Walley
    Levels of prevention *11*
    Prevention or cure? *12*
    Interventions for achieving better health for all *12*
    Public health programmes *13*
    Basic clinical services *17*
    Conclusion *20*
    Further reading *20*

3 Epidemiology in practice *21*
John Wright
    Defining a case and defining a population *22*
    How do we measure disease? *23*
    Incidence and prevalence *25*
    How do we describe disease? *27*
    Monitoring trends: Use of coverage charts *28*
    Health surveys *30*
    Evaluative epidemiology: Do treatments work? *32*
    Randomized controlled trials *32*
    Systematic reviews *33*
    Further reading *34*

4 Assessing health needs *35*
John Wright
    Health needs *35*

Health needs assessment *36*

Routine information *38*

Community appraisals *40*

Emergency needs assessment *45*

Acting on the assessment *46*

Further reading *47*

5 Choosing the best public health interventions *49*
John Walley

Introduction *49*

When to review? *49*

How to review *50*

Assess health needs *51*

Review health services and programmes *51*

Identification and analysis of the problem(s) *52*

Review and choose the best interventions *53*

Effectiveness *54*

Organizational feasibility *55*

Gender-cultural and political feasibility *55*

Financial feasibility *56*

How detailed should a review of interventions be? *57*

Review and choice of the best service delivery approach *59*

Draft activities and action plan *62*

Budgeting *64*

Summary *64*

Further reading *64*

6 Planning, implementing, and managing interventions *65*
John Hubley, Sylvia Tilford, and John Walley

Assessing health needs *65*

Assessing resources and developing a project team *66*

Recruitment of staff *67*

Setting objectives *68*

Choose the best interventions to achieve objectives *68*

Budgeting *69*

Programme implementation *70*

Pilot in the early district sites *71*

Phased implementation *72*

Implementation according to plan *72*

Achieving sustainability of programme effects *72*

Monitoring and evaluation *80*

Implementation research *84*

Conclusions *86*

Further reading *86*

7 Understanding and using health economics and financing *87*
  Sophie Witter
    Introduction: The health economic perspective *87*
    Health financing *88*
    Taxation-based funding *90*
    Insurance schemes *91*
    User charges *93*
    Costing services *94*
    Economic evaluation *97*
    Project appraisal *99*
    Resource allocation *100*
    Priority setting and service packages *101*
    Improving the organization of services *105*
    Payment systems *107*
    Public/private mix and performance management *109*
    Conclusion *113*
    Further reading *113*

8 Health promotion *115*
  John Hubley and Sylvia Tilford
    Introduction *115*
    Components of health promotion interventions *117*
    The planning process for health promotion *117*
    Specifying the health promotion intervention *125*
    Programme implementation *127*
    Selection and implementation of communication and education methods *129*
    Monitoring and evaluation of programmes *136*
    Conclusion *137*
    Further reading *137*

9 Health policy and systems *139*
  Andrew Green
    Introduction *139*
    Key historical policy shifts *139*
    How are decisions made, and by whom, about services? *148*
    Policy and planning processes *151*
    Monitoring, evaluation, and regulation *152*
    Conclusion *152*
    Further reading *152*

10 Developing a district health care service *155*
  John Walley and Sarah Escott
    Where we are and where we want to be *155*
    What is a district health system? *156*

Developing and improving district health systems *162*

Management support systems needed by a district health service *170*

In-service training and supportive supervision *171*

Organizational values to promote in a health district *177*

Summary *178*

Further reading *178*

11 Maternal, neonatal, and child health *181*
John Walley and Nancy Gerein

Burden of disease *182*

Historical development of MNCH services *185*

The MNCH package of interventions *185*

Maternal health *187*

Access to information and services for safe motherhood *187*

Neonatal care *192*

The IMCI interventions *195*

Nutrition *199*

School education and health *203*

Population and family planning *204*

Ensure quality of MNCH services *210*

Conclusion *211*

Further reading *211*

12 Essential drugs *213*
Kathleen Holloway

Introduction: How medicines fit into public health – a responsibility at all levels *213*

Medicine selection and the essential medicines concept *214*

Access *218*

Rational use of medicines *224*

Medicine quality and medicine regulation *231*

National medicine policy *233*

The role of government in the pharmaceutical sector *235*

Summary *237*

Further reading *237*

13 Communicable disease control principles and toolkit *239*
Martin Schweiger

Major killers *239*

Relationship between individual health and the health of the community *240*

Balance between the host and the invader *241*

Nosocomial infection *244*

Communicable disease toolbox *246*

Outbreaks *254*

Objectives *255*

Conclusion *257*

Further reading *257*

14 Controlling major communicable diseases *259*
John Walley, Roger Webber, and Andrew Collins

Transmission, control, and classification *259*

Water, sanitation, and hygiene-related diseases *260*

HIV and sexually transmitted diseases *270*

Insect-borne diseases *277*

Zoonoses *284*

Integration within district health systems *284*

Conclusion *285*

Further reading *285*

15 Non-communicable diseases *287*
Kamran Siddiqi

Introduction *287*

Global impact of non-communicable diseases *287*

Causes and determinants *291*

Prevention and control *294*

Conclusion *308*

Further reading *308*

16 Quality control, safety, and better practice *309*
John Wright

Part 1: Health care quality assurance *309*

Part 2: Patient safety *312*

Part 3: Improving quality and patient safety *315*

Further reading *318*

17 Future trends in global public health *319*
John Wright and John Walley

The global burden of disease *319*

Changes in the burden of disease 1990–2020 *321*

The social determinants of health *323*

Primary health care *323*

An agenda for action *324*

The challenge of implementation *328*

Future challenges: Mega-problems *330*

Conclusion *331*

Further reading *332*

Glossary *333*

Index *345*

Contributors

Andrew Collins
Medical Doctor & General Practitioner,
Part time Lecturer in Global Health,
Department of Epidemiology and
Public Health,
University College Cork,
National University of Ireland,
Ireland

Sarah Escott
Honorary Senior Lecturer,
Academic unit of primary Care (AUPC),
Leeds Institute of Health Sciences,
University of Leeds,
Charles Thackrah Building,
101 Clarendon Road,
Leeds LS2 9LJ,
UK

Nancy Gerein
Senior Lecturer,
Nuffield Centre for International Health &
Development,
University of Leeds,
Charles Thackrah Building,
101 Clarendon Road,
Leeds LS2 9LJ,
UK

Andrew Green
Professor of International Health Planning,
Nuffield Centre for International Health &
Development,
University of Leeds,
Charles Thackrah Building,
101 Clarendon Road,
Leeds LS2 9LJ,
UK

Kathy Holloway
Medical Officer – Policy, Access and
Rational Use,
Dept Essential Drugs and Medicines Policy,
WHO,
Avenue Appia 20,
1211 Geneva 27,
Switzerland

John Hubley
International Health Promotion Consultant/
Senior Lecturer in Health Education & Health
Promotion,
Leeds Metropolitan University,
21 Arncliffe Road,
Leeds LS6 5AP,
UK

Martin Schweiger
Consultant in Communicable
Disease Control,
West Yorkshire Health Protection Unit,
HPA Laboratory,
Bridle Path,
Leeds LS15 7TR,
UK

Kamran Siddiqi
Clinical Senior Lecturer,
Nuffield Centre for International
Health & Development,
University of Leeds,
Charles Thackrah Building,
101 Clarendon Road,
Leeds LS2 9LJ,
UK

Sylvia Tilford
Professor in Health Promotion,
Leeds Metropolitan University,
UK

John Walley
Professor of International Public Health,
Nuffield Centre for International Health &
Development,
University of Leeds,
Charles Thackrah Building,
101 Clarendon Road,
Leeds LS2 9LJ,
UK

Roger Webber
Formerly of the London School of Hygiene &
Tropical Medicine,
London,
UK

Sophie Witter
Health Economist & Research Fellow,
Department of Public Health,
School of Medicine,
University of Aberdeen,
Foresterhill,
Aberdeen AB25 2ZD,
UK

John Wright
Consultant in Clinical Epidemiology and
Public Health,
Bradford Hospitals NHS Trust,
Bradford Royal Infirmary,
Duckworth Lane,
Bradford BD9 6RJ,
UK

Acknowledgements

The editors would like to thank especially Lynn Auty and Carolyn Clover for formatting and proof reading etc, and the following for their helpful contributions: Sarah Escott (Chapter 1); Jennifer Parr, University of Leeds (Chapter 6); Reinhard Huss, University of Leeds (Chapter 10); Martin Schweiger, Leeds Health Protection Unit (Chapter 14); Marthe Everard, Policy, Access and Rational Use, Department of Essential Drugs and Medicines Policy, WHO, Geneva, Switzerland (Chapter 12); Dr Hans Hogerzeil, Coordinator for Policy, Access and Rational Use, Department of Essential Drugs and Medicines Policy, WHO, Geneva, Switzerland (Chapter 12); Philippa Saunders, Essential Drugs Project, London, UK (Chapter 12); Keith Hurst, University of Leeds (Chapter 16); Owen Johnson, University of Leeds (Chapter 17). The following are acknowledged as sources:

Chapter 1: Figs 1-1.3, Daphne Paley-Smith, Leeds.
Chapter 4: Fig. 4.1, David Gifford (from Lankester T 1992 *Setting up community health programmes*, Macmillan).
Chapter 12: Table 12.3, *Health Reform and Drug Financing*, WHO/DAP/98.3. Fig. 12.2, Quick *et al., Managing Drug Supply* (1997), Kumarian Press, ISBN: 1-56549-047-9. Fig. 12.3, As 12.2. Table 12.1, Kafuko J, Zirabumuzale C, Bagenda D (1996), UNICEF, Uganda. Table 12.2, Chaudhury R (1999) *Essential Drugs Monitor*. Box 12.1, *Health Reform and Drug Financing*, WHO/DAP/98.3. Box 12.2, *How to investigate drug use in health facilities,* 1993. WHO, Geneva. WHO/DAP/93.1. Box 12.3, WHO *Geneva*, WHO/HTP/MAC(11)99.6; WHO/EDM/QSM/99.3; WHO/DAP/95.3; WHO/PHARM/94.568. Table 12.4, Hogerzeil *et al., Lancet* 1989, **333**, 141-2. Table 12.5, Holloway K, Gautum B (1997), http://www.who.int/dap-icium/posters/4e2-Text.html. Table 12.6, Hadiyono *et al Interactional group discussion. Social Science and Medicine,* 1996, **42**, 1177-83. Table 12.7, Paredes *et al. Applied Diarrhoeal Research Project,* Lima, Peru, 1996. Box 12.4, *Comparative analysis of national drug policies.* WHO, Geneva 1997. WHO/DAP/97.6. Box 12.5, *World Bank Flagship Centre,* Module 7 *Towards improved efficiency in the pharmaceutical sector,* finalised by Marthe Everard, EDM/WHO, 1999. Box 12.6, WHO 1997, Public-Private roles in the pharmaceutical sector. Implications for equitable access and rational use, DAP series no.5, WHO/DAP/97.12.
Chapter 14: Figs. 14.1, 14.2, 14.7, Table 14, Webber R 1996 *Communicable disease epidemiology and control*, CAB International, Oxford.
Chapter 17: Fig 17.2, David Gifford (from Lankester T 1992 *Setting up community health programmes,* Macmillan).
Glossary: Extracts from Witter S, Ensor T, Jowett M, Thompson R 2000 *Health Economics in developing countries: a practical guide*, Macmillan, Basingstoke.

Chapter 1

Public health and the burden of disease

John Walley

This chapter gives an overview of the following topics:

◆ What is public health?
◆ Who is involved in public health?
◆ Burden of disease;
◆ Determinants of disease.

What is public health?

Imagine yourself as a health worker in a consultation room. In front of you is a sick person who has come to be treated. As a clinician you do everything you can to make that individual better. You have a similar attitude for the other patients sitting outside in the waiting room. You are committed to your job and are very busy day to day treating those people who come for help. You give little thought to those people who haven't come to the health facility. Indeed you assume that anyone who is really sick will visit you or other clinicians and so you are not concerned about those people who have not come to the clinic. Being such a clinician, you would be taking an 'individual case management' approach to healthcare.

In reality, there are many sick people in your area who do not come to the health facilities for help. Many try and deal with the problems themselves. They may buy medicines from shops. They may visit traditional healers. They may even continue to suffer at home without taking any action. Perhaps when the disease is very advanced eventually they come to the clinic or hospital. Often it is too late by then – had they come earlier, they may have been cured of their illnesses, or the complications reduced. In fact, in many cases the disease could have been prevented completely; for example, by immunization or improved sanitation. A 'public health' approach to health care looks at this wider picture.

Public health deals with the health of the whole population. Public health programmes aim to improve the health of the population. Public health professionals work to improve the health of the population. Note that the concepts of 'public health' are the same as those of 'community health'. Some people call the 'population', 'the community'.

Public health is understanding health needs and intervening to improve the health of the population.

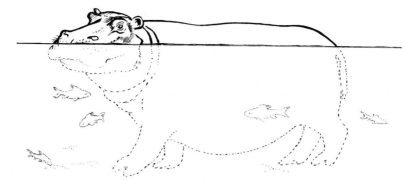

Fig. 1.1 The part of the hippo out of water is like the people and their diseases which we see in our clinics. The part under water is like the people and their diseases which don't come to our clinics.

But what is a population?

There are several different ways that a population can be defined. The population may be:

♦ An *administrative area* – such as a health centre catchment area, a district, a province, or country;

♦ A specific *population group* such as pregnant women or young children;

♦ A *disease specific* group (including people at risk of the disease) such as for STDs/AIDS or tuberculosis.

The point is that, as a public health professional, you have a responsibility to improve the health of the whole of this population, and not just the members of the most visible population who come to the health facilities (Fig. 1.1).

Now imagine yourself as a teacher with a large lecture room full of people. Because they are nearer to you it is likely that you will communicate most with those people who sit in the front. You can see them more clearly, recognize when they look confused and need more explanation, and notice when they want to ask a question. But what about the rest of the class? The people who are sitting at the back of the room are just as important, even if you can hardly see them. Teachers should be aware of this bias and put extra effort to communicate with the students at the back.

There is often a similar bias in the provision of health care in an area, as there is for a lecture. It is easier for those people who live near the health facilities to travel when they need help. Health professionals usually notice problems in their area more easily than those in the distant rural areas. To the public health professional the people living in remote rural areas or urban slums are just as important as those who live close to health facilities, and extra effort may be needed to reach these people who could otherwise be neglected.

Who is involved in public health?

Anyone who is involved in improving health services and programmes, or advocating for better living conditions, is involved in public health. This book is aimed at health professionals (qualified or in training) who are or will work in middle to senior levels in health, such as:

♦ District and provincial health offices

♦ National health programmes

♦ Health facilities (which serve the surrounding population)

♦ Health promotion programmes (outside health services) eg in the media

♦ Other sectors; water, housing, education, agriculture (nutrition)

This book is aimed at helping health professionals do a better job of improving the health of the community.

Public health is a multi-professional discipline. All people who are involved in developing programmes and services which will tackle the causes of common diseases need to have a public health perspective. This population-based view of health is required by district medical officers, health service managers, health inspectors, community nurses, nutritionists, health educationists, general medical practitioners, and many others.

Health for all

Public health aims to provide the best possible health services for everyone, everywhere in the district.

When planning health services for the population several things need to be considered:

1 How do people physically reach the health services? This is called the *access* to health services. It is especially important in areas with no clinics, bad roads, and no public transport. It is affected by the distance people must travel and the ease and cost of the journey.

2 Are the health services *acceptable* to the people? The services should be friendly, respect confidentiality for sensitive issues, and have short waiting times.

3 Do the health services deal with the right problems? Health staff should give most of their time and interest to the common diseases which cause the most ill-health in the population, rather than concentrating on a few people with rare and 'interesting' diseases. That is services should be *appropriate*.

4 Are the health services fairly available to everyone? Health service access should be equal for all members of the population: Male and female, rich and poor, Christians and Muslims. In most countries there are sub-groups of the population that have found it difficult to access health services. For example, women may not attend if there are only male health workers; people who do not speak the main language may not attend if they don't have a translator. This may mean that extra effort and resources are needed to reach the previously under-served groups. In this way we can achieve *equity of provision* of services and *equity in utilization* of services.

5 Indeed we must make sure that all areas have health service *coverage*. This means there need to be enough health facilities so that every member of the community can reach them when needed. Also that interventions such as vaccinations reach high % coverage of the target group, such as young children.

These principles apply to all public health services and programmes. For example, we must achieve equal access to vaccination. Services must be acceptable with little waiting. Where there are no health centres we arrange *outreach*, to cover all areas. As a result high vaccination coverage rates are achieved.

We have now learnt that 'public health' is about achieving health for all members of the population. Public health therefore shares the same ideals as *primary health care*.

These are easily remembered as the four 'a' words:

◆ affordable

◆ acceptable

◆ accessible

◆ appropriate

A useful tip is always to think first of those people who usually come to the health services last! There will be people or groups who will not appreciate this change in priority. Some people will be used to receiving more attention and easier access to health care. They may not previously have realized that other groups in the population are not as fortunate. Unfortunately, even when they do realize this, they are reluctant to support any change that means a reduction in the services in their area. In general the facilities in the centre of cities are more accessible and better staffed than those in rural or peri-urban slum areas. The people living in towns may have a higher overall level of education and more political influences than those in the rural areas and urban slums. In public health we have to listen and take note of the demands of the influential groups while at the same time doing our best for the poor and less influential people. With different groups having people with different demands and needs, it is hard to please everyone and we may have to make some compromises. What is most important is that we keep our 'eyes on the ball' and aim for better health for all.

Burden of diseases

Which diseases cause the most illness or death in a population?

This is an important question that must be addressed for every population. It is important to know this for the district or other area for which you are responsible. Think about a clinician seeing an individual patient who has a problem. Before treating the patient the clinician must first decide what is wrong. This is done by finding out the facts of the case, taking a detailed history, and making an examination of the patient. In public health we also need to find the 'facts of the problem' before deciding on a solution. In public health we use statistics and epidemiology to understand the problem (instead of history and examination) and plan public health interventions (instead of treatment) to solve it. See also Chapter 3, basic epidemiology.

When collecting information about the population we are concerned with both morbidity and mortality. The term *burden of disease* includes both morbidity and mortality. Morbidity can also be called disability, and can be a few days during the acute illness with measles, or *years with disability* with blindness. Mortality can also be measured in terms of *years of life lost*. That is, the number of healthy years lost due a premature death as compared to full life span. A combined measure of years with disability and years of life lost is the 'disability-adjusted life year' or DALY. *One daly is one year of life lost*, or for example two years with blindness.

The proportion of morbidity and mortality varies from disease to disease. More DALYs are lost from disability in the case of depression and leprosy. In contrast, a disease with high mortality rates, such as TB, results in more DALYs lost through lost years of life. DALYs are a useful broad guide to priority setting. However, as with all data, think about their limitations, for example, the assumption in calculating DALYs and the sources of data. DALYs use the best available data from each part of the world, but the information is very patchy in some areas, such as Africa. Ideally it would be better if we could include an assessment as to how people perceive their quality of life, and so calculate quality-adjusted life years, but these need special surveys.

The pie chart in Fig. 1.2 shows the global burden of disease attributable to selected determinants (risk factors) such as malnutrition (Murray and Lopez, 1996). The burden of disease is in DALYs, as discussed above; *one DALY is one year of healthy life lost*.

The pie chart shows that the most significant determinants are malnutrition, poor water, sanitation and hygiene, unsafe sex, alcohol, tobacco, and occupation. Others will include high salt and fat diet, lack of exercise, genetic, and many other causes. It should be remembered that there are considerable variations between regions and between men and women. Men have greater risk from alcohol and tobacco, and women from unsafe sex – including from infections and unwanted pregnancy. In sub-Saharan Africa unsafe sex is the underlying cause of around one-third of the burden of disease in women (and is a major cause in other world regions as well). Furthermore,

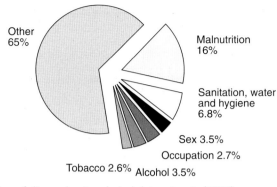

Fig. 1.2 Global burden of diease due to selected determinants (1996).

the rates are changing over time with, for example, the rapid rate of rise of tobacco use which is expected to kill many more people in future decades. The above are based on the DALYs caused by the determinants, that is, underlying causes. The burden has also been estimated by disease groups, that is, the direct cause of disability and loss of life.

HIV/AIDS and malaria are at the top of the list in the sub-Saharan African region – while perinatal conditions top the list in South Asia. Cerebrovascular, ischaemic heart, and chronic obstructive pulmonary disease are also high (– largely caused by tobacco smoking and an unhealthy lifestyle). These are at the top of the list in East Asia. Other diseases causing high disability and deaths are depression and TB.

There are also major variations in the burden of disease by age and sex, as well as world regions. For example, depression is more common in women while ischaemic heart disease is more common in men. HIV/STIs due to unprotected (no condoms) sex, affect both men and women. Unplanned pregnancy is a major factor in maternal deaths. Malnutrition and infections of childhood, such as measles and trachoma continue to cause blindness and death especially in sub-Saharan Africa.

For our own populations we will need to know what the most common causes of morbidity and mortality are, so that we can concentrate our efforts on the priority problems. We will put more time and resources towards tackling the problems that cause the most burden of disease (and have effective interventions at low cost, see Chapter 2).

Determinants of disease

Disease can be caused by many factors. Some are direct causes and others more indirect or underlying causes.

Imagine once again that you are a clinician in a health centre. You see a young child who is severely dehydrated with diarrhoea. The direct cause of his illness is an infectious agent, for example *shigella*. However, there are several underlying factors that determine his current state of health. These include

- poor nutritional status (affected by underfeeding, recurrent infections, bottle-feeding);
- inappropriate home treatments (traditional remedies and incorrectly stopping feeds when ill).

In addition, there are several underlying factors that have contributed to these problems. These include:

- large family size
- lack of land or income for food

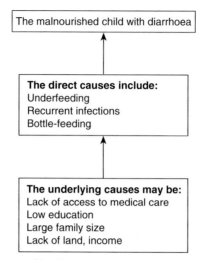

Fig. 1.3 Underlying determinants of health.

- ◆ low education
- ◆ poor access to medical care – including poor access to health education
- ◆ poverty – no access to clean water and sanitation

These underlying determinants of health illustrated contribute to death from infections and malnutrition, as in Fig. 1.3.

Maternal health also illustrates these underlying causes of illness and death. As clinicians we often fail to consider why women do not come for antenatal check-ups, or for delivery in health facilities or if developing complications, why they come to the hospital late. We do not consider the underlying causes that contribute to late presentation and diagnosis of maternal health problems such as eclampsia (Fig. 1.4).

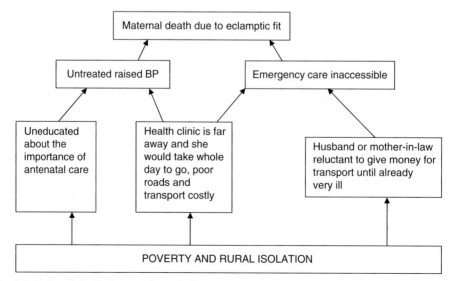

Fig. 1.4 Maternal death due to eclampsia fit.

Table 1.1 Broad patterns of the disease burden, by World Bank Region, 2001

Category	Prevalence %		
	Sub-Saharan Africa	South Asia	East Asia and the Pacific
Communicable, maternal, perinatal and nutritional conditions	70.4	44.3	22.2
Non-communicable diseases	21.2	44.4	65.8
Injuries	8.4	11.4	12.0

Note: Latin America is similar to East Asia.

Source: Mathers and others, 2005, in Disease Control Priorities, 2006.

The cause of a maternal death starts with the underlying socio-economic situation in which the woman lives. There is commonly poverty, low education, poor access to services (poor roads and transport and little money), and poor quality of services – all contributing eventually to her death (see also Chapter 11, Maternal neonatal, and child health). A similar pattern applies to deaths from other causes. We have to consider the underlying and the more direct causes of ill health and death (Table 1.1).

Not surprisingly the communicable, maternal, and perinatal conditions cause the biggest disease burden in sub-Saharan Africa. However non-communicable diseases, such as cerebrovascular diseases, are becoming more common, while communicable diseases are becoming less common. In South Asia they are now equal. While in East Asia and Latin America, non-communicable disease is now more common than communicable disease.

The demographic and health transition

Socio-economic development (including urbanization, better housing, water supply, sanitation, and access to education and health services) leads to a reduction in diarrhoea and other infectious diseases. Parents have more confidence that their children will survive. Children have to go to school, rather than help in the fields, and so having more children is costly. Couples choose to have fewer children and if modern family planning methods are accessible – the number of children born per woman declines. The number of children declines while the proportion of the population who are older increases. This is called the demographic transition. The process has occurred more in East Asia, especially China where there is economic development, strong population policies, and accessible family planning services (see also Chapter 11, Maternal neonatal, and child health). This *demographic transition* is a well-advanced in process in India, Bangladesh, and elsewhere in South Asia. In many low-income countries the time death rates (especially in children) have come down, but birth rates remain high. Economic development is limited and is not keeping pace with population growth. Population policies and family planning services are poorly implemented. At current rates, even taking into account HIV/AIDS, the populations of many countries such as Malawi and Uganda are set to increase to three or four times the existing level. Arable land and growth in food production are limited. It is difficult to migrate to other countries. Unless serious action is taken, hunger and even war may increase. Other countries with strong economies, good population policies, and good family services are progressing well through 'the transition'.

As countries go through the demographic transition and there are more older people in the population, communicable diseases become less common and there is relatively more chronic and non-communicable diseases. This is called the *epidemiological transition* Fig. 1.5.

Low and middle income countries

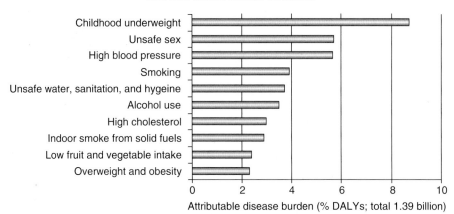

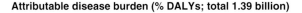

Attributable disease burden (% DALYs; total 1.39 billion)

Attributable disease burden (% DALYs; total 1.39 billion)

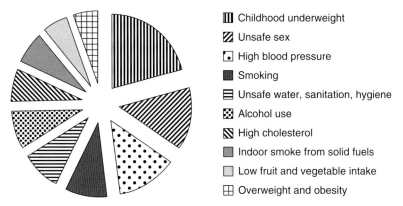

- Childhood underweight
- Unsafe sex
- High blood pressure
- Smoking
- Unsafe water, sanitation, hygiene
- Alcohol use
- High cholesterol
- Indoor smoke from solid fuels
- Low fruit and vegetable intake
- Overweight and obesity

Fig. 1.5 Demographic and Health transition.

Chronic diseases of older people, such as osteoarthritis, and non-communicable diseases, such as hypertension and ischaemic heart diseases, become more common as the population ages. Also, now, more than half the world's population live in cities. Urban lifestyle includes less exercise, more fatty food, which lead to obesity and diabetes. Tobacco use also increases, leading to cardiovascular disease and chronic obstructive pulmonary disease.

As mentioned above, the leading causes of disease burden are changing. In Africa infectious diseases still dominate and there is a particularly high burden of HIV/AIDS and malaria. In South Asia these infections also exist, but less so, with perinatal conditions and heart disease becoming more important. In East Asia and Latin America the demographic and epidemiological transitions are well-advanced with non-communicable, heart and lung conditions being predominant. In Latin America the situation is the same, except that homicide and violence are more common (the other conditions being relatively less common). But where communicable diseases have declined, these conditions become relatively more important and move up the ranking. Perinatal conditions and mental health problems such as depression are a problem in all regions of the world (Table 1.2).

Table 1.2 Leading causes of the disease burden, by World Bank Region, 2001

Rank	Sub-Saharan Africa	South Asia	East Asia and the Pacific	Latin America and the Caribbean
1	HIV/AIDS	Perinatal conditions*	Cerebrovascular diseases	Perinatal conditions*
2	Malaria	Lower respiratory infections	Perinatal conditions*	Unipolar depressive disorders
3	Lower respiratory infections	Ischaemic heart disease	Chronic obstructive pulmonary disease	Homicide and Violence
4	Diarrhoeal diseases	Diarrhoeal diseases	Ischaemic heart disease	Ischaemic heart disease
5	Perinatal conditions*	Unipolar depressive disorders	Unipolar depressive disorders	Cerebrovascular diseases

*Perinatal conditions include low birth weight, birth asphyxia, and birth trauma.

Source: Mathers and others 2005, in Disease Control Priorities, 2006.

As public health workers, we must remember the underlying as well as more direct causes. Given that so many factors can influence health, we must keep a broad view of the most appropriate ways to tackle the problems causing disease. It is all too easy to concentrate on the treatment of the most visible cases – such as acute illnesses, and severely malnourished children. But in doing so, not enough attention may be given to addressing the underlying causes. It is understandable that health workers, who are trained to treat the sick, concentrate on treatments, but in doing so we may miss the opportunity to prevent the problem in the first place. The long-term solutions are often found in areas that are often not considered under 'health'. Promoting nutritious crops, promoting clean water and sanitation projects, and advocating for change to remove the underlying causes will ultimately results in great improvements in health. Climate change (due to the release of carbon dioxide from burning oil, coal, and gas) will in the coming decades increasingly affect our lives. Warming of the atmosphere causes chaotic rainfall patterns with the rain coming at the wrong time or very heavy, reducing crop yields, and causing hunger. We need to act (intervene) on more than one level when addressing the causes of malnutrition and ill health and their causes in our fight to reduce the burden of disease. Such prevention and intervention may require working with others, such as those in agriculture or education. Where health, workers are working with other sectors to improve nutrition and health, this is called the *multi-sectoral* or *inter-sectoral approach* for example with politicians and agriculture agencies.

To achieve results it will also be necessary to work with the community. Health workers commonly think they know best, and just tell people what is good for them. This doesn't work well. Community members know the actual situation in their area. *Community involvement* means that health workers listen to the views of the community members and jointly decide on the needs and priorities as proposed in Primary Health Care (PHC). For example, communities are most likely to grow new nourishing foods and feed these to their children if they *participated* in the decisions.

Public health can also be defined as 'The process of promoting health, preventing disease, prolonging life and improving the quality of life through the organized efforts of society'.

Designing and implementing such interventions require a lot of time in listening, discussing and sharing opinions. This forms another important part of 'defining the problem' of the community. As well as collecting statistics about mortality and morbidity, the public health manager has to meet with the community members, community leaders, and officers from other sectors involved in treating the underlying causes of ill-health, see Chapters 3 and 4.

Conclusion

Public health is concerned with improving the health of the population, rather than just the individuals seeking treatment. We must make appropriate health services available to the **whole** population, especially those at risk. The demographic and epidemiological transitions affect the rankings of high burden diseases. Preventive interventions and essential health services are needed to tackle these diseases as outlined in the next chapter.

Further reading

Jamison D. et al. *Disease control priorities in a developing world, second edition.* World Bank/Oxford University Press, 2nd edition, 2006. [A very useful disease and health systems reference] http://www.dcp2.org/page/main/BrowseDiseases.html for Burden of Disease by risk factors, see www.dcp2.org/pubs/GBD

Walley, J., Lawn, J., Tinker, A. et al. (2008) Primary health care: making Alma-Ata a reality. *Lancet*, **372**, 1001–8.

WHO. World Health Report (2008) http//www.who.int/whr/2008/en/

World development report: investing in health. World Bank/Oxford University Press 1993. [A detailed explanation of DALYs and Essential PH Interventions etc.]

Chapter 2

Public health interventions

John Walley

This chapter gives an overview of the following topics:
- ◆ Levels of prevention;
- ◆ Public health programmes;
- ◆ Intervention strategies;
- ◆ Delivery strategies;
- ◆ Public health and essential clinical interventions;
- ◆ Effectiveness and cost of interventions.

Levels of prevention

Preventive programmes and clinical services reduce the burden from disease through prevention at primary, secondary, and tertiary (third) levels.

Primary prevention aims to prevent the condition from starting. This may be through control of mosquitoes, immunization, and behaviour change such as stopping tobacco smoking and eating less fat and salt.

Secondary prevention aims to detect disease at the earliest stage and to prevent the condition from progressing. *Screening* identifies disease before symptoms occur, for example smears to detect pre-cancer of the cervix and blood pressure checks to detect hypertension. *Prophylaxis* is preventive treatment given over the long term. For example, people with HIV taking the antibiotic *Cotrimoxazole* to prevent some common infections. *Cure* is a form of secondary prevention in that early effective treatment results in no remaining damage – for illnesses such as malaria.

Tertiary prevention aims at 'damage limitation' in those with established disease. This can include treatment with drugs, surgery, or rehabilitation to restore function. These interventions are what most doctors and nurses in hospitals are busy with on the wards, while much of out-patient and health centre work is primary and secondary prevention.

Examples of primary, secondary, and tertiary prevention for diarrhoeal diseases include:
- ◆ Primary prevention of diarrhoea by water and sanitation and hygiene education;
- ◆ Secondary prevention of dehydration by oral rehydration in those with diarrhoea;
- ◆ Tertiary prevention of shock with IV fluids for severe dehydration.

Another example is TB:
- ◆ Primary prevention of *infection* by improved housing/ventilation and BCG vaccination;
- ◆ Secondary prevention of active *disease* in those infected by preventive treatment with isoniazid, or once symptomatic, then cure by early diagnosis and treatment of symptomatic disease with a full course of TB drugs;

♦ Tertiary prevention by treatment and then rehabilitation of remaining damage, e.g. from TB of the spine.

Prevention or cure?

'*Prevention is the best cure*' is generally true. However, for some communicable diseases '*Cure is the best prevention*'. Treatment of pulmonary TB is secondary prevention for the sick individual but its early diagnosis and treatment also prevents transmission to others. Similarly, treatment of sexually transmitted diseases (STDs) prevents their transmission to others. While in malaria, both early diagnosis and treatment are important, together with prevention through insecticide impregnated bednets etc. in control of the disease.

Effective control of malaria, and many other diseases, depends on both curative and preventive measures. Maternal health services include antenatal care, which is both primary prevention, through education and intake of folic acid supplements, and secondary prevention, through screening for asymptomatic problems such as raised BP, syphilis and HIV infection and anaemia and treating them if found. Tertiary prevention of complications is provided through emergency obstetric care for women who have developed complications such as eclampsia (Fig. 1.4).

Compared to other medical specialties, public health is more concerned with prevention rather than cure. Nevertheless we are also concerned with the provision of essential clinical services.

Interventions for achieving better health for all

Interventions, or more correctly intervention strategies, are actions to improve health. There are different types of interventions:

♦ Immunization;

♦ Interventions that promote changes in lifestyle, – such as reducing HIV through condom promotion; reducing heart disease risk through advocating for laws against tobacco advertising; reducing malaria risk by promoting the use of impregnated bednets;

♦ Interventions that may improve the early diagnosis and treatment and in turn reduce the duration or severity of disease, – such as the diagnosis of pneumonia or teaching mothers the correct use of Oral Rehydration Solution (ORS) for their child with diarrhoea.

Public health interventions may be:

♦ *Population-based* programmes aimed at reducing specific disease groups – such as reduction of diarrhoeal diseases through water and sanitation improvement. These interventions are often multi-sectoral, that is they involve other agencies, not only health ones. They seek to remove the underlying causes of ill health – resulting in long-term reductions in occurrence of many diseases;

♦ *Personal preventive services* – such as screening for cervical cancer; and

♦ *Basic clinical services,* such as ORS for diarrhoea and antibiotics for pneumonia.

Some programmes are both population-based and personal preventive programmes. For example, the expanded programme of immunization (EPI) operates through education and outreach vaccination sessions in the community. It also acts as a personal preventive service giving vaccination to children attending health facilities as required (even if they attended for another reason).

Delivery strategies

Generally, public health programmes actively encourage the participation of population at risk, and include activity (e.g. outreach vaccination services) outside the health facilities. While personal preventive interventions are those provided within the health service alongside clinical services – for which people generally seek treatment, some such as the immunisation, are already established components of the district health system. Other interventions are not yet part of the district health system but should be incorporated, for example, adding supplementation with vitamin A to the routine immunization schedule for children.

The following section gives an overview of the range of public health programme interventions and essential clinical services. It also introduces how we review the situation and then choose the best interventions.

Public health programmes

Public health programmes are a systematic implementation of intervention (strategies) to control disease. This may be a disease or a group of diseases which share a similar epidemiology and interventions for control. For example diarrhoeal disease control interventions are the same, regardless of being caused by viruses, bacteria or protozoa. Interventions against these diseases include promotion of water, sanitation, and hygiene. Some programmes mainly include interventions which are outside the health services, such as those for water and sanitation, food fortification, and legislation against tobacco. Other interventions such as those against TB are mainly within health services. While in many others, such as the malaria programme, include both interventions within (treatment) and outside health facilities (bednets). Interventions can be delivered through various approaches. For interventions within health services, public health managers try to ensure that community, health centre, and hospital levels are effectively linked by good referral, supplies, and supervision etc.

'*Delivery Strategies*' are the way to get coverage of the target group. The most effective and feasible should be chosen (see Chapter 5). For example, bednets can be delivered (implemented) through antenatal clinics and/or by social marketing through shopkeepers. The promotion of bednets or other interventions can be through various delivery strategies (also called implementation strategies) for example, a combination of one or more of: mass media (radio, TV or newspapers), 'small' media (posters), school education, or peer-education. Each delivery strategy will require a series of *activities*, such as planning meetings, ordering drugs, training, and supervision. Examples of programmes for the high burden diseases are given below. Each programme may include various interventions and the related delivery strategies. An intervention is best implemented by more than one delivery strategy (which will in turn include a number of coordinated activities. For example vaccination (interventions) can be delivered in health facilities and at outreach sessions in distant villages.

1 **Vaccination**

Vaccination and immunization have a similar meaning. The Expanded Programme of Immunisation (EPI) aims to achieve high coverage of the target groups – young children with various vaccines (together with tetanus for women). These can be delivered through health facilities, as well as by specific outreach services. For example, the mass treatment of intestinal parasites may be by outreach service delivery through schools. Interventions include:

EPI includes a minimum of six childhood vaccines: BCG, DPT (diphtheria, pertussis and tetanus), polio and measles (as well as tetanus for women). Many countries have added hepatitis B and the *Haemophylus influenzae* (HIB) vaccine. Others have added vaccines for locally prevalent diseases such as yellow fever in West Africa. Many new vaccines are being developed and tested through trials. Some are already available but expensive, such as the pneumococcal and Human Papilloma Virus (the cause of cervical cancer) vaccines – but are likely to become cheaper and more readily available in the coming years.

2 **Screening and treatment**

Screening is of asymptomatic individuals to identify and refer for treatment those affected by disease. Screening involves individuals of a certain category such as age or sex. Examples include growth monitoring of children (screening for low weight for age), and cervical smears to detect carcinoma-in-situ of cervix. Screening is used where there are no signs or symptoms of a serious illness, but with a test the problem can be detected early and then treated. The screening may be organized as a national programme, but delivered through primary care (personal preventive) services. This may be '*opportunistic screening*' of people who attend for other reasons; for example, doing BP and random glucose checks in over-weight adults.

Case-finding is screening of people who have a particular risk factors or symptom, for example, requesting sputum smears for people with a cough of more than 2 (or 3) weeks to detect possible TB.

3 Mass treatment

Mass treatment is a strategy to control disease, such as soil-transmitted helminth (worm) infections. In areas of high prevalence of parasite infection, mass treatment programmes administer inexpensive and safe drugs to the population in the affected area. In this case testing for the presence of parasites in individual cases isn't necessary and would add to the cost. Mass treatment of worms may be delivered to under-five-year-olds together with vaccinations, and to school children (who often have higher heavier worm loads than adults). The (safe and effective) drugs include albendazole for helminths and praziquantel for schistosomiasis. While ivermectin is given in order to control onchocerciasis (river blindness). The drugs are given by community volunteers, a service delivery approach, called 'community-delivered treatment'.

4 Nutrition

Inadequate nutrition causes marasmus and kwashiorkor. It also contributes to deaths from diarrhoeal and respiratory disease. Nutrition interventions include:

- Health promotion relating to protein-energy malnutrition through:
  - Growth monitoring of weight for age (a form of screening) using a chart to identify under-weight children, discussing feeding practices and food availability with mothers, and then giving specific nutrition education based on what is realistically available to that family.
  - Health promotion through mass media, e.g. for breast feeding (exclusive breast only for the first 4 months, then continued together with 'weaning' foods).
  - Promotion of specific crops: Large-scale agricultural and small-scale home garden.

- Supplementation with food or micronutrients:
  - Food supplementation may be targeted to specific groups such as giving food parcels to underweight children or pregnant women attending health facilities. Other programmes subsidize staple foods to make them available at lower prices, or give food aid (such as food for work projects in famine areas).
  - Micronutrient supplementation includes iron for pregnant women and vitamin A capsules for children. In some areas the childhood micronutrient supplementation programmes are administered together with the EPI vaccination. In other areas supplementation is given as part of the integrated management of childhood illnesses.
  - Fortification of foods with specific micronutrients, such as iodine in salt or vitamin A in monosodium glutamate (MSG) flavour enhancer in Indonesia. This approach is highly effective if the legislation can be enforced, with quality control of the amount of micro-nutrients added at the factory, and prevention of imports of non-fortified products.

5 Fertility

- Family planning services should be accessible and acceptable for all. Birth spacing improves the life expectancy of mothers and their existing children. In the long term, nutrition depends on families being able to produce enough food to feed all the family on the land available. When populations increase, the poor families are often forced to try and grow crops in the marginal dry areas, where in dry years crops fail, or clear hill areas where soils are often washed away (And these problems are likely to increase due to climate change in the coming decades). For all these reasons fertility is a public health concern. Interventions include:

- Family planning services can be provided together with other mother and child health services at all health facilities. Another approach making family planning more accessible is community-based distribution, e.g. of oral contraceptive pills by trained local women and referral for long-term methods for women who have their desired number of children. It is important to provide a mix of methods. This should include, for example, depot injections and 'emergency contraception', oral contraceptive pills taken within 72 hours of unprotected sex.

- *Social marketing* is a service delivery approach useful for condoms and contraceptive pills, where these are provided through shops and street sellers. This is called 'social' as the product is for better health and 'marketing' as the methods used are like those of business. The presentation is researched by group discussions with clients to make sure that the name, logo picture, and leaflet are attractive and understandable. Marketing is through commercial retailers and marketed by 'lifestyle' appeal advertising (as is done for Coca Cola!).

- Family life education in schools, including sex education by teachers, is best if it is part of the regular curriculum. It must be taught at an appropriate level for each age group.

- Access to safe abortion and post-abortion care is important for women's health. The numbers of abortions are little affected by whether they are legal or illegal, because women resort to back-street abortions, often resulting in infection, bleeding, and death. It is important to provide safe abortion. The best way to minimise abortions is to provide good quality access to family planning services.

6 **Vector control and environmental health**

Most of the environmental interventions require multi-sectoral action, involving the environment health staff, together with local authorities and building regulations. Interventions include:

- Vector control: Indoor residual (household) spraying with insecticide and the promotion and use of insecticide treated bednets for protection from *anopheline* mosquitoes and hence malaria.

- Water: Provision of clean water, in sufficient quantity in or near the home is essential. Clean water to prevent water-borne diseases. Enough water to allow washing and so prevent water-wash diseases – hand washing promotion is the key to preventing diarrhoeal disease. Piped or pump water near the home, so avoiding water-contact diseases such as schistosomiasis.

- Sanitation: Promotion of low cost locally appropriate toilets, such as ventilated pit latrines (VIPs) which are popular in Africa as the vent tube control smells and mesh at the top cuts fly breeding, or 'pour flush' toilets popular in Asia.

- Housing: To provide greater space per person and regulations for builders to include ventilation, to reduce air-borne transmission e.g. of measles and tuberculosis (Fig. 2.1).

- Occupational: Many occupations expose the workers to health risks. For example, agricultural workers may be exposed to poisonous insecticides. These issues can be addressed by enforcing regulations for the provision of protective clothing and informing workers of the dangers. Occupational risks may not be obvious at first – for example, the effects of prolonged exposure to workplace noise leads to deafness only years later yet could be prevented by the use of ear protection.

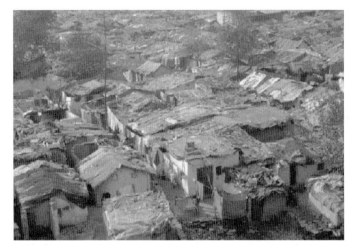

Fig. 2.1 Slum in New Delhi, India. Poverty and poor housing can be an obstacle to health.

- Air and water pollution: Interventions may include regulation to reduce *Air pollution* from lead and sulphur from car fumes in cities and *Water pollution* from industrial wastes and radioactive wastes.

- Climate change: *Global warming* is due to the trapping of the sun's heat by a build up of carbon dioxide released from the combustion of coal, gas, and oil. Climate change will become worse unless serious action is taken, such as through promotion of building insulation, wind and solar power generation and electric vehicles. Climate change has already begun to cause an unpredictable climate, with rain storms alternating with drought – already affecting food production in much of Africa and Asia, causing previously fertile areas to become hotter and drier. All of us need to advocate and act urgently to reduce use of oil & coal, protect forests and conserve soils and water.

- Road transport: The environmental health hazards of traffic may be reduced by legislation on vehicle safety (both construction and maintenance), insurance and legal liability; use of seat belts; restriction of cars in cities and residential areas; and additional road safety education.

7 **HIV/AIDS/STIs**

HIV is spreading so quickly across Africa, Asia, and elsewhere that it is important to treat it as a special priority group of diseases. Untreated STIs cause ulcers or inflammation allowing the transmission of HIV across mucous membranes. Interventions include:

- Providing information: either aiming to educate specific target groups or the general population.

- Condom promotion to specific groups such as prostitutes and their clients (for example migrant workers and truck drivers) or to the general population. Methods include social marketing.

- Reducing blood-borne transmission with screening of blood products.

- Sexual health services to promote early identification and treatment of genital lesions and inflammation (which facilitate transmission of HIV).

- Voluntary counselling and testing (VCT) provided in special clinics or regular health facilities. The counselling includes preventive counselling and condom promotion. VCT is best linked to follow-up care with preventive treatment for those infected with TB, and cotrimoxazole to prevent various opportunistic infections.

- Surveillance, such as by anonymous testing for HIV and syphilis in antenatal clinics, is critical to monitor the epidemic and to alert the authorities for the need for action.
- Care of AIDS patients (covered under clinical services) is required in order to alleviate pain and manage opportunistic infections, including tuberculosis, diarrhoea, and candidiasis.

8 **Reducing abuse of tobacco, alcohol, and other drugs**

In some countries tobacco smoking, especially by men, is widespread. In others the use of tobacco is being heavily promoted and consequently is increasing. On average half of lifetime smokers will die from heart and lung diseases caused by tobacco. It is expected that many countries will face dramatic increases in morbidity and mortality due to smoking over the next decade.

Five policies for controlling tobacco use: Smoke-free environments; support programmes for tobacco users who wish to stop; health warnings on tobacco packs; ban on the advertising, promotion, and sponsorship of tobacco; and higher taxation of tobacco.

Alcohol causes fewer deaths directly but contributes to other health problems by means of multiple unprotected sexual partners and domestic violence. In some countries, other drugs such as heroin and crack cocaine are causing problems.

Basic clinical services

The public health approach to clinical services is to ensure that clinical services are dealing effectively with the diseases which cause the highest morbidity and mortality.

As mentioned in chapter one, the services must be accessible and acceptable so that they are well utilized; the services must be available to the whole population at risk, not just to those who usually demand services. The public health approach is to:

- Systematically design the clinical services;
- Decide what can be done best at the community, primary, and secondary levels of care;
- Provide evidence-based guidelines for diagnosis and case management;
- Strengthen systems such as the drug supply management and the district referral system for ensuring the patient receives the correct services at each level.

Maternal and neonatal and child health services (MNCH) involve all levels of the service from the traditional birth attendant or community midwife, the health centre, and the district hospital. Family planning prevents unwanted pregnancy and can reduce maternal mortality by a third. Further reductions depend on basic and emergency obstetric care. Emergency obstetric care depends on avoiding *three delays in*:

(i) Recognizing complications,

(ii) transport to a health facility, and

(iii) action at the health facility.

Emergency obstetric care (as with other emergency care) depends on a well-functioning referral system. This includes good communication and referral from the community level to health centre and hospitals (see Chapter 11, MNCH). *Child health* depends on ensuring good nutrition, education, and child development, as well as quality health services. Child health interventions include the management of diarrhoeal diseases, acute respiratory infections, malaria, and other infections, together with vaccination, vitamin supplementation, and education on home care. Child spacing saves child lives by providing more mother care time and breastfeeding, before the next child comes along. These are all now implemented as part of the 'integrated management of childhood illness' (IMCI) programme (see Chapter 11). Training and supervision for staff are based on standardized case management and the use of 'essential' drugs (Fig. 2.2).

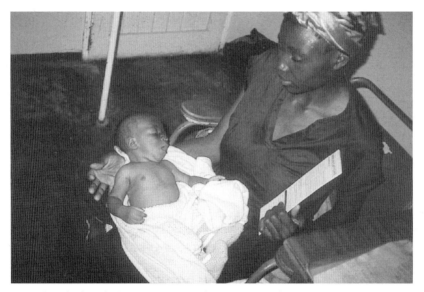

Fig. 2.2 Counting the breaths in one minute to detect pneumonia. . .

Communicable diseases are viral, bacterial, and parasitic diseases. Many of these are common, cause a high burden of disease but yet have cost-effective prevention and treatment available. Treating one person may prevent transmission to many others. Therefore, as in malaria, the clinical services as well as prevention are both key to controlling the disease. Similarly, for sexually transmitted diseases, treatment as well as prevention through education and condom promotion are important. As BCG is not very effective in preventing adult TB, treatment is the main means of control. Treating a person ill with infectious TB *disease* will prevent *infection* in many others. In these examples, ensuring early diagnosis and treatment is an important intervention benefiting both the currently sick and the general population. Delivery strategies may include strengthening the hospital, health centre, and home-based services. Activities may include ordering drug supplies, providing microscopes, and training of health workers. Health workers need to use evidence-based guidelines for common infections. Many countries have adapted the WHO 'Integrated Management of Adolescent-Adult Illness', which enables effective syndromic diagnosis and management in primary care and proper referral to hospital for severe cases. Care of HIV/AIDS includes treating opportunistic infections such as pneumonia, chronic diarrhoea, and candidiasis. Care includes preventing common infections by giving *co-trimoxazole* and (if active TB is excluded) *isoniazid* preventive treatment, as well as anti-retroviral treatment (ART) (see Chapters 13 and 14).

Non-communicable and chronic diseases include both acute and chronic diseases and injuries. Non-communicable disease control includes promotion of healthy policies, such as tobacco tax increases, smoke-free workplaces, and banning advertisements. Similarly, health promotion of exercise, and healthy low fat, high fruit, and vegetable diets is part of control of cardiovascular diseases. Most common conditions are best managed at the health centre, including the chronic care for asthma, diabetes, hypertension, epilepsy, and mental health (see Chapter 15). The more complicated cases may need to be referred to a hospital for investigation and initiation of treatment. However, they can be referred back for chronic care at their nearest health centre. Primary care facilities need to provide chronic care with regular appointments, education, and adherence support for patients – a service for people living with any of these diseases. The TB programme is a good example of a chronic disease programme. In Malawi, the TB care system has been adapted and extended for ART care. While in Swaziland, HIV/ART, diabetes, epilepsy, and mental health problems have been added to the chronic disease care service based on their community based TB programme. In chronic conditions, education on the condition is particularly important. They will need to adjust their lifestyle behaviours, for example, eating a healthy diet and adding more exercise into their daily life. Furthermore, the patients over time can become an 'expert' in their own condition. Health workers guide them to recognize significant changes in symptoms and adjust the dose of their medication accordingly.

Public health specialists work with health managers and practitioners to ensure services are designed and strengthened to deliver these essential clinical and preventive interventions.

Cost-effectiveness

Whether we are working in a high income or low income country, our health service will have to be provided within the budget allocated. This means that the cost effectiveness of alternative interventions is a very important public health issue.

When an intervention, such as a vaccine, is tested under 'ideal' research conditions, is the % reduction in incidence or severity of disease called the *efficacy*. The *effectiveness* of an intervention is how well it reduced the burden of disease under programme conditions (see examples in DCP2 in further reading below). The difference between efficacy and effectiveness is due to various operational factors which make the effect less in practice. For EPI the operational factors include maintaining the cold chain and transport.

Effectiveness is also influenced by cultural and social beliefs, for example whether sleeping under bednets is acceptable or not to the community.

Cost is a very important factor influencing our decisions on whether to include this or the other intervention (see Chapter 7, Health financing). If two interventions are equally effective but one is cheaper, then we will choose the cheaper intervention. If both interventions are the same cost we will choose the most effective. This applies to tests, drugs, vaccines, operations and other health interventions. Costs are influenced greatly by the level of care. An intervention, such as pneumonia or malaria treatment given in a hospital is usually costlier than the same given in a health centre. This is true the world over. However, in developing countries resources are particularly scarce. We have to make the most from the opportunity given by the limited resources we have. Of course, hospitals are still required, but used as a referral service for the complicated, rarer or more severe cases. While more common health problems including treating serious disease early before it is severe, is best done in health centres and community services.

Cost-effectiveness is greatest for primary prevention, then secondary prevention (screening and early treatment), and least for other tertiary prevention such as surgery. Of course surgery will always be needed for injuries and common problems such as appendicitis. However, prioritization of surgical services, as with medical services, needs to be done according to effectiveness and cost.

Interventions such as vaccination, ORS for diarrhoea, and TB treatment, cost only US\$ 1–5 per year of healthy life saved. For these reasons, communicable disease and MNCH services are priorities for public health.

If we spend money on one thing there is less for another. Economists call this the *opportunity cost*. We therefore have to make difficult decisions. We have to prioritize our limited resources. We should tackle those diseases with the most effective and least costly interventions and get the biggest improvement in health for our population, with the little we have.

Conclusion

Public health is concerned with improving the health of the population, rather than just the individuals seeking treatment. We must make appropriate health services available to the whole population, especially those at risk, as mentioned in Chapter 1.

Public health aims to prevent disease through health programmes. Some of these are within and others outside the health services. We are concerned with promoting health, such as for malaria and HIV education on the radio, and the marketing of bednets and condoms in the shops, while within health facilities we deliver services such as vaccination and malaria care.

Health services need to be prioritized, so that they tackle the causes of the greatest burden of disease using the most cost-effective interventions. The existing services can be systematically strengthened with supplies, guidelines, training, and supervision. New intervention strategies may be added if they are found by research and experience to be effective and feasible. Resources are limited and needs are great, so we must choose interventions which are both effective and affordable, when implemented across the whole district. We also need to choose for each intervention (e.g. bednets) the best delivery strategy and effectively implement according to the context in this way and achieving high coverage e.g. of children sleeping under bednets.

Moreover, we need to understand the community and their perception of ill health. We are concerned with providing services which are acceptable, accessible, and affordable to the community. To be successful we need to enable the community to participate in improving their own health. We need to involve the community in decisions about the health services. In addition, we need to involve other sectors, such as teachers and agricultural extension workers, for better nutrition. These are the strategies of PHC which are central to public health. We need to minimise climate change and protect the environment for the future of our children.

There are international and national programmes for the major diseases, such as the EPI led by WHO and UNICEF. These organizations provide documents which are adapted and used by national programmes. Guidelines and modules are included for managers, district coordinators, and health workers, for EPI, HIV/AIDS, tuberculosis, diabetes, mental health, and other diseases.

Further reading

Disease control priorities in a developing world (DCP2) (2006) World Bank/Oxford University Press, 2nd edition. http://www.dcp2.org/page/main/BrowseDiseases.html

Webber R, *Communicable disease epidemiology and control.* (2004) 2nd edition. CABI Publishing. Oxford (new edition due 2009).

World development report: investing in health. (1993) World Bank/Oxford University Press.

World Health Organization. *Health topics.* www.who.int/health topics.

World Health Organization. World Health Report 2008. http://www.who.int/whr/2008/en/

UNICEF (2008) 'Countdown to 2015'. *Maternal, neonatal and child survival: tracking progress in maternal, newborn and child survival.* http://www.childinfo.org/countdown.html

Chapter 3

Epidemiology in practice

John Wright

This chapter gives an overview of the following topics:

- What is epidemiology?
- How do we measure disease?
- Using rates in measuring disease;
- Describing disease in terms of time, place, and person;
- Defining cases and populations;
- Undertaking health surveys.

Epidemiology has always been an essential part of improving the health of populations. Its early use was in the study of infectious diseases and epidemics. Describing the distribution of an epidemic such as cholera allowed doctors to find out what was causing the epidemic. In recent years, epidemiology has been used more to find out what causes diseases such as heart disease and cancers. This has shown how factors such as diet, smoking and living conditions are important *risk factors* for causing disease. Epidemiology has also been used to find out what treatments are effective in reducing disease and ill-health.

Epidemiology is the study of the distribution and determinants of disease in human populations. It is concerned with:

- Describing which diseases occur in populations and the frequency with which they occur;
- Understanding the causes (determinants) of diseases.

Three approaches to epidemiology can be defined:

1 **Descriptive epidemiology.** This concerns the description of disease (where it occurs, when it occurs and who it occurs in). This can be as single cases of disease (case reports) or several cases (case series).

Examples: AIDS was first recognized after a case series of *pneumocystis carinii* pnuemonia in young men in the United States. Thalidomide was identified as the cause of birth defects after a case series was reported in women who had used the drug in pregnancy.

It can also be as a description of how frequent a disease is in a population (cross-sectional study) or between different populations (correlational study).

Example: A link between TB and AIDS was suspected after HIV infection was found to be common in patients with TB. A link between salt and hypertension was suspected after hypertension was found to be uncommon in developing countries with low salt diets, and common in Western countries with high salt diets.

2 **Analytical epidemiology.** This concerns the search for causes of disease. Two types of study allow an idea (or hypothesis) to be tested.

(a) Case control studies. People with a disease (cases) are compared with normal people (controls). This can show that if a suspected cause of the disease occurs more commonly in those with the disease than those without it.

Example: Smoking was shown to be a possible cause of lung cancer after smoking was found to be much more common in patients with lung cancer.

(b) Cohort studies. A group of people are studied over a period of time. Some may have been *exposed* to a suspected cause of disease and the others are not. If the disease occurs more commonly in those exposed to the suspected cause of disease, then this suggests that there is a link.

Example: A group of healthy middle-aged people was observed over 10 years. Those with high blood pressure were found to be more likely to suffer a stroke than those with normal blood pressure. This supported the suggestion that hypertension causes strokes.

3 **Evaluative epidemiology**. This concerns the study of how effective a treatment (or preventive measure) is. It uses intervention or clinical trials to find out how a disease can be treated or prevented. These are commonly *randomized controlled trials* to make sure the evaluation is objective or *unbiased*.

Health professionals will rarely take part in analytical or evaluative epidemiology studies. However, it is very important to understand them. When we choose a treatment for an individual patient we need to know if it will be *safe* and *effective*. When we choose a public health intervention for a population (for example health education, or a vaccine) information on their effectiveness is essential if we are to use resources efficiently. These studies provide the *evidence* for the treatments we use in health care. This will be discussed at the end of this chapter.

For district health teams, descriptive epidemiology will be their main approach. It allows health workers to describe and monitor the frequency and changing patterns of disease in the district. An understanding of these is essential to provide the necessary care and also take action to reduce the problem. It allows the *health needs* of a population to be identified so that health services can provide effective and equitable health care.

Defining a case and defining a population

Before patterns of disease can be described, the person with the disease (the *case*) must be defined. The absence of a common case definition will lead to confusion.

Example: In District A all people with a systolic blood pressure of greater than 150 mmHg are recorded as being hypertensive. In District B all people with a systolic blood pressure of 160 mmHg are recorded as being hypertensive. District A has a higher prevalence of hypertension than District B, but only because District B is using a stricter case definition, which does not include those people with a blood pressure of between 150–160 mmHg.

For some diseases, the case definition may be simple, for example, defining high blood pressure as being greater than 160 mmHg can be understood by all health workers. However, some diseases can be diagnosed with less certainty. If the case is defined by clear criteria then it is possible to describe how certain the diagnosis is. For example, pulmonary TB could be defined in three groups:

- Possible TB – patients with a 3-month history of cough and fever.
- Probable TB – patients who also have cavitating lesions on chest X-ray.
- Definite pulmonary TB – patients who also have acid fast bacilli (AFB) seen on stain or culture.

In addition to defining a case, it is important to recognize that there may be differences in how cases are detected or *ascertained*. Some cases will nearly always be detected, for example, deaths from suicide or patients with a fractured humerus. Others are less obvious and variations may be due to differences in case ascertainment (case finding) rather than real disease variation. The accuracy and quality of the reporting of cases should always be considered before comparisons are made.

Example: Schizophrenia is found to be twice as common in District A than District B. However District A has a psychiatric unit, whereas District B does not. It is likely that more cases are being detected in District A because services are better and more cases are detected.

In addition to clearly defining a case, it is important to clearly define the *population*. The population will be the denominator for producing a rate of disease. So if the population is inaccurate, the rate will be inaccurate. Definition can be in terms of geography, such as a district or region. It can also be by age or sex. Differences between populations in characteristics such as age and sex should be corrected by standardization before comparisons are made.

How do we measure disease?

District A reports that in the last year there have been 10 leprosy cases diagnosed. District B reports that in the last year there have been 15 leprosy cases diagnosed. Which district has the most leprosy? It would seem obvious that it must be District B. But then we find out that the population in District A is 100 000, and the population in District B is 300 000. So, although there are more *cases* of leprosy in District B, the disease is more common in District A because there are more *cases per head of population*. In epidemiology *rates* of disease are used rather than *numbers of cases*. Rates of disease describe the number of cases (the numerator) in proportion to the population at risk (the denominator) within a stated time period.

So the leprosy rate for District A is 10 cases/100 000 population
= 0.1 case per 1000 people [or 1 in 10 000]

The leprosy rate for District B is 15 cases/300 000 population
= 0.05 case per 1000 people [or 1 in 20 000]

Box 3.1 gives the definitions of rates which are commonly used in health care to describe the state of health of the population. Rates can be *crude* which use a total population as a denominator, or *standardized* for age and sex and other characteristics of a population. For example, the crude birth rate uses the total population as the denominator. This includes men, children, and post-menopausal women who obviously cannot contribute to the numbers of births. The fertility rate uses the number of the population of *women of childbearing age* as the denominator. This gives a more accurate rate to describe fertility.

The infant mortality rate is commonly used for comparing the health of populations. It is a marker of the general health and standard of living of populations, as it indicates the many different influences on health during the first year of life. The perinatal mortality rate is used as an indicator of antenatal care.

Q.   In 1997 the infant mortality rate for your country is 95 per 1000 total births. You look at your local registration of births and deaths and find that there were 14 000 births during 1997 and 1148 deaths of children under 1 year. Does your district have greater health problem than nationally?

A.   No. Your district Infant Mortality Rate (IMR) = 1148/14 000 = 82 per 1000 total births. This indicates that the health of infants in your district is better than in the country generally.

Figure 3.1 shows how different rates can be used to describe health in one region compared to the rest of the country. This also shows how important education and progressive social policies can be.

Box 3.1 Common examples of rates used to describe the health of a population

Crude Birth Rate (CBR)
This is the number of live births per 1000 total population per year. The denominator includes men, children, and women.
Example: In 1993 CBR for the UK = 14; for Mozambique = 45

General Fertility Rate (GFR)
This is the number of live births per 1000 women of child-bearing age (between the ages of 15–44) per year.
Example: In 1993 GFR for the UK = 64; for Mozambique = 240

Crude Death Rate (CDR)
This is the number of deaths occurring per 1000 total population per year.
Example: In 1993 CDR for the UK = 11; for Mozambique = 18

Infant Mortality Rate (IMR)
This is the number of infants (children less than 1 year old) who die during a stated year per 1000 live births.
Example: In 1993 IMR for the UK = 7; for Mozambique = 164

Perinatal Mortality Rate (PMR)
This is the number of stillbirths (deaths after the 28th week of pregnancy) plus the number of deaths in the first 7 days after birth, in a stated year per 1000 total births (live births plus stillbirths).
Example: In 1990 PMR for the UK = 5; for Mozambique = 108

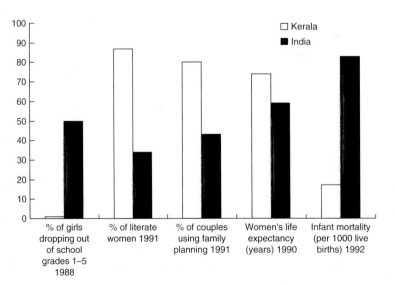

Fig. 3.1 Kerala compared with the rest of India.

Incidence and prevalence

The rates discussed above describe events such as births or deaths. There are two important ways of expressing them to describe *disease*.

+ **Prevalence** is the number of people with a disease (the cases) per total population. This can be at a defined period of time (*point prevalence*) such as a certain day. This provides a snapshot of the disease in the population. Less commonly, it is described over a defined period of time (*period prevalence = cases at start of period plus new cases during period*). Prevalence rates are useful in describing the burden of disease and planning the health service required to provide the necessary care and reduce this burden.

    Example: On 1st January 1997 there were 252 patients on the district TB register as having active TB. The population of the district is 300 000.

    So the Point prevalence = 252/300 000

    $$= 0.84 \text{ per 1000 population}$$

Box 3.2 shows the practical application of prevalence rates to case finding and its implications on health.

Box 3.2 Case finding in tuberculosis: An example of applying incidence rates to the district population

Case finding is identifying the people who become ill with tuberculosis – the incident cases – in the district. The following worked example refers to cases of *smear positive* pulmonary TB.

The WHO target, used in most countries, for new smear positive TB case finding is 70%

$$\text{Case finding (\%)} = \frac{\text{The actual number of cases}}{\text{The expected number of cases}} \ (\times 100)$$

The actual number of new TB cases can be counted in the district tuberculosis register.

But how do we know what number of people to expect?

The expected number is estimated by applying national rates to the local population, as follows:

+ Ask the national programme what the estimated annual risk of infection (found by testing the tuberculin reaction in school children) for the country.

+ The expected number of new (incident) sputum smear positive cases in a year will be the annual risk of infection × 50 per 100 000 of the population.

+ If your country has an annual risk of infection of 1.5, then the expected number is 1.5 × 50 = 75 per 100 000

+ If your district population is 200 000 then the expected number of TB cases will be 2 × 75 = 150

If there are only 75 new smear positive TB patients in the TB register in the last year then case finding = 75 ÷ 150 × 100 = 50%

Note the total TB cases is (100 per 100 000), that is, double the rate that of smear positive. Furthermore, prevalence of TB cases is roughly double that of incidence. However, in countries with a generalized HIV epidemic, the rates will be higher and this way of calculation doesn't work! This is because HIV positive people commonly develop active TB. Where available, use community survey data to make case finding estimates.

Box 3.2 Case finding in tuberculosis: An example of applying incidence rates to The district population (continued)

A case finding of 50% is not enough. Half of your TB cases are missed. Either they do not present at the health facilities, or more likely, when they do attend with a cough the health workers just give an antibiotic, forgetting to screen for TB. Indeed all patients with a cough more than 2–3 weeks should have 2 or 3 sputum smears sent for microscopy, that is, they should be screened for TB.

A sputum positive pulmonary TB case will on average spread the infection to another 10 people. Untreated half of these untreated cases will die. This should not happen as there is a cost-effective intervention available (TB chemotherapy).

Treatment outcomes. It is also important to achieve at least 85% case holding, this is calculated from the TB register in a similar way to the case finding above. The treatment outcome should have been written for each patient in the register. Count the number cured in the quarter ending a year ago (as all these patients should now have completed treatment). It is best also to look at the sputum results recorded to confirm that they were in fact cured – sputum smear positive patients who become negative at the 2-month sputum check and remain negative at the end of treatment. Divide the number cured by the number of all smear positive patients registered in that quarter. Cured/total smear positive × 100 = cure rate. Similarly calculate the other treatment outcomes; defaulted, died, relapsed. Also calculate these outcomes for all TB patients registered (pulmonary smear positive and negative and extra-pulmonary cases).

If the cure rate is not improving or less than 85% then review the TB service (see Chapter 5 and Chapter 14 'Control major communicable diseases'). Check the quality of care, in particular, the information and counselling given, treatment support in the community/family, supervision in the health facility, tracing of defaulters – that is look for the causes of poor case holding.

Monitoring. Case finding and treatment outcome results for each 3 months (quarter) are reported to the TB programme. The progress, or deterioration, in the results can be best seen by putting them on a graph – and displaying it on the wall in the health office. The results can be compared to other districts in the province. If you see the results are deteriorating or are not as good as other districts then take action.

- ◆ **Incidence** is the number of new cases of a disease in a specified period of time per total population. The period of time is usually 1 year, but can be any specified time. Incidence rates are useful in describing the occurrence of new cases. They are useful in monitoring trends and determining the cause of a disease. Incidence rates are also useful in setting targets for improving health and measuring effectiveness of treatments.

    Example: In 1997 there were 173 new cases of bilharzia. The population of the district is 300 000.

    The incidence of bilharzia in the district = 173/300 000 per year.

    $$= 0.58 \text{ per 1000 population per year.}$$

    Incidence measures just new cases. When a person develops a disease they can either recover or die. Prevalence measures all cases with a disease, whether newly diagnosed or nearly recovered, or nearly dead. The longer the duration of the illness, the greater the prevalence will be. Also the more new cases there are, the greater the prevalence will be. Figure 3.2 shows the relationship between incidence and prevalence. In acute infectious diseases, recovery

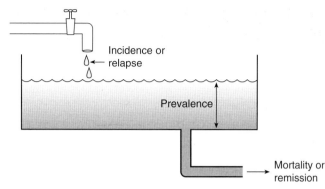

Fig. 3.2 Relationship between incidence and prevalence – the prevalence pool.

(or death) is usually rapid, so even if the incidence is great, the prevalence will be small. With most chronic diseases, recovery is rare (heart disease, diabetes etc.) or slow (TB), so even if the incidence is small, the prevalence will be great.

How do we describe disease?

Disease can be described in terms *time, place,* and *person.* This means when it occurs, where it occurs and who it occurs in.

Time – when?

Diseases can be described over the seasons of a year. This can show how certain health problems occur more commonly at different times of the year. Figure 3.3 shows the variation in admission rates for two diseases (malaria and malnutrition) to a district hospital during 1 year.

Diseases can be studied over shorter times. For example, an epidemic of cholera should be described in terms of days and weeks. Diseases can also be studied over longer times (secular changes). For example, the prevalence of AIDS in a district should be monitored yearly so that its impact on the population can be assessed and health services planned appropriately.

Place – where?

Patterns of disease can vary with geography. People may be more likely to become ill if they live in certain areas. For example, if they live in an area without clean water supplies, or if they

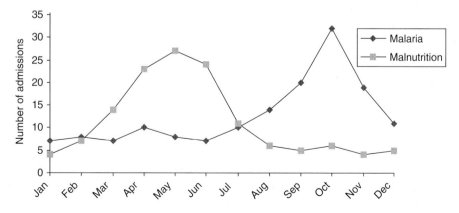

Fig. 3.3 Variation in hospital admissions over 1 year.

live in a town rather than rural dwelling. It is useful to think of three types of geographical variation:

(a) *International*. Comparison of diseases *between* countries can identify particular problems for an individual country.

(b) *National.* Comparison of diseases *within* a country can identify particular problems for an individual region.

(c) *Local*. Comparison of diseases within a region or district can identify particular local problems.

Person – who?

Certain groups of people may be more likely than others to develop a disease. If these people are to be identified then it is important to describe who they are. The common methods of describing people use the following variables: age, sex, ethnic group, occupation, social class and religious group. Most disease varies with age. Diseases also often vary with sex. Figure 3.4 shows this for admissions for accidents and violence at a district hospital.

Monitoring trends: Use of coverage charts

Cumulative coverage graphs are very useful for monitoring trends and progress, and giving an early warning of problems and the need for action to correct the problems. Most commonly they are used for monitoring vaccination coverage (see Futher reading for the downloadable EPI Mid Level Managers Course and Health Facility Manual, WHO). The coverage charts may be used for each vaccine, but are commonly used to monitor DPT3, and fully vaccinated children and the antenatal women receiving a full course of tetanus toxoid (TT). Coverage charts can also be used for other important health indicators, for example, number of women attending for her first (this pregnancy) antenatal (or attending the 4th), or women of fertile age (15–49 years) using modern contraceptives, etc. (Fig. 3.5).

Coverage charts can be used at the health facility level and district and higher levels. The vertical axis is 0–100%, and at the top right is the number of children under 1 year. This is the number if all (100%) children are vaccinated that year and this data can be obtained from national population census data (for example by using the birth rate data).

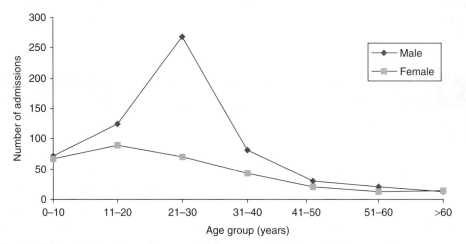

Fig. 3.4 1994 admissions for accidents and violence to a district hospital by age and sex.

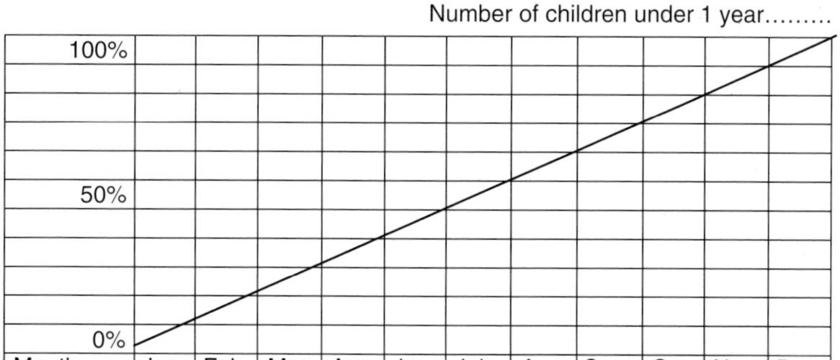

Number of children under 1 year.........

Fig. 3.5 Example of coverage graph.

Time in months (January to December) is used as the horizontal axis. Below this are recorded the number of children vaccinated that month, e.g. 25 in January. This number is taken from the health information/vaccination tally sheet where each vaccination is tallied (ticked off), or from a vaccination register. The boxes below these are for the cumulative number for that month (adding this month to the previous month cumulative total). For example, if 25 are vaccinated in January and 30 in February, then the cumulative number for February is 55. Ideally the cumulative total in December is the same as the number on the top right, which is 100% of children under 1 year.

Progress to meeting local targets can be monitored month on month and the trends displayed on a large version of the chart so that they can be easily seen by all staff involved and supervisors. If the cumulative total is falling well below the target line (and especially so if below 50%) then questions need to be asked why vaccination is below the numbers that should be happening. For example staff and parents can be asked as to about the service and why they are not attending to this task. This enquiry may uncover problems of vaccine ordering, of inconvenient service, long waiting times, non-daily vaccination service (not integrated), poor staff motivation, missed opportunities for vaccination, false contraindications, limited information given to parents, or cancellation of outreach EPI sessions. Further examples of problem analysis for EPI coverage are described in Chapter 5.

How to monitor using coverage graphs

Cumulative coverage graphs are very useful for monitoring progress, and giving an early warning of problems and the need for action to correct the problems.

Most commonly, these have been used for vaccination coverage (see reading list for the downloadable EPI Mid Level Managers course and Health Facility manual, WHO)

The vertical axis is 0–100%, and at the top right the number of children under 1 year. This is the number if all (100%) children are vaccinated that year. Many countries provide a percentage of the population under 1 year e.g. 2.5%. If not then you may get it from the population census data (is equivalent to the birth rate).

How to monitor using coverage graphs *(continued)*

On the horizontal axis are written the 12 months of the year, January to December. Below this are recorded the number of children vaccinated that month, e.g. 25 in January. This number is taken from the health information/vaccination tally sheet where each vaccination is tallied (ticked off), or from a vaccination register. The boxes below these are for the cumulative number for that month (adding this month to the previous month cumulative total). For example if 25 are vaccinated in January and 30 in February then the cumulative number for February is 55. Ideally the cumulative total in December is the same as the number top right, which is 100% of the under 1 year children.

Monitor the progress month by month. Best if a large version of the chart is displayed on the wall so is easily seen by all staff involved and the supervisors. From this chart, the progress close to the target line is seen. Or it is seen that the cumulative total is falling below well the target line (and especially so if below 50%) then questions need to be asked as to why vaccination is below the numbers that should be happening.

Ask the staff, ask waiting parents about the service, and people in the villages why they are not attending. For example there may be problems of vaccine ordering, of inconvenient service, long waiting times, non-daily vaccination service (not integrated), poor staff motivation, missed opportunities for vaccination, false contraindications, limited information given to parents, or cancellation of outreach EPI sessions. See also the EPI outreach example of using the 'but why' problem analysis method to understand the problem, in Chapter 5.

The coverage charts may be used for each vaccine, but are commonly used to monitor DPT3, and fully vaccinated children and the antenatal women receiving a full course of tetanus toxoid (TT).

Coverage charts can also be used for other important health indicators, e.g. number of women attending for her first (this pregnancy) antenatal (or attending the 4th), of women of fertile age (15–49 years) using modern contraceptives etc.

Health surveys

Some health information is available from routine sources such as hospital or census data. However routine sources are usually incomplete and lack detail, and so can provide only limited descriptions of disease. In order to provide more details, special surveys may be required. There are two main types of descriptive survey. *Prevalence* or cross-sectional surveys describe the prevalence of a disease and the characteristics of a population. This provides a 'snapshot' of health. *Longitudinal* surveys describe the incidence of disease by measuring the disease repeatedly over a period of time.

Surveys cost time and money. It is important to ensure that the information wanted is not available from routine sources. If a survey is necessary then it is important to undertake it properly. There are a number of issues to consider when undertaking a survey.

1 There should be a clear aim for the survey. What disease, or risk factor, is being measured? What is the case definition? What is the population of interest? It is important to make sure that something can be done to tackle any problems found by the survey. It is not fair to waste time and money and raise people's hopes if change is not possible.

2 Good planning is needed. Staff will be needed to carry out the survey and they will need to be trained. Resources will also be needed to cover the costs of administering the survey (postage, petrol, printing of questionnaires) and producing a report.

3 The sample size for the survey must be calculated. It is frustrating to carry out a survey of 100 people only to find one case. Estimates of expected prevalence can be made using surveys from previous times or other regions. This will guide the investigator as to how many people will need to be surveyed to find enough cases.

4 Recruitment of the sample must be considered. If the sample consists of volunteers then it is not likely to be representative of the true population. To reduce bias, a sample can be chosen *randomly* (basically tossing a coin to let chance decide who is selected) or *systematically* (e.g. every fifth outpatient, or every tenth hut). These methods need a *sampling frame* from which to select the sample. This is a list of people from the population of interest. A sampling frame can be a list of names from a local census, or a list of villages in an area. In order to select a random sample, a table of random numbers should be used. These tables are available in most statistics books. Alternatively, random numbers can be generated from computer databases such as Excel. For a low prevalence disease, for example 1% prevalence, then the sample size may need to be large, e.g. 2000, for the accuracy to be high and sampling error low. Advice on sample sizes can be obtained from appropriate books on statistics.

    Cluster samples are commonly used because they are simple and quick. An example is the '30 clusters of 7' where 30 villages are randomly chosen and in each village 7 households or people are again randomly chosen. This method has been used to estimate immunization coverage, but with a sample size of 210, it can be used to measure common health problems.

5 The measuring *instrument* must be carefully chosen. This can be a questionnaire, or a physical measure such as weight and height. For a questionnaire, questions should be simple, reliable and culturally sensitive. Leading questions must be avoided (e.g. do you think that TB is caused by AIDS?) and interviewers must take care not to influence the answers. It is important to try out (*pilot*) a questionnaire before it is used. This will allow some practice for interviewers and identify questions that are not clear.

6 It is important to achieve a high *response rate* (>80%). If there are lots of people not at home during a household survey then the results from those who are surveyed may not be representative of the local population. For example, a high rate of adult ill-health may be found because all the healthy adults were away at work.

7 Results can be *coded* so that they can be analysed easier. This involves translating information such as questionnaire responses into numbered categories for data entry. Epi info – see Box 3.3 – is a simple computer programme which can allow simple coding and analysis for results.

Box 3.3 Epi info

Epi info is a software package developed by the Centre for Disease Control in the United States. It allows easy questionnaire design (EPED), data processing, and analysis. The analysis module provides a user-friendly statistical package. It is considered public domain and may be freely copied. Its simplicity and free availability make it ideal for researchers in developing countries. (Contact: The Division of Surveillance and Epidemiologic Studies, Epidemiology Programme Office, Centers for Disease Control, Atlanta, Georgia 30333, USA).

Evaluative epidemiology: Do treatments work?

One of the key principles of a good quality health service is that medical and healthcare interventions should be effective. Effectiveness describes the extent to which treatments (such as drugs, operations, or counselling) improve health outcomes of patients in clinical practice. Most patients, and indeed doctors, assume that everything we do in clinical practice is effective – why else would we be doing it? However, it has been estimated that up to 80% of medical interventions are of uncertain benefit and continue as rituals of practice more through history than science.

In order to find out if a treatment is effective we need to evaluate its benefit (or harm) in a clinical trial. This can be a trial on a single patient, for example giving a patient with a sore throat some antibiotics and following them up the next week. This anecdotal observation is often the basis of decision-making in our clinical practice. If the patient returns the next week and reports that they feel greatly improved, it may be tempting to pat yourself on the back for your healing skills; however, there are a number of explanations that may account for her improvement.

1 Temporal changes. Sore throats are self-limiting diseases and will resolve with or without antibiotics. Similarly a relapsing and remitting disease such as arthritis may get better without any treatment.

2 Placebo effect. Every drug can exert a placebo effect, and every doctor can exert a halo effect to improve the reported health of patients. Not only can placebos lead to improvements in health outcomes, but patients will report side effects from these inactive preparations. Drug companies are never shy of advertising that 30% of patients got better on their new Fabulosa drug, but rarely admit that 20% got better on the chalk tablets in the control group.

3 Reporting bias. Patients will often report improvement to the doctor because that is what they think s/he wants to hear, and does not want to disappoint. The doctor on the other hand can exert an observation bias by recording clinical improvement in line with their prior prejudice.

Randomized controlled trials

Historically, clinical practice relied heavily on anecdotal evaluations. However, in 1948, the first randomized controlled trial was performed to find out whether or not streptomycin was effective in curing tuberculosis.

In randomized controlled trials, patients are randomized to two groups. One group receives the new treatment the other (the placebo control group) receives the old treatment or a placebo (dummy treatment). Random allocation of patients to the two groups prevents any bias or favouritism about who receives the new treatment. The control group allows the researchers to see what happens to patients not receiving the new treatment and so calculate the true benefit (effectiveness) of the new treatment. This allows us to measure temporal and placebo effects.

Example: Diazepam and phenytoin have been traditional treatments for pregnant women with eclampsia. However a randomized controlled trial involving hospitals in Africa, India, and South America showed that magnesium sulphate saved more lives than using diazepam or phenytoin.

Some interventions are so dramatically or obviously effective that observation can be sufficient to confirm benefit. For example, when penicillin was first evaluated in North Africa in the second World War medics gave it to the most severely ill patients and the healthier patients acted as controls. It was so effective that despite this selection bias in favour of the control group, the penicillin group had a lower mortality rate. Other interventions such as general anaesthesia or cardiopulmonary resuscitation are so dramatic in their effect that more rigorous trials are not necessary (or ethically feasible).

Box 3.4 Randomized controlled trials

a *Importance of a placebo effect*

Gastric freezing became a popular treatment for duodenal ulcer in the 1960s after it was shown to relieve pain in a case series of 31 patients. A subsequent placebo-controlled trial showed that the same proportion of patients in the placebo group obtained relief of their pain due to the psychological effect of the procedure.

b *Importance of choosing the right outcome*

In the 1980s patients with frequent ventricular atopics after a heart attack were found to have a high risk of death and a randomized controlled trial showed that anti-arrhythmic drugs flecainide and enconide reduced the frequency of these ectopics. After these had been put into widespread clinical practice, a subsequent randomized controlled trial showed that patients who received these drugs actually had a greater risk of dying than those who didn't. Clinical and patient-based outcomes should be used rather than physiological outcomes.

c *Importance of observation bias*

Laproscopic colosystectomy has been in a number of randomized controlled trials to lead to shorter stays in hospital and a quicker return to work. In the 1990s a trial attempted to introduce blinding by separating the surgeon in the theatre from the surgeon making the decision on the wards. All the patients were given large, blood-stained bandages to prevent the surgeon on the ward identifying who had had keyhole surgery. No difference was found in post-operative duration of stay or speed of return to work controlled trials to lead to shorter stays in hospital and a quicker return to work.

Many people would consider the randomized controlled trial as one of the greatest contributions to healthcare over the last 50 years. It provides us with the best trial evidence and has allowed us to confirm the effectiveness of many existing and new treatments, and confirmed the uselessness of others (Box 3.4).

Systematic reviews

Since the first in 1948 there have been almost a million randomized controlled trials evaluating thousands of different medical interventions. Settings range from Bradford to Borneo with many variations of patients included and the exact type of treatment given. Many of these trials have been small and have not had the statistical power to provide a definitive treatment effect. Many lie unpublished or lost in obscure journals. Some will show benefit from a particular treatment, whereas others may show harm.

If we are to find out whether or not a treatment is effective then we need to summarize the evidence from these different trials. Traditional reviews of the published evidence have usually relied on experts or researchers in the field to tell us the answer. This method has two main weaknesses however. Firstly the expert reviewer may have a particular prejudice or prior belief. They may want to push their own contribution to the research evidence as the answer, or want to put down rivals. They may want to canvass for funding for a particular research project that comes out of their conclusions. Secondly, when they search library databases such as Medline, they may miss trials. Trials that show no effect may not end up being published in journals and sitting in

Box 3.5 Example of a systematic review

Background: Antibiotic treatment of salmonella infections is commonly used to shorten illness and prevent serious complications.

Objectives: A systematic search of the research literature for clinical trials was undertaken to assess the effects of antibiotics in adults and children with diarrhoea who have salmonella.

Main results: Twelve trials involving 778 participants (with at least 258 infants and children) were included. There were no significant differences in length of illness, diarrhoea or fever between any antibiotic regimen and placebo. Relapses were more frequent in those receiving antibiotics, and there were more cases with positive cultures in the antibiotic groups after 3 weeks.

Conclusions: There appears to be no evidence of a clinical benefit of antibiotic therapy in otherwise healthy children and adults with non-severe salmonella diarrhoea. Antibiotics appear to increase adverse effects and they also tend to prolong salmonella detection in stools.

(Sirinavin, S. Garner, P. Cochrane Database of Systematic Reviews 2000)

the researcher's desk drawer. Other trials may be published in a non-English language that the reviewer does not understand, and so be ignored.

So many traditional reviews end up being haphazard and biased, and it has been shown that the majority have inappropriate or misleading conclusions. *Systematic reviews* have developed from the recognition that summaries of the evidence need to be objective and unbiased. They use careful methods to find all relevant trials and ensure that they are summarized objectively. The results of these reviews can then be used to provide a valid basis for informing clinical practice and identifying gaps in the research that should be addressed in future trials.

The Cochrane Collaboration is a group of health professionals and researchers who are trying to summarize all of the nearly one million clinical trials that have been carried out. The systematic reviews of these are published on the web www.theCochraneLibrary.com to form a single source of reliable evidence about the effectiveness of health interventions (Box 3.5).

Further reading

Barker, D.J.P. and Rose, G. (1991) *Epidemiology in medical practice*. Churchill Livingstone. London.

Vaughan, J.P. and Morrow, R.H. (1989) *Manual of epidemiology for district health management*. World Health Organization. Geneva.

EPI mid level managers course. Downloaded from: http://www.afro.who.int/ddc/vpd/epi_mang_course/index.html and "*Increasing immunisation coverage at the health facility level*, http://www.who.int/immunization_delivery/systems_policy/www721.pdf

Chapter 4

Assessing health needs

John Wright

This chapter gives an overview of the following topics:

♦ Health needs and the importance of assessing these needs;

♦ The steps to take when assessing health needs;

♦ What routine data can be used in assessing health needs?

♦ Using community appraisals to find out what local people's needs are.

♦ Assessing health needs in an emergency situation.

Most health workers are used to assessing the health needs of their own patients. Professional training and clinical experience teach them a systematic approach to this assessment before they start a treatment. Such a systematic approach has often been missing when it comes to assessing the health needs of a local population.

The health needs of patients coming through the clinic door may not reflect the wider health needs of the community. This difference between individual needs and the wider needs of the community is important to consider when planning and providing local health services. If they are ignored then there is a danger of a top down approach. This can lead to health services being provided on the basis of what a few people think to be the needs of the population rather than what they actually are (Fig. 4.1).

There are only limited resources available for health care but ever-increasing ways that they can be used. At the same time many individuals have unequal access to adequate health care, and many governments are unable to provide it for everyone. The health care resources that are available must be used carefully in order to provide the greatest possible improvement in the health of the population. It is essential therefore that the true health needs of the population are identified and addressed.

Health needs

The World Health Organization's definition of health is often used: 'Health is a state of complete physical, psychological and social well-being and not simply the absence of disease or infirmity.' (WHO 1946). This is an idealistic definition and a difficult one to achieve.

Health care needs are those needs which can benefit from health care (health education, disease prevention, diagnosis, treatment, rehabilitation, terminal care). Most health workers will consider needs in terms of health care services that they can supply. Patients however may have a different view of what would make them healthier, for example a job, a bus route to the hospital or health centre, or decent housing.

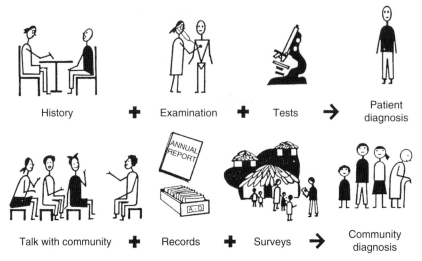

Fig. 4.1 Clinical diagnosis and community diagnosis compared.

Health needs covers the wider social and environmental determinants of health such as deprivation, housing, diet, education, employment. This wider definition allows us to look beyond the confines of services to the wider influences on health (genetic, environmental, and behavioural) (Fig. 4.2).

Health needs assessment

The historical development of health services has also been dominated by Western models of health care and health beliefs. These have rarely taken into account how local people explain illness or seek advice. This may involve consideration of traditional beliefs about illness and reliance on traditional healing methods.

However, assessment of health needs is not simply a process of listening to patients or relying on personal experience. It is a systematic method of identifying unmet need and making changes to meet this unmet need. In public health it is the needs of the *population*, for example of the district or of women of childbearing age, that need to be assessed (Box 4.1) (Fig. 4.3).

Box 4.1 A framework of questions to consider when assessing health needs

- What is the problem? (Who? When? Where? see Chapter 2)
- What has caused the problem?
- What are the current services? (see Chapter 4)
- What do people want?
- What are the most appropriate and cost effective solutions? (see Chapter 4)
- What are the resource implications on health care or other services?
- What are the outcomes to evaluate change and measure success?

Influences on Health

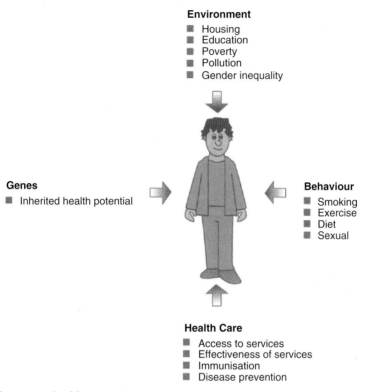

Environment
- Housing
- Education
- Poverty
- Pollution
- Gender inequality

Genes
- Inherited health potential

Behaviour
- Smoking
- Exercise
- Diet
- Sexual

Health Care
- Access to services
- Effectiveness of services
- Immunisation
- Disease prevention

Fig. 4.2 Influences on health.

If health services are to address the changing health needs of their local populations, then planners and managers need useful and timely information about the health status of these populations. Some of this information can come from routine data sources or be collected from large, one-off population studies such as surveys. Some information can be obtained from patient surveys.

Health needs assessment provides the opportunity for:

- describing the patterns of disease in the local population and the differences from district, regional, or national disease patterns.

- learning more about the needs and priorities of the local population.

- finding out the areas of unmet need and providing a clear set of objectives to work towards to meet these needs.

- deciding how best to use resources to improve their local population's health in the most effective and efficient way (see Chapter 7).

There is no easy, quick-fix recipe for health needs assessment. Different topics will require different approaches. This may involve a combination of surveys and interviews to collect original information, or adapting and transferring what is already known or available.

Example: One of the public health nurses reports that there seems to be an increase in the numbers of children with malnutrition in villages on a large sugar plantation area. What do you do?

1 *What is the problem?* The first step is to confirm the nurse's suspicion of a rise in the number of malnourished children in these villages. How is she diagnosing malnutrition? Weight-for-age charts – reliable and accurate.

2 *What is the size and nature of the problem?* Seven children under the age of five. There has been a rise in the number of cases over the past 12 months. Neighbouring (non-plantation) villages have had no cases reported during this time and the district has seen no rise in reported cases. (The problem is now described in terms of time, place, and person.)

   Interviews with mothers in the villages find that most are working at the rubber plantation during the day. The children are being bottle-fed and looked after in a nursery where hygiene is poor. Diarrhoea is common.

3 *What are the current services?* A monthly visit from the public health nurse.

4 *What do patients want?* The mothers want maternity leave, and then to return to work, but not to the harm of their children.

5 *What is the most appropriate and effective solution? Negotiate (longer) maternity leave. Also* better training of the nursery attendants in feeding, hygiene practices and nutrition.

6 *What are the outcomes to evaluate change?* Follow up weight-for-age monitoring. Incidence of diarrhoea in children.

Routine information

Chapter 3 showed how rates such as incidence, prevalence, and death rates can be used to describe disease in terms of time, place, and person. This information about diseases or use of health services can help to build up a picture of the health needs of a local population. Such epidemiological information can come from national, regional, or local sources. This can identify what the health problems are and what health services are needed to tackle these problems.

The starting point for any assessment of health needs is to find out what information is already available. This may be information from previous surveys or examination of routinely collected health information. When using routine information it is important to question how *accurate* it is; how *complete* it is; how *up-to-date* it is. Sources of information about the prevalence of disease include:

1 National census data can provide information on the age and sex distribution of a population. Social and economic indicators such as literacy levels, housing conditions, and education can provide information on the factors which influence health. Most developing countries conduct population census surveys about once every ten years.

2 Death certification and registers can provide information on the cause and place of death. Medical certificates of the cause of death usually record (i) direct cause of death and (ii) underlying illness which may have contributed to (i). Although information on deaths is usually accurate, it only describes the most severe cases of disease.

3 Disease notification systems can provide information on important infectious diseases. This can be useful in monitoring potentially epidemic diseases such as typhoid, cholera or meningitis.

4 Hospital inpatient records can be used to obtain numbers of admissions, cause of admission, length of stay. One way of presenting this information is to list the top ten most common diseases (see Chapter 1).

5 Outpatient consultations for numbers and diagnoses.

Health needs assessment includes information on existing interventions strategies and their coverage rates. Data sources for coverage of interventions may be available for health facility catchment areas, districts, provinces, and/or nationally. These include:

1 Maternal health information can include: contraceptive prevalence rates; unmet need for family planning; antenatal care uptake (proportion of mothers with four or more visits); maternal ages and parity; proportion of mothers with skilled attendants at delivery; numbers of low birth weight (less than 2500 g) babies; maternal mortality rates; proportion of mothers initiating breastfeeding early (within one hour of birth).

2 Child health indicators can include: infant mortality rates; immunization rates (measles or DPT uptake); proportion of children sleeping under insecticide-treated bednets (country data is included in the countdown to 2015 report, see further reading and other WHO documents);

3 Pharmacy information (use of essential and non-essential drugs).

4 Laboratory tests (e.g. positive sputum samples for TB, numbers of positive malaria blood slides).

5 Nutritional surveillance surveys may provide information on weight-for-height; weight-for-age or mid-upper-arm-circumference; exclusive breastfeeding rates (6 months); vitamin A supplementation rates.

6 Water and sanitation using data about the proportion of the population with access to drinking water sources and sanitation facilities.

When considered in isolation this information provides a snapshot of a population's health and status of intervention strategies. However, without comparative information, this will be of limited use in planning health services. Comparison can be with other populations (national or regional) or with the same population over time.

Comparison with other populations can identify specific health problems. However, care should be taken to correctly interpret differences which may exist for a number of reasons:

◆ Geographical (low incidence of malaria in a mountainous region compared to a low lying region)

◆ Social (higher incidence of HIV in urban compared to rural areas)

◆ Environmental (higher incidence of gastroenteritis in areas with poor water supplies)

◆ Provision of health services (higher reporting of disease due to better provision and access of health care facilities)

Comparison with the same population over time is a powerful method of monitoring health trends, identifying epidemics, intervention coverage trends, and planning health services to meet future needs.

Using reports from hospitals or clinics may just identify the tip of an iceberg of disease. People with disease who do not attend will be ignored. The other disadvantages of routine information are that it is often inaccurate and out of date. For example, outpatient records may only give the main complaint of patients attending, and will not distinguish new patient visits from repeat visits. Notifiable diseases may be missed and when they are picked up they are often not reported. It is also difficult to generalize to a local population. For example, people who attend a hospital are more likely to be more affluent and urban. Specially commissioned studies can provide more detailed, relevant and accurate information on a specific topic (see Box 4.2) but are often time-consuming and costly (Fig. 4.3).

Box 4.2 Health needs of patients with tuberculosis in southern Africa

Background: Rural African district with increasing numbers of patients with TB, rising incidence of HIV, and overcrowding at district hospital.

Objective of needs assessment: to describe changes in incidence of TB, attitudes of patients to treatment and effectiveness of service delivery.

Methods: Epidemiological data collected from review of national health data for TB and HIV, and from TB register. Interviews with patients and health professionals. Observation of TB clinic attendances. Review of current TB service and comparison with international models.

Results: Increase in incidence from 151 per 100,000 in 1993 to 280 in 2003 (86%) with resultant pressure on hospital beds. Increase highest in young males. Poor levels of knowledge about importance of completion of treatment and links with HIV. Poor communication in clinic about importance of compliance and attendance. Incomplete TB register with 33% of patients lost to follow-up. Most cost-effective model of service provision identified as community based TB care (DOTS).

Outcomes: Strengthening of TB register. Appointment of TB nurse to improve monitoring and health education. Establishment of community based, directly observed therapy TB programme in collaboration with National TB programme.

Community appraisals

Traditional epidemiological and questionnaire surveys (see Chapter 1) can be time-consuming and expensive. Community appraisals are assessments which try to involve the local people more. The assessors support and facilitate community action rather than just record information.

The information collected in these appraisals is used to develop acceptable and sustainable programmes in partnership with the community. These may be programmes of health care, nutrition or family planning that improve services for the community. The same methods can be used to monitor and evaluate the developments.

Community appraisals can provide a number of benefits:

- They can provide accurate and timely information about a health programme or one part of it;
- They are a practical tool that requires little additional resources and uses local expertise;
- They can provide information on health status, knowledge, attitudes, and behaviours of local people;
- They give communities the opportunity to participate in health planning and establish ongoing relationships with health workers;
- They allow the opportunity for team building and development and for staff to appreciate the strengths and weaknesses of services;
- They provide a foundation for more extensive quantitative assessments, e.g. surveys to find out the incidence and prevalence or death rates from a disease.

The methods used for these surveys and appraisals can include simple data extraction and questionnaires (see example of AIDS – Box 4.3). However there is a greater use of more *qualitative* techniques of interviewing and listening to people (see Box 4.4).

Box 4.3 Questionnaire survey AIDS knowledge

This survey was undertaken in a rural African health centre. Seventy consecutive adult outpatients were interviewed. The survey found that most people had heard of AIDS, through a variety of sources. Many of the informants believed that witchcraft was a major cause of AIDS and that traditional healers could cure the illness. The results also identified a fatalistic outlook on avoiding the disease, particularly among many women who felt they could not alter their husbands' promiscuity or reluctance to use condoms. These results enabled the planning and implementation of a local health education campaign to tackle misconceptions and identify coping strategies.

Knowledge and health seeking behaviour about AIDS
District: Village: Interviewer: Respondent Name: Respondent Number:
Have you heard of AIDS?　　　Y/N
Where have you heard about it? 　Friends/Family/Partner/Radio/Newspapers/Health workers/Posters/Other
How can you catch AIDS?
Is there a cure for AIDS?
How can you avoid catching AIDS?

Box 4.4 Steps in community appraisal

- Define aims of appraisal
- Identify community for assessment
- Identify study team and train in qualitative techniques
- Examine available information
- Define key questions and issues
- Pilot questions in interviews or questionnaires
- Identify key informants
- Choose and use appropriate methods
- Analyse information after each interview
- Write report and develop action plan

The assessors need to have good listening skills, a recognition that communities know their own needs, and common sense in analysing the results. Some training is necessary to provide the assessors with these skills.

This should emphasize the importance of accuracy and quality in undertaking and reporting appraisals (see Box 4.5). Training may include:

- how to design a survey form (see AIDS example);
- how to select the sample subjects;
- how to conduct interviews and focus groups (see below);
- how to pick out the key points from each interview and summarize these in the results;
- how to present results and write a report (see Box 4.6).

Assessors must also beware of generating false hopes in the community for what can be achieved.

The choice of sample for questionnaires or interviews will determine how *generalizable* the results are. If the subjects are not representative of the local population then this sampling can be done randomly, systematically (e.g. every fifth house in a village) or purposefully by selecting experts or *key informants* (see Box 4.7).

Interviews: these allow people the opportunity to give their own answers to open-ended questions. Interviews can be *structured* with a standard list of questions, *or semi-structured*, with just a list of topics that need to be covered. It is important not to bias the replies by the way questions are asked. For example 'Why is breast milk good?' implies that breast milk is good. 'What a lovely plump baby. Is he growing well with breast milk?' also introduces your own bias into the question. A more open-ended and unbiased question would be, 'Why are you giving your baby breast milk?' Follow-up questions should be used to encourage the informant to expand on simple or

Box 4.5 Methods of community appraisal

- Summarizing existing information from routine sources or previous surveys. *Example: causes of morbidity and mortality (see pie chart).*
- Exit interviews (interviewing patients after they come out of clinic) to obtain the patient's perspective on the quality of care and understanding of the health messages received. *Example: children with diarrhoea – checking that their mothers understand how to make up ORS.*
- Interviews with health worker. *Example: to assess their perception of local needs.*
- Ranking of priorities or preferences. *Example: asking local people to list their needs and then ranking these to produce a league table of needs.*
- Case note review and audit. *Example: examining the recording of tasks and health education given to patients.*
- Household survey to assess family health needs. *Example: seasonal variation in food intake and accessibility to clean water.*
- Focus group discussion to obtain the opinions of a specific population group. *Example: see below.*
- Direct observation of chosen indicators or behaviours. *Example: the performance of health workers in communication or clinical skills.*

Box 4.6 Example: Community appraisal of the factors affecting participation in nutrition, health and development in commercial farms in Zimbabwe

The workers and their families on commercial farms were one of the most disadvantaged in Zimbabwe. A Farm Health Programme was operating for 15 years in Mashonaland Central Province. This was a comprehensive PHC programme training farm health workers, monthly outreach and community including maternal and child health, family planning, preschool, nutrition, water and sanitation activities. Malnutrition in under-5 children was more common on the communal farms than elsewhere. Hence the need for a better understanding of the factors influencing nutrition, health and development.

Eight farms, ranging from well- to under-developed were selected. Permission to do the study was requested. On each farm the commercial farmer or representative was interviewed.

Participants for group discussions groups of 6–8 female, male workers with pre-school children, and seasonal workers were recruited randomly.

The research investigated:

◆ knowledge, attitudes, and practices relating to health

◆ felt needs, priority problems, opportunities, and solutions

◆ factors affecting communication

◆ factors affecting participation in health activities

◆ factors likely to assist or hinder an intervention programme

Results

Child nutrition was not viewed as a priority problem by farm workers or farm owners. Farm workers cited poor working conditions, working hours, low salaries, and lack of family food. Child health care came much lower on the priority rankings.

The workers were a fragmented community with no sense of belonging to a group. There was a tension between permanent workers, with better conditions, and seasonal workers.

An unhealthy child was described as being dirty, sick, thin, eating cold food, and having a pot-belly, and is miserable. Contributory factors included parental fighting, inadequate food, sickness, lack of child care at home or at pre-school.

Issues likely to influence participation *negatively* included *zvondo* – jealousy and mistrust amongst women. For example, not organizing a cooking roster for the pre-school, as they don't want the woman whose turn it is to cook to benefit from the food. Another example is past poor response by the commercial farmer to their efforts – having dug toilet pits, the farmer failed to provide cement and a builder to finish the job.

superficial replies (such as yes and no). However these questions should not become threatening. Patience is required; the interviewer should not be afraid of using pauses. Interruptions on the other hand, should be avoided.

Focus group: this involves a discussion with a small group of similar individuals (the ideal number is 8) on a specific topic (e.g. AIDS). It can provide insights into the attitudes, beliefs, and behaviours of a given population. An assessor guides the group of selected informants through

Box 4.7 Who to talk to? Key informants

- ◆ patients with a specific health problem
- ◆ chiefs, elders, or other community leaders
- ◆ church leaders
- ◆ shop keepers
- ◆ health workers
- ◆ government officials
- ◆ non-government organizations

a framework of questions that aim to stimulate discussion and communication of opinions. An assistant takes notes of the discussion for later analysis.

Ideally, a combination of methods should be used when assessing health needs (see Box 4.8), e.g. analysis of routine health data plus a questionnaire or focus group. This allows for cross-checking of the accuracy of results and increases their relevance or generalizability to the study population. Routine population data can be unhelpful and inaccurate, however it does allow a *quantitative* (numbers of cases) comparison with other population data. A small number of interviews may not provide opinions that represent those of the whole community; however, provided the subjects are chosen carefully, they do allow an understanding of what people really want.

Language and literacy barriers may occur when discussing complex health issues. A variety of techniques can be used to overcome these barriers in non-literate populations (see Box 4.9).

Box 4.8 Example of combining different methods of needs assessment

Bacterial and tuberculous meningitis are important causes of death and disability in developing countries despite the availability of effective treatment.

Epidemiological assessment: A national study was undertaken to describe the frequency of meningitis and the survival rate of patients admitted to hospital. The overall death rate was found to be 42% in all ages and 63% in adults. Cases were more common in periods of drought and AIDS was found to be an increasing underlying cause of cases. The study showed which age groups were being affected and what types of meningitis were being found. This allowed an assessment of the benefits of immunization programmes.

Community appraisal: Interviews were carried out on a random sample of mothers attending a health centre. A focus group discussion was conducted with a purposefully (specially chosen) selected group of health workers. These interviews found that the mothers had little understanding about symptoms. Health workers did not realize the importance of prompt referral and treatment.

Action: An effort was made to reduce the high death rate from meningitis by reducing delays in treatment. A coordinated education campaign for the public and health workers was undertaken using posters and outreach teaching sessions.

Box 4.9 Visually based methods of community appraisal

- Community mapping, where local people make maps in the ground to show the location of important local features such as water, clinics, hospitals, or the distribution of groups most at risk.
- Body mapping can be used to determine understanding of health and disease.
- Seasonal calendars, where different periods of the year are described, to show the complex relations between health and illness and annual changes in rainfall, housing conditions, food and other factors.
- Flow diagrams where connections are made with arrows to illustrate health beliefs and behaviours, e.g. what contributes to an individual's health and what choices they have when they become sick.
- Venn/chappati diagrams where overlapping circles are used to map out relationships within a community, e.g. between individuals, groups or organizations when dealing with mental health or AIDS.
- Plays in which the audience are encouraged to interrupt and participate in thinking of solutions to health problems and practising these in a 'rehearsal'.

These visually based methods provide opportunities for local people to explore and analyse their needs in their own terms.

Emergency needs assessment

Quick decisions and actions are vital after a disaster. The immediate, life-supporting needs after any major disaster are similar whether the cause is drought, flood, earthquake or war (see Box 4.9). Information must be obtained not only from government or other agencies (including, increasingly, the international media), but also from the affected community. This community will be able to help itself and any disaster response should build on these capacities (Box 4.10).

Involving the community is important in assessing the effects of the disaster and helping those most at risk (young children, the elderly, pregnant women). It is also vital to avoid cultural problems. For example, a famine relief programme ran into problems because the affected population, used to a staple of white maize, had strong traditional beliefs that the yellow maize being distributed was inedible and poisonous.

Box 4.10 Immediate needs

- Clean and adequate water and sanitation
- Food
- Shelter – including clothing and blankets
- Essential medical care
- Safety – from violence and harassment

The UNHCR have developed a simple needs assessment tool called "people-orientated planning" to help guide decisions about refugee needs (Which foods should be supplied? How should they be distributed? Who should live where? What are the critical medical needs? What are the cultural patterns of health care? How are target groups best reached?) This is approached through an analysis of the refugee population profile (numbers of children, pregnant women, elderly, undernourished etc.), activities and use of resources.

In addition to considering immediate needs, it is important to plan for the future. A community dependent entirely on donor food supplies will be in danger when these are withdrawn and normal food production is still disrupted. Good *surveillance systems* are also vital to report and monitor health and malnutrition. For example, surveys of children in refugee camps or outreach clinics, measuring weight for height or mid-upper arm circumference, can provide valuable nutritional assessments. Monitoring of infectious diseases such as measles can prompt timely immunizations.

Acting on the assessment

The hardest part of any needs assessment is translating the results into policies and practices which will provide beneficial change. The involvement of health workers in techniques such as rapid or rural appraisal will encourage changes at an individual level. Local workshops can provide an opportunity to review the lessons learnt to other health workers. If this change is going to last and be responsive to new needs, then the appraisal should be a continuous process which provides up-to-date feedback. Implementation of strategic changes (e.g. deciding how health resources are used) can be helped if the policy-makers themselves are actively involved.

Factors that will increase the effectiveness of needs assessments in securing change include:

- Careful planning and preparation with clear aims and objectives;
- Consideration of the potential resource implications of the assessment from the beginning (discussion between commissioners and assessors);
- Methodological rigour to ensure the results are valid and believed;
- Ownership of the project by relevant stakeholders from the start and effective communication during the work;
- Involvement of decision-makers even if this just involves keeping them informed during the assessment;
- Good dissemination of the results.

If needs are to be matched to available resources so that as much need as possible is met, then cost effectiveness must be considered (see Chapter 7). At a practical level this involves:

- Determining how resources are currently spent (programme budgeting).
- Defining options for change (marginal analysis) by specifying alternatives: (a) identify potential services for more resources; (b) identify services which could be provided at the same level of effectiveness but at reduced cost, releasing resources for (a); and (c) identify services which are less cost-effective than those identified in (a).
- Assessing the changes in costs and benefits for different options.

The aim of planning effective health services is to increase investment in (a) and reduce investment in services identified in (b) and (c).

Assessing health needs is the first stage in review and programming. These needs and the health and social care service that try to address them are always changing and it is important to return to the assessment work, to review it and update it, and to evaluate the impact it has had. The next stage is to review the health services and preventive programmes.

Further reading

Annett, H., Rifkin, S.B. (1995) *Guidelines for rapid participatory appraisals to assess community health needs: a focus on health improvements for low-income urban and rural areas.* Geneva: Division of Strengthening of Health Services, World Health Organization (WHO).

Chambers, R. (1994) Participatory rural appraisal (PRA): analysis of experience. *World Development,* **22,**1253–68.

Countdown to 2015: Maternal, neonatal and child survival. UNICEF 2008. www.childinfo.org/countdown. html

de Koning, K., Martin, M. (1996) *Participatory research in health. Issues and experiences.* Johannesburg: Zed Books.

Reynolds, J. (1993) *Primary health care management advancement programme: assessing community health needs and coverage.* Geneva: Aga Khan Foundation.

World Health Organization (1993) *Rapid evaluation method guidelines for maternal and child health, family planning and other health services.* Geneva: World Health Organization.

Wright, J. (1998) *Health needs assessment in practice.* London: BMJ Books.

Chapter 5

Choosing the best public health interventions

John Walley

This chapter gives an overview of the following topics:

1 Assess health needs (referring to Chapters 3 and 4)
2 Review health service and programme problems.
3 Choose the best interventions and delivery strategies to solve these problems.
4 Draft activities and action plan.

Introduction

In Chapter 1 we discussed which determinants and diseases cause the largest burden of disease (morbidity and mortality) in your area of responsibility. Chapter 2 included an overview of the available public health and basic clinical service interventions, including vaccination, health promotion, screening and treatment for these diseases.

In order to choose the best interventions for a particular situation, we have to first assess health needs. In Chapters 3 and 4 we discussed the techniques of basic epidemiology and how to assess health needs. These are methods which can be used to review the situation in your area of responsibility, such as the malaria in your district. We also need to *review* – that is describe and analyse – the existing health services and programmes and find solutions to any problems found.

The next step is to review the alternative interventions available for disease control and treating ill health, analysing which are the most effective and feasible in each situation. These interventions may include both medical *technical* strategies (such as vaccination, bednets, or improved treatment of malaria) and also the related management *support* strategies such as for improved human resource management and emergency transportation.

When the best interventions have been decided upon, the best *delivery* strategy can be considered, the necessary activities listed, a draft action plan and decide how to monitor progress during implementation (see Fig. 5.1).

When to review?

A public health review approach can be used for any public health issues. It can be used when designing a new programme or when improving existing programmes. Whether you are working at district, regional, or national levels, the programme(s) for which you are responsible will need to be periodically reviewed. Examples of different programmes that will need reviewing include any of the components of the district health system (see Chapter 10); programmes targeting specific diseases

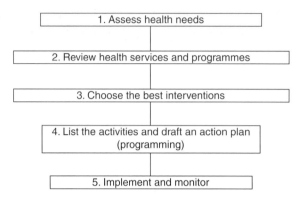

Fig. 5.1 Summary of how to choose the best public health interventions.

such as the treatment and control of TB; or programmes targeting specific groups such as EPI or maternal health services. Various situations may make you think that a review is necessary:

- A survey or analysis of the routine health information may indicate an increasing **burden of disease.** For example tuberculosis may be increasing in your district.
- There may have been an **epidemic**, for example cholera or dengue.
- There may be **new evidence** of the effectiveness of new control strategies, such as impregnated bednets for control of malaria.
- A new member of staff may have a particular **interest** in a problem.
- There may be a **request** from the Ministry of Health.
- There may be **new funding** available.
- There may have been a **critical incident,** where things that should have happened did not happen, or things happened that should not have happened – alerting you to a problem. Examples include complaints about cancelled outreach services or expiry of vaccines.

These are all **opportunities for action**. Remember that a good time to act is when, for any of these reasons, the interest of senior managers, health staff, other departments, or the community has been provoked. These are all '*stakeholders*', who have their own views and interests in the activities of the programme. These interests may be as clients wanting the best services in their locality; as staff are concerned about an increase in workload or want per diems for outreach work; or as managers concerned with not over-spending their budgets. All these groups are important and need to be consulted. Their opinions and interests should be taken into account during the review.

How to review

When you have decided to do a review, then the next step is to decide the scope of the review. This involves decisions about:

- How **broad** is the scope of the review to be – the district? the hospital?
- Which **subpopulations** are relevant to the review: children under 5, women aged 15–49, tuberculosis patients?
- How **urgent** and hence how much **time** can be given to it?
- Who is to be **involved**? – decide who to invite as members of a working group.

Box 5.1 Health needs assessment *(see also Chapter 2 and 3)*

Epidemiology

- numbers at risk, by age, sex, occupation, geographical area etc.
- incidence, prevalence etc.

Socio-economic indicators, e.g. water supply, sanitation, culture, life style, literacy rates?

Compare local situation with other areas: Worse?

Policies and programme plans, any existing? are they appropriate? are they implemented or just on paper?

Community views; visit, discuss their opinions on their health problems and services.

Assess health needs

Before making a decision about the best interventions for a particular health problem, the relevant health needs In the context of, for example, the district, must be assessed (Box 5.1). Some issues will need to be analysed in detail, if they are important for control of the disease, while other less important factors may be only briefly considered. For example, in some countries HIV/AIDS transmission through heterosexual sex is important while in many countries transmission through needles is less important (and in others, e.g. in central Asia, the opposite is the case). The best available epidemiological, social, and health service information should be used to describe the existing situation (see Chapter 3 for the basic epidemiological principles and Chapter 4 for how to assess health needs). If there is no reliable information from any particular area, then estimates for the district can be made using the figures from a similar district where there is data. Analysis includes interpretation of data, for example the trends in district coverage (%) for vaccines or HIV seroprevalence trends.

As well as the epidemiology, relevant social and cultural factors should also be included. For HIV/AIDS, this would include sexual behaviour and attitudes. Also review the health policies and plans, find out to what extent these are being actively implemented, or whether they are just 'on paper'.

Review health services and programmes

Review of health sevices and programmes should describe the existing control and care interventions, but only those which are relevant. For example you should consider the coverage, quality, and effectiveness of:

- Clinical services: Community, primary, and secondary care
- Control strategies: E.g. vector control, health promotion
- Support services: Supply of essential drugs, laboratory services, transport
- Finance: budget, 'flow' of funds, appropriate use

As with the assessment of health needs, local data should be used where they are available: This information may be supplied by the existing health information systems. Alternatively data may be obtained from programme reports or studies done by other agencies. Are there any coverage data, for vaccination coverage for example? Is there evidence of effectiveness? The best evidence is health *outcomes* data such as the tuberculosis cure and default rates (percent of patients cured or defaulted from the tuberculosis register). In most situations the best information available is that obtained by the personal observation of staff – but one must be honest about the failings of

> **Box 5.2 How effective are existing services and programmes?**
>
> As part of the health needs assessment, consider the effectiveness and gaps in the coverage, quality, and effectiveness of:
>
> ◆ Clinical services; community, primary, and secondary care
>
> ◆ control strategies; e.g. vector control, health promotion
>
> ◆ support services; supply of essential drugs; laboratory services; transport;
>
> ◆ finance: budget, flow of funds and appropriate use

existing control measures; for example if the policy of supplying condoms for use in bars and hotels may not be happening due to limited supplies, see the summary (Box 5.2).

Identification and analysis of the problem(s)

When health needs and health service delivery issues are being assessed, the existing problems must first be identified. It is worth spending some time on the analysis of these problems, so that efforts to solve them will be as effective as possible. A problem-solving method can be used to understand the problem and help decide upon the best solutions. One such method assess the strengths and weaknesses (at the present) and opportunities and threats (in the future) – the SWOT methods. Another is the 'but why' method (Cassels and Janovsky 1991) which is used to analyse the underlying causes of health and health service problems. This method is outlined in the example below.

The district health team (DHT) is concerned about an outbreak of measles, with some deaths, in children in the outlying areas of the district. The DHT decides to review the expanded programme of immunization (EPI). Their general objective is to reduce deaths from diseases which can be prevented by childhood vaccination.

The district health team discusses the outbreak. They consider whether to investigate the outbreak using epidemiological methods (Chapter 3) and the attitudes of the mothers by a community appraisal (Chapter 4). However, the District Medical Officer estimates the numbers of cases and decides that such numbers would be *expected* in these outlying areas due to the low vaccination coverage rates. The district community nurse says that mothers in these areas used to come regularly to the outreach sites, but since the previous year the outreach sessions had often been cancelled.

For now they decide to analyse the operational problems contributing to low levels of vaccination in the district. After some discussion, they identify the problem as the fact that many mothers do not bring their children for vaccination because of a lack of confidence in outreach sessions, which are irregular due to transport problems'. To analyse the problem further they ask themselves *but why?* (Fig. 5.2).

This method of problem analysis identifies the underlying cause of each problem by asking 'but why?' In this way the cause and effect relationship can be understood, enabling identification of the problems which need to be solved. Problem solving can be done as a group, such as the DHT, or on an individual basis. Write the problems, in a few words to summarize these ideas. Arrange these notes with arrows from the course to the effect. That is, causes below, leading to the effect above (which is why the arrows in Fig. 5.2 go upwards). You may draw the problem (cause and effect) 'tree' on a sheet of paper.

It is best to summarize this analysis of the problem and its underlying causes in what is called a problem statement. A problem statement is written as a long sentence or a short paragraph, such as: '*There is low childhood vaccination coverage due to lack of confidence by mothers that the outreach visit will occur. The vehicle is used by other programme officers, often visiting the same health*

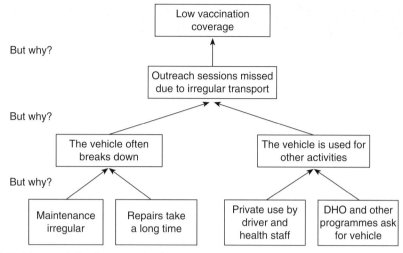

Fig. 5.2 Problem analysis of low vaccination coverage.

centre (on different days) and is used for private business by the driver and some health staff. Due to irregular maintenance the vehicle is commonly off the road being repaired or awaiting spare parts'. The steps in problem analysis can be summarized as:

◆ Identify problems;

◆ Analyze problems using the 'but why?' or other methods;

◆ Write problem statements as a summary of the analysis;

◆ Write the objectives, e.g. to increase vaccination coverage (by what % and by which number of years time).

Review and choose the best interventions

Reviewing the various possible solutions will help us avoid making false assumptions, and in doing so making the wrong choice. As with problem analysis, solution analysis can be done on an individual or group basis. The first step is to list all possible interventions that may solve the particular problems that have been identified. It is best to write down every idea so that none are missed right at the beginning. Some of the ideas listed may be obviously not very practical and can be excluded straight away – leaving a shortlist of the others to be considered in more detail.

Returning to the EPI transport example in Fig. 5.2 above, the DHT would need to list possible solutions. They may think of solutions to the irregular maintenance and long repair times, such as improving scheduling and quality control at the government vehicle workshop or alternatively contracting out the repairs to a private company. Similarly, they could list possible solutions to the uncoordinated and inappropriate use of the vehicles, for example improving co-ordination by forming a transport committee and/or controlling inappropriate use by introducing vehicle log books (recording each trip and the kilometres on the clock). They would then need to review these interventions and choose the best. How should this be done?

When reviewing the options for intervention one should decide on criteria for example to think about their:

◆ technical effectiveness

◆ organizational feasibility

◆ gender, cultural, and 'political' feasibility

◆ financial feasibility (cost)

The effectiveness and feasibility of each intervention should be considered in turn. Consider how effective and feasible each intervention would be in the situation under review. Then compare the different interventions to decide which is best. For example, in the control of malaria (see also Chapter 14, 'Major communicable diseases'), we would first need to choose our priority intervention strategies from the many available, such as:

- Reducing the breeding sites by drainage (periodically draining irrigated fields to kill larvae)
- Reducing man–mosquito contact by the use of insecticide treated bednets (ITN)
- Reducing infection in pregnancy through intermittent preventive treatment (IPT)
- Improve case management (early diagnosis and treatment) through home-based treatment of fever/malaria.

Once the priorities have been chosen, say the use of bednets and improved diagnosis and treatment, then the same criteria of effectiveness and feasibility can be used in helping to decide on the best way to deliver the service, the 'best delivery strategy' i.e. are those which increase coverage of an intervention, such as the percent of people using ITN. Bednets can be delivered by social marketing, community based distribution, distribution through health facilities, or a mixture of these strategies (see examples below). We need to choose the best delivery strategy. To do this, we can assess the technical effectiveness and feasibility of alternative delivery strategies. Feasibility includes organizational, gender-cultural, and political as well as financial factors. We will first discuss what is meant by technical effectiveness, organizational, gender-cultural and political, and resource/cost feasibility.

Effectiveness

The effectiveness of a public health intervention is how well it controls disease. How effective it is depends on how well the intervention interrupts the cycle of disease, and so reduces illness episodes and death rates. This requires knowledge of the epidemiology of the disease. In the case of drug treatments the effectiveness is compared with the usual drug, cure rates or other treatment outcomes. For infectious diseases, interventions act at different points in the chain of transmission between the vector, the host, and the environment (see Chapter 13, 'Communicable diseases principles and toolkit').

To find out more about the disease epidemiology and control interventions, search online, e.g. with Google or PubMed for published literature. Look at the abstracts and read more of the most relevant articles. Published literature should be consulted for trial evidence of the benefits (and of harms) of the interventions. For example circumcision for HIV prevention show 40% protection. Systematic reviews of ITN trials in Africa show around 17% reduction in all causes of child mortality. It is also important to know that the drug causes more good than harm. The same applies to preventive interventions. Articles may show the effectiveness of alternative delivery strategies in terms of coverage achieved. For example, the % of children sleeping under bednets after implementation of delivery strategies such as bednet promotion campaign, a voucher scheme or a social marketing programme. It is best to consult studies from the same or a neighbouring country, or otherwise from the same subcontinent, because variations in disease epidemiology etc. will influence effectiveness. For those with access to libraries, and as internet resources, such as Google, PubMed, (Medline) and BIDS (see Chapter 17, 'Future trends') this is now easy to do. The easiest approach is to read review articles which summarize the evidence from all papers on the subject or the abstracts of specific trials. Read in more detail from the papers most relevant to your context. Also ask national programme offices or research institutes who will be able to supply study reports and policy guidelines. It is vital to think critically about what is written: about whether the study was done properly and whether the context is similar or different to your own. Then decide how much of the findings and recommendations are relevant to your situation.

Similarly, for management problems, such as the EPI transport example above, the effectiveness and feasibility of delivery strategies improving the service need to be assessed. To do this reports can be consulted and people interviewed in order to find out their experience of doing what is being considered for the problem in question. Remember when reading articles do think about how similar (or not) the situation was to your own, and to assess whether the strategy would be effective in your context.

Organizational feasibility

Organizational feasibility is an assessment of how easy (or not) it is to implement the intervention. Complex interventions are more difficult to implement and scale-up. What are the requirements for managers, health workers and users. The organizational feasibility of some interventions is more dependent than that of others on the level of health facilities or the skill of health workers. For example, the syndromic management of sexually transmitted infections, as compared with the diagnosis of the specific causative organism, as syndromic approach, does not need laboratory facilities or doctors. Similarly, some delivery strategies may be easier because they fit in with existing services. For example, it is easier to add supplementation with vitamin A capsules onto the existing EPI schedule than to start working with communities to promote the cultivation of green leafy vegetables. The promotion of bednets and other healthy products through a community based approach is much easier if the community groups and CHW already exist. As with technical effectiveness, the potential advantages and disadvantages for each intervention must be considered in relation to your situation. WHO documents and guidelines and journal articles include some detail on how the implementation was done and the results. Consider how well this operational experience is relevant to your context. Articles often include some detail on the implementation done and the results. Remember that previous experience, and results in journal articles, may be from small 'pilot' projects. But consider all the organisational constraints to be overcome for scale up to full coverage.

Gender-cultural and political feasibility

Gender-cultural and political feasibility is an assessment of how *acceptable* the intervention is to the community and community leaders. For example, would sex/AIDS education in schools be acceptable to parents and religious leaders? Or would it be more acceptable if these topics were included within a broader 'family life' curriculum? The feasibility of the intervention must also be considered in relation to particular populations.

Gender. 'Gender' differences are how society creates differences (rather than biological sexual differences) for women and men (and girls and boys). Gender issues need to be considered in relation to interventions. Women are biologically more vulnerable to HIV, but there are also gender differences: for example in many countries it is difficult for women to insist on the use of condoms – even if she knows that her husband is being unfaithful. Would, for example, the intervention be accessible and acceptable to women (or men)? Or why are men less likely to accept an HIV test and so be late in starting anti-retroviral treatment (ART) culture?

Do the interventions depend on a high degree of involvement of the community and is this likely to occur. For example, as is required for interventions involving the construction and maintenance of village water and sanitation facilities.

Search online for studies done in your country or neighbouring countries. Read the documents and journal papers in the methods and discussion sections which often describe experiences and analyse how they were overcome.

Consider the 'political' constraints within organizations. It should be remembered that each type of organization (whether government, mission or company facilities) have their own long-established ways of thinking and doing things. These are likely to be country/context specific, so find out through talking to people in these organizations. Their views and interests may have to be taken into account if they are to be involved. If the proposed intervention requires other people to do things very differently than usual, they are less likely to do it or may even react negatively. To avoid negative reactions it is best to describe the merits of the strategy from their perspective.

Also consider the political constraints for community leaders. Community leaders are answerable to the community, especially at election times, and will be reluctant to accept potentially unpopular actions, such as increasing user fees. Or at national level policies such as tax rises for tobacco and alcohol. To understand these constraints, it is wise to consult politically powerful individuals. If the views and interests of the stakeholders are taken into account, they are less likely to oppose the proposed changes. Remember too to find out what motivates the other members of the health team, and take these factors into account when deciding what is feasible (and through consultation ensure their support).

Financial feasibility

Financial feasibility is an obvious further consideration. What are the costs of the manpower, money, and materials required? (The 'three Ms' is easy to remember, but really it should be 'person-power' as many if not most health workers are women!). Which of the alternative intervention and delivery strategies falls within the available budget? In public health we often advocate interventions known to be the most effective and have a relatively low cost in comparison to existing interventions. For example, hepatitis B vaccination at birth is effective in avoiding transmission and subsequent death of adults from hepatitis and liver cancer, which are common causes of death in many developing countries. There is an easy delivery strategy for Hepatitis B, given at birth, i.e. it is operationally very feasible to include it within EPI. Also there is a very low risk of harm. However, it may be difficult to convince policy makers to make the funds available, when the benefits will not be felt until decades later. What is more, it is difficult to save money from the existing health services, such as from reduced admissions to hospital with hepatitis, even though this is more costly than vaccination in the longer term.

Whether the intervention is financially feasible may depend on the flexibility in budgets. In some countries, such as Uganda and Ghana, the budget planning was decentralized after health sector reform, while in other countries the budget is fixed centrally according to budget 'heads' for salary, allowances, maintenance etc. with little local flexibility. The regulations may not allow the use of funds allocated for one thing, such as equipment, to be used for another, such as field allowances. This limits the financial feasibility of interventions depending on outreach or home visits, as these may not be feasible unless funds for daily allowances are given. If a project is started, the means for it to continue should be known, that is it must be *sustainable*. For example if field allowances are stopped then the outreach service is often not sustained.

On the other hand new funds may be available for some programmes and not for others. UNICEF may fund cold chain equipment for EPI but not equipment for obstetric services. Donor funds are usually for capital, costs for example, for construction of facilities or training courses, rather than for recurrent costs (like year after year costs such as salary). Therefore donor funds may not be relied on in the longer term.

It is best to search online for costing and cost-effectiveness studies. Therefore you should look at studies and review articles which summarize cost-effectiveness of interventions. **Cost-effectiveness** (see Chapter 7) should be conducted to help compare the various options. Then the intervention options found to have the least cost for the greatest effect on health are chosen. In practice, such data are rarely available locally. International data on the burden of disease in developing countries is presented in the *Disease Control Priorities in Developing Countries*, see further reading. These references use international data to estimate the cost-effectiveness of various interventions for specific disease groups. But these data needs to be interpreted with care when applied to individual countries. Some conclusions are not surprising, such as that heart surgery has low cost-effectiveness while, childhood vaccinations, antibiotics for acute respiratory disease and oral rehydration for diarrhoeal diseases are highly cost-effective, at US\$ 5–10 per year of life saved. Surprisingly, perhaps, treatment of tuberculosis is equally cost-effective. This is due to the benefits from the reduced transmission of disease to others as well as the benefits to the individuals treated. Remember when using this data that many interventions reduce diseases from more than one group such as water supply and sanitation interventions.

In the absence of economic analysis data, it is still worthwhile thinking about the likely costs in terms of manpower, money, and materials for each intervention, and use this to compare the cost of one intervention with the alternative(s).

How detailed should a review of interventions be?

How much time is taken to review the intervention options depends on how important and urgent the problem is. If little time is available or the issue is urgent then a review may be something that can be done in an afternoon. Or a review may require some weeks, if it is part of the preparation for a large new project, or months if it is a national policy review. In this case some time may be needed to find local data, interview stakeholders, read published evidence, and analyse how relevant the evidence is to the context. However, only spend time considering in depth interventions (and their delivery strategies) that are likely to be acceptable and workable within the scope of national programme policy and plans, and the reality of existing health services.

Then analyse the problems and write problem statements (Box 5.3):

Box 5.3 Problem analysis

Identify problems;

Analyse problems using the 'but why?' or other methods;

Write **problem statements** as a summary of priority issues.

Then review the intervention strategies to decide which are best for your situation (Box 5.4). Similarly, for each chosen intervention, review and choose the best delivery strategies.

Box 5.4 How to review interventions

- List all the potential intervention strategies for the objective.
- Assess the effectiveness and feasibility of each the possible interventions in the relation to your context.
- Compare the effectiveness and feasibility of the strategies.
- Decide which are the best – that is, are likely to be effectively implemented within the operational and financial constraints of your situation.

Preferably, a review of interventions should be done wherever there is a decision to be made, unless the decision is so obvious to make such an analysis a waste of time. Not to do the review may mean that the best intervention(s) are missed. The equivalent in clinical medicine is not to consider the differential diagnoses.

Write a summary of the advantages and disadvantages of each intervention, so that you can look at it later and remember why a particular intervention was considered to be the best. When preparing a project proposal the analysis will be useful when writing the justification for the project and the technical appraisal sections if required, or may be included in an appendix.

Example: Review of HIV/AIDS interventions

In a [fictitious] district called Salukwi, the District Health Management Team (DHMT) decided to review their HIV/ AIDS control and care activities, because 100 000 Kwacha had been made available from the AIDS control programme. The DMO asked for suggestions on how best to use these funds for HIV control or care. The following intervention strategies were proposed by DHMT members:

A Introduction of syndromic management of sexually transmitted infections (STIs) in all district health centres – suggested by the Hospital Superintendent.

B Promotion of behavioural change and condoms to all adults – suggested by the Nursing Officer.

C Expand HIV counselling and testing (HCT) and offer the test to all patients attending all health facilities – suggested by the Health Education Officer

D Expand provision of antiretroviral drugs for those infected with HIV – included by the DMO.

E Needle exchange programme for intravenous drug users – suggested by a community leader

At the suggestion of the DHO, they read up reference papers and WHO documents, and at the next meeting they discussed the effectiveness and feasibility of each of these strategies. The DHMT meeting secretary noted down the opinions about their technical effectiveness and organizational, gender-cultural and political, and financial feasibility. A summary was written in the form of an option appraisal table (see Table 5.1)

Table 5.1 includes in brief points about the effectiveness and feasibility in the Salukwi situation for each suggested interventions. The DHT decided to promote all except the last of these intervention strategy options. They decided that syndromic management of STDs, behaviour change, and condom promotion should be chosen because there was evidence of effectiveness in the published literature, and that the intervention could be organized and would be acceptable to the community. The cost of condoms and their promotion was subsidized by the national AIDS programme and was therefore considered to be affordable and otherwise feasible. The additional STI drugs were also considered affordable, as was HCT. The provision of antiviral drugs and laboratory tests would be possible at least while global funds are available. The DMO offered to draft a proposal and send to the National AIDS Committee. However they decided against introducing needle exchange because there are only a small number of intravenous drug users (drug users in

Table 5.1 Appraisal of intervention strategies for HIV/AIDS prevention and care

Strategy options	Effectiveness	Organizational feasibility	Gender cultural and political feasibility	Financial feasibility
Syndromic management of STIs	High, leading to 40% less HIV transmission in Tanzania study	Training and supervision all H centre/ OPD Drs and nurses	High for those attending, but many go to private practitioners	More drugs are used.
Condom promotion	99% effective if consistently used, also reduces unwanted pregnancy	Requires distribution system and marketing by posters etc.	Yes, as large increase in use in many countries affected by HIV	Costly to users, but now subsidized or free condoms available from the National AIDS programme
HIV counselling and testing (HCT) for HIV	Is effective entry point into HIV care and opportunity for health education	Staff available but busy; need to train them	Increasingly well accepted, most recommended a test in a clinical setting accept test (few opt-outs)	Expensive tests and uses up time of nurses to counsel.
Provision of antiviral treatment (ART) drugs for people with HIV	Very effective as long as drugs are taken regularly (>95% adherence, missing no more than 3 pills out of 60 per month)	Needs skilled medical care – risk taking staff from other work and HIV prevention work. Need to task shift from Doctors to nurses, nurses to volunteers. ART patients make good peer counselors	Demand is likely to be high. Is a risk that preventive messages e.g. condom use, may be given inadequately or ignored	Expensive lab tests and drugs provided via global funds at present, long term sustainability a concern

this area smoke drugs). The district team in this example prioritized the interventions, including which to introduce first and which later, in a phased implementation.

Review and choice of the best service delivery approach

Once the best intervention(s) have been prioritized more thought may be needed on *how* best to deliver the service. In some situations the choice of an intervention strategy is easy, but the choice of the best delivery strategy for this intervention needs more detailed thought. For example, there is strong evidence that insecticide impregnated bednets (ITN) are highly effective in preventing malaria and related mortality. The important decision then is **not whether** to use ITN, **but how** to deliver them to the whole population at risk of malaria. In this case the most effort will be put into appraising alternative delivery strategies (Box 5.5).

Information on delivery (implementation) strategies can be obtained by:

- ◆ Visiting and asking people who have implemented the approach elsewhere in the country
- ◆ Consulting the relevant national institute
- ◆ Reading about overseas experience published in journals or WHO documents found through a web search.

Box 5.5 'Delivery strategies – mass drug administration

Mass drug administration (MDA) is distribution of drugs to the entire population of a administrative unit such as district or village (though sometimes with exclusion criteria). MDA entails close collaboration between the ministry of health or other organization responsible and communities. Usually the aim is for the community to take charge; hence the term **community-directed treatment** may also be used. The most experience has been with onchocerciasis control with ivermectin (see also Chapter 14).

MDA is a public health intervention that can be implemented through a number of different **delivery strategy options**:

- **House-to-house** administration by mobile teams. The drug distributor collects the drug from a designated centre and goes from house to house to administer it – effective, but labour-intensive.

- **Booth distribution** (fixed teams). Drug distribution booths are set up at sites selected to be accessible to the community. Drug distributors administer the drugs to the beneficiaries who come to the booth. This approach is most suitable in urban situations.

- **Special population group locations.** Administering drugs to special population groups who can easily be reached at particular locations: inmates in prisons, factories, displaced persons in refugee camps, and students in schools (as used for schistosomiasis with the drug prazequantel).

- **Community gathering areas.** Marketplaces, bus and railway stations, fairs and festivals, places of worship and other sites where people congregate can also be used to reach the community.

- **Campaigns.** An intensive campaign may be organized as a focus effort, either as a national day, a week or a few weeks – depending on the operational constraints of reaching each village or other sites (as for polio vaccination campaigns).

Note: Choose the best delivery strategies, using the criteria: Effectiveness and operational, gender-cultural, and financial feasibility as discussed earlier in this chapter.

Table 5.2 illustrates various delivery strategies found in a review article on the implementation of bednets. These are not exclusive, as more than one may be needed and used in combination to achieve geographical coverage. For example health days may be used to promote bednets and bednets can be distributed to local traders to sell when they visit isolated villages (a form of social marketing).

The approach to reviewing delivery strategies is similar to that for the interventions described above – that is to consider the technical effectiveness, organizational, gender-cultural, and financial feasibility. For delivery strategies the technical effectiveness is an assessment of the merits of the strategy in terms of achieving high percentage *coverage* of those at risk. Then the organizational constraints, gender-cultural acceptability, and affordability of the delivery strategies can be assessed in relation to the context.

Doing a review of the delivery strategies (as in Table 5.3) enables you to decide on how best to implement the chosen intervention in your own context. Without doing such an option appraisal, it may be falsely assumed that a particular approach, which succeeded in delivering high coverage elsewhere, will be equally successful in your area. For example, a district in one country may successfully implement social marketing, because they can link their district to an existing national

Table 5.2 Examples of delivery strategies for bednets, from Lines J (1996)

Delivery strategy	Example
Social marketing	High profile advertising, brand image, local retailers and hawkers by PSI in Central African Republic.
Pre-natal clinics	Giving free nets or vouchers at pre-natal clinics.
Community health worker	CHW's trained to reimpregnate nets annually before the transmission season in the Gambia promote and sell nets (keeping profit as an incentive) as in Bangladesh or (BRAC).

NB: The EPI and pre-natal clinics are opportunities to deliver nets to high risk (vulnerable) pregnant women and children. In table 5.3 these delivery strategies are reviewed.

Table 5.3 Choose the best delivery strategies; appraising the effectiveness and feasibility issues for achieving high coverage with bednets

Delivery strategy	Effectiveness	Organizational	Gender-cultural	Financial
Social marketing	Geographically high coverage through shops and traders who may sell nets and packets of insecticide for re-impregnation	Make links between local distributor/shops with national social marketing organization. Promote on local radio, leaflets, posters	Willingness to pay depends on mosquito biting nuisance and awareness of risk of malaria. Translate messages into local language	Ability to pay depends on local incomes (higher after harvest) and level of subsidy for nets.
Community-based, through village groups with CHW	Coverage depends on existence of community groups and CHW. Groups can arrange with Health Office days for re-dipping nets	Environmental Health Assistants meet village leaders/ groups – but 4 officers and 400 villages in district! But can reach most areas by joining the EPI outreach	Willingness of CHWs to do work increased if they keep some profit from sale of nets. Or if free distribution, other incentive.	Daily allowance for officers. If nets sold, same issues as above. If donated are there enough for the district, and can it be maintained in future years?
Pre-natal clinics	Free nets (or vouchers for subsidized nets) given out during pre-natal clinics, reaches a high risk group	Promotion of ante-natal attendance If ante-natal attendance is high, is effective way to reach target of pregnant women and their infants (who are vulnerable to malaria)	Acceptable, though men (who are less vulnerable) may use the nets. Best if able to provide more than one net per family	Full or subsidized cost of the net depends on the government/ donor funds – possible recently due to global funds

Note: CHW, community health worker.

social marketing organization. But this may not be feasible in another district in a country which has no national social marketing organization.

Draft activities and action plan

The design of a programme includes the listing of activities and writing of an action plan. These will be required for implementation. Commonly additional resources are required, and to get these a project proposal will need to be submitted. A simple layout for a project proposal is shown in Box 5.6. Note that the objectives are easily written by rewording of the problems in the form that they are solved (as a result of the project intervention strategies, delivery strategies and activities). For example, if the problem was high transmission of malaria due to low coverage of bednets then the objective will be to reduce transmission of malaria by promotion of bednets (the chosen intervention strategy) through social marketing (the delivery strategy).

It is wise to think about and list the activities soon after deciding on the best interventions and delivery strategies. This is because in the review of delivery strategies, you will have already considered the activities that will be required for successful implementation. It is best to write out all the activities that are required to implement a particular strategy. Activities may be ordering supplies, conducting meetings, training courses and supervision visits etc. The activities should be written down in full sentences, so that the details are clear. They should be written in the order that they need to be implemented. For example, with the community-based distribution of bednets example there may be the following activities:

1 Make a bulk order for bednets and impregnation insecticide packets, by the Pharmacist.

2 A meeting to coordinate the work of the Environmental Health Assistants village visits with the EPI outreach schedule and health promotion activities by EPI nurses.

3 Training course for Health Assistants on how to conduct village meetings, and how to arrange community re-dipping days for the existing non impregnated nets.

4 Supervision by the Environmental Health Officer of the work of the Health Assistants.

5 Schedule into the DHMT meeting a review the progress of implementation issues and coverage achieved and decide how best to deal with any problems occurring.

Box 5.6 A simple layout for a project proposal

+ **The situation and problem statements** (background and scale of the problem as justification for the project).

+ **Objectives** (the problems reversed at the end of the project, coverage % to be achieved etc.)

+ **Interventions and delivery strategies** list those chosen.

+ **Activities** written in sentences and listed in the order to be implemented.

+ **Action plan** for each intervention/delivery strategy and related activities, which specifies:
  • The resources (manpower, money and materials) required, and the source of the resources;
  • The health workers responsible;
  • The approximate time required;
  • The expected outcome or target, and how monitored.

+ **Inputs/ budget**

Table 5.4 An action plan for a HIV and Sexually Transmitted Disease (STI) project

Strategies\Activities	Who Responsible	When-dates	What resources	Outcome	How monitored
1. **Schools HIV/STD education within Family health**	District Education Officer (DEO)	Q4	75 000 kW; allowance material	Reduced transmission	Knowledge of HIV and STDs in under-18-year-olds
1.1 Meet with the District Education Officer.	Health Education Officer (HEO)	Q2	Refreshments	Agree on strategy and learning needs	Minutes of meeting
1.2 Develop curriculum and learning materials	HEO and DEO	Q2	Time to adapted national materials	Curriculum and learning material drafted	Curriculum and prepared
1.3 Train teachers	DEO	Q3	Print Materials	Teacher skills increased	Teachers observed conducting a class on HIV
1.3 Start HIV/ STD education in district schools	Teachers	Q4	Learning material	Student know about HIV and STDs in tests	Written test and group discussion

The activities will be written in an action plan. An action plan is written for use at the level of implementation, such as the district. An action plan includes the list of activities and a summary usually in the form of a table as in Table 5.4.

When preparing an action plan give careful consideration to the following points for each activity: who is responsible, when it is to be done, with what resources, the outcome and how this will be monitored.

Who is responsible: Say who will be responsible to make sure that the activity is carried out. This person may also be one who will do the activity, or the person who supervises to make sure it has occurred. But it is best not to put just the DHT or DMO for each activity, rather to be more specific and name individuals. Being more specific makes it clear that the work involved is distributed fairly and avoids overloading one particular person.

Timing: State when you expect to start each activity. You should also include the date by which it should be completed. In the example in Table 5.4 the quarter (Q) in which the activity is started and finished is included, rather than the specific date. In addition, it is useful to redraft the plan in the form of a timetable. An example of this is a Gantt chart (see Chapter 6) which lists the activities according to the month or quarter in which implementation occurs.

Resources needed: Include the main resources required, and the actual cost estimate if known. You may not need to do this for resources within the existing budget, but it is particularly useful for additional resources to be requested. Resources may include any of the '3Ms' mentioned before: manpower, materials, and money.

Expected outcome: Specify what you expect to achieve for each strategy and activity. This is important, so as to avoid wasted effort, e.g. meetings with no clear agenda (see also Chapter 6) and is useful for deciding if the activity was successfully carried out and achieved its expected effect.

How monitored: Specify the means to find out whether the expected outcome will have actually been achieved. This is necessary so that you know in advance what, how and where the monitoring information will be collected.

Budgeting

The chosen interventions and related activities are likely to require new resources or reallocation of existing resources. These resources, whether manpower, money or materials, need to be translated into a budget.

Budgets usually separate the recurrent and capital cost categories. Recurrent costs are those that occur every year and include such things as salaries, allowances, drugs, maintenance, and the cost of utilities such as electricity. Capital costs, sometimes called development or investment costs, are major one-off expenditures, such as new vehicles, buildings, and training. It should be remembered to include all the recurrent cost implications, such as the salaries of additional staff employed and maintenance of equipment and vehicles (see Chapter 7).

Summary

This chapter has discussed how to review of the health services and programmes, and so understand the existing situation and analyse problems. Then how to review and choose the best intervention strategies and delivery strategies, by assessing their effectiveness and feasibility. Lastly how to draft a list activities and action plan.

The next chapter discusses how to plan, implement, and manage services and programmes, and then Chapter 7 is about the economics and financing.

Further reading

Method

Cassels, A. and Janovsky, K. *'Strengthening health management in districts and provinces'*, Handbook for Facilitators. WHO/SHS/DHS/91.3

McMahon, Barton and Piot. (1980) *On being in charge: a guide for middle-level management in primary health care*. WHO, Geneva.

Green A. *'Introduction to health planning for developing countries'*. Oxford University Press. Oxford.

Interventions

Disease Control Priorities in a developing world (DCP2). World Bank/Oxford University Press, 2nd edition, 2006. http://www.dcp2.org/page/main/BrowseDiseases.html

Jamison D et al. (2006) *Disease control priorities in a developing world*, second edition. World Bank/Oxford University Press, 2nd edition. [A very useful Disease and health systems reference] http://www.dcp2.org/page/main/BrowseDiseases.html

Webber R (2004) *Communicable disease epidemiology and control*. 2nd edition. CABI Publishing. Oxford 2004. (new edition due 2009).

UNICEF (2008). 'Countdown to 2015' *Maternal, neonatal and child survival: tracking progress in maternal, newborn and child survival*. http://www.childinfo.org/countdown.html

Chapter 6

Planning, implementing, and managing interventions

John Hubley, Sylvia Tilford, and John Walley

This chapter gives an overview of the following topics:
- ◆ The programme planning process
- ◆ Stages of planning, implementation, and evaluation
- ◆ Key management processes needed to support programmes
- ◆ Give examples of programme implementation and issues for specific health programmes.

Various public health planning models are available, some of considerable complexity. The simplest type of model is shown in Fig. 6.1, and it includes the key elements required in programme planning. The activities are presented in a linear sequence with feedback from evaluation being fed back into earlier stages leading, where necessary, to programme revisions. In practice, the progression through stages is less clear cut. It is often helpful to think quickly through all programme planning tasks at the outset before detailed consideration of the early stages. For example, thinking about evaluation at the outset can influence the early stages of planning. Initial specification of all aspects of a programme will often be needed in order to produce a project proposal to secure funds for implementation. More detailed planning can follow the gaining of funds. For ease of discussion we will consider the stages in order but readers should not assume that the process has to be as clear and straightforward as this when carried out in the real world.

Assessing health needs

The first stage of planning is a health needs assessment (review of the situation) and an analysis of the problem to be dealt with. An appropriate programme can then be designed. Chapter 4 considered assessing health needs in detail and can be referred to again at this point. As a reminder assessment may draw on existing data on mortality, morbidity, and use of services, augmented by further data needed to gain a full understanding of a situation. While professionals may lead this process it needs to involve fully the communities in which a programme will take place. Although professionals may consider that there is strong evidence of the need for a programme, communities may have very different assessments of need. Adequate time needs to be allowed for involvement of the community in discussion on needs and solutions. The methods used can include those which are time intensive, such as surveys, as well as rapid appraisal methods. You will need

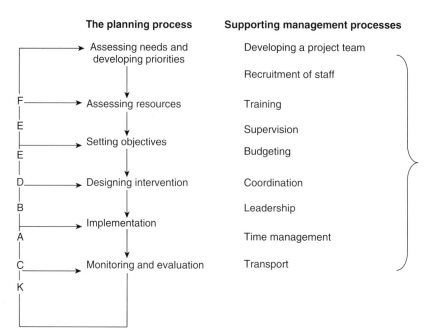

Fig. 6.1 Planning and management of public health programmes.

to understand the determinants of the health issue which the programme is going to address. To do this you will need to consider:

◆ Environmental factors – physical and socio-economic;

◆ Health and other service influences; and

◆ Health behaviours and the factors which influence them.

Chapters 4 and 5 describe how to review the situation and choose the best interventions and delivery strategies. Chapter 8 gives further details on understanding health determinants and health promotion. From the problem analysis programme priorities and the target population for action begin to emerge. Priorities should be set on the basis of the impact of the issue on the health of the community (incidence, prevalence, mortality, and morbidity) and assessment of the feasibility of your programme having an impact. The feasibility will depend on the nature of the health issue (for example the scope for prevention), the resources at your disposal, and whether it is perceived as a serious problem by a community.

Assessing resources and developing a project team

The resources available, both human and material, will determine the priorities that can be addressed. Depending on the scale of programme that is being planned, additional resources are often required and to get these a project proposal will need to be submitted, as noted earlier, summarizing key features of the proposed programme. Where major funds are needed, the case for securing them can be strengthened by evidence from an evaluation of a small pilot of the planned programme. Once the resources are obtained, planning can go ahead in detail.

Putting together the right team for a programme is important for success. You may be able to do this from existing staff or may need to recruit new staff.

Recruitment of staff

It is important to have clear agreement of the job description from all involved (see Box 6.1) for any new post(s) including the tasks, responsibilities, and experience required and any other special characteristics required. In looking at candidates you will need to assess their suitability, including experience, qualifications, previous performance, attitudes, personal qualities, and acceptability to the community. Recruitment and selection have to be carried out in a way that is fair to everyone. This means letting as wide a number of persons know about the existence of the post and using a selection process which is open and does not discriminate against anyone on the basis of their gender, tribe, or background.

Once you have recruited good staff, it is important to keep them. A high turnover of staff is one of the reasons for programme failure and can represent a serious problem – especially when scarce resources have been used to recruit and train valuable field staff. People may leave for many reasons including dissatisfaction with pay and work conditions, attractive work conditions elsewhere, and personal circumstances such as the need to be near family, schools, and spouses' employment. Although not all of these can be influenced by you, remember that salary is important but job satisfaction can play an even greater part in decisions to leave. Overall, good leadership that is responsive to the needs of staff is vital.

Where existing staff will deliver a programme, there may be training needs that have to be met. For example, if the programme will have an element of peer education undertaken by community

---

Box 6.1 Job descriptions

One of the most important parts of any plan is to specify the roles of the different persons involved including both field and management level. This involves consulting all interested groups including management, field staff, and members of the target audience to ensure that the proposed additional functions are acceptable and fit in with existing workloads.

Job descriptions are required for:

- Volunteers operating at the community level, e.g. peer educators, volunteers
- Field staff involved in delivering essential services, e.g. STD care
- Persons carrying out a supervisory role
- The key person managing the intervention

In order to:

- Ensure that the responsibilities for important tasks are defined
- Make sure that everyone is clear about their roles
- Prevent overlap of activities as well as gaps
- Define lines of authority and supervision

A job description consists of the following:

- Job title
- Qualifications
- Job summary and list of duties
- Relationship with other persons – authority and communication

members, staff may need some in service training about this method in order to be able to train peer workers. Training is discussed in a later section.

Setting objectives

The term 'Aim' is usually kept for general statements of intent or purpose for a programme, e.g. to reduce maternal mortality, control diarrhoea or lower deaths from accidents. A general statement of intent is useful for bringing people together to agree on the broad purpose of a programme. However, planning of activities requires a more precise statement of purpose. The term 'objectives' – sometimes called specific objectives – is used for precise statements of what a programme plans to achieve over the time scale of the project. The purpose of management is to ensure that a programme achieves its objectives.

Planning an activity involves making the following decisions:

◆ *Where are we now?* (baseline)

◆ *What do we want to achieve?* (objectives)

◆ *How do we plan to get there?* (strategy)

An objective that is specified in a precise and measurable way is called a 'target'. More information is provided on setting of targets in the later section on monitoring and evaluation. Decisions on objectives for a programme are made on the basis of the assessment of needs, consultation with communities, and available resources. Targets can be set at the beginning of a programme and used to monitor and evaluate progress. A useful guideline is that targets should be SMART:

Specific to the needs of your programme – this involves moving from vague aims such as using condoms to very specific and measurable outcomes such as shipment to field of condoms, ability to demonstrate correct usage through a demonstration.

Measurable by simple and objective methods with a baseline level at the beginning and a target level for achievement at the end of the programme.

Achievable – it should be possible to achieve the change during the time scale of the project with the resources available.

Relevant – the target is relevant to the programme you are carrying out.

Time limited – The time scale for the change is specified.

The objectives are best made 'SMART' adding targets, only after the intervention strategies have been chosen.

Choose the best interventions to achieve objectives

Chapter 5 discussed in detail the selection of the best interventions and their delivery (implementation) strategies. Interventions (and their delivery strategies) need to be carefully thought through. A new intervention must be appropriate to the objectives set for a programme, the programme situation and the people to be involved and take into consideration the factors discussed in the earlier Chapter 4, including local policy statements and the evidence of what is known to work. In addition to finding any evidence from local studies, various methods can be used to find existing evidence from elsewhere. Look up, for example, on www.who.int/topics and click on the health topic and publications of interest. Also you can search with key words typed into Google or Google Scholar for review articles or specific trial publications. In some cases there may be systematic reviews of the type of interventions you are interested in. Read, at least, the abstracts and summaries of studies identified. These provide evidence for what is effective in other countries. But do also consider the differences between those contexts and your own. Think about the effectiveness and feasibility of alternative interventions in your context and choose the best. For the chosen interventions decide the best service delivery approach, list the activities and prepare an action plan (as described in Chapter 5 'Choose the best intervention'). Even if the senior levels have decided the intervention and the delivery strategy to be adopted (for example, promoting vaccine coverage through social mobilization), you should still analyse how best to do it in your local context, decide the activities required and prepare an action plan. Remember, that one of the options to consider may be the strengthening of an existing intervention and delivery strategy, for example EPI outreach. Indeed it may be poor implementation or lack of continued attention to the existing strategy that is the reason for poor effectiveness. Whether you decide to strengthen the existing and/or add a new strategy, these will need to be implemented systematically. Each delivery strategy will include a number of activities.

The planned intervention may be approached through a single delivery strategy such as social mobilization, or creation of healthy settings (see Chapter 8, Health Promotion) or may involve a mix of strategies, for example, mass media, public education in primary health care, and changes in health care delivery. Whatever is selected, detailed planning of actions and their timing needs to be completed, as well as budgeting of the programme. A useful approach is to set out your objectives as a table or a 'time chart' (sometimes called 'Gantt' chart, see Table 6.1) for a particular programme on which to show dates for completing planned activities.

You can also set out a work plan as a table that sets out for each planned activity: The person responsible for carrying out the activity, the date for completion, how you will measure achievement, and cost. When the activities are displayed on a chart it will become obvious when you have planned too many activities during the same period or have put an activity at the wrong time! The time chart is also a valuable tool for monitoring your activities.

Budgeting

The chosen interventions and related activities are likely to require new resources or reallocation of existing resources. These resources, whether human, money or materials, need to be translated into a budget. Sound financial management is essential for the running of public health programmes. Preparation of a budget involves specifying the anticipated costs of planned inputs and activities. Costs normally have to be separated into:

- *Capital costs* which take place once during the life of a project: Purchase of equipment, vehicles and buildings; and
- *Recurrent costs* which take place regularly including: Purchase of consumables such as drugs, leaflets and batteries; printing of educational materials, fuel/maintenance, salaries and allowances of staff.
- Costs should allow for inflation and include a general contingency fund to cover unexpected expenses. When preparing a budget as part of an application for funding, it will be necessary to take into account any special requirements of the funding body. It is also necessary to include some justification for expenditures (why you need particular equipment, staffing, training etc.)

A suggested checklist for a budget is listed below:

Capital expenditure
- *Construction:* Health units; training facilities, latrines/washing facilities, water supply, staff housing;
- *Commodities*: Equipment, furniture and vehicles.

Recurrent expenditure
- *Personnel*: Health workers/other technical staff, administration and other support staff, consultants, casual labour.

Table 6.1 Example of a 'Gantt' chart showing timings for a community-based project using volunteers for health promotion activities

Specific activities	Jan	Feb	Mar	Apr	May	Jun	Jul	Aug	Sep	Oct	Nov	Dec
Meeting of key agencies to discuss project	▓											
Community meeting to discuss needs	▓											
Set up community health committee		▓										
Baseline survey in commuvnity		▓										
Prepare plan with community			▓									
Recruit volunteers				▓								
Develop learning materials				▓								
Train volunteers					▓							
Health promotion by volunteers						▓	▓	▓	▓	▓		
Supervisory visits by health workers							▓	▓	▓	▓		
Monitoring meetings with community								▓		▓		
Evaluation Survey											▓	
Design of next phase of project												▓

- *Training*: Workshops, refresher courses, study visits, manuals, and other training materials.
- *Travel costs*: Bus, train, and air fares; per diems for personnel including training;
- *Supplies*: Medical supplies including drugs, training supplies, office supplies including stationery, printing, and photocopying, vehicles;
- *Maintenance*: Of equipment, buildings, and furniture
- *Vehicle running and maintenance*: Operation and maintenance of vehicles, fuel, vehicle insurance and, tax.
- *Other costs*: Utilities (water, electricity, rent, fuel), communications (e-mail, telephone, and postage), insurance.

(Checklist adapted from Janovsky 1987 – see recommended reading)

Programme implementation

Implementation is the main part of a public health manager's work, yet often they have little knowledge of what makes for effective implementation. A number of components of implementation, such as training, are mentioned in various chapters. Here, we briefly bring together and describe the components which, from experience, lead to effective implementation.

When planning the implementation there are some general questions that need to be considered:

- Will the intervention be piloted on a small scale and then scaled up?
- How will implementation be phased?
- How will implementation according to plan be achieved?
- How will the sustainability of programme and its effects be achieved?

These will be discussed in turn.

Pilot in the early district sites

Piloting is trying things out on a smaller scale before expanding to everywhere else. If the intervention is to be nationwide, then the piloting may be in a number of districts. If the intervention is a new initiative of the district health team, then the piloting may be in some sub-district or health centre catchment areas. The important thing is to try out the new approach and revise based on experience, before scaling-up. Unfortunately 'piloting' has a bad name, because it has often been done badly. Indeed an expression the 'pilot project trap' is used because development projects frequently do not get beyond the pilot stage. The pilot project may achieve good results while well resourced by a donor, but fails when donor funding ends – that is, it wasn't *sustainable*. Or this level of resources isn't available when implemented in the scale-up sites, and so isn't *replicable* to other areas. So when planning and piloting a new intervention we should always be realistic – design in a way to be sustainable and replicable. That is, design the pilot according to the likely level of human, material, and financial resources that will be available during scale-up. Ensure that the intervention (and the related service delivery approach, activities, and inputs) are piloted before scaling-up.

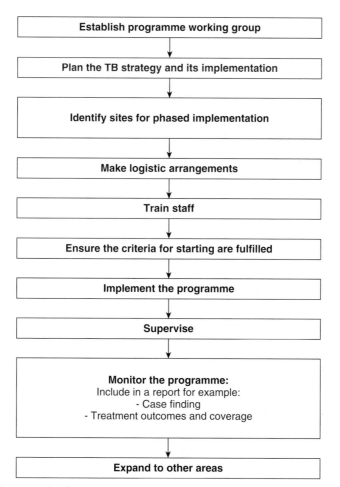

Fig. 6.2 The 10 steps to implementation.

Phased implementation

Do not attempt to implement everywhere at once. This sounds obvious, but too often the higher level just sends out an instruction to the next level *telling* them to implement. But effective implementation requires thinking through the details, and then drafting the guidelines and materials. Based on the initial (pilot) site experience, revise the guidelines and materials, helping to ensure quality when moving to the next group of district sites. Implement step-wise, systematically scaling-up to all the district sites.

Implementation according to plan

It can happen that programme objectives are not achieved, not because the chosen intervention was wrong for the purpose but because of shortcomings in implementation of the programme protocol. These shortcomings could include:

- ◆ Implementation of only part of the programme;
- ◆ Poor implementation, for example, using inappropriate methods in a component of a programme;
- ◆ Subversion of a programme; for example, health workers using education methods they are comfortable with rather than the ones which were required to achieve effectiveness, or the diversion of programme resources, thus undermining effectiveness.

Good monitoring and process evaluation should expose shortcomings promptly so that they can be remedied.

Achieving sustainability of programme effects

Sustainability refers to the continuing achievement of project objectives after a funded period. We will only know if programme effects have been sustained if some follow up evaluation is built into the programme. Some programme effects are difficult to sustain especially where human behaviours are involved. The motivation of individuals or communities to sustain behaviour changes is known to be difficult and can be even more so where there are many barriers to maintaining the changes. Thinking carefully when choosing interventions about what changes are more likely to be sustainable is very important.

The factors which promote sustainability have been studied in a number of public health projects. For example, factors identified as influencing the sustainability of community nutrition programme in the Gambia and a village health care project in Cameroon (Eliason 1999 and Aubel 1996) included:

- ◆ Community responsibility and ownership;
- ◆ Compatibility with community norms and values;
- ◆ Building on existing social units and roles;
- ◆ Motivation, training, and supervision of community actors;
- ◆ Community contribution of resources;
- ◆ Less complex interventions;
- ◆ Support from key male and female community leaders;
- ◆ Collaboration with community development agents;
- ◆ Adequate knowledge;
- ◆ Relevant follow up support.

To achieve sustainability the necessary actions must be identified and in place well before a funded programme finishes. For example, a well building programme will need to ensure that training of community members to maintain wells is effective during the funded programme and also that some after support is organized to maintain motivation and skills. In addition, the access to spare parts should be organized. We will now consider the practical elements of implementation.

Implementation in practice

For an intervention to succeed there are many things that need to be in place. Training, for example, is necessary but not sufficient for success. If staff are trained to use a guideline and new drug regime, but the drugs are not ordered and ready in time, then the health workers will forget what they have learned by the time the drugs arrive. Similarly if the right clinical record card is not provided, then the health worker will not be able to do the job and be discouraged. Everything required for implementation needs to be planned, ordered, and be ready in time for when any training courses, if needed, start. It is best to hold an implementation planning meeting. Include all the relevant people in the meeting, including the (e.g. malaria) programme and general health managers, pharmacist, laboratory, or health information officer as relevant. You may include representatives of NGOs, company, and private providers in the planning activities, if the intervention includes them.

Working group process

Choose a small group of the most able and experienced people to develop programme materials. Between 4 and 8 people is a manageable group, who can sit around a table to discuss and agree on details. Make sure the roles of the group are clear. Meet regularly, for example once per week, until the task is completed. One member will chair, another will be the facilitator who prepares the first draft and edits in the agreed changes. Others contribute according to their particular technical roles, for example, a specialist in that subject, knowledge of participatory training methods, or front-line experience of delivering care. The group works through each stage of the care or management processes. The group edits each of the materials to make sure they are compatible (say the same thing); for example that the case management, training modules, supervisory tools mention the same drug regimen or follow-up care procedure. The working group members can be the facilitators for the training of trainers.

Draft guidelines and other tools

Managers should not just send out a directive to people telling the next level to do something. If only receiving an instruction, but no details, then they are may not know what to do and make a mess of it. Guidelines (also called manuals, protocols, procedures) and other tools for implementation, such as supervision checklists, are usually necessary. Guidelines should be based on the available research evidence. They also should 'capture' on paper the experience of able people who have already implemented effectively. These guidelines and tools make possible quality implementation by less experienced or less able people, so effectively scaling-up the programme. Case management guidelines are adapted from the best available source materials, e.g. WHO generic guidelines. This can be done through a working group, as above. The group adapts the guideline or material to fit with the local / country context, for example editing the:

- Epidemiology, e.g. edit according to the level of malaria risk
- The diagnostic process
- Treatment regimens recommended by the national programme
- The names and roles of the health facilities and workers

- The initial and follow-up care process
- Recording and reporting procedures

Training

Most public health programmes require some training activities to provide field staff with any additional skills they need for successful implementation (see also District Health Systems chapter 10). Training can take place in different ways. Many people receive their initial training through a pre-service course such as a nursing or medical course, others through training in post. The initial training of many health workers has been heavily biased towards curative medicine and training is an important part of a strategy for reorientation of health workers towards community-based approaches involving prevention and health promotion. Newly-recruited staff may need an induction course to orient them to the additional skills they may need for a particular post.

Even after they have qualified, field staff need to be updated on new procedures or understandings of health and disease required for specific programmes. In-service training, also called continuing education, can be carried out through training workshops, on-the-job training, or supervised practice. It can also be done through distance learning – correspondence courses, self-instruction manuals. Some of the decisions involved with training are shown in Table 6. 2

Conduct effective training

Training should be performance based, teaching the skills needed to do the job. For each worker, write down the tasks they have to do. The tasks are included in the guidelines, mentioned above. The training course and modules should include all these tasks. For in-service training, first assess the training needs; find out which tasks have already been taught and practiced effectively. Focus the training on the needs and the tasks not previously taught or found not to be done well.

Prepare training materials

Training materials may already exist, either in the country or from WHO. Select the most relevant parts. Unless done already, adapt the material to the local context. It is too easy to leave in all the facts. Don't. Prioritize the essential skills, and only include the knowledge required for these skills. To help you, think about a target and aim for the red central spot – the essential skills and related knowledge. If you include more, then there may not be enough time for developing the skills, and performance will not improve (Table 6.2).

Table 6.2 Summary table determining the training requirements of the intervention

Components of training	Procedures/factors to be considered	Comments
Objectives	• Orientation to the programme and the role that the persons are required to fulfil in implementation and overall approach e.g. empowerment, participatory etc. • The acquiring of the specific competencies (and necessary knowledge, skills, and attitudes) that the persons require to undertake their role in intervention.	The starting point for planning training is defining the job descriptions/functions of key persons in the proposed implementation. Those activities in the job description that the person requires training to undertake form the objectives for the training

Table 6.2 *(continued)* Summary table determining the training requirements of the intervention

Components of training	Procedures/factors to be considered	Comments
Selection of participants	◆ Persons requiring training might be field staff, volunteers and peer educators. Persons selected should be the ones who will actually be doing the work. ◆ When using volunteers and peer educators the characteristics required must be clearly defined e.g. the educational level, age, sex, position of trust/respect in the community, ability to move freely in the community, and future residence in community.	◆ It is important to ensure that the people who come for training are those who will actually do the work. ◆ It is often useful to have a multi-disciplinary mix of participants, e.g. teachers, health workers, and community workers to encourage sharing of understandings. ◆ Wherever possible the community should be involved in the selection process.
Organization of training	◆ *How long* – e.g. afternoon, day, few days, weeks etc. ◆ *In one block or as a series of sessions* spread out over a time period e.g. weekly. ◆ *On-the-job training* e.g. under supervision of field staff. ◆ *Distance learning* – e.g. with tasks/reading to be completed at home.	◆ It is often a good idea to spread training out and use subsequent sessions to review experiences in the field. ◆ Pressure of work may severely restrict the time that people can spend away on training. You have to use sessions to cover what is really essential and consider including distance learning methods that the participants can follow from their workplace.
Location of training	◆ At a training centre, field centre, or in the project location. ◆ Accessibility of target audience for practical work.	The training location should be similar to the situation in which the participants will be performing their future tasks.
Selection of teaching methods	◆ Talks/discussions with suitable learning aids e.g. slides, overhead transparencies, flip charts, flannelgraphs etc. ◆ Participatory learning activities e.g. exercises, games, problem-solving exercises. ◆ Role plays and practice teaching/counselling sessions. ◆ Field work/field exercises/supervised practice with real patients.	◆ Educational methods should be appropriate to the learning objectives especially for communication, manual and decision-making skills. ◆ There should be opportunities to practice skills with each other and in test communities. ◆ Participants should be exposed to educational methods that they will themselves be expected to use in the field.
Evaluation of training	*Short-term evaluation* through observation/feedback questionnaires immediately after the course e.g. have they acquired the knowledge, skills that were taught in the course. *Long-term evaluation* through follow-up visits and supervisors' reports 3–6 months afterwards – are they putting into practice what they learnt during the training?	Evaluation can be linked to supervision/monitoring activities and also be part of follow-up teaching sessions.

Teach skills

A programme will often require decision making, practical, and communication skills. Decide the *decision-making skills*, such as how to diagnose a case or district programme, and write case studies for these. Decide the *practical skills*, such as completing and analysing patient register data and also write exercises for these. Decide the *communication skills* required with patients, health workers, and managers, and write role-plays to teach these. Include the case studies, exercises and role-plays in the training material. These case studies, exercises and role-plays may each last for 5–15 minutes each. Minimize what is said by the trainers, participants don't want lectures. Indeed it is best to prepare notes for the 'facilitator' of the course. For each section of the training programme, ask the participants to read the text (essential knowledge) and then do the exercise or case study. For communication skills such as counselling, divide into groups of three. Two people read the case study and one role-plays the health worker and the other the patient, behaving as a patient would. The third person observes, and at the end of the role-play comments firstly on some points done well and (only then) comments on parts that 'could be done better' according to the guideline. That is, starting and finishing on a positive comment encourages the participants and helps them to accept the 'could be done better' points. During a course the participants take turns playing each of these roles.

Train in a practice setting

All the health workers who are involved in specific programme tasks should be trained. For example, all those who care for young children need to have training on IMCI. Don't assume that if you train the nurse in-charge the rest will be taught by her. It is best to conduct training in the same type of health facility or other setting where the work will be done. Train and supervise the resident staff in this health facility so they are confident doing the tasks, are competent, and can supervise course participants before using the facility as a field practice site. There should be a mix of class sessions and practice sessions. First the participants observe the experienced health worker in action. Then the trainee is observed while they practice. After each case or session, the supervisor comments on the work.

Follow-up after training

Schedule to visit within a week of the end of training. Ask to sit in and observe the health worker, and see whether they do what they were trained to do. It may be that they don't have the required materials. Maybe they need help to reorganize the flow of patients or re-arrange the consultation room. Help them do these things. Whatever else, the follow-up visit convinces the health worker that you are serious about them actually putting into practice what they have been taught. Thereafter this new practice can be integrated within routine supervision.

Supervision

This is the process of assessing the performance and activities of field staff. It is carried out in order to ensure satisfactory job performance by field staff and to help them improve performance. Unfortunately supervision, if done at all, is often more like policing, and is commonly a de-motivating experience. You may be familiar with a car-full of supervisors descending on a health centre, each looking at the register, drugs, or fridge as relevant to 'their' programme, criticizing the defects and then disappearing over the hill until next time. Make sure that your own, and others' supervision is supportive. As with training, the supervisor should focus on observation of performance and reinforcement of skills. Supervision can take place through field visits, direct observation of performance, self-evaluation reporting forms filled out by the field worker and group meetings with field staff. The supervisor should take time to sit in on consultations and observe preventive services where these form part of a programme. The most important part of supervision is noticing what is done **well**. Make sure that supervisors complement the good points before they comment on what could be done better. Good supervision involves being supportive, establishing rapport with staff, taking time to listen to problems, successes, and questions, praising good performance and never criticizing in front of others. Wherever possible supervision should be a learning process with opportunities for the field workers to analyse their own performance and find their own solution to problems.

Before leaving they (and you) should discuss and agree a plan of action on what should be done before the next supervision visit. These records should be referred to before the next supervision visit. As a manager, practice good supervision with your team members – quality implementation depends on it.

Programme coordination

Coordination of the various activities within a programme is essential. The implementation plan will have set out clearly the ordering of programme activities but guaranteeing these are properly coordinated has to be ensured. Coordination of a new programme with already existing activities in a community must also be considered. This can be more difficult when there are several organizations working within a community, especially if they have different objectives or adopt alternative approaches – for example, on treatment strategies, advice on personal behaviour or on equipment designs. This can be a role for the working group or for the overall programme manager.

Leadership and facilitation

The difference between success and failure of a programme can often depend on the quality of leadership. Leadership depends on an individual's ability to make decisions and solve problems. It also depends on the ability a person has to command respect, to show understanding of others and to build a team.

In looking at leadership a common approach is to consider leadership styles. A relaxed 'laissez-faire' style of leadership where a leader leaves decision-making to others may not get the task accomplished. An 'authoritarian' leadership style involving top-down management with giving of orders or even bullying may get the job done but stifles creativity and responsibility among staff who may be afraid to take decisions for themselves. The best approach, often labelled as 'democratic' is somewhere between the two. A leader consults programme participants and shares decision making. The leader acts as a facilitator but when necessary can bring pressure to bear to move actions along.

One of the important – and most difficult – skills of leadership is delegation to others. This spreads the workload, develops responsibility, and shows trust for others. A good leader understands the motivation of the persons being led, recognizes and rewards achievement, and is responsive to their needs. A programme manager can be the major programme facilitator but someone else can have this key role. Understanding what is involved in facilitation is important.

Facilitation is the art of helping others to do a better job and to be a catalyst for change. The facilitator may be someone from the health office, an NGO, a research team, or other organization. The facilitator has the ability and time to carry out developmental work in collaboration with the responsible general health service or specific programme manager. The facilitator will help, but not take over, the work done by the health manager. The facilitator may propose and contribute to meetings, trainings, and workshops. S/he may prepare draft versions, and revise them, after receiving the comments from the manager and health workers. The facilitator will encourage the process through to successful completion, in this way the health manager will learn to trust and appreciate the support from the facilitator.

Intersectoral collaboration

Many programmes require the active collaboration of other sectors and agencies working in a community if they are to be fully successful. You need to identify these and work out the best ways of working with them. Possible government agencies might include: Schools, adult literacy, community development, agricultural development, environmental health, water, and sanitation. NGOs working in your community may be involved in health, women's affairs, water, and sanitation, cooperative and income generation, old persons, pre-school facilities, youth, sports. You need to decide on the degree of collaboration that is required and plan activities to achieve this. You can have informal meetings with key agencies on a regular basis or more formal coordination committees taking into account the points below on meetings. Effective collaboration is influenced by many things, for example:

- The support of all agencies and sector workers involved for a programme's goals and its activities;
- Understanding and sharing of the cultures of different sectors and professionals;
- A positive attitude towards working together;
- Establishing and agreeing roles and responsibilities;
- Clear agreement about the way that collaboration will take place;
- An agreed timescale for collaboration;
- Working to secure interim goals and achievements to sustain the alliance;
- Sensitivity to process issues and mechanisms for resolving conflict (Box 6.2).

NGOs take a back seat

The ownership by the health service and programme managers is key. So other organizations such as NGOs, involved in strengthening health services/programmes should keep a low profile – and make sure the credit for the work goes to the programme. Guidelines, training modules, and other products should be printed with ministry of health/national programme name top of the list.

Community participation

We emphasized the importance of working with communities in assessing priorities. Involvement of communities is also an essential part of programme delivery and gaining acceptance for programmes. This can take place when either your staff or you hold meetings with community members, by attendance at meetings of community groups, primary health care committees, or school committees and holding public consultation meetings. If you are seen to be someone who is interested in and supportive of their activities, they are more likely to support yours. It is important to involve all sections of the community in decisions, including both men and women and from different social groups. This can take time – especially when there are different views and possible conflicts to take into account.

Meetings

Meetings may be necessary at all stages of programme development and implementation. They are an important way of working with colleagues, other sectors, and the community. Meetings need to be carried out well in order to achieve their objectives. Meetings can fail because of different priorities, personality differences/clashes among the members, lack of information, unbalanced membership/exclusion of key persons and poor leadership. In the setting up of a committee

Box 6.2 Fortification of wheat project in Pakistan – an example of intersectoral collaboration and a public-private partnership for health

Fortification of wheat flour Initiative in Pakistan

Micronutrient malnutrition has been a public health problem in Pakistan. Anaemia is found amongst half of non-pregnant mothers and about a third of pre-school and school-age children. More than a quarter of maternal deaths each year are related with iron deficiency anaemia. Wheat is the major food staple in the country. The Ministry of Health decided to address the iron and folic acid deficiency through countrywide fortification of wheat flour. There are about 600 flour mills in the country. A series of 'production trials' and 'stability and acceptability' studies informed the selection of the fortification mix.

The strategies and implementation details were agreed between the stakeholders, which were the Ministry of Health Nutrition Department, the Pakistan Flour Mills Association and the technical partner the Micronutrient Initiative Pakistan. These included the: (a) import and distribution of mixers and fortification mix, (b) capacity building needs and arrangements for public and private sector partners, (c) millers' role in food control and monitoring, (d) regulation and support of millers through the Pakistan Flour Mills Association, with assistance of public sector and partners, (e) subsidy and pricing mechanisms, (f) demand generation measures, (g) consumption and impact measurement modalities, and (h) sustainability beyond project support, mainly through a mix of public and private inputs.

The project has been successfully implemented. This is an example of addressing a national level public health issue through an effective and sustainable public-private partnership. It is also an example of intersectoral collaboration.

it is important to create a climate of trust among the members, share expectations and to agree on the objectives for the meeting. Once a group has formed it will need to take action which might include gathering information and making decisions and deciding future objectives.

Good leadership can greatly improve the functioning of meetings. Some of the ways a good chairperson can help to encourage decision-making is through:

- Focusing on the agenda/purpose of the meeting
- Introducing new information
- Recognizing when more information is needed to make a decision
- Clarifying points of confusion
- Summarizing the position reached
- Inviting suggestions from members
- Dealing with difficult group members
- Encouraging quieter members to participate
- Dealing with conflicts
- Seeking consensus
- Pushing the group to make a decision
- Trying to find new ways around a problem

Time management

We have already noted the importance of time management for effective implementation. In more detail the timing of activities will depend on the following:

1 *The logical sequencing of activities including dependencies of some activities on completion of others.* Some activities will need to take place earlier in a programme and some later. Some activities will depend on the successful completion of others, for example improved STD services will need to be in place, staff trained and drugs procured before communication activities are carried out to encourage people to use these services.

2 *The availability of staff and other resources.* Timing will depend on when the staff are available. You will need to find out other demands on their time. Activities in your intervention that require the same people for implementation should be separated in time. Timing may also be determined by availability of equipment.

3 *Seasonal factors.* – The timing should take into account public holidays, busy times of the year e.g. planting season for rural communities, accessibility of community in rainy season.

At a personal level it is useful to make up a 'to do' list of tasks you need to carry out. This will prevent you becoming distracted by other demands on your time that are less important. Another simple approach is to write intended activities on a calendar and circle important days. You can buy or draw for yourself a 'year planner'. This is a large sheet with a square for each day of the year on which you can write key activities using colours to show particular tasks. Time is a precious commodity and you need to ensure that how you spend your time reflects your priorities.

Transport

Transport is essential for the operation of many activities within health programmes such as field visits, delivery of supplies, supervision, and training. The cost of vehicles, maintenance, and fuel can be a big part of a programme budget. Problems in transport include high costs, competing demands from different persons for the same transport, breakdown of vehicles, and misuse of vehicles for non-programme activities.

These problems can be overcome through an effective transport policy which sets out guidelines for:

- ◆ Priorities for use of vehicles that are publicized and implemented in an open and fair way;
- ◆ Anticipating transport needs when setting up a new activity and ensuring that costs of fuel and maintenance are included in budgets;
- ◆ Encouraging the use of low cost transport wherever possible – public transport, bicycle, motorcycle and animal transport;
- ◆ Ensuring that drivers are trained to drive safely, seatbelt use is enforced and that vehicles are properly maintained; and
- ◆ Efficient scheduling of travel so that different activities are combined, e.g. delivery of drugs combined with supervisory visits.

Monitoring and evaluation

Monitoring

Most people are convinced that what they are doing is useful. Managers often want to get on with implementation and not waste time and money on monitoring and evaluation. But often the programme isn't working as well as you think! There is nothing more wasteful than finding out late that something isn't working well. So it is important to systematically monitor indicators.

Monitoring is the collection and recording of data in order to track a project's progress and ensure quality of the activities in a programme. It is carried out from the beginning of any activity and should identify early on any problems and successes in order to be able to make corrections immediately. Monitoring can also identify any short-term results for the activity.

The most efficient way is to decide which are the most useful and available indicators to monitor, and make sure this information is collected properly from the start of implementation, that is, collected prospectively. Make sure that the recording and reporting of the essential indicators are covered within implementation guidelines, materials, training and supervision. This is the case for example in the TB DOTS package, with a standard TB card and district register. The name and details of each new TB case are recorded in the register and the number counted and reported at the end of every 3 months (each quarter). The initial and later sputum microscopy test results are recorded. Someone who was sputum positive but then becomes and stays sputum negative is 'cured'. From the register other 'treatment outcomes' for the quarter are calculated, including the number and percent (of all registered in the same quarter) who defaulted, died, or relapsed are reported. If the cures are increasing and defaulting is decreasing, then the programme is working well. But if the indicators are getting worse, or are not as good as in similar districts, then you have to find out why.

Evaluation

Evaluation is the process by which we assess whether an intervention has been effective in achieving its stated objectives and leads to an improvement in the situation. A good evaluation strategy will obtain feedback from the field so that you can continue to improve your intervention. Evaluation is concerned with the effectiveness and efficiency of an intervention and also with its process:

- *Effectiveness* – whether or not a programme achieves its stated objectives at the end of the programme, i.e. did it work?
- *Efficiency* – the amount of effort in terms of time, manpower, resources and money required to reach the objectives – was it worth the effort?
- *Process* – recording information during a programme which helps in understanding why a programme has succeeded or has not succeeded as well as expected. It is closely related to monitoring. The advantage of process evaluation is that information is collected as the programme develops so it is possible to make changes and adjust the activities.

Methods that can be used in monitoring and process evaluation are shown in Table 6.3.

So evaluation involves showing that: A *change* has taken place, the change took place as a *result* of the programme, and the amount of *effort* required to produce the change was worthwhile. The results of evaluation can then be fed into decision-making about programme changes. Critical decisions in choosing an evaluation strategy are:

- *What changes* should you look for including both expected and unexpected changes?
- *What data collection methods* should you use to find out what changes have taken place?
- *Who* should do the evaluation?
- *What evaluation design* can you use to show that the changes were a result of your intervention?
- *How* can you involve the target audience in the evaluation process?

Table 6.3 Summary table data collection methods for monitoring and process evaluation

Main categories of Sources of data	Specific sources of monitoring data	Characteristics of the data source
Routine information sources *Sources of data based on on-going activities and not requiring special inputs above normal programme implementation*	*Clinic records:* (either as part of case management or surveillance)	Useful for measures of service utilization, behaviour change, and treatment efficacy. However, value depends on the quality and consistency of record keeping. Data in records is a measure of utilization of services, not of prevalence in the community. Using records for monitoring requires revising record sheets, training health workers and supervisory visits to ensure accurate data entry
	Stock records: e.g. condoms, drugs, needles	This is a useful measure for measuring delivery of materials. However, it needs to be supplemented by other sources of monitoring data to provide information of the quality of condoms use needles etc.
	Field worker contact sheets: notes completed by field workers/peer educators on activities, educational sessions	This can be a valuable source of data on delivery of intervention, impact, and problems experienced. Persons with low education e.g. peer educators may find difficulty in completing forms. There may be a risk that workers may make up data for forms. Simple forms for data entry need to be developed and training provided on using them. Data from self-completed forms need to be supplemented by supervisory visits
	Notes on supervisory activities: notes completed by supervisors following meetings with individuals or groups of outreach workers and observation of them working in field setting.	This is one of the most important sources of monitoring data. It can identify problems experienced by field staff and is especially useful when peer educators find it difficult to fill out forms. Forms should be developed for supervisors to record their visits. In addition to discussing progress, supervisors should observe field activities in practice. To cross check the information given, the supervisor can set up surprise visits, send 'dummy' patients to tryout a service or carry out exit interviews (see below)
Non-routine data collection sources	*Focus Groups:* discussions carried out by a trained facilitator with groups of 6–8 persons from the target audience.	This is a particularly useful method as it can be undertaken quickly and cheaply and gather valuable insights into problems and solutions. Care needs to be taken to use a trained facilitator and in selection of the composition of the focus groups. It needs to be supplemented with quantitative data from other sources such as records, supervisory visits.
Sources of data which require additional programme effort above that of ordinary implementation	*Exit interviews:* Interviews with persons immediately following encounter with programme e.g. the STD service, counselling session etc.	This can be a useful method for obtaining information on the quality of the intervention – and can be combined with supervisory visits and observation of intervention activities.

Table 6.3 *(continued)* Summary table data collection methods for monitoring and process evaluation

Main categories of Sources of data	Specific sources of monitoring data	Characteristics of the data source
These are usually more appropriate for evaluation rather than monitoring.	*Rapid assessments:* surveys using a mix of qualitative and qualitative data on small samples of the target audience and key informants.	This is a low cost alternative to a full survey (see below) and provides data on the current situation, problems and causes. Care is needed to ensure that it is carried out properly and the data collected is not biased.
	Surveys: structured data gathering with questionnaires and/or observation schedules and large samples.	Surveys are mainly used in monitoring when the programme is trying out radically new approaches or tackling difficult problems.

A good monitoring strategy will generate some of the data you need to evaluate your pro-gramme. However, if you are trying develop new methods to tackle a problem you will need to gather additional data that will identify the factors contributing to success or failure and show that the methods you used were the cause of any changes and exclude other possible explanations for the changes you observed. Process evaluation will provide such information. You should also consider whether to set up *control* communities who are not exposed to the intervention that can be compared with your target community.

Indicators and targets and data collection

One of the most important tasks in monitoring and evaluation is to design suitable indicators that can be used to measure progress and achievements. This has to be done at the beginning of a programme when setting the priorities and objectives (see discussion in earlier section). Indicators can be designed for:

Project inputs: Field visits, number of training sessions completed, leaflets produced, drugs procured, budget spent;

Activities completed: Number of consultations, drugs/condoms dispensed, leaflets given out, educational sessions held, home visits carried out;

Short-term results: e.g. Persons coming for treatment, changes in community knowledge, changes in practices, e.g. self medication, use of oral rehydration, latrine construction, contraceptive use;

Long term results: Gains in health, reduction in morbidity and mortality.

Choice of indicators is often a compromise between what is desirable and what is possible. For example, distribution of condoms to sex workers is easy to measure but not an indicator of whether the condoms are used properly. Decisions on targets depend on the local needs, the resources at your disposal and how easy or difficult you think it will be to achieve progress. Actions on health topics are more likely to be successful if they are in response to the felt needs of the community. A useful guide is to see what has been accomplished by programmes in communities that are similar to your own.

The processes of collection and handling of data have to be carefully organized and carried out. Key points on these processes are shown in Box 6.3.

It is worth emphasizing the importance of prompt analysis of any qualitative data that may be collected from interviews or focus groups. When such discussions have been recorded in writing

Box 6.3 Data collection and handling

◆ Data collection should be accurate and reliable. Use a standard data collection form. Make sure the people collecting data are properly trained. Check the accuracy of data at regular intervals.

◆ Data collation should be simple and accessible. Information should be kept up to date in one central location. Collation can be in the form of a filing system, indexed cards, a register book, or a computer database.

◆ Data analysis should be undertaken at regular (e.g. monthly) intervals to provide summaries of information for feedback. Analysis can be by manual counting (for frequencies or incident cases) or by computer programmes (e.g. Epi Info, Excel) for more complex analysis or large numbers.

◆ Data storage. It is important to ensure that any patient details are stored securely and that confidentiality is maintained at all times. Health information is sensitive information and patients have a right to confidentiality.

◆ Data dissemination. There is no point collecting information that does not get used to plan, monitor or change services. Summaries of information should be fed back to relevant health professionals and regional or national agencies.

analysis is easier when the meeting is still fresh in the mind. Even when possible to tape meetings the quality of tapes can differ. Immediate transcribing of tapes while the memory is fresh helps in filling in any gaps and going back to people to check information. Staff need to be given adequate time to complete these activities.

Dissemination and communication of evaluation results

It is important to communicate your experience and results to others. These include funders, agencies, workers, and local communities. This can be through presentation in meetings or through publications. Communication should be with the public through the local media and community and political leaders. Communicate the key points and distribute guidelines and materials through health team meetings to your local and national colleagues. If you can write up as a journal article for publication to inform the wider audience (and they look good on your CV). It should be noted that many journals now actively seek to publish papers based on experience in parts of the world which have not previously had wide coverage.

Implementation research

When trying out new intervention strategies, the opportunity can be taken for implementation research. Another name for this is operational research, i.e. finding out the best operational approach to most effectively implement a new strategy. The simplest approach is to compare the indicators (such as TB treatment outcomes) before and after implementing the new approach. But there may be other (confounding) reasons why the indicators improve. So better to choose similar district/ sites where the existing approach has been implemented for comparison (control sites). Then if the results are significantly better in the intervention compared to the control sites, then you can be confident that the new approach is better. It is even better, and fairer, if the intervention and control sites to be the first to implement the new approach are chosen at random. To do this, list all the sites first- to last and use random numbers from the computer to decide, or just write down the name of each site on a piece of paper and pick out from a hat which will be the intervention and which the control sites. Randomization avoids both known and unknown causes of bias.

The creation of integrated MNCH and Family Planning Services is an example of implementation. There is great variation in how MNCH interventions are delivered in health facilities. New service delivery approaches may need to be introduced to improve coverage or quality. Perhaps new vaccinations or family planning methods would improve existing services. New approaches need to be developed, perhaps initially in one health facility and then replicated. This approach is illustrated with a case study of implementing daily, integrated MNCH services in Ethiopia, see Box 6.4. This case study also brings out the importance of helping workers to accept and manage change.

There are many constraints to integration, and scaling-up from small successful pilot studies is difficult. Implementation of more integrated MNCH services depends on all the staff knowing what is required and being given the medical and technical means to carry out their function. However, the major constraint is frequently overcoming the simple organizational changes required. The following are some of these constraints and how they may be overcome (as done in Ethiopia).

Winning over the staff. People tend to resist change, as they are comfortable with the familiar routine. In order to accept the introduction of changes, staff will need be persuaded that the new approach will be more varied and interesting for them, as well as more beneficial to the patient. They need to see for themselves – and participate in – a well-functioning service incorporating the improved approaches.

Simplicity of the work and workload. It is obviously easier to do one task at a time especially when dealing with large numbers of women and children. Integrated services require health workers to take longer for each consultation. On the other hand, fewer contacts will be required with each mother and child. Integration, therefore, requires that procedures be simplified using checklists so that treatment and the relevant preventive interventions are provided effectively and quickly.

Case records. The case recording system may need reorganizing. The separate case notes, vaccination cards, weight charts and ante-natal cards are best redesigned as integrated into child and

Box 6.4 Daily integrated MCH services in Ethiopia

Prior to integration the adult and children's curative and preventive services were provided separately. A mother would walk long distances for treatment of her child sick with a respiratory infection, only to be told to come back on another day for vaccination, ante-natal case, or family planning. After integration all these services were provided daily, and most by the same health worker in the same consultation.

Kombolcha health centre schedule before integration

Type of service	Schedule	Frequency
Curative care	Daily	
Vaccination of children	Tuesday a.m.	×1/week
Ante-natal care	Wednesday a.m.	×1/week
Family planning	Thursday a.m.	×1/week
'Sick baby' (treatment and weighing of ill infants)	Friday a.m.	×1/week

women's health cards. This requires national level action. In the absence of this the separate cards can be stapled together or put in a family folder.

Patient flow. If you are to organize integrated services, then you may need to re-arrange the flow of patients. The usual approach is to have a common registration point with patients directed to the examination room or vaccination room etc. depending on what they request. In a more integrated MNCH services introduced in Ethiopia all the patients are seen in integrated consultation rooms.

When the health worker has first provided the curative care the mother is then receptive to advice on preventive services. This integrated approach provides a more personalized service with fewer missed opportunities. Only those with more complex illness need to be referred on to the doctor, who then has time to properly assess and treat these cases.

For integrated MNCH and other services a well functioning district health system and referral system is required, see Chapter 10. Good management is required to implement effective daily MCH services. These include coordination, training, supervision, and community involvement. In addition, changing the health seeking behaviour, and care practices with sick children and pregnant women requires effective health promotion, see Chapter 8.

Conclusions

Programme development and implementation is the biggest and most important part of a public health manager's job. This starts with a review of the existing situation and so knowledge of the health needs. Effective implementation depends on choosing and prioritizing the best interventions and their delivery strategies. The activities and an action plan are prepared. This programming should be done by a small group of the most experienced people. Realistic objectives are set. The programming is designed in a way to be effective, sustainable and replicable. A working group process can be used to adapt guidelines, training modules, supervision, and other materials. Implementation is usually best done in a phased way. Piloting is useful for refining approaches and materials, and this can be done in the early implementation sites.

Indicators are chosen and monitored, gaps identified and activities are adjusted as required to maintain progress. The subsequent chapters cover health economics policy, promotion, the district health systems, and essential drugs, which include important issues relevant to effective programme design and implementation.

Further reading

Abbatt, F. and McMahon, R. (1985) *Teaching health care workers - a practical guide*, London: Macmillan.

Abbatt, F. (1990) Personnel development and training. In: Streefland, P. and Chabot, J. (Eds.) *Implementing primary health care: experiences since Alma Ata*, pp. 41–50. Amsterdam: Royal Tropical Institute.

Amonoo-Lartson, R., Ebrahim, G., Lovel, H.J. and Ranken, J. (1984) *District health care - challenges for planning, organisation and evaluation in developing countries*, London: Macmillan.

Green, A. (2007) *An introduction to health planning for developing health system*, 3rd edition. Oxford: OUP.

Hubley, J. (2005) *Communicating health: an action guide to health education and health promotion*, 2nd edition. Basingstoke and London: Macmillan.

Janovsky, K. (1987) *Project formulation and proposal writing*, World Health Organization, Geneva

UNICEF. EPI mid level managers course, including the modules on monitoring and supervision.http://www.afro.who.int/ddc/vpd/epi_mang_course/index.html

Webber R, Communicable Disease Epidemiology and Control CABI Publishing. Oxford, second edition, 2004 (a third edition due in 2009).

WHO. On being in charge. A guide to management in primary health care: By R. McMahon, E. Barton and M. Piot, in collaboration with N. Gelina and F. Ross. WHO Geneva, 1992, ISBN 92-4-154426-0.

Chapter 7

Understanding and using health economics and financing

Sophie Witter

This chapter gives an overview of the following topics:

- What is health economics? Why does it matter?
- Health financing options, focussing on health insurance and user fees;
- How to cost a health programme;
- The uses of economic evaluation;
- Financial sustainability and project appraisal;
- Designing a formula for resource allocation between areas;
- Rationing and essential service packages;
- Measuring performance and efficiency of services;
- Public/private mix issues;
- Payment systems for health care staff and institutions.

Introduction: The health economic perspective

Economists in general have a poor public image. They are associated with unintelligible graphs, people who are obsessed with making savings and a lack of concern for the suffering of the poor and sick.

Nothing should be further from the truth. Health economics, like public health, takes a population perspective, and asks the fundamental question: How can we get the best results, in terms of better health, from the resources which are available in this community? In pursuing this question, health economists use public health information about, for example, the effectiveness of a health programme and combine it with information about resources (money, staff time, equipment etc.) in order to advise on whether that programme should be pursued.

Why bother about resources? Quite simply, because money spent on one programme means less available for another. This is what economists call '*opportunity costs*'. Pursuing an ineffective programme, or running a badly managed one, means that people will remain ill or die who might otherwise have been saved by that money, if it had been spent on a more effective programme. Similarly, a programme which relies on financial contributions from patients will take away money which families might have used for other important needs, such as food or education. That is why we cannot make judgements about services without taking into account how much they cost, and how they are to be paid for.

What are the types of questions which health economics can help to answer?

1 What resources are available for improving health? Are they adequate to sustain the services which are most needed in a given context? How can we increase them in a way which is fair or equitable, taking into account the different needs and ability to pay of different social groups? This is the area of health financing, which we will tackle first.

2 Given these resources, which services should be provided or expanded, and which diminished? This involves a series of issues, including costing services, assessing benefits, and then combining the information with local needs, preferences, and priorities to plan the most appropriate mix of services. This area – what we should do, or *allocative efficiency* – will be discussed next.

3 Given these resources and this plan, a series of questions can be asked relating to implementation. Who should provide the services (e.g. public or private sector?)? In which kind of health facility are the services best delivered? How should services best be bundled, taking into account both provider and user needs? How efficient are existing services? Could they be improved by reorganization or changes to budgets, staffing etc.?

These questions (Fig. 7.1) – not what we do, but *how* we do it, which economists call '*technical efficiency*' – form the last section of this chapter.

Health financing

Introductory comments: Options and issues

There are many different potential sources of funding for health services. These include, for example:

- Government funding, taken from central taxation;
- Local taxes, on incomes, services, sales, land etc.;
- Compulsory insurance schemes, usually set up by the government;
- Voluntary insurance, either profit- or non-profit-making;
- Official user fees, for public or private services;
- Informal payments, in cash or kind;
- Community payment schemes;
- Individual savings accounts;
- Aid funds.

Health financing is concerned with how much can be raised through these different sources and the efficiency (value-for-money) and equity (fairness) of the different methods.

Typically, financing systems which 'pool risk' tend to be more equitable than those which do not. By risk pooling, we mean that the costs of prevention and treatment are shared across a group of people, regardless of who is actually using the services. Poorer households generally suffer from worse health and are less able to afford healthcare. If they have to pay directly for health care (e.g. through informal payments a major source in many low and middle income countries today) then there may be a number of negative effects for them, such as having to delay treatment, not being able to afford treatment, falling into debt, or having to reduce consumption of food and other important goods. On the other hand, if their risks are pooled, through, for example, a national financing scheme, then families with higher health needs may be subsidized by those who are less needy and/or more able to pay. For this reason, a transition from low risk-pooling systems (such as user fees) to high risk-pooling systems (such as taxation-based public finance or social insurance) is generally recommended.

To achieve this cross-subsidy, we need to look at who is paying for services (e.g. in the case of central taxation, who is paying the taxes: on which groups in the population does the highest burden fall?) but also, crucially, at who is using the services. If public funds are concentrated on services which are mostly used by a relatively affluent urban elite, then increasing those finances will have an adverse effect on poor rural populations.

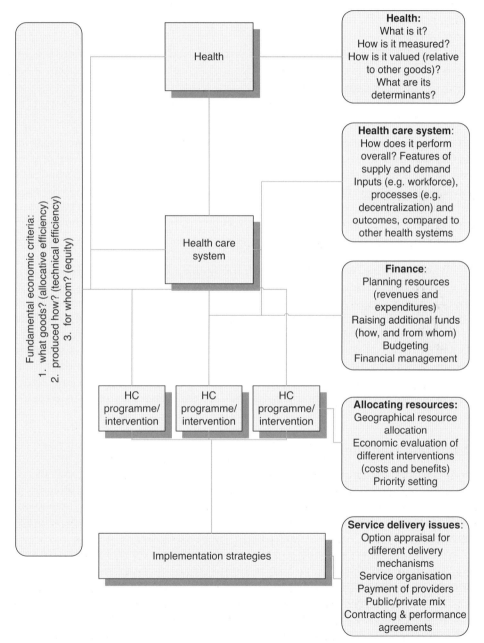

Fig 7.1 Health economics questions.

Table 7.1 Global health financing overview, 2005

	GNI per capita (current $, Atlas method)	Health expenditure per capita (current $)	Health expenditure (% GDP), 2005	% Health expenditure private	% Health expenditure from external sources	% Private payments paid out of pocket
Low income	583	27	4.6	75	6	92
Middle income	2,646	162	6	49	0	75
High income	35,014	3979	11	38	0	37

Source: World Bank, HNP Stats, 2008.

Is there an easy rule-of-thumb about the right level of financing for a given area? Sadly not. Comparisons with other similar areas will tell you whether you are relatively well or poorly financed, but nothing about optimal (or ideal) levels. The optimal level depends on many factors, such as the level of health needs; other priorities for spending in the area; income levels; and the effectiveness of health services. More is not always better – for example, health may be better improved through increased funding for infrastructure (e.g. water supplies, or schools) or rural development. Health services can sometimes deliver poor value-for-money, or even be harmful to people's health.

Generally speaking, funding for health care should rise as health needs increase, as income levels rise, and as effectiveness of services increases. In most developing countries, the level of financing is rightly regarded as too low, and the key issue is therefore how to increase it. Average expenditure on health care in low income countries in 2005 was $27 per person (under 5% of GDP), while for developed countries it was almost $4000 per person (11% of a much higher GDP). In addition to being too low overall, expenditure in low income settings is unequally distributed and dominated by private contributions, and those private contributions are largely out-of-pocket (see Table 7.1). In this short chapter, we cannot go into great detail on different funding mechanisms, but will make a few comments about some of the most common methods.

Taxation-based funding

Funds which the government collects through taxes and passes on to health services in the form of budgets and staff payments are the main source of public finance in developing countries, and also the main source of health finance globally. They are, however, declining as a proportion of overall spending in the health sector, which means other funding channels have been growing in importance.

Tax-based funding has the advantage of pooling risks over a large group (as taxation is compulsory, at least in theory), and it can be *progressive,* if taxes take proportionately more from the richer in society and services are used proportionately more by the poorer. In practice, however, in many developing countries taxes may fall more heavily on the middle class and poorest, and services are often used most by the relatively better off. Furthermore, although everyone has theoretical entitlement under this system, if the collection system is poor, or if the allocation

The challenge of coordinating aid

Donors are an important channel of health financing, particularly in low-income countries. There are over 40 bilateral donors, 26 UN agencies, 20 global and regional funds and 90 global health initiatives. All of them operate different projects, with different funding mechanism and goals, which can undermine the development of strong national health systems. One approach to harmonizing aid in the 1990s was the development of SWAps – **sector-wide approaches**, in which donors would pool funds to support the health budget, subject to agreed planning and review processes. This has been successful in some contexts, but many donors and global programmes are unable to join SWAps, which undermines their effectiveness. Indeed, the emergence of large disease-specific global funds (such as the Global Fund for AIDS, Tuberculosis and Malaria) threatens to re-fragment health systems which were integrating funding and service provision.

The **Paris declaration** of 2005[1] focused on improving the quality of aid and aid coordination. All host countries and donors are now supposed to be working towards agreed targets, including strengthening national development strategies and systems, aligning aid with national priorities, increasing the predictability of aid, mutual accountability, and sharing of common operating procedures.

In some countries, donors are moving to **multi-donor budget support**, which implies even greater pooling, in that funds are not allocated to any particular sector, but become available for the government to allocate inter-sectorally, subject to jointly agreed indicators.

[1] http://www.oecd.org/document/18/0,2340,en_2649_3236398_35401554_1_1_1_1,00.html

to health is low, then the reality can be a semi-privatized system, relying substantially on contributions from households.

Insurance schemes

Insurance schemes differ from government funding in that there is usually a specified package of benefits (e.g. free or reduced price services, and sometimes drugs) and eligibility is limited to those who have contributed to or have been enrolled in the scheme. Setting up an insurance scheme raises a number of important issues.

1 *Individual or group premiums?* Private insurance schemes usually operate individual *risk-rating*, which means that a high-risk individual (e.g. who smokes, or has a history of medical complaints) will be charged more to join than a low-risk individual. This may attract low-risk individuals to join the scheme, but it pools risk less, and is also more complicated to operate (as information on lifestyles etc. must be obtained for applicants).

   By contrast, a group premium is simpler to set, but runs the risk of '*adverse selection*', which means that only relatively high-risk individuals or families choose not to join. This will cause premiums to rise, if this scheme is to remain financially viable.

2 *Setting premium levels. How much should be charged?* The simple answer is: enough to keep the fund solvent. Assuming that the premium is fixed-rate, this means working out:

   ◆ The cost of the benefits which are covered by the scheme (based on utilisation rates and cost of services);

   ◆ The number of people who you think will join;

- ◆ How much it will cost to administer;
- ◆ A reserve to cover difficult times (and profits, if the scheme is profit-making);

$$\frac{\text{community premium} = \text{expected benefits} + \text{administrative costs} + \text{reserve} + \text{profits}}{\text{number insured}}$$

3   *What to include in the benefits package?* There are all sorts of considerations here, including whether services are of high priority (see below), whether there is high demand for them (i.e. whether they will attract people to join the scheme) and whether they are affordable.

These considerations do not always match. For example, from a public health point of view, you may wish to include programmes with knock-on positive effects, such as TB treatment, which limits the spread of a disease to others (this is known as a 'positive externality' by health economists). However, popular demand may focus more on what are perceived as urgent needs, such as accident and emergency services. There may also be a high demand for free drugs, for example, but including this in the benefits package may violate the last principle of affordability, as costs tend to escalate if users face no charges for drugs.

All three principles are important and have to be balanced against one another, so that the scheme achieves some measure of all – attractive, affordable, and making a contribution to improving community health.

4   *Dealing with moral hazard.* '*Moral hazard*' is the term which economists use to describe a situation where consumers do not bear the direct costs of services and so are encouraged to behave in a way which increases the use of those services. For example, they may take risks or fail to take preventive measures if they know that the insurance company will pay for all future treatment. In the medium term this raises the cost of premiums, which is undesirable, and insurance schemes need to find ways of limiting moral hazard. One option is to set up copayments, so that use is not entirely free to users. Another is to risk-rate individuals, as described above.

5   *Achieving high coverage.* The smaller the scheme, the higher will be the costs of running it (as a proportion of revenue) and the smaller the risk pool (implying less stability, and/or the need for a bigger reserve). Schemes will want to achieve economies of scale (lower costs, because of being larger), but this can be difficult if membership is voluntary.

A well-run and attractive insurance scheme can combine the advantages of risk-pooling with providing a clearly specified, relatively high quality service. However, insurance is not a panacea.

Overall sources of health finance and composition of health expenditure: The role of national health accounts

All countries raise finance for health care from a variety of sources, and spend them through a variety of channels. Often decision-makers do not have the full picture of how health care is being financed (particularly private contributions and private sector activities). A tool called national health accounts has therefore been developed to help map the flow of funds through the health care sector as a whole, and to provide a uniform measurement tool which can allow for comparisons across regions and countries. A full guide to how to develop a National Health Account is provided by WHO (http://www.who.int/nha/docs/English_PG.pdf). An equivalent tool for mapping health expenditure at the district level has been developed in Tanzania (http://www.idrc.ca/uploads/user-S/10936340001TEHIP_Discussion_Paper__-_District_Health_Expenditure.pdf).

If income levels are low, affordability will be a problem. If membership is voluntary, coverage levels can be disappointing. If benefits are over-generous, schemes can go bankrupt quickly. The establishment of a parallel bureaucracy to collect funds and make payments also generates costs. All of the issues raised above need to be considered before starting up.

User charges

User charges were widely implemented in the health sector in developing countries in the 1980s and some general lessons have been learnt from that experience.

1 User charges can add useful small amounts of income at the local level, but rarely re-coup a large proportion of costs. (They should therefore be seen as a supplementary channel, rather than the main one.)

2 They may limit 'excessive demand' (unnecessary use of services), as originally argued by organizations such as the World Bank, but they also limit legitimate demand, especially by poorer families, and can force households into poverty (see Box 7.1).

3 Exemption schemes for the poorer are rarely well-implemented, so the equity effects of charges have to be considered carefully in advance (see Box 7.2).

4 In addition to creating financial barriers for users, user fees have the potential to distort supply, encouraging facilities to provide services which are profitable, rather than necessarily appropriate.

5 By reducing demand for public health services, user fees can reduce the efficiency of service provision (most of the costs for staffing and buildings are fixed, so lower utilisation automatically increases the cost per case).

It is now recognised that user fees are the least desirable health financing mechanism, although many countries continue to rely heavily on them.

Box 7.1 Out-of-pocket payments and catastrophic expenditure

There has been increasing concern about the extent to which households have to make direct payments for health care – not just fees, but also payments for travel, food, accommodation, drugs, accompanying relatives, etc. – and the impact of these payments on the household economy. A recent WHO report found that around 6% of the population in 89 study countries were pushed under the poverty line by health care payments. Other impacts can include:

◆ Having to reduce essential expenditures, such as food and clothing

◆ Having to withdraw children from education and send them to work

◆ Getting into debt, with long-term implications for future spending

◆ Mortgaging productive assets, such as land

◆ Reduced access to treatment, with potential long term health consequences

◆ Social and emotional impacts, including family break-down and increased risk of depression

Catastrophic costs are closely correlated with user fees and measures to reduce them focus on extending other forms of health financing which pool risk more, with a particular emphasis on providing financial protection for the poor and marginalized populations.

Box 7.2 Reducing the impact of user fees – recent trends

It is generally recognized that user fees are a regressive method of raising funds for the health sector (one that hurts poor families and prevents them accessing care). This led a number of health systems to develop waiver systems, which state that poor families should be exempted from paying user fees. However, as these waiver systems are usually not funded, they have been found to be ineffective in general. Facilities need to fund their services, and unless the revenue is being replaced, will continue to charge patients for services. In addition, identifying the poor is not straightforward, and health staff may face conflicting pressures to increase facility (or personal) revenue.

In response to these difficulties, governments have taken a variety of approaches to increasing access to care. These have included:

- Identifying priority services to provide at no cost to users. These typically include services with high positive externalities, such as vaccination and TB treatment
- Identifying priority population groups, such as mothers and young children, who are exempted from paying for health care
- Using geographic targeting of exemptions, for example by making certain services free in poorer or more marginalized areas of the country
- Using external agencies (such as NGOs) to assess eligibility for exemption and to provide financial support to the poor
- Providing subsidies for poor households to join prepayment, community health insurance or social insurance schemes
- Removing fees as a whole for whole categories of care (e.g. primary care) or for all health care

Some have gone beyond removing fees to providing additional financial support to enable households to access essential care (including costs such as transport). For example, cash might be given to households if they bring their children in for vaccination, or if they deliver in facilities, rather than at home. These 'conditional cash transfers' have been shown to be effective for preventive services, though they can be expensive to administer.

Informal charges of various sorts currently play a large part in funding health care in many developing countries. There is a debate about whether these should be 'legitimized' into official user fees. The argument in favour is that it would be easier to control these funds and use them appropriately and that the cost would be more predictable for customers. Where customers feel that they are able to use additional payments to secure quality, and practitioners have an entrenched interest in receiving them (this tends to be more the case amongst urban secondary specialists), it may not be easy to ban informal payments. The risk is that user charges are added onto, rather than replacing, informal charges.

Costing services

In order to advise on how to use the available funds to achieve the best results for the health of the population, we need to be able to measure and compare the costs and benefits of different health programmes. Costing services is therefore an important task, which allows us to draw up contracts for services, carry out economic evaluations and identify ways of improving the organization of services.

Many people assume that we already know how much it costs to provide the main health services, but that is rarely the case. Let us imagine that you want to know how much it costs to run the village health worker (VHW) programme in your district. What information would you need to find; where would you find it; and how would you put together an overall figure?

1 **Allocating costs.** The first person to ask would probably be the district finance officer. You ask for the health budget. It arrives (if you are lucky!), broken into headings such as maintenance, staffing, transport, and supplies. Budgets tend to be structured by inputs (e.g. salaries, training costs etc.), rather than outputs, so the first task is to assign the right amount of each type of expenditure to the programme which you are costing.

   For example, how many staff work on the programme, and for what proportion of their time? How much of the vehicle mileage is attributable to the programme? What proportion of the supplies are used by the programme and how much clinic or office space? Using whatever information is available (or carrying out independent surveys, if necessary); you can work out roughly how much is spent on the VHW programme.

   In a hospital setting, you will need to allocate the costs of administrative departments and support services (such as diagnostics or lab services), either exactly, if you know how much of that service has been used by your programme, or using some proxy such as number of patients (relative to the total) or number of bed-days in that department.

2 **Capital costs.** These cover items such as major equipment and vehicles, or other items which are not replaced every year. They are usually costed separately because their total cost has to be divided by the number of years that they are likely to last. That figure can then be added to the recurrent costs listed above.

If we are using costing for some relatively simple purpose such as establishing a budget for the programme, then we may be able to stop at this level of analysis. However, if we wish to compare costs with other programmes, in order to decide whether to increase the VHW activities, then we should ideally include a wider range of costs.

1 **Higher level costs.** Do not forget to include costs incurred in supporting or developing the programme by other parts of the health system. For example, time by managers or training activities – all of these are real costs to the health system which should therefore be included.

2 **Other agency costs.** Similarly, other government departments, or non-governmental organizations, may be making inputs into the VHW programme (such as training). Although these do not affect the health budget, they are resources which could be used for some other purpose if this programme was not running, and should therefore be included if you can get estimates for them.

3 **Patient costs.** Health service personnel are rarely concerned about the costs of patients. These may take a number of forms. First, there may be *direct costs*, such as user fees or informal payments, or payments for drugs and transport to access services. These are 'direct' in the sense that the patient (or their relative) actually hands over money for them. Collecting information about these types of costs usually requires a survey of patients. Where informal payments are semi-legal, it may be hard to get accurate figures for how much is being paid.

   In addition, most patients face *indirect costs*. For example, if they take time off work, they may lose income. Women may have to trade favours with a neighbour to get them to look after the household while they are away. In such cases, a real cost is faced, although it is harder to estimate. One of the simplest approaches is to use the hourly wage rate as a proxy for the

Web-based resources for costing, planning, and economic evaluations

There are now many web-based tools which provide assistance on costing services and packages of services, and on estimating the costs of scaling up (and sometimes cost benefit and cost-effectiveness ratios). See, for example:

- The WHO Choice website (http://www.who.int/choice/en/) for unit cost information and tools for conducting cost-effectiveness analysis

- CorePlus, a tool for bottom-up costing of health care packages. Also available from dcollins@msh.org.

- Marginal budgeting for bottlenecks (MBB) (http://mdgr.undp.sk/PAPERS/MBB%20 Concept%20Paper.doc) – a tool developed by a number of organizations to assist planners in projecting the resource requirements to meet MDG goals.

- UNDP Integrated Health Model – a tool for comprehensive costing of the resources needed to meet the MDGs (www.undp.org).

- Reproductive health costing tool, developed by UNFPA. Available from: weissman@ unfpa.org

- Making pregnancy safer-integrated healthcare technology package, a resource planning and costing tool developed by WHO and the MRC, Cape Town. Contact issakova@who. intfor details.

- Resource Needs Model, which is an Excel worksheet that calculates the funding required for an expanded response to HIV/AIDS at the national level (http://www.constellagroup. com/international-development/resources/software.php).

- GOALS, a resource allocation tool for HIV/AIDS programme (RNM website above)

- Planning, costing, and budgeting framework for HIV/AIDS programme. Available from dcollins@msh.org.

- PMTCT evaluates the costs and benefits of intervention programmes to reduce transmission of HIV from mother to child (RNM website above)

- FamPlan projects family planning requirements needed to reach national goals for addressing unmet need or achieving desired fertility (RNM website above)

- BenCost compares the monetary cost of family planning programmes to the monetary benefits in terms of reduced levels of social services required at lower levels of fertility (RNM website above)

- The malaria cost estimation tool, developed by WHO to estimate the resource implications of proven malaria interventions over a period of time (http://www.rbm.who.int/docs/ malariaCostingToolUserManual.pdf)

- Planning and Budgeting for TB – developed with the Stop TB programme in WHO to support planning the resource implications of implementing Stop TB policies in-country. Contact floydk@who.int.

- cMYP – a costing and financing tool for childhood immunization, developed by WHO. Available from lydonp@who.int

value of one hour's time. For further details of this technique see the Drummond book, referenced at the end of this chapter.

4 **Other opportunity costs.** Are there any other costs, such as volunteers' time, which we have not yet included? The question to ask here is: What was the next best use of that resource? So, for example, if the VHW would otherwise have been working in agriculture, then their likely earnings from that represent the value of the time they spend on the health programme.

5 **Marginal costs.** If cost information is being collected in order to decide whether to expand or reduce a service, then what is required, ideally, is not the overall (or average) costs of running it, but how much costs would increase or decrease as service activity increases or decreases. This is what is known as 'marginal costs'.

    The reason why marginal costs may differ from average costs is that some costs are fixed, which means that they do not vary with output (e.g. one clinic building must be maintained, no matter how many patients come in to be seen). Others are variable: Each extra person seen will need forms, drugs, tests, for example. Other costs again are semi-variable: A certain amount of increase in activity, for example, may be carried out by existing staff, but beyond a point new people will have to be recruited.

    If the bulk of costs are fixed, then increases or decreases in activity will not make much difference to expenditure. This should influence decisions about the optimal size of programmes.

Economic evaluation

Economic evaluation combines the information on costs which we have described above with information on benefits of programmes. The purpose of this is to inform decision-making about which activities to fund, to expand or to contract.

    Cost-minimization is the simplest type of economic evaluation. If there were two options under consideration (e.g. drug A versus drug B), both with the same effectiveness, then naturally we would choose the cheapest one. By carrying out a careful costing, we should be able to advise which one to use.

    Life is rarely so simple. More commonly, we need to consider two options which offer the same type of benefits (e.g. prolonged life), but to differing degrees. In this case, we also need to look at how much extra life is gained by each option, relative to their costs. This is called a *cost-effectiveness analysis* (CEA).

    Typical cost-effectiveness measures are cost per life saved, cost per added year of life, or cost per case averted (in the case of preventive measures). Which measure you choose will depend on the nature of the programme which is being evaluated, and how much information is available. Some evaluations have to use activity data rather than outcome data, for example if information on the effectiveness of an intervention is lacking. In this case, we may end up with figures for cost per family visited, or cost per case treated. This is less than ideal, as we are left guessing how much impact the visits or treatments have had. This may be the case for our village health workers, especially if they are carrying out multiple functions.

    A few points about CEA:

1 It should be used to compare options whose benefits can reasonably be reflected in a single index. If one programme primarily reduces pain, and another primarily increases life expectancy, then their benefits cannot easily be reflected by one outcome measure, and some form of cost-utility analysis (CUA – see further on) may be needed.

2 As with all such calculations, the result will only be valid if the right information is used. Have all appropriate options been considered? Are the cost and benefits calculations accurate? etc.

3 The decision rule about which programme to choose is not as simple as with cost-minimiza-tion, where the cheapest option is automatically the best. A programme with a higher cost-effectiveness ratio (CER) may still be chosen if (a) high coverage is important; (b) it is affordable and (c) it is still efficient relative to other possible uses of the funds.

As noted under costs (above), marginal benefits may be a more useful measure than the overall, or average, benefit. What is the marginal CER of expanding this vaccination programme? The answer will depend on how costs are affected by increasing coverage. Costs are likely to rise as outlying groups are serviced.

Where costs and benefits occur over a number of years, it is accepted practice to 'discount' them. Discounting reflects the fact that individuals, and society as a whole, prefers a benefit now rather than later. This 'time preference' varies, but commonly discount rates in the range of 3–5% per year are used. This allows us to compare costs and benefits which occur at different points in time on an equal footing.

Sometimes we want to compare options which have very different outcomes. For example, should we invest in improved ante-natal care, or in school health programmes? What are the outcomes here? We might wish to include lives saved, reduced maternal and child morbidity, reduced anxiety and improved attendance at school. How can these all be captured and compared in a single index? One option is to try to create a multi-dimensional index which can reflect improvements in quantity and quality of life. This approach is called *cost utility analysis (CUA)*.

A basic example of CUA is the disability-adjusted life year (DALY), which the World Bank commonly uses in priority-setting exercises. Gains in morbidity are counted as fractions of a 'full' year of life, according to expert assessment of the degree of disability caused by a disease. These can then be added to life years gained by programmes which avert death.

All of these indexes are complicated to compile and depend on a number of assumptions. We generally assume, for example, that one life year is of equal value, no matter who gains it. This assumption will not be true, of course, but it is a useful and egalitarian assumption. We may or may not assume that one life year is of equal value, no matter at what age it is 'gained'. The World Bank World Development Report of 1993, for example, age-weights DALYs to reflect the impor-tance of the productive adult years. We also have to make assumptions about life expectancy. Should we use the local level (which may be relatively low, thus reducing estimates of potential gains) or an ideal level (e.g. Japanese life expectancy of 81, used in the World Development Report)? All these assumptions should be spelled out, as they may make a significant impact on the results.

A more complicated system is the quality-adjusted life year (QALY), which uses assessments of quality of life by patients or doctors. Different dimensions can thus be incorporated – not just reduced physical disability but also other factors which are very important to patients, such as pain, mobility, social functioning etc.

All of the measures mentioned so far give a relative indication of cost to benefit ratios. Is it worth pursuing this programme, in comparison with the other options? The only measure which gives an absolute indication of whether a programme is worth pursuing is *cost-benefit analysis* (CBA).

In CBA, all costs, appropriately valued in monetary form and discounted, are taken away from the benefits, appropriately valued and discounted, and if the net present value (NPV) is positive, then the project is worth pursuing, in absolute terms. Health projects are treated in the same way as any other investment project – i.e. requiring a favourable comparison of the stream of benefits, relative to the costs, with both expressed in monetary terms.

In a constrained budget situation (i.e. real life!), we should ideally assess all possible invest-ments, calculate NPVs, and then fund them in order of size of NPV until the budget is exhausted.

Public expenditure review – a tool for assessing efficiency and equity

Public expenditure reviews are often carried out at national level to assess trends in health financing and overall sector performance. However, they can also be conducted at district level as part of management and planning processes. They investigate patterns and trends in relation to the following questions:

- What is the composition of financing sources?
- What is the overall relationship between income and expenditure?
- How are funds allocated, by region or district?
- How are the funds allocated, by line item?
- How are funds allocated, by level of service delivery (or programmes, or agencies, depending on the structure of the sector)?
- How are infrastructure and staffing distributed?
- Does the allocation of resources reflect data on needs (e.g. poverty maps, or information on burden of diseases)?
- What proportion of funds is spent (by budget categories)?
- Do funds arrive on time?
- What is the expenditure per person (overall, or broken into more detail, according to the information available – e.g. for primary care, for hospital care (in-patient/ out-patient) etc.)

This recognizes that where resources are constrained, not all projects with positive NPVs will be funded.

The problem lies with valuing health benefits in monetary terms. Some people see this activity as unethical (how can you reduce life to mere dollars?), but that argument should be rebutted. As explained at the beginning, if you ignore costs you may be causing needless loss of life and quality of life through inefficiency, poor services, and lack of access for those in most need. Ignorance, not analysis, is unethical. The problem is more practical and methodological how can we value the different benefits?

Some benefits will be easily expressed in monetary form. Future patient or health service costs averted (the direct benefits) can be estimated. To this can be added estimated productivity gains from programmes which allow people to return to work or to be more productive at work. Wage rates can be used to value these. The problem lies with *intangibles*: How much is life, or the relief of pain, worth to the patient? Various techniques have been developed to elicit patient estimates (such as contingent valuation or conjoint analysis) and debated and are complicated to calculate but these are still being refined.

Project appraisal

Appraising a project or programme should include an economic evaluation in order to assess the net benefit to society of investing in the project. However, other considerations also have to be looked at before proceeding. We will focus on the question of financial sustainability here. Even if a project is cost-effective, there may not be sufficient money to fund it. In that case, the project will not be financially sustainable.

To assess sustainability means first estimating *how much it will cost to run the service.* This depends on cost per person, and the likely coverage of the service. How many people are likely to attend? What are the projected capital and recurrent costs? If there is high wastage or low turnover, this should be reflected in the estimates. Relying on cost estimates taken from another context may be misleading as input costs (notably staff), levels of efficiency and usage rates may vary greatly.

If the programme involves investments over a period of years, *what is the projected pattern of expenditure?* When will the costs fall, over time? Will some costs rise by more than or less than the rate of inflation? Will any savings be generated by the project? For example, improvements to primary facilities may relieve workloads at secondary level. If costs are variable, we may be able to reduce expenditure at the secondary level as a result. If costs are fixed, however, then reduced workload may not affect costs much.

How will these costs be covered? If the programme is to be publicly funded, *then how do the estimated costs compare with the amount in budget?* How is the budget anticipated to change over the project period? Clearly we do not usually know the precise answers to these questions, but will have to rely on educated guesses (e.g. the budget will grow at the same rate as projected growth for the economy as a whole, or some such explicit assumption).

If patients will pay some or all of the costs, *how does the cost per person compare with disposable income, or with current private expenditure on health?* If patient contributions are needed to finance the programme, then you need to estimate how much demand there is likely to be for the service. Normally, the higher price of the good, the lower the demand – so setting a price too high may reduce your overall revenue from patients. On the other hand, if quality is high and alternatives are expensive, and then demand for your service may be maintained, despite significant user fees.

There is no one rule-of-thumb for affordability, but we need to consider the impact of proceeding with the programme. What other activities would have to be cut to fund this programme (i.e. *what are the opportunity costs?*) etc.?

If estimates suggest that there may be problems of sustainability for a project, then there are a number of options, which may be pursued separately, or combined:

- Scrap the project
- Redesign the project, if possible, to reduce costs
- Reduce the scale of implementation
- Seek additional funds. This might be achieved by arguing for an overall increase in allocation to health sector spending; by prioritizing this programme within the health budget; or by any of the supplementary funding options outlined above in the health financing section. The financial analysis and the analysis of expected benefits will help to make your case and demonstrate that you have thought through the resource implications of the programme.

Resource allocation

Another important issue on which health economics can advise is how health budgets are divided between regions or districts. This is known as geographical resource allocation.

Typically, money and staff are currently distributed from central budgets downwards according to (1) historical patterns and (2) political bargaining. This tends to mean that those institutions and areas which have been powerful will get a disproportionate share of the resources, reinforcing inequity in access to services. Similarly, if funding follows indicators of capacity (number of facilities, staff etc.) or even utilization (patient visits, bed-days etc.), it will tend to favour institutions which have been well-funded in the past.

In contrast, most health economists would argue that money should follow health needs. There are two reasons for this: First, because of the principle of equity, which suggests that money should be spent on the sickest and most vulnerable, who are often the poorer members of society. Secondly, because of the principle of efficiency: Spending on those in less need reduces the potential for health gain.

How can we measure need on a population basis and develop a formula which is fair and objective? The answer will depend largely on what information is available in the local context. However, the following are desirable:

1 *Population size.* Very crudely, the more people, the higher the need, on average, so the population of a district or region should be the starting point for needs-based formulae.

2 *Age and sex profiles.* Utilization patterns are generally higher for certain ages (e.g. young children and the elderly) and sexes (e.g. reproductive age women), so age and sex profiles of a population – where available – can be used to weight the population data.

3 *Morbidity.* Some areas may have higher morbidity than others, even allowing for age and sex variation, and this will create legitimate health care needs. Indicators such as infant mortality rates, where these are available for different regions or districts, could be used as a proxy.

4 *Social deprivation indicators.* Because of the connection between poverty and ill-health, some formulae include an indicator of general socio-economic deprivation, such as unemployment rates or proportion living in poverty.

5 *Cost weightings.* If some areas face increased costs in providing services (e.g. because of higher salaries in that area, or transport costs to remote regions), then it is legitimate to compensate these to some extent in the formula.

With all of these indicators, we have to ask a number of questions:

- How well does it capture the relevant feature (e.g. using possession of a television as an indicator of relative wealth: Is there a 'good fit' here?)
- Is the data available and regularly updated?
- Is it accurate?
- Is it as simple and transparent as possible?
- How much weight should be given to each of the above types of indicators: what is their relative importance in contributing to health needs?

Devising a geographical resource allocation formula is one thing, and putting it into practice is quite another, especially if it will result in big shifts from historic funding patterns. Issues to consider include how to phase in changes in funding so as to allow for adjustment, both in areas which may have to cut facilities and others which may have to develop a larger capacity. If some regions have greater external donor investments, that should also be taken into account. One option is to use the results of the formula to induce greater donor interest in areas of high health need. Introduction of the new system of resource allocation can also be used to stimulate discussion of service patterns. In South Africa, for example, changes in the resource allocation system went alongside the attempt to shift funding from secondary to primary care.

Priority setting and service packages

By priority setting, we mean that not all needs or desires for health care can be met. All countries ration health care. No matter how rich, no country can meet all health needs. Health needs are limitless, as we try to prolong life and increase the quality of life with increasingly expensive technologies and drugs (see Fig. 7.2).

The question then is not whether but how to ration. In privately funded systems, like the US, rationing takes place by ability to afford insurance coverage. Those without coverage have reduced access, especially to high quality care. In tax-funded services, like the UK's, which are free at the point of delivery for patients, the rationing has taken place historically through waiting lists for certain services (especially elective surgery, such as hip replacements).

In many systems, rationing is implicit, not explicit. The criteria for rationing are hidden, and unclear, rather than being publicly stated. For example, a vague notion of clinical need underlies UK rationing, but exactly how services are prioritized, and how the access of different groups (such as the elderly) is ranked is not clear. Moreover, systems with implicit rationing are likely to

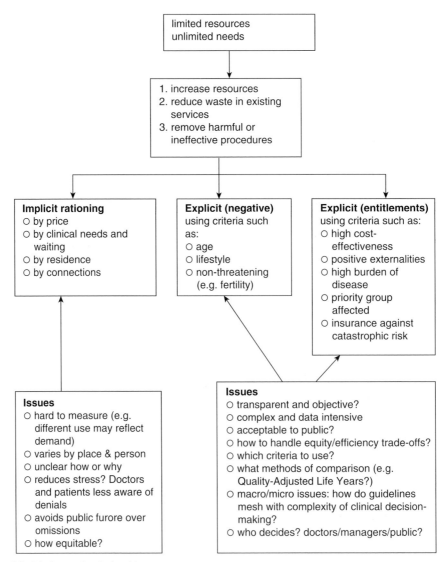

Fig. 7.2 Priority setting in health care.

have large variations from region to region, as local health staff and managers work without clear guidelines as to how to set priorities.

What are the advantages of 'implicit' rationing (see Fig. 7.3)? It avoids difficult, high-profile, political issues, such as stating categorically that a certain service will not be provided as part of the publicly-funded health care. It also allows for flexibility at the local level in assessing health needs and allocating resources. However, it also has major disadvantages. In particular, it means that it is hard to examine and compare how and why priorities are being set. It also places stress on individual clinicians and managers, who take day-to-day rationing decisions about patients.

Explicit rationing can be carried out on a negative or positive basis. Negative means that all services are provided unless they meet some exclusion criteria. An easy example is excluding all procedures which are ineffective or harmful to patients' health. More controversially, age limits could be imposed (e.g. no major surgery for over-75s) or restrictions related to lifestyle. All of these have to be interpreted in practice, and once stated are open to challenge by patients and lobby groups.

In contrast, a positive rationing system is a bottom-up approach, adding services which meet the inclusion criteria to the package which will be provided (or which will be publicly funded).

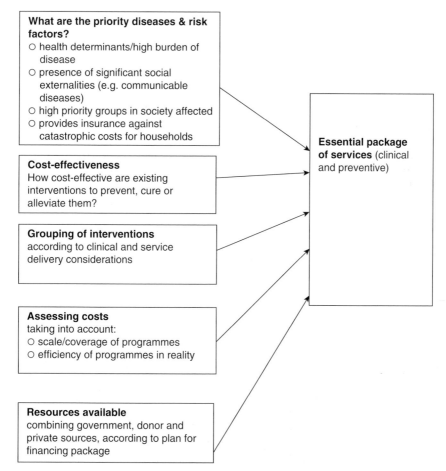

Fig. 7.3 Designing an essential package of services.

An example of this is the World Bank 'essential service package' idea, contained in the 1993 World Development Report. The criteria which were used to select services here included:

◆ High burden of disease caused by the condition in developing countries

◆ Cost-effectiveness of intervention

◆ Positive externalities associated with the treatment or prevention (see above: knock-on effects of reducing transmission etc.)

The World Development Report preventive package included the following items:

◆ Immunization (EPI Plus)

◆ School-based health services

◆ Health promotion and selective services for nutrition and family planning

◆ Alcohol and smoking reduction programmes

◆ Regulation, information and limited investments in the household environment

◆ AIDS prevention

It also suggested that a minimum clinical package in each country should include five groups of interventions:

◆ Pregnancy-related care

◆ Family planning services

◆ TB control

◆ Control of STDs

◆ Care for serious childhood illnesses, such as diarrhoea, ARI, measles, malaria, and malnutrition

The cost of the public health component was estimated at $4.2 per person per year for low income countries, and the clinical package at $7.8, bringing the total to $12. The equivalent for middle income countries was $21.5 per person per year, for both elements (1992 prices). A decade later, the Commission on Macroeconomics and Health revised and costed an essential package of cost-effective health care for low income countries and suggested that an average of $34 per capita would be required to provide it.[2]

The essential service package approach is controversial. There are two main groups of objections. One is political/philosophical, focussing on the ideal of primary health care, with its holistic and grassroots-based approach to health. The problem here is that in the absence of greatly increased public funding, health systems in most developing countries are struggling to provide even minimum services and the current pattern is arguably neither efficient nor equitable. A low-level subsidy is being provided to public services, which are predominantly used by the better-off or better-connected members of society. The main burden of paying for health care falls on individuals and families. Rationing is, therefore, implicit and based on ability to afford health care. High priority diseases, such as STDs, get underfunded, and the poor face much higher real costs than the rich. In that context, prioritization by service, however clumsy, appears attractive.

There are, however, many practical issues about how such packages are assembled and used.

1 *Universal solutions*. There are no universal solutions, given the different disease patterns and also costs which health services face. Local priorities and criteria should also be established. All of this takes information and analytical capacity, which are often in short supply.

---

[2] http://www.who.int/macrohealth/infocentre/advocacy/en/investinginhealth02052003.pdf

2 *Measurement problems.* There has been a lot of debate about approaches to measuring the burden of disease. There is no one correct tool, but some quantification will be necessary.

3 *Resource shortfalls.* Many developing countries are currently unable to fund even a minimum essential package of services, such as the one outlined above. Priority setting clearly does not fill the resource gap in that situation. However, it could serve to outline to donors the nature and size of the need and act as a co-ordinating framework for aid.

4 *Maintaining current gains*. It is important not to overlook the health gains which are already being achieved through cost-effective interventions. For example, if a country has an effective immunization service in operation, then low mortality from those infectious diseases may lead to the suggestion that they are not priority areas (and hence to withdrawal of funding from the immunization service). That would clearly be a mistake. A comparison with similar countries which have low coverage rates may allow a calculation of the cost per DALY gained by the established programme.

5 *Future disease trends.* Similarly, it would be a mistake to base prioritization purely on the current burden of disease without taking into account the likely future trends. For example, in many developing countries smoking is predicted to become the major cause of premature deaths within the next two decades. Given the lag time involved, present day figures do not present it as such a major public health target. Nevertheless, prevention now is likely to be highly cost-effective, even with discounting of future benefits. The same point applies to control of the spread of HIV, which has even larger positive externalities in the form of reduced onward infection.

6 *Public/political acceptability*. It is likely to be politically controversial to focus public resources on a limited range of services. Even though a comprehensive free service probably did not exist in reality before, it is still hard to explicitly exclude services. Politicians, health professionals and the general public have to be won over to this approach and the view that it may be the least bad option.

There are no easy answers when it comes to prioritizing health care. Prioritizing between programmes means taking politically charged decisions. The decision to focus on key primary health care interventions, for example, may be a decision to withdraw public funding from other important sections of the public (those benefiting from cancer treatments, for example). The decision to divert funds to the village health posts may mean cutting jobs at regional level. For every winner there is likely to be a loser, and so political skills and determination are called for. The timing and sequence of reforms are likely to be crucial to their success. Deciding how much to undertake is also very important. Where there is considerable political will (e.g. a new government, committed to change), change can be dramatic. More commonly, incremental changes are introduced.

An important point is that a small positive change is better than no change at all, even if it falls short of the wholesale change which the situation seems to demand. For example, if detailed data is lacking with which to calculate costs, use rough estimates. Involve local communities in setting priorities (as discussed in Chapter 4). Priorities are not set once and for all, but require continual information gathering, dialogue and decision-making. The initial outcome is therefore less important than starting a process in which key players reflect on what they are trying to achieve, and how best to do so within the real constraints.

Improving the organization of services

Having prioritized the right mix of services, we also need to ensure that we are providing those services as efficiently as possible. That is the theme of this last section. Let us start by clarifying what is meant by efficiency? How can it be assessed and improved? Let us take a simple example.

The Millenium Development Goals & priority setting

In 2000, the world's leaders committed to a series of targets to be reached by 2015 (http://www.un.org/millenniumgoals/index.html). The eight targets included three specifically relating to health:

◆ MDG 4: To reduce by two-thirds the mortality rate among children under five

◆ MDG5: To reduce by three-quarters the maternal mortality ratio; and achieve, by 2015, universal access to reproductive health

◆ MDG6: To halt and begin to reverse the spread of HIV/AIDS;to achieve, by 2010, universal access to treatment for HIV/AIDS for all those who need it; and to halt and begin to reverse the incidence of malaria and other major diseases.

Such international declarations can bring helpful pressure to bear on national and local leaders to take seriously neglected areas, such as maternal health. However, they are crude tools, as they apply across-the-board goals regardless of local context and needs. The resources which are brought to bear in support of these targets by donors can also distort local planning and priority setting. It is critical that national leaders plan based on local needs, local priorities, and local opportunities, while taking advantage of the international support that the MDGs and other global initiatives can generate.

Imagine a doctor running a private village clinic, with two assistants. He sees 20 patients per day, and makes a small profit, after paying his assistants and the costs of running the building etc. Is he operating his business efficiently?

There are a number of options for him to look at:

1 He might be able to offer the same service using fewer inputs – e.g. could he do the same with just one assistant? That would reduce his costs and so increase his overall profit.

2 He might be able to obtain the same inputs at a lower price – e.g. getting a cheaper source for his supplies. This again would decrease his costs.

3 He might be able to use the same inputs but increase his output – e.g. seeing more patients, for example, by working at times more convenient to most clients. This would generate more revenue from their fees, and so increase profits.

4 Alternatively, he might have the same costs and see the same number of patients but provide a better quality of service. This should enable him to keep his clients from visiting rival clinics, and might also allow him to increase his charges.

All of these strategies would increase efficiency, which means minimizing inputs for a given output, or maximizing output for a given input. Note that quality should be an integral part of assessing efficiency. If an increase in activity is accompanied by a decline in quality, then the service may become less, not more efficient.

In practice, there is often no absolute measure of whether a service is operating efficiently, so studies tend to rely on relevant comparisons. How do the costs of this hospital compare with the neighbouring hospital? What are the average costs for ante-natal care in this district, compared with that district?

These comparisons are imprecise, because no two hospitals or districts are going to be exactly the same. If the comparison is to be meaningful, we need to ensure (a) that the conditions affecting service delivery (such as utilization, input costs and case mix) are as similar as possible between the two areas being compared; and (b) that the quality of service provided is comparable.

If we find that the cost of providing a procedure is higher in one facility or area than another, and we are satisfied that the quality and the conditions are comparable; this indicates that efficiency improvements might be possible. The next step is to identify the causes of low efficiency and agree strategies for dealing with them.

What are common barriers to efficiency in developing countries? The following are just some of the most frequent problems:

1 *Poor incentives* – for example, budget systems which claw back savings, or payment systems which encourage doctors to see patients frequently, rather than treating them effectively (see below).

2 *Lack of control over resources* – for example, poor financial systems, so that funds are unpredictable and inadequate, or poor human resource management, which allows staff to leave work early to do private practice and so not work their full hours in official duties.

3 *Over-centralization* – for example, where local managers are unable to use staff or monies to meet local needs, but have to follow a central plan.

4 *Financial shortfalls* – underfunding itself can cause inefficiency as the health service focuses on its own short-term survival rather than providing the best service possible with the resources available.

5 *Lack of service ethic* – particularly with public services, there is often a problem of staff treating patients without consideration. This reduces utilization of services, and decreases the effectiveness of the clinical interactions which do take place.

6 *Poor management* – for example, lack of supervision of staff or poor organization of services so that clients are inconvenienced and staff are less productive than they could be.

7 *Lack of information* – it is hard to plan services, or to assess their performance if even routine cost and activity information is lacking.

8 *Lack of coordination of services* – this is an endemic problem which is often made worse by donor funding, with its different funding sources, priorities and reporting requirements, often operating side-by-side within the same area.

9 *Poor training* – if clinical skills are weak and/or out of date, then it will be impossible to provide a high-quality, effective service to patients.

In analysing problems and drawing on stakeholders' ideas for solutions, it is worth distinguishing between two issues:

1 Is there the motivation to tackle the problem? – i.e. what are the incentives which staff or managers face, and how could these be changed to improve performance?

2 Do they have the tools to do so? – i.e. they may wish to tackle a problem, but lack the skills, or be restricted by bureaucratic rules.

Payment systems

Health care providers are in a powerful position to influence demand for their services, given that most patients are unaware of the causes of ill-health and of how to treat themselves. Patients have to trust health staff to recommend appropriate action for them. The way in which staff and institutions are paid is therefore important, as this will be a major influence on what sort of health care is provided.

What are the different types of payment systems (see Table 7.2)?

1 Some are based on the volume of service provided. For example, fee for service links payment to the number of visits to a doctor, or the number of procedures carried out in a hospital, or some other unit of measurement, such as number of bed-days spent in hospital.

Table 7.2 Main types of provider payments

	Individual practitioner	**Medical institution**
Time based	Salary	Fixed budget (based usually on historic allocations)
Service based	Fee for service Fee for patient Target payments	Fee for service Fee for patient Budget based on case-mix/utilization Cost and volume contracts
Population based	Capitation payment	Block contract

2 In contrast, there are payments which are fixed for a period of time, no matter what activity is performed. A salary remains the same, no matter how many patients you see. A fixed annual budget operates in the same way. (It may vary in practice, in unpredictable ways, such as if funds are not paid in full, but this does not relate to how much work is being done.)

3 An intermediate approach is to link payments to population. For example, family doctors can be paid according to the number of patients registered with them ('capitation payments'), and hospitals can be paid according to the population for whom they provide a service.

Payment systems which are based on population rely on competition between providers to create quality incentives. For example, capitation payments assume that patients can choose with which doctor or primary care clinic to register, and that they have a number to choose from. If these conditions are absent, then the incentives will be similar to fixed payment methods. Generally speaking, primary care services tend to be more competitive than secondary, and urban areas more than rural ones.

There is no one ideal payment system: Different payments systems tend to create different incentives, and the right one will depend on the context and what the local priorities are. For example, if keeping overall costs down is an important priority (as it has become in most Western health systems recently), then payments linked to activity should be avoided: There is a proven relationship between fee-for-service and higher numbers of visits to doctors, tests, readmissions etc., which leads to cost escalation. Alternatively, if it is a high priority to improve the quality of services, then historic budgeting and salary systems need to be at least amended to stimulate higher performance.

The local context is all-important in designing payment systems. For example, if management capacity and information technology are scarce, it would be a mistake to choose a payment system which requires complex charging per individual case and detailed monitoring (such as Diagnosis-Related Groups – DRGs – in which payments are made according to a fixed tariff per category of condition). These need regular updating and controls against cheating (e.g. wrongful classification of patients, to increase the payments made to the institution).

Some of the simplest payment systems can be made to work better if used differently. For example, salaries are associated with absenteeism and poor quality services. This is particularly likely if:

◆ Staff are paid below subsistence, or below comparable payment levels in other sectors (such as private practice).

◆ There are no promotion prospects, or promotion is not based on merit, but some other criteria.

◆ There is no chance of losing your job through poor performance (e.g. no supervision; no managerial flexibility to sack or demote staff; no short-term contracts).

If bureaucratic rules can be changed to allow poor-performers to be disciplined; if hard work and skill can be rewarded by promotion or bonus payments; if staff payments can be increased to realistic levels, then we should be able to increase standards and efficiency without necessarily changing the type of payment.

Similarly, fixed budget systems can be made to work better by making a number of important changes. For example:

1 Budgets could be set according to more rational criteria than 'what you got last year plus inflation', or some such rule-of-thumb. Note, however, that if a measure of workload is used, then we need quality checks too to ensure that quantity does not rise at the expense of quality.

2 Having set budgets and targets, managers should have flexibility to deploy resources within them. In a low-trust culture, there is reluctance to do this as managers fear that funds will 'walk'. For that reason, careful auditing is also required.

3 Perverse incentives should also be removed. For example, if a district makes savings, will it lose that money from next year's budget? If so, there is no incentive to make savings. Instead, there should be clear rules about how savings can be used – e.g. a certain proportion in staff bonuses; the rest reinvested in facilities or supplies etc.

In developing countries today staff and institutions generate a varying, but often large, proportion of their revenue informally, from illegal or semi-legal payments by patients, private practice during work time and creative uses of public facilities, equipment and supplies. While this informal economy is not well documented, it must be taken into account when designing or changing official payment systems. How those will work will depend largely on how they add to or replace informal sources of income.

Public/private mix and performance management

There has been a lot of dogma flying about over the past decades about the relative merits of public and private sectors. The private sector, it is generally believed, is more efficient and provides higher quality services. Some organizations have given the impression that the private sector offers all the answers to public health problems in developing countries. Others, on the other side of the political divide, see private sector operators as evil profiteers, contributing nothing to the public good.

When we discussed financing, above, it became clear that there is a strong case for public financing of health systems – at least, a substantial minimum portion of them – to ensure social solidarity, risk-sharing and access for the poorest. When it comes to provision, however, there are less consensus on public and private roles. Perhaps more than public or private status, what matters is the context, the incentives and the management framework which governs a facility. Staff who are nominally in the public sector are perfectly capable of acting in an entrepreneurial, profit-seeking manner – indeed, that is how most of them currently make their living. Similarly, given the right incentives, private practitioners are able to deliver core public services at a reasonable standard (Box 7.3).

The emphasis in recent years has therefore been on developing tools which set the right incentives for staff and institutions, regardless of ownership status. We will look briefly at a number of alternative or supplementary strategies which have been adopted recently in developing countries.

'Internal markets'

Some countries in the West and some developing countries, like Indonesia, have attempted to bring the virtues of the private sector into their public sectors by making public institutions, such as hospitals, into autonomous provider units which have to market their services to public sector

Box 7.3 Public–private partnerships for health

Public–private partnerships (PPPs) is a term used for a collaboration between private sector organizations or medical practitioners and a health programme. The partnerships can be organized at international, national, and sub-national levels.

International

WHO has arranged PPPs with pharmaceutical companies to develop drugs, vaccines, and laboratory tests for neglected tropical diseases such as leishmaniasis and TB. PPPs include a public subsidy for the development and production, as otherwise there wouldn't be enough profit for a drug, vaccine or test used mainly in developing countries (www.who.int).

National

In Pakistan, for example, a micronutrient fortification project has been successfully implemented. The partnership is between the Ministry of Health nutrition programme and the Micronutrient Initiative (providing policy and resources) and the Pakistan Flour Mills Association members who are implementing the policy. The flour mill factories are fortifying the wheat with the correct amount of iron and folic acid. The project should reduce anaemia in women and children by a third (www.micronutrient.org).

Sub-national

In the main cities of Bangladesh and Nepal, the national TB programme has a partnership with the local NGOs and private medical doctors. The doctors are trained, follow the national policies and refer people with chronic cough to approved laboratories to be screened for TB by sputum smear microscopy. They report cases diagnosed to the TB programme and refer patients for treatment support and supervision by NGO community-based workers until confirmed cured. Doctors do not get a fee for this work, but benefit from an enhanced reputation for giving high quality care amongst the patient's family and friends. The initial sites have greatly improved case finding and cure rates, and now the PPP is being expanded nationwide (www.comdis.org).

In many countries contraceptives, bednets, and other healthy products are socially marketed by companies such as PSI in collaboration with the Ministry of Health. In Pakistan the PSI 'Greenstar' (www.greenstar.org.pk) programme increases access to family planning through franchising private medical practitioners to provide family planning services. This PPP provides around 27% of all modern contraception being practiced in Pakistan.

purchasers (e.g. health authorities) and others. This has had varying results. There are a number of general points to bear in mind here:

1 While there is a potential for gain, in terms of creating incentives to operate efficiently and attractively, there will also be new costs, notably the 'transaction costs' (costs of negotiating, setting up agreements, monitoring and enforcing agreements), which did not used to exist.

2 A strong public management capacity is needed to regulate the new market, which is being established. Without good systems and good information transfer, fragmentation and confusion may ensue.

3   There may a tension between the need for central planning and coordination of services and individual bargaining at the local level.

4   Issues of competitiveness and local power relations become (even more) important. So, for example, a weak health authority may not monitor and enforce contracts effectively, even if in theory it has the financial strength to do so.

5   Where public finance is anyway only a small part of the revenue base of an organization, the purchaser's leverage is even more limited.

Subsidies or incentives to the private sector

Where government facilities are lacking, it has been common, particularly in parts of Africa, for non-governmental organizations (usually non-profit-making, such as churches) to provide basic health care in an area with funding from the state. This often takes the form of the state providing recurrent costs, with capital costs being met from the provider's funding sources. This might be called 'implicit contracting', where the full costs of services are met, or a subsidy, where the costs are only partially covered by the state. Unlike in formal contracting out of services, there is rarely a clear specification of what services are to be provided, at what quality etc.

This system offers advantages in spreading the financial burden, where government capacity to build and run facilities is poor. However, there can also be problems of coordination and consistency between government-run and NGO-run services.

Another approach has been to use incentives or subsidies of various kinds to influence private sector behaviour. This follows from the recognition that private providers are the first point of contact for so many patients, including for diseases with significant externalities, such as tuberculosis. Rather than trying to curb private practice, many Ministries of Health have focused instead on the more positive question of how to increase private practitioners' awareness and use of cost-effective approaches.

For example, training and equipment can be offered to clinics providing preventive services or services with substantial positive externalities (e.g. treatment of sexually transmitted diseases). Alternatively, subsidized goods or tax breaks could be provided to private clinics which meet minimum standards of quality, or which comply with reporting standards, for example. In some countries, voluntary accreditation of private providers, which involves meeting certain minimum standards, has been linked with benefits such as eligibility for reimbursement by the insurance fund. This is a type of regulation, but one which offers positive incentives rather than the threat of sanctions (the carrot rather than the stick) (see Box 7.4).

Another way of keeping private providers informed about government policies is to 'contract in' private specialists to provide a specific service in government hospitals, for example. In Zimbabwe and Malawi, governments allow private doctors to use public facilities for their patients in return for seeing government cases requiring specialist treatment free of charge.

Contracting out of services

This is mostly used for non-clinical services, such as cleaning, but contracts for clinical services are also becoming more widespread in developing countries. Again, as with internal or quasi markets, gains are dependent on the public sector having sufficient competence to manage the relationship effectively. The essence of a contract is that it states clearly certain specifications – such as the nature of the work to be done, the price, the minimum quality standards etc. – and any efficiency gains will depend on the contract being carefully monitored and agreements enforced. To do this requires bargaining power by the purchaser, the will to enforce, the capacity to do so, and alternative possible providers to whom the work could potentially be shifted.

Box 7.4 Distribution of insecticide-treated bed nets for malaria control – social marketing versus free distribution

Insecticide-impregnated bednets (ITNs) are a recognized cost-effective strategy for control of malaria, particularly in the young. However, a debate has been raging about the most effective strategy for increasing the uptake of bednets, which are expensive for poorer families and require regular re-treatment.

One approach has been to use 'social marketing', which means the use of advertising, branding and selling of essential goods with social value through local distributors. This approach can aim at cost-recovery and sustainability (including the incentives for the local retailers) or can be carried out at heavily subsidized prices (or heavily subsidized for specific groups, such as pregnant women and children under five, sometimes using vouchers schemes). Considerable investment has gone into establishing and extending social marketing programmes for bed nets and other public goods.

Some have argued however that this approach penalizes vulnerable groups and fails to deliver the high levels of coverage which are needed to reduce the spread of disease. They have called for universal free distribution of bednets. They dispute the claim that freely distributed ITNs are less likely to be used effectively by households. WHO's Malaria programme calls for ITNs to be considered a public good in high-burden areas (www.who.int/malaria).

Most national malaria plans try to address this equity-sustainability dilemma by emphasizing integration of public and private markets for ITNs, using the dynamism of the private sector as well as the subsidies which the public sector can offer to increase access for the vulnerable. Integration with other malaria control strategies, such as access to treatment, is also recognized as a key component in reducing morbidity and mortality.

Within the public sector, the use of 'performance contracts' is increasing. This involves setting explicit standards and volumes of work for public employees, together with rewards for over- and sanctions for under-achievement. This is sometimes known as "performance-based payments". As this assumes that managers can control the factors leading to achievement of the targets, it needs to be complemented by policies such as decentralization and changes to budgeting and resource allocation which give local managers more autonomy over resources. As with contracting out of services, it is important to avoid 'perverse incentives', such as paying per person treated, which is likely to lead to an increase in volume but a decrease in quality.

Regulation

Whether dealing with the private or the public sector, each country needs a set of rules which protect patients against malpractice or incompetence by health staff. Some of this *regulation* is carried out by the medical profession itself – self-regulation. However, as medical associations represent their members, they are likely to put members' interests first when there is a clash between their interests and the interests of their patients. For that reason, independent government regulation is required, and most countries have rules about minimum training standards, registration requirements, poor practice, and/or excess provision and overcharging.

The problem in many developing countries is enforcement. Regulatory bodies are often poorly funded and face a diverse private sector, with many small operators. This is particularly true of the drugs market, which may have a lot of small, part-time sellers whose activities are hard to monitor. Furthermore, there is always a potential problem of corruption between regulators and the providers. For this reason, independent consumer organizations and an active media will be an important third force in regulating health markets, and one which should be fostered in developing countries.

Conclusion

This has been a very brief introduction into some topics covered by health economics. More broadly, health economics is a way of thinking which is of general use in planning, managing and evaluating health services. It encourages you to ask certain systematic questions of any health programme or policy decision. For example:

- ◆ What are the objectives?
- ◆ What are the options for meeting those objectives?
- ◆ What are the costs of different options; how do they compare with the benefits (taking the broadest societal perspective, where possible)?
- ◆ How are costs and benefits distributed (the equity angle)?
- ◆ Are they affordable and sustainable?
- ◆ What would be the next-best use of the resources?

It is an analytical approach which encourages being explicit about what the goals are and what the implications are of meeting them. This does not always fit well with an environment where decisions are personal, political, or ad hoc. However, it can provide a useful discipline. It does not dictate health goals, but does assist in clarifying goals and their implications.

Further reading
Health economics generally

Jack, W. (2000) *Principles of health economics for developing countries*. Washington, D.C.: World Bank.

Witter S. et al. (2000) *'Health economics in developing countries: a practical guide'*. Basingstoke: Macmillan.

Health financing

WHO: *Mapping of available tools to help strengthen health sector financing*. Geneva: WHO, (2007). http://www.who.int/choice/HSF%20Road%20map%20±%20tools.pdf; http://www.who.int/health_financing/mechanisms/en/

Abel Smith, B. (1994) *'An introduction to health policy, planning and financing'*. Harlow: Longman.

Conn, C., Walford, V. (1998) *'An introduction to health insurance for low income countries'*. London: Institute for Health Sector Development.

Software package to model introduction of health insurance: http://www.who.int/health_financing/tools/simins/en/index.html

Costing

Creese, A., Parker, D. eds. (1994) *'Cost analysis in primary health care: a training manual for programme managers'*. Geneva: WHO. See box 7.5 for web-based costing tools.

Economic evaluation

Drummond, M., O'Brien, B., Stoddart, G., Torrance, G. (1997) *'Methods for the economic evaluation of health care programmes'*. Oxford: Oxford University Press.

WHO Choice website, with costing and cost-effectiveness tools and information http://www.who.int/choice/en/

Project appraisal

Over, M. (1992) *Economics for health sector analysis.* Washington, D.C.: World Bank.

Adhikari, R., Gertler, P., Lagman, A.(1999) *Economic analysis of health sector projects – a review of issues, methods and approaches.* Asian Development Bank. http://www.adb.org/Documents/EDRC/Staff_Papers/ESP058.pdf

Purchasing and health sector performance

WHO: World Health Report. (2000) *Health systems, improving performance.* Geneva: World Health Organisation.

Cassels, A. (1994) 'Health sector reform: key issues in less developed countries'. *Journal of International Development,* **7(3)**,

Bennett, S., McPake, B., Mills, A. (1997*) 'Private health providers in developing countries'.* London: Zed.

Barnum, H., Kutzin, J., Saxenian, H. (1995) 'Incentives and provider payment systems'. *International Journal of Health Planning and Management,* **10**,

The Tanzania Essential Health Interventions Project. IDRC Canada (2008) website www.idrc.ca/tehip includes various resources including District Health Accounts which is a tool designed to help district teams analyse their budgets and expenditures.

Chapter 8

Health promotion

John Hubley and Sylvia Tilford

This chapter gives an overview of the following topics:

♦ What is health promotion

♦ Components of health promotion interventions

♦ The planning process for health promotion

♦ The stages of developing and implementing health promotion programmes: Situation assessment and development of priorities; specifying interventions; implementation; and evaluation

♦ Selection of education and communication methods.

An important function of health promotion is prevention of disease.

Introduction

Health promotion

Health promotion is concerned with all those activities which promote health, prevent disease, and enhance wellbeing. Health promotion was a key part of the Health For All 2000 strategy. This focussed attention on the multiple determinants of health and so the need for multi-component actions to improve health. Health promotion combined activities to develop health knowledge, skills, and behaviours in individuals and communities – together with changes in social, economic, and environmental conditions designed to make health easier to achieve. In 1986, the Ottawa Charter on Health Promotion was drawn up and this document was a key one in specifying the principles of health promotion. It identified three main strategies for health promotion:

> *Advocacy* for health;
> *Enabling* all people to achieve their health potential; and
> *Mediating* between different interests in society in pursuit of health.

In addition The *Charter* set out five key components for health promotion:

> Building healthy public policy;
> Creating supportive environments;
> Strengthening community action;
> Developing personal skills; and
> Reorientation of health services.

These component parts have subsequently been explored in a series of Conferences in Sundsvall, Jakarta, Bangkok, and Mexico (see further reading). A formula which presents the key elements of health promotion is shown below. Health education activities can focus on developing individual and community health knowledge and skills or on encouraging advocacy actions to secure policy and environmental changes. Health education broadly covers 'developing personal skills' and 'strengthening community action' in the Ottawa Charter.

Health Promotion = Health Education × Appropriate Services × Healthy Public Policies

Healthy public policy is–policy designed to create a supportive environment to enable people to lead healthy lives. A widely adopted slogan is that healthy public policy enables 'the healthy choice to be the easier choice'. You should note that the term health promotion is not always used to refer to this combination of health education, health services and policy actions but is used simply to describe health education activities directed towards individuals' knowledge, attitudes, and health related behaviours. The policy element of health promotion is not included.

The relationship between health promotion and public health

Since public health and health promotion both claim to be concerned with promoting health and preventing disease you may wonder in what ways they actually differ. It isn't possible to state a clear distinction that will apply in all countries because of the different ways that both health promotion and public health are understood. Where the term health promotion is used to mean health education only, it forms one activity within public health as defined in this book. Where health promotion is understood to combine health education, services, and public policy for health, it overlaps public health. The differences can be small and lie mainly in the relative emphases on certain specific activities, most particularly educational and advocacy ones in the case of health promotion (Box 8.1) and disease control activities in public health. Both support the common values of:

+ A population perspective;
+ The importance of policy actions to address the determinants of health;
+ The development of multi-sectoral partnership working to secure health;
+ Community participation in promoting health and preventing disease;
+ Building capacity of communities, organizations, and professionals to work for health.

Box 8.1 Specific emphases of health promotion

+ Like public health it has a population focus but can also include activities directed towards individuals
+ It pays particular attention to the health education (information, education, communication) process within public health
+ It stresses the promotion of positive health as well as the prevention of disease
+ Support for a number of key values: Empowerment, equity, participation, advocacy, reduction of inequalities
+ The importance of developing health in the settings in which people live and work
+ Use of qualitative as well as quantitative methods in evaluating interventions and the involvement of communities in evaluation activities

In the countries where you are working you will need to check how the two activities are defined and the relationships between them are understood. This will facilitate communication and collaboration in practice.

The promotion of health and the prevention of disease

Health promotion is mainly focussed on primary preventive activities, in addition to secondary and tertiary prevention. The kind of actions relevant to the three levels of prevention include:

Primary: The encouragement of practices which promote health and reduce the risk of disease e.g. diet, exercise, breast-feeding, immunization, moderate drinking, avoidance of tobacco, hygiene behaviours, lifestyle change.

Secondary: Action to detect early signs of disease and take appropriate action to minimise risk of permanent damage to health e.g. attendance/uptake of screening services, oral rehydration of children with diarrhoea, home management of acute respiratory infections, early detection and self-referral for leprosy, sexually-transmitted diseases and malaria.

Tertiary: Actions at late irreversible stages of a disease to rehabilitate and improve quality of life. e.g. exercise, dietary changes and foot care with diabetes; education to promote rehabilitation after trauma.

Components of health promotion interventions

We need well-planned programmes which take into account the many factors which influence the health of a community and the transmission of disease. Programmes will need to include the three components within our health promotion definition:

- ◆ The *health education* component,
- ◆ The *services* component; and
- ◆ The *structural* (*enabling factors*) component which focuses on policy and environmental changes.

The balance of activities between these three will depend on the nature of the health topic and the extent to which it is influenced by lifestyle factors, appropriate health services, or the wider social/ political environment. It also depends on the extent to which any programme is able to work on each of the three components. For example, working for changes in policy may seem more difficult than undertaking public education but the success of the latter will often require some efforts directed towards policy. Table 8.1 gives some examples of the kinds of interventions that might be possible for a range of common topics.

The planning process for health promotion

The sets of decisions required for planning a health promotion intervention are shown in Fig. 8.1 You may find it helpful to refer to Chapters 4 and 5 for further details on the planning process. We will look briefly at each of the main stages of the planning process as relates to health promotion.

A review of the situation and the development of priorities

Many interventions have failed because the many factors that influenced the issues under consideration had not been analysed and inappropriate interventions had been selected. For example,

Table 8.1 Examples of health promotion strategies for education, service improvements and policy

	Education to individuals/communities	Improvements in services	Advocacy/agenda setting for policy change
Road safety	Public education on road safety	Improved emergency services	Road safety laws Compulsory seat belts Crash helmets for motorcyclists Improved car safety design
Breast feeding	Public education on benefits of breast-feeding and dangers of bottle-feeding Education of husbands to support breastfeeding	Establishment of baby-friendly health facilities Training of health workers in breast-feeding counselling Setting up ante-natal classes for fathers	Control of advertising of infant formula International Code for marketing of breast-milk substitutes
Lung cancer	Public education to persuade people not to start smoking and to persuade smokers to quit	Establishment of quit smoking clinics	Control of tobacco advertising Taxes on price of cigarettes Bans on smoking in public areas
Malaria	Public education on mosquito control, avoidance of biting, and the need for treatment of malaria and prophylaxis	Vaccine development. Improved case detection and case management Environmental mosquito control activities	Government support for malaria control measures Policies concerning environmental hazards/mosquito breeding sites
AIDS	Education of general public and specific groups e.g. truck drivers, sex workers, youth on safer sexual behaviours Mass media campaign	Counselling services. Social marketing of condoms. Voluntary testing facilities. Home care services Combination therapy/treatment of ante-natal cases Setting up a peer education programme	Legislation safeguarding human rights Patents/pricing of drugs Employment protection in the workplace Legal protection of sex workers and injecting drug users

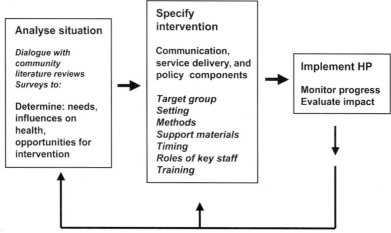

Fig. 8.1 Programme planning for health promotion.

a programme which focuses on behaviour change but fails to recognize and act on the environmental barriers to adoption of behaviours is likely to be unsuccessful.

You will need information on:

- The size and nature of health issues and who is affected by them
- Community views about the health issues
- The three components of health promotion:
    (i) Health related skills and behaviours and skills and the factors influencing them
    (ii) Existing policy and environmental measures
    (iii) Level and quality of service provision
- The kind of community you will be working with – people, structures, and processes

We will comment on each of these.

The size and nature of health problems and who is affected

If you know that a programme has to work on a defined issue, for example malaria, or child health, the extent of the problem may have already been assessed. If you are starting out to assess the range of health issues in a community you will need to review the available epidemiological data (as described in Chapter 3). In short you will need information on the specific problems and the size and nature of each of them. You can draw on available data on mortality, morbidity and use of services but may need to undertake further data collection in order to obtain a fuller picture. You will need to do a rapid (or more thorough) community assessment as described in Chapter 4.

Community views about health issues

It is essential to find out what a community itself thinks are its health problems. If it has formal organizations, such as women's groups, trade unions, transport workers' associations, or youth organizations you can contact these and consult the members. You can also try to find out if these organizations have recorded feelings about health concerns in minutes of meetings, reports in the newspapers and petitions/requests to officials and politicians. In addition it is important to bring people together in groups to discuss their problems and possible solutions. The various techniques for rapid appraisal discussed in Chapter 4 can be used in finding out about health concerns. It is unlikely that there will be one agreed view about health needs. Extensive discussion will be needed to bring out a single agreed view on what should be done. When you aim to develop a social mobilization intervention, described later, the work with communities at this stage is central to the developmental process and the main starting point for the rest of the process. Individuals from communities can be recruited to work in partnership with workers and researchers to carry out the situational assessment.

The three components of health promotion

For the specific health issues that are described you will then need information on the influences of social, economic and environmental factors, health related skills and behaviours; and health and other services. Important influences to consider are listed in Fig. 8.2., while Fig. 8.3 illustrates one particular environmental influence, commercial advertising.

1. Socioeconomic and environmental factors   Depending on the problem to be addressed the information required might include:

- *Economic factors*: Poverty, purchasing power, low earning power, unemployment.
- *Status and power relations:* The ability of poor people to insist on their rights, obtain proper services, etc.

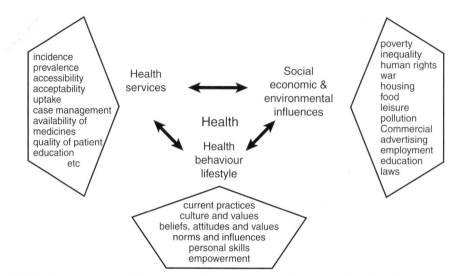

Fig. 8.2 Information required from a situation assessment to determine role of health promotion.

- *Gender relations* – The position of women in society, for example, whether a woman can realistically insist on her partner using condoms, power over household decisions such as use of latrines, family size, female genital mutilation (female circumcision).
- *Discrimination*: Prejudice against homosexuals, drug injectors, and sex workers.
- *Laws* which affect the feasibility of an intervention, e.g. the legal status of sex workers, housing standards, factory safety measures.

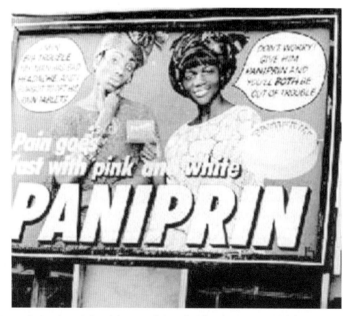

Fig. 8.3 Photograph caption: Advertising medicines in Nigeria – commercial pressures can influence community decision-making.

When the specific socioeconomic and environmental factors related to a specific health concern have been identified some further analysis of each will usually be required if you are going to attempt to change any of them in your intervention. For example, if district and national policies on tobacco control are needed understanding the reasons why policies have not been developed in the past and knowledge of the policy making processes with which a programme will need to engage, will be necessary. Alternatively, policies which impact on a health issue may exist but have never been properly implemented. You need to find out why this is the case and consider what could be done to improve implementation.

2. Health related skills and behaviours and the influences on them   Many people involved in health promotion give priority to empowering individuals and communities to take actions to improve health. To be empowered people need:

- Beliefs that they can take action – self efficacy;
- Positive feelings about themselves described as self esteem;
- Skills, including – advocacy, communication, decision making and critical literacy.

The empowerment of individuals can be assessed through dialogue with them or through the use of formal measures. Empowered communities will have a record of past actions that you can assess. Many others in health promotion, while recognizing the importance of empowerment, prefer to focus directly on health related behaviours in order to change these where necessary with the aim of achieving early impact on health. It is important, therefore, to obtain as detailed a description as possible of the important behaviours in a community which might affect any specific health problem Different kinds of behaviours that are important for health and disease are summarized in Box 8.2. For every health topic there will be specific behaviours that are important, for example:

> *Sexual health*: Number of partners, frequency of intercourse, type of sexual intercourse (vaginal, anal, 'dry sex'), use of condoms, drug injection, STD care-seeking behaviours, self medication;
>
> *Maternal and child health* – Immunization, feeding practices, breastfeeding, bottle feeding, home treatment of diarrhoea, fevers, and respiratory infections;
>
> *Parasitic diseases:* Mosquito control practices, use of mosquito nets, water contact/swimming habits for schistosomiasis, use of latrines, self medication, and care seeking behaviours for early symptoms.

Once the behaviours have been identified we need to gain a deeper understanding of the influences on those behaviours. It has been widely assumed that if people are simply provided with relevant information they will adopt recommended behaviours. This is very rarely the case. Although knowledge and awareness *are* important they are only one of many factors which influence the behaviours that people adopt. It is necessary to gain some understanding of these other factors and decide which are the more important ones to focus on in an intervention. A quick reflection on the factors that influenced a recent health behaviour decision in your own life will reveal the multiple influences. These factors can be broadly grouped into:

1 **Individual and cultural factors** and
2 **Enabling** factors which can either be within, or outside the individual's control

Individual and cultural factors   Key factors that have been identified in research and specified in health education and psychological models include:

1 *Beliefs* There are many kinds of beliefs that can influence decisions on health behaviours including:
   - beliefs about a specific health topic. People may have information about the health topic but may not believe it. It is the beliefs that are more likely to determine health decisions.

Box 8.2 Human behaviour and health

Human behaviours – also called actions or practices – are an essential but often neglected component of improving the health of the community. Some key behaviours include:

- ◆ Community action: Actions by individuals and groups to change and improve their surroundings including community participation in health decision-making

- ◆ Health behaviours: Actions that healthy people undertake to keep themselves or others healthy and prevent disease e.g. exercise, good nutrition, breast feeding, weaning, latrines, child-spacing, hygiene practices, tooth brushing, taking anti-malaria drugs; reduction of health-damaging behaviours such as smoking, bottle-feeding, excessive alcohol consumption, and accidents. These behaviours may be based on decisions or are done regularly and have become habits – or routines

- ◆ Utilization behaviours: Utilization of health services such as ante-natal, child health, immunization, family planning, and screening programmes

- ◆ Illness behaviours: Recognition of early symptoms and prompt self-referral for treatment such as oral rehydration, leprosy, and sexually transmitted diseases

- ◆ Compliance behaviours: Following a course of prescribed drugs such as for tuberculosis

- ◆ Rehabilitation behaviours: What people need to do after a serious illness to prevent further problems

The process of identifying the behaviours that are necessary for the prevention and control of specific diseases or for the promotion of health is called the behavioural diagnosis. When this is not carried out properly effort can be wasted persuading people to change behaviours that are harmless or failing to influence the behaviours that really could have an impact on disease in the community. While the behaviours of individuals and communities are important determinant of their health, the factors that influence behaviours frequently lie outside the individual's control and are influenced by economic, social and political factors operating at the district, national and international level.

- ◆ beliefs about whether people feel at risk of a disease and whether the disease is believed to be serious;

- ◆ beliefs about whether the benefits of adopting a recommended behaviour outweigh the costs. For example, I may believe that wearing a crash helmet when riding a motorcycle can prevent head injuries but the financial cost may be high and it is not seen as macho to wear a helmet;

- ◆ self-efficacy beliefs. People may be willing to adopt a recommended behaviour but do not feel they have the 'self efficacy' to do so. For example I may know what appropriate weaning foods are but don't believe I can put these into practice in my family context.

The beliefs that a person holds in relation to a behaviour will lead to a positive or negative attitude to adopt it.

2 *Social and community norms governing behaviour*

Norms are beliefs, perceptions, and behaviours that are shared by groups of people. When they are shared by many people they are part of the culture. When they are shared by small groups of persons, such as sex workers or street children, the term sub-culture is used. People's beliefs about social and cultural norms and the extent to which they want to conform to them are often a very important influence on behaviours.

The various beliefs and attitudes relevant to a specific health behaviour will interact to generate a chance of people deciding to adopt a new behaviour or change an existing one. Other factors described as *enabling factors* influence the chance of the intention being carried out and the behaviour sustained. Frequently it is a failure to consider the enabling factors that is the cause of programme failure. Enabling factors can be individual or structural.

Enabling factors

Individual

<u>Knowledge:</u>   This may be needed to translate an intention into action. Young people, for example, ready to adopt condom use will need to know where condoms can be acquired.

<u>Skills:</u>   A key factor in many cases would be the level of skills of an individual or community to perform an action required. Skills could include:

  (i) *Performance skills*: E.g. building latrines, using condoms, sterilizing syringes, impregnating mosquito nets with insecticide;
 (ii) *Communication skills* e.g. a woman negotiating safe sex with her partner, parents discussing health issues with their children, a sex worker insisting that a client uses a condom, a young person overcoming embarrassment to ask a pharmacist for condoms.
(iii) *Literacy skills* – people may lack the necessary skills to understand information required to implement health behaviour.

Structural factors

These can include any of the factors identified in the socioeconomic and environmental situational analysis. For example:

- Having sufficient money to acquire material things such as impregnated bednets required to adopt a preventive health behaviour;
- Lack of social support for the adoption of a new action;
- Social censure of women taking responsibility for sexual health.

In some situations there may be time and resources to research the influences on health skills and behaviours in order to identify what may need to be changed. You can, however, get a good sense quite quickly of what are the key influences through discussions with individuals and groups and in using participatory rapid appraisal methods.

3. The level and quality of service provision   This involves critically examining the existing provision of health, social, and other services as they relate to the specific health issues. Typical information required might include:

- The existence of services: For example, if you are going to promote higher uptake of child immunization, are services available, accessible, and acceptable to a community.
- The balance between prevention/curative activities and between clinic and community activities. The Ottawa Charter emphasized the importance of reorienting services towards prevention.
- The provision of appropriate communication and patient education and counselling activities.
- Involvement with other sectors both formal, for example schools, social services and informal, for example traditional healers, within the community.

- The availability of supplies to support the adoption of practices, for example, oral rehydration solution, condoms etc.

Once you have analysed all the information that you have gathered, priorities for a programme can be established. Before planning the specific interventions you will need some general information about the people you will be working with and the ways that you are going to be able to communicate with them.

WHO? – General background information on the programme community or population

You need an accurate picture of the numbers of people to be reached, where they are located (see, for example, Fig. 8.4), their ages, educational level, language, occupation/income, cultural group and religion. You will need to find out if the community is split into groups with distinct needs which have to be reached through the use of different methods (see Box 8.3).

HOW? Information on communication channels

This final set of information includes data on entry points and channels of communication that you might be able to use in your intervention. This would include information on:

- Media habits of the target community: What radio, television programmes, newspapers, and magazines are listened to, watched, or read.

Box 8.3 Different kinds of education and communication objectives

- *Awareness/knowledge* – specific information that people may need to make decisions for themselves
- *Decision-making /problem-solving skills* – the ability to make decisions based on available information
- *Beliefs, attitudes and values* – motivational elements – often rooted in culture – that can influence decision-making
- *Communication skills* – e.g. participation in community meetings, negotiating safe sex with partner, refusing to take part in risky behaviours
- *Empowerment* – the confidence to put decisions into practice and improve one's situation
- *Individual and community action/behaviour change* on health issues

Key decisions

WHO the communication should be directed towards – the target group? This may include members of the community directly involved in the community or persons with influence such as influential persons in the family or community.

WHAT is the purpose of the communication, including the objectives and content of any messages?

HOW, WHEN and WHERE is education to be carried out?

WHO is to carry out the activities?

- Leadership structures and social networks, for example persons in the family or community who have influence or are trusted by the target community.
- Community associations that might be mobilized e.g. women's associations, market traders' associations, trade unions, church groups.
- Non-governmental organizations that are working among the programme community that might become involved in your intervention.
- Health and other services that are already working among the community and are trusted.

Specifying the health promotion intervention

Considerable time and effort can go into the situational analysis but the effort is repaid if it leads to the development of an intervention which focuses on the most important priorities in a community or population. The priorities can include any mix of the three components of education, services and structural/ enabling factors. (refer back to Table 8.1)and the actions for each need to be carefully specified. The chosen intervention should be: Relevant to the health issues and needs in a community; based on available evidence of effectiveness, and realistic and feasible to implement in the specific community. We will comment in a little more detail on specifying these components.

Specifying the policy and environmental actions needed – the enabling component

The situation analysis will have indicated the policy and environmental actions needed. As noted earlier in some cases there is a need for new policy, or frequently there is a policy or law in place but it is not implemented. For example, policy may exist on motorcyclists wearing helmets but is not enforced by the police.

Depending on the health issue you are working on examples of changes that might be considered include:

1 Income-generation: Employment, cooperatives, income support, subsidies for latrines, specific foods.

2 Supportive legislation: For example, improvement in housing standards to ensure proper construction methods such as earthquake resistance, safety standards in the work place and reasonable working hours, road safety laws including speed controls, wearing of seat belts and motor cycle helmets, environmental and planning controls, human rights legislation to prevent discrimination, legalizing prostitution so that it can be regulated and made safe, ensuring inheritance rights for women.

3 Policies affecting service provision: For example new policies on education and health services, collaboration between services etc.

4 Taxes that support health goals: Prices of alcohol and tobacco, subsidies for nutritious foods.

The enabling component of an intervention will usually consist of a mixture of **shorter-term** and **longer-term** activities: Short-term activities are those which may be achievable during the time scale of the intervention and which will have some impact on improving the situation. These might include income-generating activities, subsidies on essential supplies, for example condoms or medicines, changes in specific laws (or if not the laws themselves, at least the interpretation/ enforcement of laws by the police).

Long-term activities are those through which the intervention initiates a process of debate and discussion that in the long term might lead to changes in policy and law.

Enabling factors such as improving the status of women, removing discriminatory laws, improving economic status, and tackling prejudice are among the most difficult factors to influence in an intervention. Many of them are determined at the regional, national, and even international level and are not easy to influence by activities at the community level. There may also be opposition from sections of the community to the social, economic, and legal changes necessary to provide enabling activities. Because they are difficult to change, many interventions leave out tackling the enabling factors. However, when making a situation assessment it becomes obvious that enabling factors are important influences in communities and must be tackled if your interventions are to have an impact on the community.

Deciding on the service delivery component of the intervention

This involves changes in services to make them more appropriate. This might involve improvements in:

1 Effectiveness: Availability of condoms, appropriate balance between prevention and cure, integration of health education in services including one-to-one, group education and outreach, links with other services such as schools and community groups.

2 Acceptability: The improvement in attitudes of health workers to patients and community, community participation in the management of facilities and establishing of special services such as 'baby-friendly hospitals', 'youth-friendly clinics', and outreach/peer education activities in the community.

Three decisions are involved when specifying the service delivery component of an intervention

1. What changes in service provision are needed?

You will need to specify as to what exact changes in service provision you wish to introduce. What you include in this will depend on the nature of your intervention, for example the setting up of counselling, social marketing of condoms, or treatment support for tuberculosis. How will you obtain institutional support for change and overcome any barriers. These barriers might include objections from persons in senior/middle management or from the field staff who have to implement those changes. It is important to hold discussions with both field staff and persons in management and find out any objections that they may have. These might be due to prejudice against the target community, a reluctance to take on additional work, or lack of confidence to change their methods of working. You should try to involve field staff in planning the improvements in service delivery that you wish to introduce as this will make them more likely to support you.

2. What are the implications of your proposed changes for staffing?

This will involve deciding if additional staff are needed to implement the proposed changes in service delivery or whether the work can be achieved through redeployment and changes in work-patterns of existing staff. You will also need to specify any orientation and training required by different kinds of field staff in order to implement those service changes.

3. What additional requirements will you have for equipment/materials?

This will involve specifying any additional equipment or supplies that are needed, for example condoms, drugs for STDs, supplies of disposable syringes etc.

Determining the communication and education component

This component includes all activities that have traditionally been called health education, public education, information, education, and communication (IEC), or simply communication.

The use of these terms varies between countries and between NGOs and international bodies. A serious weakness of many programmes has been an over-emphasis on factual knowledge. As shown in Box 8.3, an effective education and communication component usually has to go beyond just giving facts according to the factors revealed in the situation analysis. The activities specified will be influenced by the health promotion approach that is preferred in a particular situation. Do you want to prioritize empowering individuals and communities to take health related actions or do you want to focus directly on providing knowledge, developing attitudes, and changing behaviours identified in the situational analysis. As you read reports of health promotion programmes you will see examples of these alternative approaches. The former is more consistent with health promotion as represented by the Ottawa Charter and the principles outlined earlier. On the other hand where there are serious health issues that need to be tackled quickly the empowerment approach might not be seen as appropriate and direct actions on behaviours should be undertaken.

Once the various elements of the intervention have been clearly defined specific programme objectives need to be written. These will include:

◆ Educational objectives;
◆ Service provision and delivery objectives – the specific changes to be introduced in the intervention;
◆ Enabling activities objectives – those enabling factors that you wish to modify as part of the intervention in order to create a supportive environment for the behaviour changes and improvements in service. (see Chapter 6 for details on writing objectives.)

Programme implementation

The appropriate methods for achieving the different objectives have to be identified and the strategy for implementation of the programme decided and appropriate methods chosen for the different parts of a programme. Depending on the nature of an intervention implementation may be within whole communities or within specific locations such as schools, workplaces, primary health care or hospitals etc. Broader implementation strategies include the use of a settings approach and the use of social mobilization.

Settings approach

The Ottawa Charter advocated that health promotion should adopt a settings approach to programme implementation where all aspects of the setting – policy, environment, services provided and education are concerned with the promotion of health. This is more ambitious than simply using settings as convenient locations for providing health education. Common settings that have been used are the school, hospital, workplace, primary health centre, village, and city (see Fig. 8.4). The World Health Organization and other international agencies have given support to movements intended to encourage health promotion within settings including the Healthy Cities Movement, the Health-Promoting School (Fig. 8.5), the Health-Promoting Hospital and The Baby Friendly Hospital Initiative.

The kinds of activities and structures that you might want to find in specific health promoting settings include:

◆ **The workplace:** Workplace health policies, education of the workforce and employers, health facilities; and safety standards; first aid, absence of bullying and discrimination.
◆ **The hospital:** Education of patients, policies, for example on food and on patient education as a key component of care, balance between prevention and cure, links with primary health care and a good working environment for health care workers.

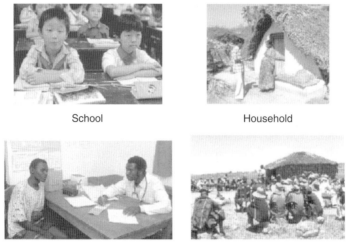

School · Household

Health facility · Community

Fig. 8.4 Some common settings for health promotion.

- **The school:** A healthy school physical and social environment including buildings, clean surroundings, water and sanitation and gardens; good relationships and actions on bullying and violence; health education in the curriculum; school health services including screening, first aid; and school-community collaborations for health, for example on road safety or improving environments to reduce malarial transmission.

- **Primary health care:** First line treatment/prevention services, community-based services such as village health workers, links with the informal sector such as traditional healers and health education within clinic and community.

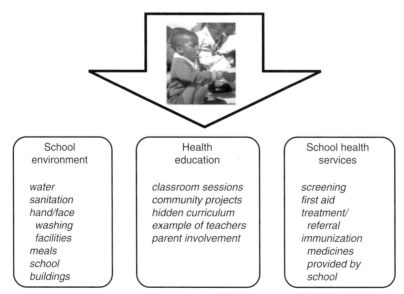

A health-promoting school

School environment	Health education	School health services

water
sanitation
hand/face
  washing
  facilities
meals
school
buildings
	classroom sessions
	community projects
	hidden curriculum
	example of teachers
	parent involvement
		screening
		first aid
		treatment/
		  referral
		immunization
		medicines
		provided by
		school

Fig. 8.5 A health promoting school.

Developing a health promoting setting

How do you go about developing a health promoting setting? You can consider all aspects of a setting from the outset and decide what is needed to improve health in the setting. You can then develop an intervention which is comprehensive. Alternatively, you can identify a small starting point for development and expand to other activities over time. Health promoting hospital developments have frequently selected small starting points for settings developments such as improving all aspects of the out-patient clinic, while smaller settings such as schools have often taken 'whole school' approaches from the outset. Whatever the approach selected all those who have a 'stake' in the settings development need to be informed and involved. It is usually efficient to have a small representative working group to organize the development. In some countries there are national or regional networks that are useful to refer to for support in development. Internationally, the World Health Organization publishes documents to support settings development, including criteria than can be used by schools and hospitals in carrying out a baseline assessment of their health promoting status (see WHO website).

Social mobilization

Another delivery strategy is social mobilization. The process is described by UNICEF as a comprehensive approach that emphasizes political coalition building and community action. It consists of bringing together allies from various sectors with an interest in a specific health problem in order to raise awareness and stimulate demand for a particular programme, and assist in strengthening community participation to achieve sustainability and self-reliance. Social mobilization is closely akin to what others have labelled community development: A process through which community members become aware of a problem, identify it as high priority for action and decide on steps to take action with the added emphasis on the process of coalition building and communication The empowerment of individuals and communities is central to social mobilization. This will require raising awareness of health issues through dialogue and knowledge building, developing trust and confidence plus agenda setting and advocacy skills, and enabling communities to participate in decision making processes. A social mobilization strategy ensures that new ideas and practices come to be owned by communities rather than be seen as imposed from outside. It should be apparent that social mobilization is very similar to health promotion as presented in the Ottawa Charter. Programmes with very similar elements may at times be described as health promotion and at other times as social mobilization. The strength of social mobilization interventions is that they typically offer a strategic and well-organized response to the issues under consideration. Social mobilization has been used in a number of major public health and development programmes, including immunization, TB, child labour, and water and sanitation. Initiatives differ in the emphasis given to differing components with some, for example, giving greater attention to top-down communication to populations and lesser attention to raising critical awareness in communities about the issue in question and achieving genuine participation. Two examples of social mobilization projects are shown in Box 8.4.

Selection and implementation of communication and education methods

These will depend on the nature of the objectives set and the resources available to a programme. They can include advocacy for public policy, mass media and interpersonal methods for communication and education activities. These will be discussed in turn.

Box 8.4 Social mobilization projects

Youth Net and Counselling (YONECO) takes a multi-sectoral approach to tackling TB in Malawi and encourages community based educators, market vendors, and theatre artists to take an active role in disseminating information to their communities. Educators and artists have training on TB prevention and treatments. Advocacy meetings were held with district health officials and district assembly leaders to encourage the dissemination of information in communities and to advocate for increased access to treatment for people living with TB and AIDS. The project expects to create a stronger demand for TB and HIV treatment and more effective services through increased TB and HIV literacy at community level, improved treatment adherence through better drug supplies and active follow up by community volunteers.

Malawi Anti Child Labour Programme addressed the problem of exploitative child labour which is damaging physically and mentally to their health in the short term. Girls are particularly affected. When labour impacts on school attendance and educational achievement it can lead in the long term to trapping people in a cycle of poverty and disadvantage. UNICEF campaigned against child labour in 2000 through a series of workshops resulting in a steering committee of all stakeholders and a number of intervention projects. 'A 2-year intervention "Strengthening the Fight Against Child Labour" used a human rights framework and aimed to strengthen the creation of an enabling environment to protect the rights of children involved in child labour'. The project worked closely with the media to disseminate information and communication materials on child rights using participatory approaches.

Advocacy is the process of overcoming major structural (as opposed to individual and behavioural) barriers to public health goals though influencing decision-makers to change their policies. Examples of advocacy campaigns include:

◆ Local communities working together to get enforcement of road safety laws to protect children selling food by roadsides;

◆ Campaigning for tobacco control policies and effective implementation. See Box 8.5 for illustrations of tobacco related advocacy actions at an international level. There are a number of activities that are central to the advocacy process:

1 Defining the policy issues to be addressed and setting the agenda

2 Deciding the target audience – the policymakers you are trying to influence, e.g. MPs, local officials etc.

3 Building support: Forming alliances with other groups or individuals who are committed to supporting your issues

4 Message development – statements designed for different audiences that define the issue, state solutions and list actions that need to be taken

5 Communication channels. The means by which a message is delivered to the various target audiences, e.g. meetings, radio, TV etc.

6 Fund raising – depends on the scale of an advocacy campaign but funds may be needed for implementation

7 Implementation of the planned activities using lobbying, media advocacy, direct action etc

8 Monitoring and evaluation and revision of campaign as necessary

Selected aspects of this process are discussed further under mass media.

Box 8.5 Advocacy in action – the framework agreement for the control of tobacco

Global action to control the tobacco epidemic:

According to the World Health Organization, 4 million people die each year as a result of tobacco use. Forward projections suggested a major epidemic with 10 million deaths a year in 2030, most of them in developing countries. This is more than the combined deaths from malaria, tuberculosis, AIDS and several major maternal and childhood conditions.

Tobacco causes one-fifth of all deaths due to cardiovascular diseases. In 1999, cardiovascular diseases accounted for about 1 in 10 deaths in Africa; 3 in 10 deaths in South East Asia; 33 percent of all deaths in the Americas, as well as in WHO's Eastern Mediterranean and Western Pacific regions; and 50% of all deaths in the European region.

Tobacco causes one in three cancers deaths worldwide. Cancer accounts for 1 in 20 deaths in Africa; 1 in 14 deaths in South-East Asia and in the Eastern Mediterranean region; and 1 in 5 deaths in the Americas, Europe and the Western Pacific.

The continued marketing of tobacco products to the youth of today means millions of deaths in 30 to 40 years' time. Surveys in developing and transition countries show that about 20% of school children aged 13–15 are already current users of tobacco products.

In resolutions unanimously adopted by the World Health Assembly in May 1998 and 1999, Member States gave themselves the political mandate to negotiate a Framework Convention on Tobacco Control. Actions proposed include a combination of:

- increased taxes to discourage smoking,
- bans on tobacco advertising, sponsorship, and marketing,
- controls on smoking in public places,
- expanded access to effective means of quitting,
- tough advertising to discourage smoking, and
- tight controls on smuggling of tobacco.

In attempts to implement this framework, it is likely that there will be considerable opposition from the tobacco industry.

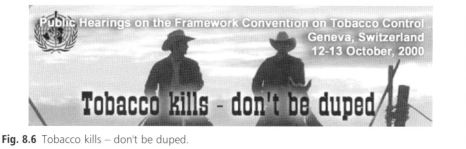

Fig. 8.6 Tobacco kills – don't be duped.

Mass media and interpersonal communication methods

The range of these are described in Table 8.2.

Table 8.2 Different kinds of communication methods used in interventions

Approach	Approach examples	Advantages	Disadvantages
MEDIA	Television	◆ Reach can be broad ◆ Cost per person reached can be low ◆ Can reach both literate and illiterate people ◆ Combines visual dimension with spoken word ◆ Can influence behaviours that are not deeply entrenched ◆ Message can be accurately controlled	◆ Television ownership often mainly high income urban population ◆ High initial investment in production ◆ Difficult to meet needs of specific groups ◆ Lack of feedback
	Radio	◆ Very broad reach ◆ Regional radio provides opportunity to broadcast in local languages ◆ Easy to include content from interviews/music recorded in local communities ◆ Simple to make programmes ◆ Can record programmes on cassettes and play to local audiences	◆ Similar problems as TV from difficulty of making content specific to different local communities and obtaining feedback ◆ Lacks a visual dimension ◆ Depends on appropriate timing of broadcasts, quality of reception and availability of electricity or batteries
	Newspapers, posters	◆ Reach can be broad ◆ Can be distributed to highly targeted group and influential persons ◆ Can include pictures ◆ Can provide information	◆ Written material not suitable for non-literate communities ◆ Reach of newspapers may be limited
INTER - PERSONAL	**Outreach** using field staff, volunteers, peers, drama in community settings e.g. bars, road-side, markets and public places	◆ Takes the education out to where the community live and therefore good for difficult-to-reach groups ◆ Allows the education to be made specific to the needs of the audience, taking into account their special needs ◆ Persons from the target community (peers) will be trusted and believed by others in their community and be effective communicators ◆ Can be very effective at influencing beliefs, attitudes and behaviours providing specific skills and generating empowerment	◆ Requires resources – field staff, time and transport which may not be available ◆ Takes longer to reach audience ◆ Depends on quality/training in communication of field staff ◆ Peer educators/ community health workers require support and supervision. They may leave and need to be replaced

Table 8.2 *(continued)* Different kinds of communication methods used in interventions

Approach	Approach examples	Advantages	Disadvantages
	Facility based e.g. clinics workplace	◆ Allows the education to take into account special needs ◆ Can be very effective at influencing beliefs, attitudes and behaviours providing specific skills and generating empowerment ◆ Educational method can be delivered efficiently and combined with treatment/delivery of preventive services	◆ Only reaches those people who utilize services ◆ Space and time available can make it difficult to use participatory methods ◆ Time available for education may be limited because of pressure of work ◆ Depends on the quality of training of clinic staff in communication methods
	Large Meetings public meetings drama productions	◆ Capable of generating a large amount of interest ◆ Can lead to community participation ◆ Good approach for advocacy	◆ Without advance preparation and follow-up will not lead to lasting change

Mass media

These can be used as a means of providing information to large numbers of people, in efforts to change attitudes on health matters, agenda setting and for media advocacy as an element of advocacy campaigns. The decisions involved in preparing a mass media programme are made on the basis of the media habits of your audience and whether you have access to mass media. The mass media should only be used if the situation assessment shows that the mass media are used in a community. The actual choice of mass media including timings and the kind of programme content will also depend on the information you have on readership of newspapers, listenership of radio programmes, etc. If you are working at the community level you may not have the resources or influence to develop a mass media component in your programme.

Agenda setting is communication directed at raising the profile of a topic among communities and decision makers so that it is a subject of public debate and heightened awareness. This can be carried out through national or local media and it can also be carried out through face to face methods of community drama.

Media advocacy is increasingly popular with health promoters trying to get action on health issues. This is using the media in a strategic way to reach key decision makers, legislators and community groups in order to highlight the structural and environmental determinants of health, rather than individual behaviours. Examples include bringing to public attention the activities of baby milk companies in persuading mothers to use artificial formulas or the tobacco companies in persuading young people to take up cigarettes. A tactic in some countries has been to change the messages on tobacco posters to messages on the dangers of smoking. Fig. 8.6. illustrates a WHO image on smoking.

Social marketing A delivery strategy that uses mass media is social marketing. Essentially this consists of using the methods used in marketing and applying them to selling of health ideas but with no intention of making financial profits. In commercial marketing, consumers get a product that they want, at a price they can afford and the producer gets a profit (the 4Ps). In marketing health the consumer gets the promise of improved health and quality of life at the possible cost of giving up a pleasure or making some physical or psychological effort. Social marketing has been used in health programmes across the world and a specific example is discussed in the next chapter.

Interpersonal communication and education

This can take place within any of the settings used in health promotion. In schools it will be an integral part of the curriculum as well as a part of other activities in the school as a health promoting setting. In health facilities, where it may also be called patient education, it is a good approach to use for reaching people who come for treatment or preventive care. The education can be available for the patient and his or her partner or children. It can be carried out as part of the consultation with the health worker or by a specialist educator/counsellor. It can also take place through group teaching sessions or through home visits. One useful way of remembering the basic principles of one-to-one communication is the word GATHER (see Box 8.6).

Some people do not use health facilities very often. The workplace can, for example, be a good place to reach men. However, in most situations you will need to go out into the community. An effective community-based approach will involve dialogue with the community, and various educational activities using those popular with any community. Drama is often a popular means

---

Box 8.6 GATHER approach to one-to-one communication

G *Greet the person.* Put them at ease, show respect and trust. Emphasize the confidential nature of the discussion.

A *Ask about their problem.* Encourage them to bring out their anxieties, worries and needs. Assess their present degree of risk behaviour. Determine their access to support and help in their family and community. Find out what steps they have already taken to deal with the situation. Encourage them to express their feelings in their own words. Show respect and tolerance to what they say and do not pass judgment. Actively listen and show that you are interested and paying attention. Encourage them through helpful questions.

T *Tell them any relevant information they need.* Provide accurate and specific information in reply to their questions. Give information on how they can reduce of their risk of becoming infected again. Demonstrate any preventive measures e.g. use of condoms, mixing oral rehydration solution. Explain any medical procedures and tests being used. Keep your language simple, repeat important points and ask questions to check that the important points are understood. Provide the important information in a leaflet that they can take away.

H *Help them make decisions.* Explore the various alternatives. Raise issues they may not have thought of. Be careful of letting your own views, values and prejudices influence the advice you give. Ensure that it is their own decision and not one that you have imposed. Help them make a plan of action.

E *Explain any misunderstandings.* Ask questions to check understanding of important points. Ask the person to repeat back in his/her own words the key points you have made.

R *Return to follow up on them.* Arrange for a follow-up visit or referral to other agencies. If a follow-up visit is not necessary, give the name of someone who they can contact it they have need for help.

through which community education can take place. If you want to give communities a major role in providing educational activities you can facilitate community members to provide activities that they select. Alternatively, you can recruit persons from the community as educators in order to use a peer education approach.

Peer education   This is the sharing of health information or provision of further educational activities and counselling between members of similar age, interest, or status groups. Peer education is particularly useful in working with hard to reach groups such as young people who are out of school, and with sex workers. It has also been used as a core activity within a major project implemented in more than 80 countries, Child-to-Child. Peers are typically seen as credible sources of information, and they can be more effective educators than professionals. If they have contact over a longer period they can be effective in reinforcing education and they can be positive role models for behaviour change.

To make peer education effective it is necessary to:

◆ Select peers who will be acceptable to those they will work with;

◆ Ensure that peer educators have understanding of the health topic in question, can clarify the knowledge of others and know how to find further knowledge when required;

◆ Provide initial and continuing training to enable peer educators to use the variety of counselling and education skills needed to achieve programme goals;

◆ Ensure peer educators have the confidence to work in situations where they may be challenged. An example of a programme using peer methods is shown in Box 8.7.

Support materials

These include leaflets, charts, flip-charts, flannelgraphs, films, videos, and cassettes. You can use what is easily accessible and simple materials can be as effective, or more effective than more complex ones. Support materials can be useful for: Explaining difficult points, ensuring that key messages are correctly put across by field staff and providing a focus for participatory learning and triggering discussion. They are also an essential component of advocacy activities. When working with groups of people participatory learning materials such as games, discussion

---

Box 8.7 EntreNous Jeunes Peer Education (Cameroon)

This is a peer based adolescent reproductive health intervention designed to increase contraceptive use and reduce the prevalence of unintended pregnancy among sexually active adolescents. The programme uses a large number of existing community based youth services, clubs and sports and religious associations. Volunteer peer educators are recruited and receive one week's training in knowledge about reproduction and contraceptive methods, facilitating group discussion and the skills to negotiate condom use. Further training takes place every 3 months to reinforce knowledge and skills and resolve concerns and conflicts. The educators work with their own communities and refer young people, where necessary, to reproductive and health care. They arrange discussion groups and also work one-to-one. In addition they distribute materials including comic strips, calendars and posters. Peer educators receive travel expenses and special promotional materials. During a 2-year intervention they organized 353 discussion group sessions attended by 12 000 young people and had 5000 one to one contacts.

Box 8.8 Effective communication

- ◆ Promotes actions that are realistic and feasible within the constraints faced by the community. Builds on ideas, concepts and practices that people already have.
- ◆ Repeated and reinforced over time using different methods.
- ◆ Adaptable, and uses existing channels of communication – for example songs, drama and story telling.
- ◆ Entertaining and attracts community's attention.
- ◆ Uses clear simple language with local expressions and emphasizes short-term benefits of action.
- ◆ Provides opportunities for dialogue and discussion to allow learner participation and feedback on understanding and implementation.
- ◆ Uses demonstrations to show the benefits of adopting practices.

pictures, flip charts, trigger videos, or models can be used. You will need to **pre-test** both the messages and the support materials. Pre-testing involves showing the media/materials to samples of your intended target audience to find out their opinions. You should find out if the messages are acceptable, relevant, understood, and do not contain confusing words or pictures give rise to misunderstandings, or raise anxieties and fears (Box 8.8).

In implementing programmes the various factors discussed in Chapter 6 should also be taken into account including: Training; formation of partnerships and inter-sectoral collaboration and management of time and other resources. Of particular importance is the use of relevant theory on implementing different strategies and methods. Health promotion theory draws on various disciplines and a useful web based guide to some of this theory is listed in further reading.

Monitoring and evaluation of programmes

Monitoring as discussed in earlier chapters is essential to assess whether an intervention is being implemented according to plan. Mechanisms for monitoring need to be planned from the outset. With good mechanisms in place any emerging difficulties can be picked up quickly and responses made. In the spirit of health promotion efforts should be made to involve participating communities in evaluation activities. Data from monitoring can feed into evaluation. Evaluation should provide the necessary information to measure impact of the programme and identify ways in which future activities can be improved. It should seek to measure both the intended and unintended consequences of the health promotion. It is important to carry out short-term evaluation to measure immediate impact and process of an intervention and medium and longer-term evaluation:

- ◆ Immediate impact: Reach/coverage of programme, changes in knowledge, awareness, specific skills, service improvements
- ◆ Medium-term impact: Changes in behaviour after 2 or 3 years, utilization of services, sustained improvements in service provision, implementation of policy changes, health status (only for health issues where impact can be expected in this time scale)
- ◆ Longer-term impact: Changes after 5–10 years, for example sustained behaviour changes or health status

◆ Process: The collection of information during the implementation of an intervention which can 'illuminate' and help to explain the success, or lack of success, of an intervention. This will draw on monitoring data and other evaluation activities.

The amount of change you might be able to expect will depend on the health topic, its complexity, and the resources at your disposal. For example, an immunization programme might be expected to have an impact in the short term on the incidence of specific diseases while more complex topics, such as maternal mortality and lung cancer would require longer to demonstrate an impact. See Chapter 5 for a more detailed discussion of evaluation.

Conclusion

This chapter has provided a flavour of health promotion and discussed the components of holistic health promotion interventions. Health promotion practitioners differ in the goals they prioritize – some emphasizing empowerment, others behaviour change. Many people may feel most comfortable carrying out health education activities but can nearly always begin to take some actions on the other components which, if unattended, will diminish the impact of health education activities. There is a growing body of evidence on how to implement effective health promotion interventions and access to this evidence is getting easier. By ensuring that we disseminate the results of our own interventions we can contribute to developing practice.

Further reading

Adam G., Harford N. (1998) *Health on air – a guide to creative radio for development*. London: Health Unlimited.

Dhillon H.S., Philip L. (1994) *Health promotion and community action for health in developing countries*. Geneva: WHO.

Hubley J. (2003) *Communicating health: an action guide to health education and health promotion*. 2nd edition. Basingstoke: Macmillan.

Hubley J., Copeman J. (2008) *Practical health promotion*. Cambridge: Polity Press. Designed predominantly for the UK market but its accessible style should make it very useful for readers elsewhere.

Hope A., Timmel S. (1995) *Training for transformation*. London: Intermediate Technology Publications/ Teaching Aids at Low Cost.

Rifkin S., Pridmore P. (2001) *Partners in planning – information, participation and empowerment*. London: Macmillan.

Websites

International Journal of Equity in Health www.equityhealthj.com

National Institutes for Health, National Cancer Institute (2004) Theory at a glance – a guide for health promotion practice. http://www.cancer.gov/cancerinformation/theory-at-a-glance

World Health Organisation – www.who.int

Cochrane Public Health Field – for evidence on effective health promotion interventions http://www.cochrane.org

Chapter 9

Health policy and systems

Andrew Green

This chapter gives an overview of the following topics:

+ Key policy shifts historically;
+ What are health and health care systems?
+ How are decisions made, and by whom, about services?
+ Policy and planning process;
+ Monitoring, evaluation and regulation.

Introduction

For many health professionals, the terms 'policy' and 'health systems' may be unfamiliar; indeed some may consider them alien.

Policy may be seen as the province of government bureaucrats or external consultants and far removed from the reality of professionals' day-to-day life. Indeed policies may be seen as barriers or constraints which they need to find ways of circumventing. Whilst of course there are many examples of poor, unworkable, or non-implemented policies, there are also examples where policy shifts have had important positive effects on the way health care is viewed and provided. Perhaps the most well-known of these are the policies related to the Primary Health Care movement initiated at the Alma Ata Conference 30 years ago.

The other term in the chapter title – 'health systems' – suffers from an additional problem; it is often used differently by different people. National policy makers may use the term to refer to how the processes (*the system*) such as finance, human resources, medical supplies, interact. Public health programme managers may have a more practical view and use it to refer to the logistics that underpin their daily activities.

In this chapter we introduce you to some of the key policy issues related to health systems that face you as public health managers. This is important both in terms of understanding the 'bigger picture', and also in seeing how you can get involved in influencing them. Having given this broad overview of global policies we will then look at what is meant by a health system and what are its key elements.

Key historical policy shifts

We first examine a number of the policy shifts that have taken place over the last 30 years and which have a particular impact on national health systems.

Alma Ata Declaration and Primary Health Care (PHC)

We start with the Alma Ata Declaration. This was signed in 1978 by health ministers from around the world committing them to a particular approach to health called Primary Health Care (PHC).

The PHC approach is often viewed at two levels. First, it calls for emphasis on the *primary* level of care – clinics, health stations and health centres – as the bedrock of any health care system. This primary level is seen as being able to respond to the majority of the needs of individuals and populations in a cost-effective, easily accessible and appropriate fashion. It includes a number of key elements such as immunization, family planning, and treatment of common diseases. Such emphasis on primary care does not however suggest no role for hospitals – but rather a supporting role.

The second important aspect of the PHC approach, however, is the importance it places on the following key principles as critical to the success of a health system:

♦ The need to work towards equity in health and health care

♦ Inter-sectoral action to respond to the determinants of health

♦ The importance of preventive and promotive approaches to health

♦ Use of technology which is appropriate to the specific context

♦ Participation of individuals and communities in decisions about their health

Health reform policies

The Alma Ata Declaration provided the basis for much of the specific country health policies in the 1980s. There was, for example, increasing interest in community health workers, essential drug lists, and the development of rural health facilities. However, by the beginning of the 1990s there was a sense in many countries and in international agencies that health gains were not being achieved, or at least as fast as was hoped. Attention shifted to a series of related policies that were led by the World Bank labelled as 'health reforms' (see World Development Report, 1993) summarizes the elements of what were typically included in reform initiatives (see Box 9.1).

The World Bank brought significant resources as 'leverage' (influence) on weak health systems. The general approach, and in particular the introduction of user fees, has often been seen as driven by wider neo-liberal market-driven agendas. Linked to this was a more general policy of

Box 9.1 Common elements of health sector reform

Structure and governance

♦ Changing role for public sector away from provision to policy, commissioning/contracting and regulation of health care

♦ Enhanced provider role for private sector (often called the public-private mix)

♦ Decentralization including hospital autonomy

♦ Integration of vertical programmes

♦ Private sector management approaches in public sector

Priority-setting approaches

♦ Cost-effectiveness

♦ Essential Health packages

Financing mechanisms

♦ Shift from collective to individual financing (emphasis on user charges)

reducing the size of the public sector; as part of a wider economic Structural Adjustment led by the International Monetary Fund.

The subsequent decade was dominated, in policy terms, by these issues and by a belief held by a number of international agencies that existing health system structures were a major obstacle to improving health. However, increasing doubts were expressed about this reform movement. Such doubts related to specific policy aspects. For example, there was growing concern about the use of user fees and their impact on equity. For public health managers, the reforms often appeared to be the result of narrow 'economic' thinking rather than responding to the needs of the services for which they were responsible. Underlying some of these criticisms were worries that the reform agenda assumed a *blueprint* solution which was seen as appropriate to *any* health system irrespective of the social, economic, and political context. Lastly, there was considerable unease that such policies were not generated by national policy makers but imposed by external agencies. We return to the whole question of how policy is made, and by whom, in the section below on policy and planning process.

The focus on health reforms, had to some degree, meant that other policy concerns were neglected. However as the new millennium approached four areas began to emerge as key for policy.

Health funding mechanisms and levels

First, the very low levels of funding available to the health sector were recognized as a major constraint. The WHO Commission on Macro Economics and Health led by Jeffrey Sachs, estimated that a minimum of between $30–40 per capita was needed to provide *basic* health care. A number of health systems, particularly in sub-Saharan Africa, continue to fall below this. Various initiatives were developed to raise the levels of funding. Within countries alternative financing forms were explored and these are discussed in Chapter 7. At the international level, mechanisms were set up to encourage additional funding for particular diseases. Perhaps the best known of these is the Global Fund to fight AIDS, Tuberculosis, and Malaria. This is one of a number of Global Public Private Partnerships (GPPPs) which combine in a single fund, resources from governments, multilateral agencies and the private sector. There are various difficulties associated with such GPPPs; the one of most interest in this chapter relates to the way in which they stress responses to particular diseases thus leading to the charge that they ignore, or even aggravate, the wider needs of the health system – the platform underpinning all service delivery indeed the Global fund for AIDS, TB. and Malaria (GFATM) has introduced the funding of health systems strengthening alongside programme specific elements to respond to this concern.

Closely linked to this is the role and mechanisms for international support (or 'aid') to the health sector. This may be provided in many forms. It may be as:

- General support to the economy (e.g. IMF loans)
- Funding of projects
- Funding of programmes
- Technical assistance provided directly
- Training provided directly
- Support to NGOs

One particular area where public health managers may interact with international support is in the use of consultants who may be invited to provide technical expertise on particular issues. Such consultants can be very useful, but can also be time-consuming and indeed may on occasions have less expertise than you (Box 9.2).

Box 9.2 Checklist for use of consultants

- ◆ Be clear on what you want from them – set up clear Terms of Reference
- ◆ Include within this the type of deliverable that you are seeking such as:
  - ● A draft report presented to a group of key stakeholders
  - ● Length and focus of final report
- ◆ Insist on seeing, and approving, a full CV of the consultant, and ideally choosing between alternative candidates
- ◆ Set a clear but feasible timeframe
- ◆ Specify what processes you expect them to follow such as:
  - ● Whom to meet
  - ● Which documents to consult
  - ● Workshops to conduct

Aid may be provided by a variety of organizations including:

- ◆ bilateral organizations representing a high income country (such as the Department for International Development of the UK)
- ◆ multilateral organizations which represent broader groupings of countries such as organizations falling under the UN umbrella such as WHO, UNDP, UNICEF, and the World Bank
- ◆ Global Public Private Partnerships such as GAVI
- ◆ International NGOs such as Save the Children Fund

'Aid' is often criticized on a number of grounds. These include:

- ◆ The lack of co-ordination between donors, and with government
- ◆ The levels of monitoring and bureaucracy associated with it
- ◆ Its 'projectized' nature often linked to vertical disease programmes
- ◆ The disproportionate power it gives donors in determining national policies.

Increasing recognition of the negative aspects of aid, has led to a commitment by key donors to a number of principles of aid support which are set out in the Paris Declaration. It has also led to attempts in a number of countries such as Bangladesh, Ghana, Mozambique, and Uganda to develop mechanisms for pooling funds from both government and international sources into a single 'basket' which is then used to support a clear national health policy. This approach is known as the Sector Wide Approach (SWAp).

Staffing

The second broad emerging area for policy focus was that of staffing, and in particular the availability of health professionals. The encouragement to the private sector, the increasing ability to migrate to jobs in wealthier health systems such as the UK, coupled with the poor working conditions in many health systems led to a critical shortage in some countries of doctors, nurses and midwives (see by WHO region in World Health Statistics, 2005, pp. 45).

The health sector is extremely dependant on human resources and the long time required to train health professionals has meant that many health systems continue to struggle with the policy dilemma of how to staff their services. The WHO annual report of 2006 gives a good introduction to these issues and potential strategies.

Millennium development goals

The Millennium was marked with agreement on a set of eight goals adopted by UN member states. Each of these (see Box 9.3) has a set of monitorable indicators which are seen as targets for 2015. Whilst three of the MDGs relate directly to health, the others also have clear health implications. In particular the first of the MDGs reminds us of the critical importance of poverty in the fight for better health. This has been linked to health through the mechanism of Poverty Reduction Strategy Papers which set out a government's intersectoral approaches to poverty reduction. Other MDGs are also critical for health, and in particular, the role of education and the importance of gender equity. The role of the public health manager in these health-related areas can be very important.

Whilst there are some regions and countries that have already achieved, or are on the path to achieving, the targets, there are others, and in particular countries in sub-Saharan Africa, for which the predictions are less optimistic.

Box 9.3 Millennium development goals

Goal 1: Eradicate extreme poverty and hunger

Goal 2: Achieve universal primary education

Goal 3: Promote gender equality and empower women

Goal 4: Reduce child mortality

Goal 5: Improve maternal health

Goal 6: Combat HIV/AIDS, malaria, and other diseases

Goal 7: Ensure environmental sustainability

Goal 8: Develop a Global Partnership for Development

Social determinants of health

The most recent policy area of interest to health systems takes us firmly back to the foundations of public health – the wider determinants of health, as discussed in Chapter 1. The Alma Ata Declaration clearly saw the need for inter-sectoral action. However health ministries continue to focus largely on curative services or personal prevention. Public health professionals should be well aware of the wide range of factors that determine ill-health – as discussed in Chapter 3 and illustrated in Fig. 9.1.

How to support such wider activities is discussed in various chapters including Chapter 6 (health promotion). At the international level two important initiatives led by WHO show the potential importance of wider strategies. The first focuses on the ill-health effects of tobacco with their Tobacco Free initiative (see http://www.who.int/tobacco/en/) which includes the WHO Framework Convention on Tobacco Control (see Chapter 14). The second is more recent and is the Commission on the Social Determinants of health whose report came out in 2008.

Taking a broad view of the determinants of health raises issues in a number of field. For example:

- Transport policy and its effects on road traffic accidents: this may suggest the need for legislation requiring use of seat belts, motorcycle helmets and improved provision of ambulance and accident and emergency services

◆ Climate changes and their effects both on disease incidence and on food availability: this may suggest the need for policies to promote alternative sources of energy such as solar, and wind power, and energy saving, together with discouraging the use of petrol, gas and coal (which release CO_2 and cause global warming) through, for example, taxation.

Public health professionals have a role to play in developing all of these policies and ensuring that the health effects (positive and negative) are considered.

What are health and health care systems?

Within this policy overview, you will have seen the term 'health system' appear at various points. We turn now to explore what is meant by this, and what are the key aspects that are important for a public health practitioner to understand.

There are various definitions of 'a health system' and you are invited to explore these. For example, a particularly well-known one is that of WHO (WHO, 2000). Fig. 9.1 provides a graphical representation of the elements that go to make up a health system, and which we will use in this chapter. Arising from this framework are some key questions.

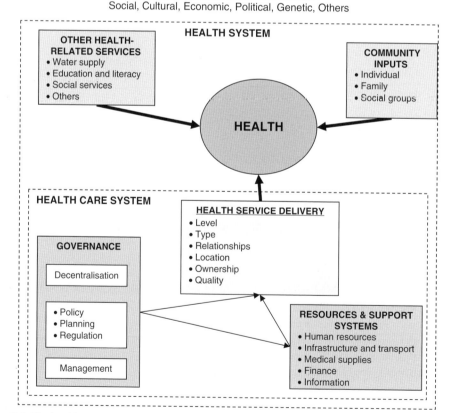

Fig. 9.1 The health system.

What is the purpose of the health system?

The starting point is the *purpose* of a health system which, at first sight, is to improve and maintain the health levels of the populations and individuals. Our diagram places health firmly in the centre to reinforce this. However, closer examination suggests that it is not quite as simple as this. First, there are questions as to how we view, define, measure and indeed prioritize different aspects of health, as discussed in Chapters 1, 3, and 4. The policy and planning processes need to have a clear understanding of this. Secondly, though populations are, of course, made up of individuals, there are differences in how a health system will respond to the needs of populations (through for example, public health programmes) compared to the clinical needs of individuals. Lastly, of course, health systems operate within a wider political and economic environment. There may be pressure on them, for example, to reduce staffing levels in response to wider public expenditure controls.

How do we improve health?

The figure above suggests three broad ways in which health can be improved. The one that health professionals naturally think of is health care – we return to that later.

For public health managers there are challenges as to how, in practice, to contribute to a coordinated multi-sectoral response to wider factors (as discussed in other chapters, including Chapters 1, 2, 8, and 15).

The third broad area is that of the actions of individuals and communities which can have a major impact on health, both in terms of life-style decisions and in terms of treatment of ill health (see Chapter 8, health promotion). Again, for the health service there are important considerations as to how to work with communities and involve them in decisions about the type of health care and how it is provided.

What kind of health services are provided and by whom?

We return now to the contribution of health services to health – the bottom half of the figure. This is often called the 'health *care* system' to distinguish it from the wider health system. For many public health practitioners this is where their energies are focussed, though of course, they should also be seeking ways to work at the level of the wider determinants of health.

Each health care system is different for a variety of reasons, often as a result of the differences in history and socio-economic contexts. In understanding them, there are some key questions we need to consider:

- What balance should there be, and relationships between, the different levels of health care and in particular between primary, secondary, and tertiary care?
- What should the balance be between promotive, preventive, curative, and rehabilitative services?
- Where should we locate health care outlets (hospitals, clinics etc)?
- What trade-off should there be between the level of quality and the 'spread' of health care given our stretched resources?
- What are the relative roles of the public and private sectors?

Some of these are issues that country health policies and plans need to deal with explicitly. A critical one for the health care system and, as we have seen, one that formed part of the agenda of the health reform movement, concerns the role of the private sector in health care provision. In most countries the public sector has a primary role in both setting policies and delivering heath care (and particularly public health). However many countries also have a significant private sector ranging from individual practitioners, through to church-operated clinics and hospitals which are found all over Africa and Asia, to large commercial hospitals, common in India and parts of South-East Asia. This suggests important questions which policy makers and public health practitioners need to address:

- How can we ensure that private practice quality is of an acceptable level?
- How can we maximize co-operation (for example in areas such as referral) and minimize duplication, whilst also ensuring that individual patients are not disadvantaged by, for example, high fees?
- How can we ensure the private sector contributes to wider costs such as training staff?

In some health systems, reforms led to the development of contracting mechanisms. This may involve the 'purchase' of services by the public sector from 'providers' such as private or NGO sectors. This had occurred in some countries for many years through annual grants to church hospitals for provision of services (Tanzania is a good example in its designated District Hospitals). Elsewhere, more complex mechanisms were set up to reimburse specific services. Examples of more complex arrangements are the contracting out of primary care services in Afghanistan and Pakistan and the contracted provision of hospital services under the Social Insurance policy of Thailand.

One particular issue is that of regulation of the private sector, to which we return later.

Which inputs are needed and how are they provided?

In order to provide health care, *inputs* are needed such as staff, vehicles, buildings, medical supplies and, underpinning all of these, finance. The last of these, finance, is covered separately in Chapter 7. We examine below three others that bring particular challenges to the health sector.

Staffing

Planning and management of health professionals is critical for the success of the health system. Box 9.4 sets out the key tasks.

Box 9.4 Elements in staff planning and management system

- Planning the numbers and types of health professionals needed in the future
- Training the health professionals including:
  - Identifying the core competencies needed
  - Developing and delivering curriculum
  - Assessing student performance
- Ongoing management including:
  - Recruitment including the development of job descriptions and person-specifications, and selection processes
  - Deployment
  - Payment
  - Supervision
  - Staff review, promotion, and discipline
- Ongoing continuous professional development and in-service training

In order to ensure health professionals are well-motivated and fully productive, the health care system needs to pay attention to all of these. In some areas there will be specialists (for example, educators and human resource planners). However one of the key functions – that of management – is likely to be shared between specialist personnel managers (who should be well-versed in the legal and equal opportunity obligations of a recruitment and management process) and health professionals who carry out both technical supervisory and general management roles.

Modern methods of management have moved away from top-down, rigid hierarchical approaches and recognize the importance of motivation. Good managers are leaders rather than drivers. Mentoring, (where a senior guides and supports a junior staff member), and staff review systems can be positive motivators. Mentoring and staff reviews can also ensure that staff understand the needs of the system, and that the system understands their concerns and development needs.

Medical supplies

The second key resource is that of medical supplies. This is covered comprehensively in Chapter 12. Ensuring that health care professionals have access to appropriate high quality supplies is another critical management function. Box 9.5 sets out the key elements of this. As with human resources, management of medical supplies is carried out by a combination of specialists (including procurement specialists and pharmacists) and facility or programme based professionals for whom this in one of a number of responsibilities. For such people there are key issues including ensuring a stock control system to ensure that ordering is done sufficiently far in advance, security to minimize improper use or theft of such supplies and appropriate storage conditions (such as the Cold Chain for immunizations).

Information

Information is critical to the well functioning of a health system, contributing to planning and day to day management. For example, information on disease incidence can be critical to ensure early response to a developing epidemic (see Chapter 13). Information can be provided from surveys, specific research and the health information systems.

Health Management Information Systems provide routine and regular information, often based on the services provided. In many health systems this information is collected by primary care workers and sent to the central level for processing and analysis. Increasingly, it is possible for analysis to take place at the level of collection. This is likely to encourage staff to ensure data is accurate, and to recognize the importance and use of such information. It is important to remember that facility-based data does not measure the health status of the wider population, but only

Box 9.5 Elements of a medical supply

- ◆ Specification of medical supply needs
- ◆ Purchase of medical supplies
- ◆ Quality assurance of medical supplies
- ◆ Central and intermediate storage including security, inventory, and shelf-life control
- ◆ Distribution of medical supplies
- ◆ Facility level storage
- ◆ Dispensing of medical supplies

that of people who use the service, where, as is the case in many rural areas, access is a constraint to use of services. This may give an inaccurate picture of health patterns.

How are decisions made, and by whom, about services?

The final question concerns how services are organized and managed. This is often labelled the *governance* or *stewardship* functions of a health system. Here we examine three key parts of the governance.

First, any health system needs national policies and plans to give overall direction and shape to the health sector. The development of these is usually the responsibility of the Ministry of Health, though it may share this responsibility with other key ministries such as Planning, Finance or the Prime Minister's Office.

Secondly, decisions are needed as to where the authority lies for day-to-day management. In particular this relates to the level and form of decentralization – which decisions are made at the national level, which at the provincial/regional level and which at the district level or below.

Each health system will be organized differently. Some will have very decentralized systems with District Health Officers or their equivalent being given considerable authority over financial or staffing decisions. Elsewhere such decisions will be made at the provincial or national level. Some health systems will have services organized around vertical programmes with strong lines of control from national programme heads down to the service delivery level. In more integrated systems, the national, and provincial programme heads will have technical leadership roles; with the day-to-day decisions on service delivery being made by local general health managers.

Lastly, some systems will have very strong public sector structures whilst others will have significant private sector roles. In each of these cases, there will need to be structures appropriate to the particular public–private mix which sets and regulates standards. In this section of the chapter we explore these issues ending with a more general look at the roles of programme managers, general managers, users, and communities.

Decentralization types

As already indicated, decentralization refers to a process where authority to make decisions is given to lower levels within a health system. This gives power to the managers and professionals who are close to the services being provided, hopefully getting more appropriate and efficient decisions without bureaucratic delays. There are three key models of decentralization (see Fig. 9.2).

The first, and perhaps most common, is known as *functional deconcentration*. In this model, the health ministry passes power down to officers employed at 'lower' levels in the ministry such as District Medical Officers to make decisions in defined areas such as finance or hiring and firing of staff. The key advantage of this form of decentralization is that control of health care staff and decisions remain with the health sector. The ministry itself may retain powers in areas such as budget approval, or national strategic planning. A common variant of this is *integrated deconcentration* where services at the local level are co-ordinated by an officer (often formerly known as a District Commissioner) who is appointed by, and responsible to, central government.

The third approach to decentralization is when power is *devolved* to an elected local government. In this situation there may still be a local District Medical Officer, but s/he would be responsible to a District Chief Executive and through him/her to local representatives. The potential strength of such an organizational configuration is that there may be greater coordination between different sectors, with the possibility of achieving a stronger and broader public health agenda. The potential weakness is the lack of direct managerial links with the health ministry with the potential for less effective technical support and career development and mobility for

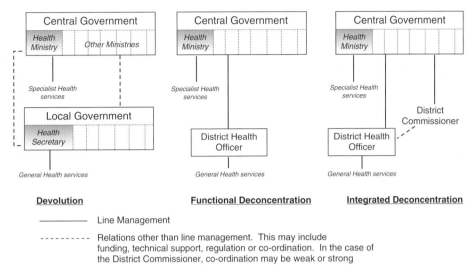

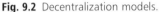

Fig. 9.2 Decentralization models.

Source: Reproduced from Green A. (2007) with permission.

health professionals. You are encouraged to identify the form of decentralization in your own health system and assess its strengths and weaknesses.

Whilst the above sets out different models for power sharing between the centre and the local level, there are, of course, numerous variations as to what type of decisions can be made at different levels. Box 9.6 gives some examples in three different areas. Again, you may find it helpful to try and identify exactly what powers are given to different levels in your health system.

Box 9.6 Examples of areas of authority in decentralization

Plans and polices
- Setting policies
- Developing plans

Budgets and finance
- Setting budgets
- Approving budgets
- Raising income through financing methods
- Incurring expenditure (within given limits)

Staff management
- Hiring and promoting staff
- Levels of pay
- Dismissing staff
- Posting staff

Semi-autonomy

Closely related to the above is a specific approach to governance known as semi-autonomy, particularly for hospitals. This can be seen as a form of decentralization in that it allows specific institutions to make decisions analogous to those of decentralized organizations. It was developed in recognition that hospitals often were constrained by central rules and regulations and unable to take local decisions quickly and in response to the specific conditions they were facing. Again the degree of actual autonomy will vary depending what is allowed. One area that has been controversial relates to the power to set salary levels for individual hospitals, with concern raised as to whether it leads to hospitals being able attract staffing through offering higher salaries. This in a situation of scarce health professionals, may reduce the number available for primary care and public health services.

Integration versus verticalism

Decentralization and autonomy refer to where the vertical lines of authority lie. The second broad issue concerning governance relates to how particular services are structured and managed. For a number of diseases and public health initiatives, there has been a history of developing programmes with their own management structures, often run from the national health ministry. In part this is a result of external agency support to particular programmes with funding being channelled and protected in these areas. These may include for example TB control, HIV/AIDS and EPI. The strong argument for such vertical programmes is that it allows a concentration of expertise and focus on a particular technical area. The arguments against it are that it may be an inefficient way of using resources (such laboratory services) which could be 'shared' and that it may affect adversely the links between general health care and specialist disease control, thus reducing for example, case-finding and referrals between them. Increasingly international funding mechanisms such as GAVI and GFATM are financing support to the general health system alongside specific disease control in recognition of this. In many countries previously vertical programmes, (such as TB in Pakistan), have integrated delivery within the general health facilities and care is provided by general clinicians; ensuring that key functions are maintained, such as district coordination and national policy-making. Whether particular functions can be integrated depends on how well the general systems, such as central drug procurement and distribution, are functioning.

The district team: Roles of managers and communities

The preceding has introduced issues related to different ways of structuring health systems. Of course, within each of these, there are a number of different types of managers and their inter-relationships are often critical to the smooth functioning of a health system. There may, for example, be the following with a management function at a district level:

- District medical officer
- District nursing officer
- Specific district health experts (e.g. disease control, health education etc)
- District general manager or administrator
- District pharmacist
- Accountant

Each of these will have a specific role and set of responsibilities which should be laid out in their job description. Unfortunately these are often not well-specified and may be outdated (perhaps predating decentralization policies). For the district to function effectively it is important that a team approach is developed. This should specify both the areas of specific responsibility and joint responsibility. Leadership of the team is essential to its wellbeing and is further discussed in Chapter 6.

The district team will need to work with a variety of other key actors – officials in the health sector above and below the district, other sectoral officers, and crucially the community. Mechanisms for discussing and agreeing district level strategies, such as a District Health Committee are needed.

Involvement of the community in key decisions brings with it various advantages – in particular team decisions are likely to be based on a better understanding of the community's view of health and healthcare. However, it can take real skill and time to involve the community in a way that reflects all elements of the community and not just the vocal and well-connected. The governance structures may require or allow this to happen through, for example, District Committees, or consultation processes around plans. Local representation may also be already available in the form of elected representatives, particularly in the case of devolved decentralization.

Policy and planning processes

At the beginning of the chapter, we looked briefly at the importance of policies. Policies are the way in which the priorities and intentions of a health system are expressed. They may, in fact, occur in a number of formats of which legislation and formal polices are the most obvious. Others include circulars, resource allocation, or guidance. Unfortunately, in some cases, policies are not clearly articulated, leading to confusion on the part of those people expected to implement them.

In many health systems, policy making is seen as being the responsibility of senior national level 'policy makers'. Increasingly however it is recognized that involvement of key 'actors' will make the policy more realistic and feasible, as different views are expressed. Such involvement will also increase the chances that policy will be implemented as expected.

There are various models for understanding how policy is made. A useful one is that of Walt and Gilson, who suggest that there are three key considerations we need to think about in developing the content of a policy:

◆ Who are the key actors who should be, involved in making the policy? For example should key stakeholders such as communities and the private sector be involved?

◆ What are the decision processes by which the policy is determined? For example is there a working group set up of key stakeholders? And is there a wider consultation process?

◆ What is the wider context within which the policy is being formulated? For example, what are the health needs that the policy is trying to address? And are there social, political or economic constraints that will affect the policy? For example Nigeria and India have a strong private health care sector; in contrast, the health system of Tanzania is predominantly public.

Closely linked to policy formation, are national strategic planning processes (see Green 2007). Many health systems will have national health plans or strategies, which set out, in broad terms how health policies are to be achieved. They are likely to have targets attached, such as levels of planned immunization coverage. Such national plans thus provide the framework against which district level or programme plans are made, and may be assessed.

Even where there are explicit transparent processes for the development of policies, they are still inevitably the result of a set of forces and interests. Increasingly there are attempts in many health systems to get policies rooted in good evidence; this requires research evidence to be presented in a format that is understandable by health policy makers – such as research briefs – and to respond to the issues such policy makers see as key. There are signs that both researchers and policy makers are improving in this regard. However, policy formation will always have a 'political' element alongside the evidence base. Different stakeholders will have different interests, values and ideologies which will affect their view on a particular policy. A policy on tobacco control is likely to receive, for example, different reactions from a hospital based respiratory clinician, a public health practitioner and tobacco companies. A useful technique in helping to understand these forces is that of *stakeholder analysis* (Varvasovsky 2000).

For public health practitioners, it is important to understand the policy and planning processes in order to interact with them and contribute field level experience. At a minimum they should try and get hold of any national level policy and strategy documents. They should also try to, find out about emerging policies and the processes for these, about the planning timetable and how they can interact with them. Public health practitioners also need to be familiar with the evidence, ready to commission new research where there are gaps, and able to synthesize and communicate evidence to policy makers. They can then contribute to effective policy making. They can provide an important bridge between researchers and policy makers.

Monitoring, evaluation, and regulation

Finally, an important part of the governance function relates to monitoring and evaluation of the services provided. Monitoring and evaluation are key managerial functions and the District Medical Officer or Programme Manager should spend a significant amount of time on these, ensuring that the services planned are being carried out. In order to do this effectively, it is essential that, at the planning stage, key SMART (Specific, Measurable, Attainable, Relevant, and Time bound) indicators are developed which will form the basis of the monitoring.

Regulation of the private sector is also, as we saw earlier, a key function of the public sector. It has often been neglected and under-resourced. However, with the growth of the private sector in some health systems, it is increasingly important in terms of ensuring that quality is maintained and that relations between the public and private sectors are positive.

Conclusion

This chapter has introduced the idea of the wider health system within which public health practitioners work. Inevitably it has been broad, and the interested reader is encouraged to pursue their interest in the various books and journals available that cover this area.

It is hoped that the chapter has demonstrated the complexity of health systems and the importance for a health practitioner in seeing where they fit into the wider system. It is also hoped that it has shown that there is no single, correct model for a health system; there are a multitude of different ways of organizing health care. How a particular health system organizes its healthcare provision will depend on a number of variables and in particular the wider social, political and economic context of the country. Furthermore, it is also important to recognize that countries may change their responses to these questions as the context changes. Health systems are dynamic and public health practitioners have a responsibility to engage with them and with developing health policies to ensure they are geared up to promote the population's health.

Further reading

Gerein N., Green A., Mirzoev T., Pearson S. (2009) in Ehiri J.E., Meremikwu, M. (eds) Health System Impacts on Maternal and Child Health *International Maternal and Child Health* Springer.

Green A. (2007) *An Introduction to Health Planning for Developing Health Systems* 3rd edition OUP: Oxford.

OECD (2005) *Paris Declaration on Aid Effectiveness, ownership, harmonisation, alignment, results and mutual* Available from http://www.oecd.org/dataoecd/11/41/34428351.pdf Accessed 17 June 2008.

Varvasovsky Z., Bruigha R. (2000) How to do (or not to do) a stakeholder analysis *health Policy and Planning*, **15(3)**, 338–45.

Walt G., Gilson L. (1994) Reforming the health sector in developing countries: the central role of policy analysis *Health Policy and Planning*, **9(4)**, 353–70.

WHO (2000) The World Health Report 2000 Health systems: improving performance WHO, Geneva http://www.who.int/whr/2000/en/index.html

WHO (2001) *Report of the Commission on Macroeconomics and Health: Macroeconomics and Health: investing in health for economic development*, WHO, Geneva http://whqlibdoc.who.int/publications/2001/924154550X.pdf

WHO (2005) World Health Statistics 2005 WHO Geneva http://www.who.int/whosis/whostat2005/en/

WHO (2006) The World Health Report – working together for health WHO, Geneva http://www.who.int/whr/2006/en/

World Bank (1993) *World Development Report: Investing in Health* OUP._ New York WHO (2008) Commission on Social Determinants of Health-final report. http://www.who.int/social_determinants/thecommission/finalreport/en/index.html

Chapter 10

Developing a district health care service

John Walley and Sarah Escott

This chapter gives an overview of the following topics:

- Where we are and where we want to be.
- What is a district health system?
- What strategies can be used to improve the district health service?
- What managerial support systems can be used to improve the district health system?
- What shared organizational values should be promoted within the district?

Where we are and where we want to be

Everyone who has studied and worked in the health system in their own country will be used to their own system. Unless one has experience of working in another country you may not be familiar with alternative ways in which health services could be organized. Although we may feel that the health service is running satisfactorily, there is always room for improvement – changing to a better system of organizing the health service.

Some people have been trained as clinicians working in hospitals and may therefore not have much understanding of the work that goes on in health centres, health posts, and the community. They may look from the perspective of the health worker rather than that of the patient. It can be very frustrating when patients present very late in the course of a disease, but we must consider the difficulties patients have in getting the care they need or in gaining access to the service. We may be totally unaware of those people who never actually consult the health service.

In this chapter we will consider the benefits of a well-functioning district health system. There are good referral linkages between community-based services, health centres, and hospitals. Fewer patients bypass the health centres by going direct to hospital because people have confidence in the health centre and know that when necessary they will be referred to the hospital. When patients are referred to hospital the necessary specialist service is provided. Hospitals also support the work of the health centres with training and supervision. Health centres support the work of the community health workers, who in turn support family members to care for sick people. Preventive interventions, such as nutrition and HIV education is given in the health facilities and the community.

So how do you get from where you are to a functioning district health system? It is best to apply the general approach of health needs assessment, selecting the best interventions, and planning and implementing better services as covered in the earlier chapters. In this chapter we discuss the specific strategies and management systems for a better district health system.

What is a district health system?

The term 'district' refers to the most peripheral unit of local government and administration that has comprehensive powers and responsibilities. It is the level at which the staff of government district offices (for example for health, agriculture, water, education) come into regular day to day contact with representatives of the community. Hence it is a level where 'top-down' government policies meet 'bottom-up' local initiatives. The district is often the level where plans and budgets are prepared and implemented. Health is influenced by water, agriculture, and education etc. departments, and the wider district health system includes coordinating with these other departments.

Typically a health district is a defined geographical area with a population of between 100 000 and 300 000 people, and may spread over 5000–50 000 square kilometres. The existing health services may depend on the population density, but also ethnic, historical and political factors. Within the area of the district, primary care is provided by several 'health centres' or 'health posts'. There is also a first-level referral hospital, often called the district hospital. As well as these physical buildings where healthcare is provided, government services may also include community programmes such as Expanded Programme of Immunization (EPI) and mother, neonatal and child health (MNCH) outreach (Chapter 11), school health services and community health worker programmes.

The district hospital is often in the main town of the district. The district health office is usually also in this town, sometimes within the hospital itself.

The district health team

A team of health workers is responsible for managing the health services in the district. This is often called either the district health team (DHT) or the district health management team (DHMT). This team typically includes the district health officer, public health officer, community nurse, environmental health officer, the hospital and district administrator, and other specialized staff such as the district pharmacist and mental health officer. It has six main areas of responsibility:

- Overall district health planning and management including specific health programmes such as EPI.
- Overall district health administration and regulation including the private sector.
- Management of the district hospital, outpatient, and referral services including quality improvement.
- Health workforce development including training and supervision.
- Maintenance of equipment and infrastructure.
- Facilitation of civil society participation.

The district health team traditionally manages only government health facilities and staff. However, a district health system includes all services, and so the DHT could also include representatives of non-government health (NGO) providers, such as mission hospitals and company clinics. In some settings the DHT may be extended to include representatives of other sectors such as education; as in Box 10.1 from Uganda.

The district health team will also be concerned about public health interventions and related health promotion activities which mainly take place outside the health facilities. These include the preventive health interventions such as vaccination (EPI) outreach as well as health education for the community e.g. through local radio. The public health interventions are summarized in Chapter 2 and health promotion in Chapter 8. This chapter will concentrate on the district health services provided by the district hospital, health centre, and community-level.

Box 10.1 District health teams – Uganda

In Uganda the district health teams are made up of full-time public servants (district health officer, public health officer, environmental health officer, and hospital administrator). They are responsible for the overall planning and coordination of all the district health services. However, quarterly and annual reviews also occur in which a wider, multi-sectoral view is taken. These are undertaken by the 'extended DHT' which includes the heads of non-governmental organizations and representatives of other key sectors such as the department of agriculture, water services, etc.

Many people influence the health of a population. Different people are concerned with health at different levels. Figure 10.1 shows the health care pyramid, with most care and prevention of disease happening at the family and community level, less at the primary level and least occurring at the secondary and tertiary levels. Despite the importance of the community and primary levels, they typically get the fewest resources, while district hospitals get more. Moreover, too high a proportion of resources are consumed at the central (tertiary level) hospitals.

Different countries often have different names for the various facilities that provide healthcare at different levels. Sometimes the same word is used to mean different things in different countries. For this reason each level will now be considered, and the term written in bold will be used to refer to such a facility in the rest of this chapter.

Community care – the community, family, and patient

It is sometimes easy to forget that the community and families are an essential part of health care for a district. By 'community' we are actually referring to both individuals in the general population and several different subgroups of people. Examples of such groups include:

1 Religious groups – religious beliefs often influence ideas about health and the causes of disease.

2 Traditional leaders – cultural practices and the organization of society may influence whether or not people accept the explanation of their illness and hence the recommended treatment.

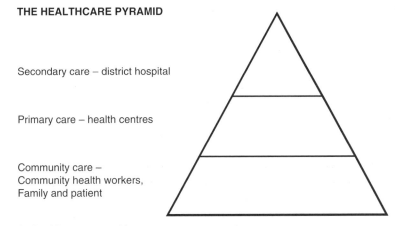

Fig. 10.1 The health care pyramid.

3 Traditional healers – many societies have well-established systems of healers whose work is often based on a different model of health belief than the one followed by the district health system. Advice from different healers may be in conflict with advice from the hospital or clinics.

4 Local government – the politics and local government of an area can influence health in many ways. The policies of local departments of welfare, water, and agriculture can all have a profound influence on the population's health. Also, local church, women's and youth groups can contribute to health promotion activity.

5 Other providers of health care – for example, private practitioners who often do not follow nationally agreed programmes and management policies.

Successful DHTs are often those who work closely with communities and encourage their participation in planning and implementation. This may take the form of consulting specific groups, open community meetings, or an institutionalized approach with district and facility boards of community representatives. It may include interventions such as education campaigns and adaptation of proposed health policies to ensure implementation is acceptable and effective. In Chapter 3 we discussed how to assess health needs using various methods of community appraisal. In Chapter 5 we discussed how to take into account the felt needs of the community and social-cultural issues when choosing the best interventions and delivery strategy.

People compare the first symptoms of an illness with their own and others' previous experience of illness which determines their explanation and health-seeking behaviour. Most people take advice from within the family before seeking help from a health care worker. Depending on relatives' knowledge and experience this advice may be beneficial, neutral, or detrimental to the sick person. Education of patients and their families by the health services therefore affects not only patients but also influences the disease episodes of others in the future.

The family is important in providing care for a sick person. We are all used to family members, often the mother, being involved in the care of children. They will consult the health worker with the child, give the medicines, and decide if the child is continuing to improve or needs to return to the health facility. This is because the child may be too young or too sick to make his or her own decisions. The same may often be true for adult patients who are too sick to care for themselves or who need help in maintaining motivation to continue treatment of chronic diseases.

Community health workers

Community Health Workers (CHWs) have great potential to promote health in the community. Other names for community health workers include village health workers and community-based volunteers. In general, CHWs are local men or women who have been selected by the community. They are trained to provide information to individuals and groups (see Fig. 10.2) about:

♦ Prevention of illness and promotion of health

♦ The causes of common diseases

♦ The signs and symptoms of diseases

♦ The action that should be taken in cases of illness

CHWs are commonly trained to assess common symptoms such as fever and treat for malaria and, if rapid breathing, treat for pneumonia. They refer more severe cases and those with chronic problems such as cough for TB screening by sputum microscopy. They provide oral rehydration solution for children with diarrhoea and provide condoms, contraceptive pills, and promote other products protecting health such as bednets. In some cases (e.g. BRAC Bangladesh) CHW's sell these products and keep e.g. a 10% margin as their pay.

With additional training some CHWs are now involved with the continuing care of patients with certain illnesses. Examples of this include being a treatment supporter of tuberculosis patients and supporting the family carers of people with AIDS and other long-term diseases. CHW schemes are often government funded; some are established by non-governmental organizations such as BRAC.

Good quality CHW programmes are running in countries such as Iran, Pakistan, and Swaziland. In these countries, CHWs are paid by the government. CHW programmes have been very successful. Other programmes such as in Uganda, have failed, especially where CHWs were unpaid volunteers and so there have been problems with high dropout rate. Analysis of several CHW type programmes has shown that programmes are most successful if:

- The CHWs have clearly defined roles.
- The CHWs are identified and chosen by the community and maintain strong community links.
- The CHWs are paid.
- There is a clear connection with the formal health services.
- There is ongoing support including supervision and training for the CHWs from the health service. This factor seems to be the most crucial of all (see Box 10.2).

Primary care – the health centres

Other names for **health centres** include health posts, clinics, treatment centres, and basic health units.

These facilities are mainly concerned with walking outpatients who come for a variety of curative and preventive health services. They should provide basic maternity and emergency services and may have some observation beds. Health centre staff should include well-trained professionals,

---

Box 10.2 The farm health worker scheme, Zimbabwe

In the mid 1980s labourers on the large commercial farms and their families were very poor and were among the least healthy groups in Zimbabwe. They often lacked access to health centres. To improve their health the farm health worker scheme was started by the provincial medical officer of health, the local government, and the support of the Save the Children Fund (UK).

Farm health workers (FHWs) were local women chosen by the community and responsible to the village committee. They were trained for 1 month and then received follow-up training for 1 day per month thereafter. They were supplied with basic drugs (such as paracetamol, an antibiotic, an anti-malarial and anti-scabies drugs) and were able to treat minor injuries. They also acted as preschool teachers. A mobile outreach mother and child health team visited each farm monthly. The nurse in charge of the programme was the main trainer as well as the supervisor of FHWs during outreach visits. With the participation of workers and funds from the commercial farmers, toilets were built and water supplies were improved. In addition, over the years a much broader range of development activities was added. The FHW programme had provided a foundation for inter-sectoral collaboration through extension workers of other ministries and non governmental organizations. As a result vegetable gardens, adult literacy classes, women's clubs, and farm development committees have been started on many farms. The scheme was replicated throughout the country. The FHW scheme has shown that a community health worker programme can be sustainable – in this case it was still providing good health services 17 years after it started (now sadly no longer, due to the general political and economic collapse of the country).

because it is the first contact of a sick person with the health care system. They assess the patient by history and examination, diagnose the problem, and if possible manage the case at the health centre. This includes conditions such as malaria, pneumonia, diarrhoea, and preventive services such as vaccination and family planning, and the provision of pre-natal, intranatal/delivery, and post-natal care. A well-equipped health centre should have a small laboratory for on-site investigations such as urinalysis and microscopy of malaria slides and TB sputum smears. Unfortunately, many health centres lack such facilities.

Health facility construction and staffing has not kept pace with the population growth, especially in the peri-urban slums. Most people get drugs directly from drug shops. Others visit private practitioners, formal or informal. These are often unregulated, not linked to the health system and quality of care is often poor. In some countries such as Thailand, private practitioners are linked to a hospital. These 'health maintenance organizations' provide care for people registered with the organization. In this way people get the benefits from primary care as appropriate and referral as needed by the hospital.

It is important that health centres treat common acute and chronic diseases and also provide personal preventive interventions such as vaccination. The integration of services, such as the integrated management of childhood illnesses (IMCI), is covered in Chapter 11. If the staff at a health centre are unable to manage a patient they refer the patient on to the next level of care – the district hospital. This can either be routinely, urgently, as in the case of major trauma or severe illness. In Asia and Latin America, health centres have doctors and paramedical staff. In Africa, commonly, health centres are staffed by clinical officers or nurse practitioners. Where there is no doctor, visits by the district supervisory team should be made monthly or at least regularly to support the health centre staff. The visiting doctors can see non-urgent referrals and patients with chronic diseases, in case there is a specific problem, at the clinic.

The exact nature and size of a health centre may vary both between countries and within a district itself, and this may affect the exact range of services available. Box 10.3 describes a typical health centre. In areas with poor access to static facilities, outreach MNCH services such as ante- and post-natal care, immunization, and family planning can be provided. They can also provide follow up care for chronic diseases. At outreach visits, the management of acute cases can be provided if the illness coincides with the mobile team's schedule.

Box 10.3 A typical health centre

- Total population served: 10 000
- Children under 1 year (2.5–3% of the population): 250–300
- Women aged 15–49 (20% of the population): 2000
- Children aged less than 15 years (40–50% of the population): 4–5000

Package of services provided:

- Maternal services: Ante-natal, delivery and post-natal care, breast-feeding advice.
- Family planning information and contraceptives.
- Child health services (integrated management of childhood illness) including acute illness care, growth monitoring, vaccination, and micronutrient supplements.
- Adult care for malaria, diarrhoea (integrated management of adolescent/adult illness), including for sexually transmitted infections, tuberculosis, and HIV/AIDS.

Primary care has been defined, described, and studied extensively in well-resourced countries such as the UK and Canada, where doctors specialize in general practice (in the USA and Canada called family medicine). In these developed countries general practice cares for most acute and chronic health conditions that people have. General practitioners may refer patients requiring specialist knowledge or tests to hospitals. The specialist then sends a letter to the general practitioner summarizing the investigations, diagnosis, and proposed treatment. Follow-up care remains the responsibility of the health centre. This is in contrast to the more limited role of primary-care in many low-middle income (LMIC) countries, where primary care is often seen as low tech care for the rural poor. However, according to WHO (2008) primary care should:

- Cover a wide range of health problems – not a few 'priority diseases';

- Be the place from which patients are guided through the health system – not a stand-alone health post or isolated community health worker;

- Be a long-term relationship between patients and clinicians, within which patients participate in decision-making about their health and health care; it builds bridges between personal health care and patients' families and communities – not a one-way delivery channel for certain health interventions;

- Open opportunities for disease prevention and health promotion as well as early detection of disease – not just be about treating common ailments;

- Be a team of health professionals: Doctors, nurse practitioners, and assistants with specific and sophisticated medical and social skills – not being synonymous with low-tech, non-professional care for the rural poor;

- Ensure that primary care requires adequate resources and investment, and can then provide much better value for money than people by-passing and going to hospitals – it is not acceptable that people have to pay for primary care out-of-pocket.

Secondary care – the district hospital

Other names for the district hospital include first-referral hospital and secondary care.

These facilities are concerned with dealing with more difficult cases and with the diagnosis of more complicated medical conditions. Box 10.4 describes a typical district and district hospital. District hospitals should deal with patients who are referred by the health centres and ideally should not provide the same services as the health centres. It would be better if they did not provide primary health-care services, but rather they should support the health centres in providing these services (as explained later in this chapter). Acute medical and surgical emergencies are managed here and the hospital will also provide emergency obstetric care, including blood transfusion and caesarean section facilities. They have the facilities for x-ray and comprehensive laboratory investigations.

In hospital, patients will be assessed and diagnosed and their treatment started by the doctor and other health workers. Sometimes, this will involve admitting the patient for investigation, at other times the tests can be done on an out patient basis. In districts with poor transport infrastructure, waiting shelters for pregnant women before their delivery may be provided at the hospital. Very sick patients will need admission for treatment and nursing until they are well enough to be able to walk and fit enough to be discharged. However, many patients who are admitted could have been managed as out-patients. Admission of TB suspects to a general ward may lead to (nosocomial) transmission of TB to others, especially those who are HIV positive. Unnecessary admission is expensive, uses up scarce resources and overloads beds. What is more, most patients prefer to be treated at home.

Box 10.4 A typical district and district hospital

Population served:

- All ages, referral support for around 15 health centres: 150 000
- Children under 1 year (3%of the population): 4500
- Children aged less than 15 years (40–50%of the population): 60–75 000
- Women aged 15–49 (20% of the population): 30 000 Referral and emergency care: Obstetrics and gynaecology
- Paediatrics
- Medicine/infectious disease
- Surgery (limited).

If illness is to be well managed on an outpatient basis the hospital staff must carefully explain to the patient and visiting relatives about the illness and the treatment. Once the diagnosis is made and the patient started on regular treatment they can usually be referred back for follow-up care at the health centre. In this way the health centre staff can provide continuity of care over time. Health centre staff are likely to know their patients, better understand their problems and (if trained and supervised), they will be better able to monitor care. If there is a relapse of the illness then the patient can be referred back to the hospital for further assessment and revision of treatment. Unfortunately, there is often little communication between hospital and health centre staff, such that the referral system doesn't work well. This is bad for patients and is an inefficient use of health services.

The designated district hospital can be a missionary, non-government, or private hospital. This may be especially so in rural districts where the next government hospital is far away. In other places there can be competition between the government facility and faith based and other non-government hospitals.

It may be decided that the referral system and other components of the district health system need to be improved. How to do this will be addressed in the next section.

Developing and improving district health systems

For a district health system to work most effectively, various strategies need to be adopted. These include:

- Defining the roles of health facilities;
- Integration of health care;
- Building and strengthening a referral system;
- Decentralization of management;
- Participation of civil society.

Defining the roles of health facilities

For a district health service to work there must be clearly defined roles for the different levels of health facilities. Confusion often exists over the roles of the health centre and district hospital in the area of primary care, as is illustrated for the case of Hlabisa, South Africa, in Box 10.5. Health centres are the best places for common illnesses and preventive services such as vaccination.

Box 10.5 The consequences of overlapping primary and secondary care roles

Hlabisa hospital is a district hospital in a rural area of South Africa. Primary health care (PHC) services are provided by 12 peripheral clinics and two mobile/outreach teams. The district covers a population of 220 000 people.

For several years the hospital had received complaints about the outpatient department. These complaints centred on the fact that the outpatient department was often very crowded and people waited many hours to be seen by the doctor. Public transport stopped at dusk and people who had been seen late in the day, or who were awaiting results, often had to sleepover on the floor of the outpatient department. There was no bedding and insufficient sanitation for this.

In theory, the outpatient department was supposed to provide facilities for:

1 Emergency cases (who had direct access to the hospital).

2 Referral cases from other practitioners (i.e. general practitioners, peripheral health centre staff).

3 Hospital follow-up for specific difficult cases – usually those requiring follow-up investigations not available at health centres.

A simple study was done to look into the problem in more detail. The outpatient register was reviewed and it was discovered that 60% of patients attending outpatients were doing so because the hospital was in fact the nearest health facility to their home, i.e. there was no primary health centre in the Hlabisa town and local area. Although in the hospital OPD such patients were seen initially by a nurse, many were still referred on to the doctor for a 'second opinion'. This was partly due to the fact that many of nurses had not yet completed their primary care certificate and were not confident about their abilities to work independently. In addition patients with chronic diseases who lived locally were often sent to see the doctor at each visit, rather than being managed by the nurse according to the agreed nurse protocols and only seeing the doctor as necessary.

The study focused attention on the different roles of the hospital and health centres. Discussions were held to try and establish criteria for which outpatients needed to see the doctor. There was acknowledgement that patients attending hospital often felt entitled to see the doctor and put pressure on the nurse. This aspect could be difficult to manage. Short-, medium-, and long-term solutions were suggested are implemented:

1 Short-term: Reorganizing and strengthening existing services by training of hospital outpatient department nurses in the use of basic protocols – that gave clear criteria for nurses to manage common, acute and chronic complaints.

2 Medium-term: Arranging for more nurses to be trained as nurse practitioners (and ensuring that they are not all reallocated to other duties)

3 Long-term: Building a health centre for the people of Hlabisa town area, geographically separate from the hospital. This would act in the same way as all other primary health centres; including the fact that its services would be free to patients (a fee is charged for hospital services). All patients would get primary care from their health centre, and can only access hospital if referred. While direct access was to be only for accident or emergency cases.

In developed countries such as Britain, people see their general practitioner or nurse practitioner at their local health centre. Most illnesses including pneumonia can be managed by the general practitioner. Patients who are severely ill or with complex conditions are referred. For example ill, newly diagnosed diabetics are referred to hospital specialists. Only accident and emergency patients can go straight to hospital. Patients know that the quality of primary care is good and prefer to see a doctor or nurse who knows them. Health centre professionals, who know their patients, are better able to assess new symptoms and so provide care. When patients are referred to hospital specialists, they are properly assessed and initiated on treatments. The hospital specialist advises on how best to continue treatment in a letter sent back to the patient's general practitioner. For example, adult diabetics will be followed up and get their tablets and check ups by the nurse practitioner and doctor at the health centre. See Fig. 10.2.

In an earlier section of this chapter we outlined the structure and activities of hospitals and health centres. We will now look in more detail at their roles in providing primary care services. It is important that health workers, managers, and administrators at all levels of the district health service understand these differing roles.

Let us consider the provision of primary care services to a district. In an integrated district health system the role of the district hospital and district health office is to support the health centres and enable them to deliver primary care services to the community. A district hospital that supports the health centres is not one that delivers primary care services itself. Such a district hospital would be acting in competition with the health centres. A district hospital that supports the health centres is one that provides the necessary technical expertise to deal with difficult cases that are referred by the health centres. Ideally, as in Britain, patients should not have direct access to the hospital as this will only serve to encourage them to bypass the health centre and overload the hospital. In addition, hospital staff should educate the general public on the roles of the different health facilities, and on where to access the services when required. They should specifically promote a positive image of the health centres.

At present there are many reasons why patients bypass the health centre:

1 Unequal distribution of health centres means that for some areas there is no health centre available. This is a particular problem if there is no separate health centre in the area of the hospital itself (as in the example, Box 10.5).

2 Lack of qualified and experienced staff and adequate equipment and supplies at the health centre.

3 The 'glamour' of the high-tech image of the hospital leads to the belief that services are better than those provided at the clinic. This is a particular problem if different management policies are used. For example if a patient being followed up for tuberculosis receives a chest X-ray at the hospital but a patient at a clinic is followed up with a sputum test alone; patients will consider the clinic to be an inferior service (when in fact an X-ray is usually unnecessary in sputum positive TB cases).

4 The perception that a patient will always be seen by a more qualified person if seen at the hospital.

5 There may be no difference in cost to the patient.

Unwanted effects of patients bypassing the health centres include:

1 Undermining of the service provided by the clinic and the morale of the staff.

2 Higher 'invisible' costs to the patient – in the form of transport and travel time.

3 Higher costs to the health service – the wider range of drugs (and tests) available often results in over-prescribing at the hospital when a condition is treated just as well by simple clinic medicines.

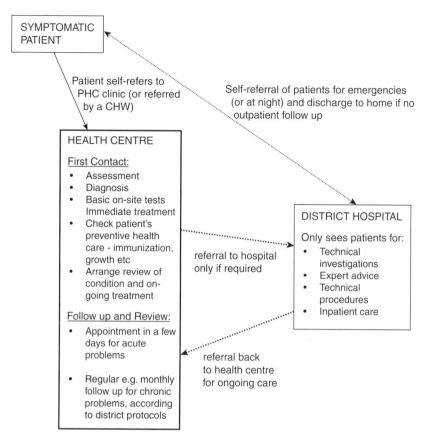

Fig. 10.2 Roles of health centres and district hospitals.

4 Over-loading of the hospital with doctors seeing a lot of non-referred patients (better dealt with at the health centre) and then having little time left for the more serious cases.

5 Unnecessary exposure of patients to hospital-acquired infections, for example the exposure of HIV positive patients to tuberculosis when in hospital.

Once the different roles of the hospital and health centres have been considered, it is worth reviewing measures that can be used to strengthen these roles:

♦ Improving the quality of care, including the use of guidelines such as the WHO Integrated Management of Childhood Illness (IMCI) and the Integrated Management of Adolescent-adult Illness (IMAI).

♦ Training and supervising of staff at health centres and outpatient departments.

♦ Improving the availability of drugs and supplies at health centres – patients will not trust the health centres if they are forever running out of drugs.

♦ Nurse practitioners and clinical officers see non-referred patients in outpatient departments of hospitals and refer to doctors as necessary, i.e. as in health centres.

♦ Introducing differential user fees in different facilities – for example a non-urgent hospital attendance would cost more than a health centre consultation.

The above actions are just some of the many things that can be done to improve the quality of care in health facilities.

The roles of health centres and district hospital are illustrated in Fig. 10.2. The integration of care is also a way of improving the quality and so outcomes of care.

Integration of health care

Integration of health care can be considered in different ways, all of which interact with one another. The different aspects of integration are outlined below.

1 Integration of government and non-government health care providers. Health care within an area is often provided by facilities run by different organizations that may not be under the direct managerial control of regional or provincial government department of health. This does not prevent such providers from working together where their services overlap. Integrated planning of these services will help prevent duplication of health care provision in some areas and allow resources to be directed to areas of need. Integrated planning should cover both the area of work and the content of the service provided to ensure common policies and health education messages.

2 Integration across time. This refers to the **continuity** of care an individual patient will receive over a period of time. In others words the patient is seen at the same health centre (preferably by the same health workers) for as long as health care intervention is needed to provide a beneficial impact on health. For example, an infant will have several contacts with health services from time of birth for immunization, growth monitoring, and treatment of childhood illnesses. Continuity of care would mean that all these events would take place at the same clinic, with the same health workers (see Chapter 11 on maternal, neonatal and child health).

3 Integration of curative, preventive, and promotive services as **comprehensive** care. Traditionally, curative services have been regarded as separate from issues of preventive and promotive health care. Clinical care and preventive care may be the responsibilities of different health workers, or the various services may all be provided on different days. Integration means, for example, that if a mother brings a sick child for care, immunization is checked and provided if needed. She is also offered pre-natal contraceptive or family planning services and education about nutrition, rather than being told to come back another day. The WHO integrated management of childhood illness (IMCI) is an example of such integration.

4 Integrated acute and chronic care. Until recently, in many countries, health centres have done little chronic care. Now routine fellowship care is done at the health centres and increasingly other chronic diseases such as epilepsy, mental health, diabetes, and HIV antiretroviral treatment care can be done at the health centre. Integrated case management means that the person is considered as a whole – the immediate problem and the ongoing chronic situations are considered. For example when treating an adult for a chest infection the health worker looks at the case record, sees that he is hypertensive and checks the blood pressure. Or, when treating a patient with recurrent diarrhoea, the health worker considers the socio-economic situation and may recommend an HIV test.

The integrated care of chronic disease patients within a district health service is illustrated in Fig. 10.3 and the way in which chronic care and support for tuberculosis and other HIV/AIDS related diseases is illustrated with a case study from South Africa in Box 10.6.

Strengthening quality of care and the referral system

Ideally patients will be managed within the district health system using an integrated model of care. For this to operate it is crucial that a good system of referral exists between the different health care providers. There must be:

◆ Case management guidelines

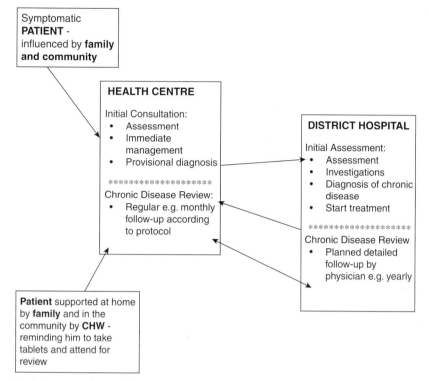

Fig. 10.3 The integrated care of patients with chronic disease.

- Clearly defined circumstances that need referral
- A reliable way of passing information about patients between different health care workers in different facilities.

These first two points can be best addressed by establishing **protocols** for the management of different clinical cases. Another name for a protocol is a **case management guideline** (see also Chapter 16). A protocol is a concise description of the steps in the assessment; classification, treatment and follow-up of care, as in the integrated management of adolescent/adult illness (IMAI) guidelines and IMCI (see Chapter 11). Some protocols are presented as flow charts, as with the WHO sexually transmitted disease (STD) guidelines. Summaries of these guides can be put on the desk or wall of the consultation room. Guidelines are adapted in country with input from experienced district and national health workers. They need to be regularly updated to summarize the actual evidence for different settings. The guidelines can help identify training needs if a deficit in knowledge or skills is identified. Such management guidelines may be adapted from WHO international guidelines, for example IMCI, tuberculosis, and STDs. They may be locally prepared guidelines, for example the case management hypertension.

Such protocols must be simple and easy to use, kept in consultation rooms and used by health care workers of all levels. It can be difficult to persuade clinicians in developing country facilities to use such protocols as they are not used to using them and may be perceived to conflict with their autonomous decision-making role of doctors. Such clinicians may need education and support in the use of protocols. Health professionals need to understand guidelines as the best available evidence and a means to ensure the quality of care. Guidelines should specify signs and symptoms when a patient requires urgent referral as 'severe' or need to be referred for tests

Box 10.6 Integrated health care (for TB-HIV)

Nthombi is a 28-year-old woman. She goes to the health centre with a persistent cough and fever that she has had for 5 weeks. She is a single mother and brings her 9-month-old child with her. The health worker at the health centre uses the IMAI case management guidelines, 'Integrated management of adolescent/adult illness (IMAI) care' cough page and realizes that Nthombi may have tuberculosis. She tells Nthombi to go the hospital for sputum tests the next day. Before the family leaves the health worker also takes the chance to check the immunization and growth of the child. He is growing well but has missed his measles vaccine. She gives this to him.

Nthombi goes to the hospital and is diagnosed with sputum-positive tuberculosis. She receives health education about tuberculosis and its association with HIV. She is counselled and accepts to have an HIV test, she is HIV positive.

- she is counselled on using a condom
- seeking advice early in the event of illness
- taking the antibiotic cotrimoxazole to prevent many infectious diseases related to HIV

In order to treat her tuberculosis Nthombi is started on a community-based TB treatment. It is arranged that her community health worker will supervise her tuberculosis treatment. Every month Nthombi visits the health centre for a check up. At 2 months she is reviewed by the hospital doctor and her TB has improved, but she needs treatment for chronic diarrhoea. After 6 months the doctor says she is cured of tuberculosis. She is reviewed every 3 months for ART.

Nthombi brings her husband along and and he is found to be positive. He also starts on treatment. Over the coming months Nthombi tells the rest of her family about her diagnosis and asks for their support. By then she is well and remains well. She is introduced to other people with HIV/AIDS in her area and through this contact is able to join an income generation project. She also becomes a peer counsellor explaining to others the benefit of having an HIV test, behaviour change, and use of condoms.

e.g. for TB. Developed country doctors and nurses are used to referring to evidence based guidelines. Good examples are the BNF (British National Formulary) for medicine treatment and the UK NICE (National Institute for Health and Clinical Excellence) guidelines to promote health and prevent and treat ill health according to the best available evidence.

The sharing of relevant information can be addressed in a variety of ways. The best solution depends on the local situation and on what system of record keeping is currently used. For example, in many places patients have a 'patient-held health card'. This is kept by the patient at home and is brought to the health worker whenever the patient accesses care. All relevant information is recorded on this card. Workers at different health facilities can read each other's notes and hence information is shared. This system has the advantage of involving patients in their healthcare by giving them responsibility for record keeping. Disadvantages include the problems that arise when patients lose their cards, or bring them intermittently. Incomplete records will result if some health workers fail to complete and return the card. As well as a patient held card there are health facility record cards and registers. When a patient is referred between facilities information should be sent between facilities, either as hand-delivered letters, letters delivered by the postal system, by telephone or by email, if available. Problems can arise, however, if referral and discharge letters and messages fail to arrive, leading to a breakdown in the integrated management of patients. Thus it is important that the system of record keeping and sharing of information is chosen to suit the local situation. Whichever kinds of records used, it is important to make sure the communication between health facilities works well. The records kept at the health facility can be used for record review to assess the quality of care. Refer Chapter 6, Table 6.1 (case audit). It is important that all management systems work well and so support quality care. These support systems are crucial to the functioning of a district health system and will be considered in the next section.

District health management

A district health system will function best if there is some degree of decentralization of management from the higher levels of the health system. Decentralization involves giving the district the power it needs to make decisions affecting the service it offers. This enables the DHT to plan, budget, and organize care for the population under their control. It allows for local prioritization of needs and local adaptation of policy to address those needs. The district should work within national policies, while implementing the policies in accordance with the local situation. Policies should be explicit about the mandatory national framework such as the immunization schedule of the National EPI (Expanded Programme of Immunization) policy or the essential medicines list of the national medicines policy. Policies should also be flexible and provide a decision-making space for district managers to achieve the planned targets such as high vaccination coverage for EPI. This may be achieved through partnerships with the private sector, inter-sectoral collaboration, or specific incentives for peripheral health workers.

In the past many disease control programmes were set up in a 'vertical' structure. They were (and some still are) vertical in that the decisions and money flowed vertically down from the national to the provincial to the district and to the local workers employed by the programme. Vertical programmes are often not very well coordinated with other programmes and the general health service. This leads to poor integration and a narrow focus on targets of one specific programme. Many countries have successfully integrated these programmes within district health services. With integration the person responsible for the programme in the district is managed by the District Health Officer and is part of the DHT. This helps in the coordination of, for example, supervision, transport, and supplies. However, responsibility for the technical policies and guidelines remains with the national programmes.

The decentralization to the district of decision-making about the budgets and operations of programmes and basic services enables the integration of activities. For example, each DHT member can learn to observe and discuss the objectives of a wider set of services, not just the one programme they are responsible for such as EPI, but for the wider services e.g. Maternal, Neonatal and Child Health (MNCH).

The principles of decentralization can also be applied to the financial management of a district. The DHMT would be responsible for specified areas of the budget that they could use without clearance from the province or ministry of health. This enables local needs to be addressed. An example is shown in Box 10.7.

Civil society participation

Active and well-informed citizens are an essential factor to improve health services and achieve the common good of 'health for all'. Community participation is one of the principles of the primary health care concept, and has been described as the institutionalized participation of civil

Box 10.7 Decentralization of limited budget to the district

An example of decentralization of part of the budget occurred in an African country with high HIV seroprevalence. Previously the budget for HIV education was managed by the region. Plans for a health education event had to be approved by the regional office and educational materials and other goods purchased by them. This created long delays – such that sometimes material arrived after the event. After decentralization of this part of the budget, the coordinating team was able to purchase health promotion and teaching materials locally. In this way they were able to support their local economy and local income generation projects. They employed a local craft cooperative to make wooden condom demonstrators and print health education T-shirts. They employed local women to prepare and serve refreshments at educational events. Where more technical material was needed, for example leaflets and posters, these were still purchased via the regional office, ensuring discounts for bulk orders.

society in policy development, implementation, and accountability mechanisms. Community boards at district and facility levels may assist with the management of programmes and facilities assure transparency and mediate in the case of conflict with communities.

However, such participation may also give rise to several conflicts. Board members may not represent the interests of all groups in the community; especially women, young people, and ethnic minorities are often underrepresented. Political parties and influential groups may try to influence the decision-making process in their favour. Elected or appointed board members may also require training so that they are able to fulfil their role effectively.

Functioning boards can monitor the provision and quality of services and prevent mismanagement and corruption. At a national level civil society may even influence policy decisions. The South African organization 'Treatment Action Campaign' is a good example how active citizens can use the constitutional law of a country and change a government policy, so as to make widely available anti-retroviral medicine nevirapine for the prevention of mother-to-child transmission of HIV infection to some pilot sites. It ordered the state to ensure that the use of nevirapine be made progressively available throughout the public health system.

The Tanzania Essential Health Interventions Project (TEHIP) has demonstrated how to match health expenditure to the packages of care which cover the main burden of disease. That is, strengthening health care by reallocating funds to cost-effective interventions that address the greatest contributors to the burden of disease. The TEHIP website www.idrc.ca/tehip, includes various practical tools and resources.

Management support systems needed by a district health service

In order for a district health service as a whole to be effective and efficient, various support functions need to be in place and running. These support systems include the:

- Information system
- Transport and maintenance
- Logistics and supplies
- Training and supervision
- Finance.

These support functions (see also Chapter 7) are important for the implementation of the various health services and programmes. For example, strengthening the transport system – which may include integrated planning of the schedule for outreach visits, maintenance of vehicles and introduction of logbooks – will be helpful for all programmes. Outreach visits for vaccination in villages far from health centres were originally only for EPI, but other MNCH, family planning, and health education activities may be added. The environmental health assistant can use the scheduled outreach trips as a way of getting to the villages to work on water and sanitation activities, or to follow up with defaulters for tuberculosis treatment.

The district nurse responsible for mother and child health can use the schedule to supervise child health (e.g. including IMCI, EPI and nutrition) maternal and activities in the health centre. If strengthening of the transport systems includes the hospital ambulances then acute referrals will be strengthened. Thus all technical functions in the clinical and preventative programme can be affected by improvements to transport. Table 10.1 shows a matrix for the relationship between general support functions and technical functions. In a district health system the strengthening of support functions will improve all the health services/programmes. As shown with the example of transport, in Table 10.1, but equally well the example could have been health information, showing how improvements in the health information system would benefit all the programmes.

DHTs need to ensure that all initiatives to improve technical functions such as EPI or HIV are designed in ways that help strengthen the district health system in general. For example, ensuring that per diems for training or outreach are paid according to the same procedures as for everything else. This is in contrast to 'vertical' programmes which were set up with their own different procedures and administrative systems. Having many different systems, for example different finance and accounting procedures, is likely to be confusing, time-consuming, and inefficient. On the other hand, if the procedures are integrated, then investments in a particular programme will help to strengthen general support functions, to the benefit of all programmes. In summary, efforts made to strengthen a particular programme should be done in ways that strengthen the general functions and hence the district health system in general. In this way time and effort spent strengthening the support functions will benefit all the programmes.

Similarly, health system strengthening, to improve general management (support functions, such as human workforce or medicines) should take into account the technical needs of each service or programme see Box 10.8, for example the pharmacist orders the appropriate drugs regimen according to the TB Programme policy. Similarly the transport system includes the needs of transporting TB sputum samples to the district hospital laboratory and the results back to the health centre. Also, coordinating supervisory visits of district officers to ensure regular supervision of MNCH, TB, HIV, malaria, mental health, and other services provided at health centres and in the community.

In-service training and supervision are commonly major components of public health programme activity. These activities are an opportunity to improve the quality of services and the functioning of the referral system, and are discussed in more detail below.

In-service training and supportive supervision

Training and supervision are important aspects of any health care system. No one can depend only on what they learnt during their basic training. Everyone needs to be learning throughout their professional life (see Chapter 6 'Plan, managing and implementing interventions' and Chapter 16, 'Quality and safety'). Training must be built into the district health system, and is especially important for those working in health facilities geographically distant from the main centres. Health workers need to feel that they have enough skills to perform the tasks required of them, and to know that they have the opportunity for further training if required.

Table 10.1 Technical and general support function in a direct health system (including community, health centre, hospital levels). Example Transport and supervision strengthening, and support to the various programmes/services

Management support function	Technical function/programmes						
	General Medical/ adult care	Child Health, Nutrition EPI	Maternity/family planning	Water sanitation and Hygiene	Communicable diseases, malaria, TB, STI, HIV/ART	Non communicable/ chronic care, Diabetes, Epilepsy, mental health	Surgical, A & E TL, vascetomy
Transport Supervision	Ambulance, Supervision of health centre care	Outreach	Emergency obstetric via ambulance	Water pump maintenance, Sanitation promotion	Health/bednet promotion. TB, HIV samples	Review clinics in health centre	Ambulance
Training							
Health information							
Logistics, Supplies							
Finance							
Other: personnel, health promotion							

Supportive supervision means noticing when a worker has done a good job – to encourage them – and also helping the worker to identify areas where knowledge or performance can be improved.

Training can be done in a variety of ways, depending on the aims of the training:

1 Programme implementation training. If the aim is to train a group of workers with the skills needed to implement a new programme (e.g. IMCI or HIV/ART) then the best approach is probably to run a specific course. This is usually away from the workplace. However, such training should include field practice in a facility similar to those of the participants. Participants can then practise the skills they have learnt during class sessions, while being observed and supported by the trainers. This is covered in more detail in Chapter 10 (Table 10.3).

2 Addressing identified learning needs. Sometimes an individual health worker (or group of staff at a specific health facility) has learning needs which are not shared by others. The workers should feel able to request training if they identify these learning needs themselves. Alternatively a review, or audit, of health service performance may highlight areas where extra teaching is needed. They should rather be encouraged to address such needs and hence improve their performance. The best approach may be to hold a special training session at the place of work.

3 Continuing professional development. The aim is to develop a system of ongoing support and training, which are regular, planned training events. This can be incorporated into the timetable of the health facility and the agenda set by those attending. This type of system is an excellent way of strengthening the district health system. This is achieved by combining support and training with feedback of information between the different levels of the health service. This may contribute to the health service working as a team. Fig. 10.4 and Box 10.8 illustrate this.

There are advantages in combining in-service training, supervision visits, and communication about specific patients. The main one is that workers at different levels begin to experience the reality of their colleagues' work. They gain useful insight into difficulties experienced. These advantages can be realized by building up a regular system including:

◆ Regular meetings of health workers at the next level up;

◆ Regular supervision visits by doctors and district health officers.

The supervision of health centres will commonly be the responsibility of more than one person. The district health office may allocate someone to be responsible for a group of health centres.

This person, such as the community nurse, will take responsibility for supervising the various programmes, EPI (checking the fridge temperatures, vaccination procedures, etc.), nutrition monitoring and education, drug supplies, etc. She may also observe the clinical care for adults and children, such as the use of the protocol for integrated management of childhood illness and sexually transmitted infections. It must be remembered that health centre staff carry out a broad range of functions for various diseases and so the person supervising must also be trained to address all these roles. The supervisor will often be informed of problems at the health centre. For example, an irregular supply of drugs, failure of the telephone or radio communications, and conflict between staff or late payment of wages. These issues contribute greatly to the performance of the health centre and the supervisor must aim to solve these and/or report the problem back to the DHT for help.

In addition, the hospital doctors may be allocated a group of health centres to visit. The doctor will visit on a regular day each month and have three main roles on each visit. S/he should see non-urgent referrals that the health centre staff have identified (by using disease management

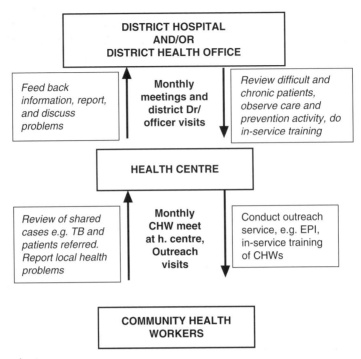

Fig 10.4 Flowchart.

protocols) as needing medical review. Then the doctor should also observe the clinical work and consultations of the health centre staff and give in-service training based on these consultations. When doctors and hospital staff carry out supervisory work they sometimes take over the treatment of the patient and the health centre staff become just spectators. Instead they should work with the health centre workers, observe practice and give advice and encourage better practice.

This method of in-service training is especially useful for training on the use of written case management protocols. Such protocols, for example the WHO STI flow charts and IMCI guidelines, can be easily referred to in the consultation room and make possible a big improvement in the quality of curative care and patient education. The protocols must be well written and user friendly. Unfortunately, the use of such protocols is unfamiliar to many health workers. They may feel uncomfortable referring to a guideline during the consultation. The patient may get the impression that the health worker doesn't know his or her job. Consequently the health worker has to be trained and encouraged to use the protocols and supervision, and in-service training is important for their effective implementation. Finally the visiting doctor can provide in-service training in the form of a tutorial tackling specific issues. However, it must be realized that technical knowledge is often not the most important issue affecting performance of the health centre. The issues mentioned above (drug supply, and other "support" functions etc.) can be much more important and also need strengthening, see Box 10.8.

Supervision and in-service training are equally important for the CHWs. These may be provided by the health centre staff holding teaching sessions at the health centre or by the CHW coordinator (see Box 10.9).

Supportive supervision means helping people to do a good job. This includes:

♦ Discussing the tasks that should be undertaken for quality care and prevention

♦ Observing and noticing when the work is done well

Box 10.8 Technical and support function strengthening, TB example

District health managers ensure that:

- The pharmacist orders the appropriate drug regimens according to the TB Programme policy.
- The transport manager includes the transport of TB sputum samples to the district hospital laboratory and the results back to the health centre.
- A District health officer is given resupervisory visits include TB, as well as other technical programmes such as MNCH, HIV, malaria, mental health.
- Community health workers are trained and supervised to provide treatment support for TB patients, as well as their MNCH, family planning, malaria, and other tasks.
- TB case finding and treatment outcomes (quarterly reports, based on the TB register) are included in the health information system.

The national/provincial TB programme managers:

- Ensure that TB guidelines and training include about testing for HIV, giving cotrimoxazole and antiretroviral treatment.
- Daily allowances given during training are according to the regular rates.
- Donor funded drugs are distributed through the general stores, district pharmacy system
- TB microscopy quality assurance strengthening is also applied to malaria microscopy, and contribute to general laboratory strengthening.
- Training on performance monitoring (assessing trends in case finding and treatment outcomes, gaps, and solution analysis) are also designed to be also applicable to other programmes.

In this way strengthening of support functions benefit all programmes, and all programmes contribute to systems strengthening.

- Discussing points which could be done better
- Agreeing on what should be done
- Observing and discussing progress on these points during the next visit.

People accept and appreciate supervision when it is supportive. That is, if the supervisor **is** checking up on the quality of the work done. However, the way the supervision is done must not be threatening, and must be helpful to the health worker being supervised. In-service training is most effective when it is based on the needs of health workers and their existing performance. The training may be a mix of off-site and on-site training. Training is most effective when linked to supportive supervision. The supervisor can help the health workers introduce their new skills acquired during training.

When planning in-service training and supervision, the following points should be remembered:

1 The District Health Authorities should stop assuming that the doctor knows everything about health.

2 The selection of a supervisor should be appropriate. It is less appropriate for a hospital-based nurse to supervise health centre nurses, better for the senior nurse of a well-functioning health centre to supervise them. The supervisor should be more experienced, with experience in the

Box 10.9 Integrated management of community health workers and health centre staff

Our district hospital is based in an area with 11 peripheral health centres which provide primary health care to the population. In addition there are two community health worker (CHW) teams that work in programmes in the two halves of the district. These CHW programmes were initially set up by different non-governmental organizations. Every month the CHWs of each programme report to their managers and receive pay. At present there are few links between the CHWs and health centres.

The DHT is strengthening community integrated management of child illness (cIMCI) interventions, including promotion of bednets and early treatment of malaria with the new national drugs regimen. The DHT wants to make sure that the child health/malaria work will help strengthen the general health system, especially communication, supervision, and in-service training.

The DHT meets including the community nurse responsible for child health, the health centre supervisors, and the managers of both CHW programmes, to discuss ways to implement this. One aspect that they discuss is the ongoing support and training of staff at all levels. They proposed and implemented the following:

1 Training of health centre staff – who then train the CHWs – on child health and malaria treatment before starting the new service.

2 Reorganizing the monthly payday meetings of the CHWs to be done at the health centres.

3 Initiation of regular monthly meetings of CHWs at the health centres. CHWs who live in the catchment area of a health centre meet together every month at the health centre and facilitated by the health centre nurse or paramedic. During the meeting, one session will be for in-service education, another for the CHWs to report back on general health issues from their area, and the third for discussion of individual cases, e.g. of malaria, that are being jointly managed by a CHW and the health centres.

4 The two CHW programme leaders will work closely to plan a common timetable of issues to be covered. Initially these sessions will be to train the CHW on child health and malaria, but later on other relevant topics such as water, sanitation, and other community-based interventions and TB, HIV, and epilepsy care.

5 Every month each health centre receives a visit by a doctor from the district hospital. During this visit the doctor sees patients who according to the management protocol need to be seen by a doctor. Then the doctor will facilitate in-service education of the health centre staff.

6 Each month a health centre in-charge attends a district meeting. This too will include a report and discussion of activities. These meetings will provide 'peer group' support for health workers from similar peripheral health centres, with frank and open discussion of problems and joint problem-solving, with the support of their supervisor, the community nurse coordinator. The meeting will include an up-date education session.

7 The community nurse coordinator already makes visits to the health centres to monitor the various programmes. She will now expand her supervisory role by observing child health consultations using IMCI during the visits, and discuss progress on issues raised at the monthly district meetings.

same setting and type of work. In some cases it may be appropriate for her to be seconded to a poorly functioning clinic for a period of time to share her knowledge and skills.

3   Supervisors should be trained in integrated support supervision and orientated in the concepts of primary health care. In the past supervision has not been supportive – often due to traditional and cultural issues. Training must address these issues. It may be helpful to separate supervision and control activities.

4   Supervisors should have comprehensive and well-designed checklists. Without these they will be unable to compare different health centres or compare performance of a health centre over time. Such checklists also help compare the findings of different supervisors.

5   Supervisors should be empowered to take actions within written guidelines and limitations. This will enable supervisors not only to provide technical teaching but to be able to solve some management issues as they carry out the supervision.

6   Supervisors need to have clear procedures for reporting problems and taking action following supervision visits.

7   Supervisors will need to address motivation. Increasing motivation by offering financial reward is not an available or feasible option. Using set criteria that measure performance, competition can be introduced between health centres to improve performance. An annual ceremony could be held for the prize giving.

Organizational values to promote in a health district

In the preceding sections of this chapter we have discussed the structures, strategies, and systems needed for the implementation of a district health system. Providing a quality service to the community depends on more than just ensuring the existence of the basic constituents of a system. A quality service also depends on the attitudes of those people who are delivering the service. If a patient receives the correct treatment but this treatment is delivered without concern for privacy, and without compassion, then the patient will not have received a quality service.

We will now consider some of the core values that contribute to improving the quality of care delivered.

A patient-centred service

When providing a health service it is easy to forget that the most important people in the service are the patients themselves. Systems should be organized to facilitate accessibility, acceptability, and privacy for patients. Failure of the provision of health care is usually due to a failure of the system rather than due to a fault of the patient. For example, if a patient with a chronic disease defaults from treatment this is most often due to reasons such as a failure of patient education on the importance of continued treatment in chronic diseases, or due to an inconsistent supply of drugs. This said, the patient does have an important role to play. The patient should be encouraged to take responsibility for his or her health, for example by adopting lifestyle changes and adhering to appointments and regular tablet taking. There should be shared decision-making between provider and patient.

Teamwork

Who is the most important member of the district health team? The CHWs? The laboratory staff? Doctors? Stores manager? Health centre health worker? Pharmacy staff?

The answer is that they are all important. The district health service must work as a team. Every person within the service acts as a link in a chain. If each component of the health service is strong – if each link is strong – then the delivery of health care to the community will be successful. If just one link is weak then the whole chain of care breaks down and the delivery of the service fails.

Responsibility

The above analogy of the health service as a chain made of separate links also illustrates the importance of the ideas of individual and collective responsibility. Individuals in the health service are responsible for the standard of service delivered by their link in the chain. Collectively, everybody is responsible for the overall functioning of the service, for helping to identify possible weak links, and for working together to strengthen these links.

Flexibility

With an underlying sense of collective responsibility comes the concept of flexibility. Chapter 7 discusses the importance of allocating health service personnel to jobs for which they are best suited. There will, however, be occasions when these allocations come under pressure, for example due to staff illness. If the other workers are rigid in sticking to their job allocation then a task will not get done and the chain is broken.

A holistic service

The whole health service should understand the four main aspects of health care, and ensure that these are carried out in an integrated manner. These are:

- Health promotion
- Disease prevention
- Curative services
- Rehabilitation services.

All are of equal importance. This fact should be recognized within the district, and there should be a distribution of resources, health worker time, and managerial attention given to all four (see also Chapter 6).

Summary

The district health system is a model for delivering an integrated and holistic service of health care to the community. The district health system needs to provide coordinated services at the community, health centre, and hospital levels. The DHT should coordinate NGO and private facilities together with the government services. The DHT and hospitals support the work of health centre staff, who then support the community health workers. The strategies and systems involved in delivering such a system need to be strengthened. Finally we have looked at the core organizational values that contribute to a high-quality district health service.

Further reading

Amonoo-Lartson, R., Ebarhim, G., Lovel, H.J., Ranken, J. (1984). *District health care – challenges for planning, organisation and evaluation in developing countries.* Macmillan, London.

Lerberghe W., Lafort Y. (1990). *The role of the hospital in the district: deliver-ing or supporting primary health care?* WHO/SHS/CC/90.2.

World Bank (1993). *Revitalizing national systems of health care.* In: Better health in Africa, ch. 4.

WHO. World Health Report (2008). http://www.who.int/whr/2008/en/

The Tanzania Essential Health Interventions Project. IDRC Canada (2008) website www.idrc.ca/tehip includes slide presentations, case studies, videos, research reports, books about TEHIP.

UNICEF (2008). *'Countdown to 2015' Maternal, neonatal and child survival: tracking progress in maternal, newborn and child survival.* http://www.childinfo.org/countdown.html

Walley, J., Lawn, J., Tinker, A. et al. (2008) Primary health care: making Alma-Ata a reality. *Lancet* **372**, 1001–08.

Chapter 11

Maternal, neonatal, and child health

John Walley and Nancy Gerein

This chapter gives an overview of the following topics:

- Burden of disease
- Historical development of MNCH services
- The MNCH package of interventions
- Maternal health
- Neonatal health
- Integrated management of childhood illness (IMCI)
- The expanded programme of immunization (EPI)
- Nutrition
- School health
- Family planning
- Quality of MNCH services

One woman dies from the complications of pregnancy and childbirth every minute. Usually, birth is a positive experience, but too many pregnancies are unplanned and many women suffer needlessly. Globally, a jumbo-jet airliner full of babies is born each minute and every hour one crashes.

Maternal health refers to pregnancy, childbirth and the post-partum period. Complications arise in roughly equal proportion in each of these stages, but the vast majority of maternal deaths occur at the time of delivery. The direct causes of maternal death include haemorrhage, infection, high blood pressure, unsafe abortion, and obstructed labour. Most of these deaths could be prevented if women had access to quality family planning services and to skilled care during pregnancy, childbirth, and the first month after delivery. An estimated 15% of pregnancies and childbirths need emergency obstetric care because of risks that are difficult to predict. Post-abortion care and safe abortion services can also prevent many deaths.

Every day parents seek help for their sick infants and children – from hospitals, health centres, and community health workers. Private sector providers, drug stores, and traditional healers are also consulted.

Figure 11.1 shows that fever, cough, diarrhoea, and ear problems are the main presenting complaints. Yet these are preventable by improved water, sanitation, vaccination, health, and nutrition promotion, and a package of facility care and community intervention – such as those included in the 'Integrated Management of Childhood Illness'.

A well-functioning health system with skilled personnel is the key to saving the lives of pregnant women, their infants, and children. The weak health systems in many low-middle income countries

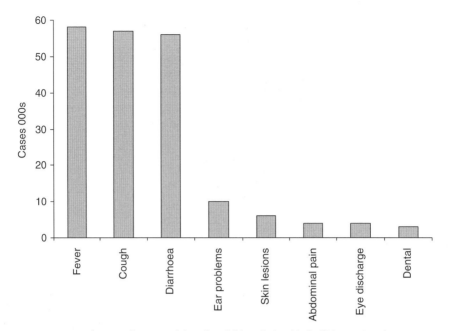

Fig. 11.1 Frequency of presenting complaints for children in health facilities at Gondor, Ethopia, 1994.

contribute to a huge gap in coverage of provision of MNCH services. The 'coverage gap' is an aggregate index of the difference between observed and universal coverage in four intervention areas: family planning, maternal and neonatal care, immunization, and treatment of sick children. Estimates from the most recent surveys showed that the mean overall gap is 43% in the 54 countries which account for 90% of deaths in the world (UNICEF 2008 Countdown to 2015).

Burden of disease

The burden of disease is the mortality and morbidity due to a particular group of diseases (see Chapter 1). The Disability Adjusted Life Year (DALY) is a measure of the years of life lost following death and/or the time spent suffering from morbidity (disability). A DALY is one healthy year of life (lost due to a disease or avoided due to an intervention). Six causes accounted for 73% of deaths in children under 5 in 2000-3: pneumonia (19%), diarrhoea (18%), malaria (8%), neonatal pneumonia or sepsis (10%), pre-term delivery (10%) and asphyxia at birth (18%). Fig. 11.2 shows the main causes of deaths in neonates. Causes related to MNCH are responsible for around half of the total burden of disease in developing countries.

For pregnant women, a high proportion of the disease burden is due to ill-health, such as anaemia, with a smaller proportion due to deaths. In the case of neonatal and childhood disease, the large majority of the disease burden is due to deaths. Every year worldwide an estimated 12 million children aged under 5 die, accounting for 36% of the total disease and injury burden in the world in 2004.

The burden of non-fatal disease is also particularly high in those aged under 5. Acute respiratory infection (ARI), diarrhoeal and perinatal illnesses, EPI-preventable diseases, malnutrition, and malaria are the most important. The picture shown in Fig. 11.3 is for sub-Saharan Africa as a whole. However, details vary from country to country.

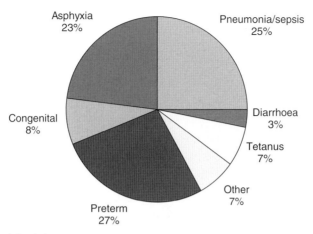

Fig. 11.2 Causes of death in neonates.

Source: WHO World Health Statistics 2007.

For example China has a very large population but relatively little malaria, whereas in Africa, malaria causes a far higher proportion of disease in pregnant women, infants, and children under 5, as does HIV/AIDS. Generally HIV/AIDS is under-recorded, as a factor in under five mortality as many deaths will be recorded under the HIV-related infection which causes the death. In these figures, malnutrition-related deaths are included within the direct causes of death, e.g. pneumonia. Malnutrition is an underlying cause of death in up to 50% of under-fives deaths. Malnutrition is common in Africa, but is more so in south Asian countries such as India and Bangladesh (Fig. 14.4).

Young children are more vulnerable to infectious disease and under-nutrition. There are fewer healthy years of life lost for children aged between 5 and 14 though the **causes** of years lost are similar, including EPI-preventable disease, ARI, malaria, and nutritional factors, as for the under 5s. However soil-transmitted helminth (worm) infections, tuberculosis, and epilepsy start to

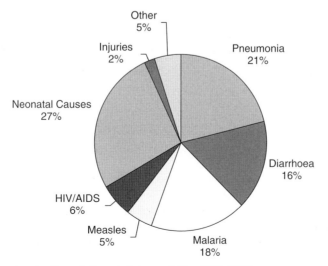

Fig. 11.3 Causes of under 5 mortality sub-Saharan Africa 2000–2003.

Source: World Health Statistics 2007.

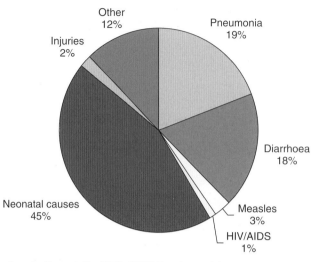

Fig. 11.4 Causes of under 5 mortality 2000–2003 Southeast Asia.
Source: World Health Statistics 2007.

become important. Worms become more common because of the increased mobility of the child and contact with environmental contamination and soil. Playing away from the home also increases the risk of drowning, road traffic and other accidents.

These figures show the deaths and disability directly due to the main groups of diseases. Remember though, as discussed in Chapter 1, that the **underlying** causes of disease include landlessness, unemployment, and lack of access to education, health services, and family planning. Put another way, poverty predisposes to disease. In turn, disease causes poverty – through reduced potential at school, at work and in the household, and having to pay for health care. Public health aims to interrupt this cycle of poverty, disease and more poverty.

Programmes and services for MNCH focus on a few effective and low-cost interventions against these diseases. As discussed in Chapter 1, there are various types of programmes and services:

- **Population-based interventions** include those for better nutrition, education, housing, water, and sanitation. These interventions are multi-sectoral. They seek to remove the underlying causes of ill health, resulting in long-term reductions in many diseases.

- **Personal preventative services** such as immunization. These services are provided at health facilities and outreach services.

- **Essential clinical services**, such as oral rehydration therapy for diarrhoea and antibiotics for pneumonia. They also include maternity and family planning services, leading to reduced perinatal as well as maternal mortality.

These MNCH interventions are highly cost-effective. They can be delivered for less than US$50 per year of healthy life saved. Some, such as vaccination and oral rehydration therapy for diarrhoea, cost only US$ 1–5 per year of healthy life saved. MNCH services are therefore a priority for public health.

The World Health Organization, UNICEF, and UNFPA support programmes to improve MNCH services. These programmes include those for vaccination and the provision of oral rehydration and family planning services. Programmes provide guidance which is simple and systematic. The biggest effort is in supervision and training of health workers. Strengthening

MNCH services is a major part of a district health officer's work (see District Health Services, Chapter 10). This leads to an improved standard of preventative and curative services.

Historical development of MNCH services

In the past, MNCH services were very variable. Most health workers concentrated on treating the presenting illness. In the 1970s, clinics for the under 5s were started. These provided both treatment and preventive interventions such as immunization. In the 1980s, after the Alma Ata conference, primary health care (PHC) was promoted. PHC includes an emphasis on providing services which are accessible and acceptable to all. UNICEF's priority was to ensure coverage with a selected package of 'child survival' interventions: growth monitoring, oral rehydration, breastfeeding and immunization ('GOBI'), but the mother's role and nutrition were missing. So female education, family planning and supplementary feeding were added ('GOBI-FFF'). The trend has continued towards more comprehensive PHC. This includes integrated services, with curative and preventive services available at the same time. In maternal services, emphasis was placed on ante-natal care and the training of Traditional Birth Attendants (TBAs) to provide delivery care. Now the focus is on skilled birth attendance and emergency obstetric care, a referral system to link the various levels, together with family planning and growing emphasis on neonatal care.

The MNCH package of interventions

MNCH interventions include:

- Maternal health: Ante-natal, delivery, post-natal, abortion, and post-abortion care services.
- Neonatal health relies on skilled care during childbirth and postnatal home visits and treat sepsis, pneumonia and birth asphyxia.
- Integrated management of childhood illness (IMCI) including the improved diagnosis and treatment of ARI, ear infection, diarrhoeal diseases, malaria, and measles.
- The expanded programme of immunization (EPI) with the standard six childhood vaccines.
- Nutritional assessment and advice on feeding of young children, promotion of breastfeeding, and vitamin A supplementation.
- School health programmes, including health education and mass treatment for worms.
- Family planning.

These interventions can be delivered at low cost most of them at first-level facilities. Together these interventions have the potential to reduce the overall burden of disease by about one-third–10–30% of maternal deaths, 20% of newborn deaths, and 30–40% of all postnatal deaths in children under 5.

The grouping together of these interventions makes sense as it cares for the mother and child as a whole, and makes best use of the mother's time. After dealing with the presenting illness, appropriate preventive interventions should also be offered. Each visit to the health worker is an opportunity to give vaccinations, assess growth, and give health and family planning information. Too often only the presenting problem is treated, with **missed opportunities** for prevention of future illnesses. Ensuring accessible, acceptable, efficient and good-quality MNCH services is one of the main responsibilities of public heath professionals.

The achievement of high coverage (percentage of the target population) for MNCH interventions is essential. Many of the key interventions for MNCH have been tracked and reported in the 2008 'Countdown to 2015' report, see figure 11.5. Although there has been considerable progress, the coverage of many of these indicators is not sufficient.

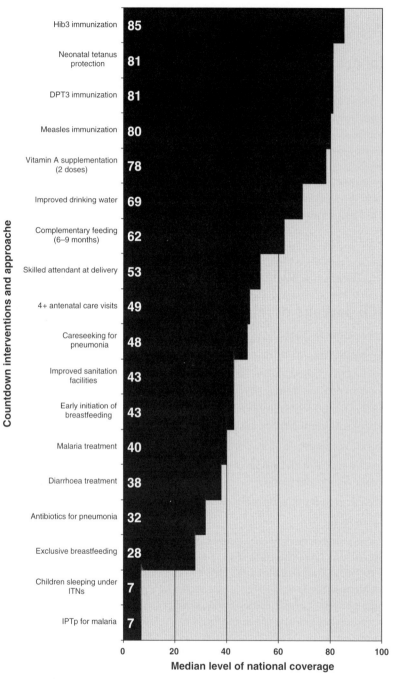

Fig. 11.5 Coverage (percentage) of key MNCH interventions.

Source: Countdown to 2015 MNCH survival.

Maternal health

Worldwide, an estimated 60 million acute complications in pregnancy occur annually. Of these 23 million require higher-level care. In total, 40% of pregnancies are affected, 98 % of these being in developing countries. A maternal death is any death while pregnant or within 42 days of the end of pregnancy. Worldwide, approximately 500 000 women die each year from causes related to pregnancy and childbirth (WHO 2005). The causes are:

- Haemorrhage (25%)
- Indirect causes (e.g. malaria, hepatitis) (20%)
- Sepsis (15%)
- Unsafe abortion (13%)
- Eclampsia – high blood pressure leading to seizures (12%),
- Obstructed labour (8%),
- Other direct causes (8%)

HIV/AIDS is having a main effect on MMR in Africa in particular. While these are the direct causes of maternal deaths, a major underlying cause is unavailable, inaccessible, unaffordable, or poor-quality care.

An estimated 55 million unwanted pregnancies are terminated each year, about half the terminations being illegal. Induced abortion is common (whether legal or illegal) where access to contraception is limited. Unsafe illegal abortions are one of the major causes – in Latin America **the** main cause – of maternal death.

In addition to those women who die, huge numbers of others are affected by infertility, ectopic pregnancy following sepsis, uterine prolapse, and fistulas following complicated deliveries.

Maternal health care consists of pre-natal, delivery, post-natal, abortion, and post-abortion care and family planning services. Women and newborns may suffer complications at any stage in the pregnancy, and family planning also reduces them. See further reading from WHO's Integrated Management of Pregnancy and Childbirth (IMPAC).

Each of these stages is also important for child health:

- Pre-natal care and improved nutrition during pregnancy reduces the numbers of vulnerable low-birthweight babies.
- Delivery care decreases the risk of congenital injury, such as cerebral palsy and tetanus infection.
- Post-natal care is an opportunity to provide preventive care to the mother and baby.
- Family planning allows the mother to space births, increasing the chance of survival for existing and subsequent children.

Access to information and services for safe motherhood

There is usually a chain of factors influencing a woman's access to services and hence the outcome of a complicated pregnancy or delivery. These include:

1 Women's isolation due to socio-economic factors:
- Low access to schooling
- Little access to information and money
- Lack of mobility
- The need to seek permission to use health services

2 Women's limited access to key maternal services:

- Family planning
- Health centre nurse-midwife for ante-natal and post-natal care
- Skilled attendance at delivery – doctor, midwife, or if they are accessible, a traditional birth attendant (trained or untrained)
- Emergency obstetric care
- Post-abortion care and safe abortion services

Together these underlying and more direct determinants may lead to maternal and perinatal mortality.

The delivery of maternity services

There are two main elements in safer maternity. The first is to provide a good quality of delivery care, with specialist care for any woman who develops an obstetric complication. The second is the identification of women with problems or at risk of complications, and the provision of treatment and/or referral. In recent decades, there has been a lot of emphasis on identification of risk. However, the criteria used, such as young and older women, previous complications, small stature, etc., meant that a large proportion of women were included as at-risk. Most of these did not develop complications, and many of the women who did experience complications had not been identified as being at-risk. In other words, the screening criteria were neither sensitive nor specific.

Instead, WHO now recommends that women should be advised that every pregnant woman has a risk of developing complications. However, complications cannot be predicted, which means that all women should be helped to plan, during ante-natal care visits, to have a safe delivery, whether at home or in a health facility.

Pre-natal care

Too often pre-natal care has consisted of routine procedures without effective actions taken. WHO now recommends focussed pre-natal care. In four visits, women should receive: At least two doses of tetanus toxoid vaccination, management of STIs, management of pre-eclampsia, intermittent preventive treatment (IPT) for malaria in pregnancy and advice on the use of bednets. IPT is a dose of the recommended anti-malaria drug (such as 'Fansidar', SP) given twice, once in early and again in later pregnancy. The pre-natal care should include PMTCT in places with a generalized HIV epidemic (where more than 1% of ante-natal women have HIV).

Information about birth and emergency preparedness is a new addition to ANC. In the four visits, the mother, and preferably her family as well, should be taught:

- to arrange for delivery care, preferably by a skilled birth attendant, but if this is not possible, a trained traditional birth attendant
- to recognize the signs of danger which indicate that she should seek professional care
- how to get to a health facility which can provide good delivery care
- about planning for transportation to the health facility
- about saving money to pay for transport and emergency care
- about the importance of postnatal care: breast feeding and birth spacing

These messages can be included on the mother's ante-natal card, using pictures which everyone in the family can see and discuss. In Bangladesh, this resulted in a higher level of recognition of danger signs and greater use of professional delivery care.

Care during childbirth

Childbirth care includes: Skilled attendance at birth (a health worker with midwifery training, supported by adequate equipment), a companion of the mother's choice at birth, emergency obstetric care, and a referral system.

Good quality delivery care is critical in preventing mortality and morbidity in the newborn as well as in the mother. If the service is affordable and acceptable, mothers will be more likely to choose to give birth with a skilled birth attendant, in a health facility.

Some characteristics that attract mothers are:

- Health workers who are kind and welcoming as well as technically competent
- Allowing mothers to have their chosen birth companion with them
- Giving birth in a position that they find comfortable (rather than on their backs with legs in stirrups)
- Not doing routine episiotomies
- Giving adequate pain relief
- Dealing with the placenta according to local beliefs, and other local wishes that health workers can determine by asking mothers and families what they find important

Although most births are uncomplicated, health facilities need to be able to deal with obstetric complications promptly, i.e. provide basic and comprehensive emergency obstetric care.

Basic emergency obstetric care has six requirements

- Antibiotics IV/IM
- Oxytocic drugs IV
- Anticonvulsants IV/IM
- Manual removal of the placenta
- Removal of retained placenta
- Assisted vaginal delivery (through vacuum extraction)

Comprehensive emergency obstetric care has all of the above plus

- Surgery (e.g. caesarean delivery)
- Blood transfusion

Where birth occurs without a skilled birth attendant, it is important to help mothers have a clean birth. This means teaching the mother and local birth attendant during the ante-natal period about hygiene (hand-washing, clean bedding, clothes, and perineal pads), and using a clean delivery kit containing soap, a sterile blade, cord thread, a plastic sheet, and pictorial instructions about clean delivery practices and neonatal care.

HIV positive women should be given a dose of ART (e.g. nevirapine) to take during labour/immediately after birth to prevent HIV in the newborn. Better still, the woman (and her partner if also HIV positive) should be started on long-term three-drug ART.

The referral system

As most obstetric complications cannot be foreseen or prevented, it is important to provide prompt emergency care for complications, as one of the main methods to reduce maternal and perinatal mortality. This is achieved through a referral system which links the community to first-level facilities and first-level facilities to secondary- and tertiary-level facilities.

The first requirement of a referral system is to have functioning referral facilities which can provide basic and comprehensive obstetric care, as described above. Transport to move the patient is necessary, and this can be organized by the community or the health service. Women can be moved on carts equipped with a mattress and umbrella, pulled by bicycles or animals. In Nigeria, private truck drivers and car owners agreed to participate in a community-organized system to ensure that transport was available at all times for emergencies.

Also important in a referral system is a means of communication, so that first-level health workers can inform the referral facility about an emergency patient, and the referral facility has time to prepare to receive her. Health personnel at all levels need training to identify and manage complications, as well as clear guidelines about when to refer. The health records of the mother should move with her, so that all levels of care know her history and what treatment has been given. Finally, mechanisms to encourage people to use the most appropriate facility are helpful in reducing the over-use of referral facilities and under-use of first-level care. For example, fees for first-level care can be lower, and exemptions from high referral-facility fees can be given, if the mother has been referred by a lower-level facility. If the nearest health unit does not have emergency obstetric care, however, families should be informed to go directly to the facility that does have this capacity.

Post-natal care

PNC is important for prevention of illness or its early identification and referral for care. During the ante-natal period, mothers should be informed of the importance of PNC and asked to attend for care within a week of birth if possible, or as soon after that as they can. The importance of attending for their baby's vaccinations should be included in this message. If the mother is HIV positive and delivers at home, the health worker should stress that, as part of preventation of mother to child transmission, the mother should attend within 48 hours of birth, so that the baby can be given ART e.g. nevirapine drops. (Some systems give the medicine to the mother to use at home.) Mothers also need to be taught to recognize danger signs (e.g. a fever after birth, or excessive bleeding). If home births are common, and mothers are confined to the home after birth, a system where the health worker visits them in the home may need to be organized.

During the post-natal visit, the health workers should check the mother to see how she is recovering from birth, and advise about caring for herself. The health worker should:

◆ Assess and check for bleeding, and fever

◆ Support breastfeeding, checking the breasts to prevent mastitis

◆ Manage anaemia, promote nutrition and insecticide treated bednets, give vitamin A supplementation

◆ Complete tetanus toxoid immunization, if required

◆ Provide counselling and offer a range of options for family planning, and initiate

◆ Refer for complications such as bleeding, infections, or post-natal depression

◆ Counsel on the danger signs and hygiene (requiring urgent hospital care)

The baby should also benefit during the post-natal visit through giving the mother information about exclusive breastfeeding, umbilicus care, hygiene, warmth, sleeping under bednets and signs of illness in an infant. The baby can be given eye gonorrhoea prophylaxis and immunization according to the local schedule especially in HIV-prevalent areas, this can also include advice on safer infant feeding practices, such as exclusive breast feeding until 6 months and then adding other foods.

'The pathway to survival'

'The pathway to survival' consists of the recognition of a problem, making a decision regarding care and providing access to quality care. This pathway to quality care applies to all life threatening illness. It should function correctly to reduce maternal and neonatal complications. The whole referral system needs to be functioning to ensure the pathway to survival (see Fig. 11.6).

Identifying problems and taking action

The effective delivery of services requires that patients and health workers not only recognize problems, but that they also make appropriate decisions regarding care. Pre-natal, delivery, and post-natal care (and other MNCH procedures such as growth monitoring) are often done as a **ritual**, which means, going through the check-up but without recognizing problems or, if problems are recognized, not taking action. In Ethiopia a women's card was designed which included the key parts of pre-natal care in a table which included a 'threshold for intervention': For example, if the BP rose by 20 mm of mercury or if the haemoglobin level falls to below 10 g, then oral iron and folic acid should be given.

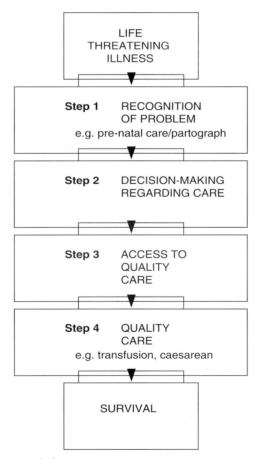

Fig. 11.6 'The pathway to survival'.

Similarly, during labour a **partograph** allows systematic monitoring of the progress of labour. Dilatation of the cervix and the frequency and intensity of contractions is regularly monitored, and an alert and action line drawn to aid decision-making for intervention/referral, such as caesarean section for obstructed labour.

Safe abortion and post-abortion care

Abortion is common where family planning services are poor, whether or not abortion is legal. Where illegal, then unsafe abortion is common. Globally about 13% of maternal deaths are due to unsafe abortion. These can be prevented by providing good quality post-abortion care and abortion services, if abortion is legal. Surgical abortion is by manual vacuum aspiration in early pregnancy. Abortion can be done by dilation and curettage, though this isn't the best method. Medical abortions through the use of the drugs mifepristone with misoprostol are also safe and effective in early pregnancy (for details see www.fwhc.org/abortion/medical-ab.htm). The dose depends on the length of the pregnancy. Access to quality family planning services is of course the best prevention, including emergency contraception; see the family planning section at the end of this chapter.

Post-abortion care consists of emergency treatment of complications of spontaneous or induced abortion; family planning counselling, services and referral for women and their partners; and linkages to other services, such as STI clinics. Mid-level health workers, such as midwives, can be safely trained in vacuum aspiration and pain and infection management. Where abortion is illegal, they may need special support for improving their counselling skills and interactions with women.

Training of traditional birth attendants

It is commonly assumed that training of traditional birth attendants (TBAs) will ensure pregnant women's access to care and an effective referral system. However, experiences with TBA training indicate that:

1 Training TBAs is not enough to influence maternal mortality, as they still need the support of skilled midwives and referral health facilities that can provide emergency obstetric care.

2 TBAs should be trained to recognize complications of pregnancy or delivery as they develop and refer women. They should be supported to do this with a transportation system (organized by the community or the health service). TBAs should be welcomed at the referral facility, where they can be taught improved knowledge and skills.

Although it is safer to have all women delivered by a skilled birth attendant (midwife, doctor with training, obstetrician), it will take years for many countries to train and employ a sufficient number to reach all pregnant women. Also, many women do not see the need for professional care and are uncomfortable with being assisted in childbirth by strangers, far from home, at considerable expense. As the use of skilled birth attendants increases, an appropriate role for TBAs needs to be developed in each country. In some countries, they have helped to reduce neonatal mortality, by learning how to resuscitate newborns, keep them warm and encourage breastfeeding from birth.

Neonatal care

Care of the newborn

The causes of death in the first month of life are included in Fig. 11.2 above.

It has been argued that nearly three-quarters of all neonatal deaths could be prevented if women were adequately nourished and received appropriate care during pregnancy, childbirth, and the post-natal period. This includes prevention of asphyxia and problems related to prematurity. Tetanus is prevented by avoiding contamination of the umbilical stump and giving tetanus vaccination to the mother and infant.

All newborns need to be dried, kept warm and clean, and breastfed as soon as possible after birth, so that they benefit from antibodies in the colostrum. Exclusive breastfeeding for 4–6 months is the most effective way to prevent infections such as diarrhoea. The baby should stay with the mother, in her bed or in a cot next to her, not separated in a hospital nursery. Health workers are often not well prepared to resuscitate newborns and special training efforts may need to be organized to prevent deaths from this common problem.

Babies who are premature or low birthweight (LBW, less than 2500 gm) are especially vulnerable to the main causes of death in infants. They should be closely observed and referred for any signs of infection or inability to breastfeed.

Kangaroo Mother Care

Kangaroo Mother Care is an effective way to meet the needs of premature and LBW babies who do not have an illness, but mainly need to feed and grow. The infant is placed between the mother's breasts, skin-to-skin and tied securely with a cloth or specially designed carrying pouch. The baby should wear a nappy, hat and socks and a shirt in cool areas. The mother then covers herself and the baby with her usual dress. Fathers can also participate, replacing the mother for skin-to-skin contact with the baby, so that she can get some rest.

Kangaroo Mother Care provides continuous or at least prolonged skin-to-skin contact between the mother and baby, warmth, exclusive breastfeeding, stimulation, protection from infection, safety, and a loving bond between the infant and parents. It is especially useful where situations where incubators for newborns are unavailable or unreliable. It also allows parents to take the baby out of hospital early and care for it safely at home, although it is desirable to support them through home visits from a nurse. Health workers need to be trained in this method, to support the mother to gradually take over the care of her small baby. Further information can be found in WHO's 'Kangaroo Mother Care a practical guide' (see further reading below).

Management of neonatal illness

Pneumonia, umbilical cord and other infections (sepsis), as well as diarrhoea are major causes of neonatal deaths. The early diagnosis and treatment of the sick infant up to 2 months is included within the WHO package of care called the 'Integrated Management of Childhood Illness'. The health worker asks the mother about the infant's problems, asks about convulsions and any feeding difficulty. They count the breaths in one minute and look for severe chest in-drawing, grunting, reduced movement, or fever. If any of these are present, the child needs IM antibiotics, management of low blood sugar and urgent referral to hospital. If these are not present but the infant has redness or pus of the umbilicus or skin pustules, then they are given oral antibiotics and seen again in 2 days. An infant with diarrhoea and the signs of severe dehydration is rehydrated and referred. If the infant has some dehydration they are given oral rehydration and followed up in 2 days. The details are included in the IMCI chartbook, as for childhood illness below.

Child health

The Integrated Management of Childhood Illness (IMCI)

Pneumonia, diarrhoeal disease, malnutrition, measles, and malaria cause an estimated seven out of ten deaths in those aged under 5 in low-income countries, as well as comprising the majority of non-fatal illnesses.

Interventions for sick children were previously introduced separately, in programmes such as those for acute respiratory illness (ARI) and control of diarrhoeal disease (CDD). Previously these programmes had their own procedures, and training modules, and courses. The WHO and UNICEF have developed a programme for the integrated management of childhood illness(IMCI). The initiative focuses on improving the performance of health workers through training and support.

The signs and symptoms of diarrhoea, pneumonia, measles, and malaria overlap, so recognizing the cause of illness can be difficult. But fortunately the treatment of these conditions also overlaps. This is the basis of the syndromic approach. The starting point is the symptoms and signs, rather than the disease. The child is assessed for the main symptoms of cough or difficult breathing, diarrhoea, fever, and ear problems. Then the child is assessed for nutritional and immunization status. Finally, the mother is asked about her own health, need for family planning (or, if pregnant, ante-natal care), and given tetanus vaccination.

The health worker carries out the following procedures with the aid of a case management guideline (see Fig. 11.7):

♦ Assess the sick child – asking questions, examining and checking immunization status

♦ Classify the sick child – using a colour-coded system for either urgent referral, specific treatment and advice, or simple advice on home management

♦ Treat the child – according to the classification. If the child is being referred then only the urgent treatments are given

♦ Counsel the mother – on how to administer drugs, increase fluids and the signs indicating the need to bring the child back to the clinic – also in countries with HIV, about the need for an HIV test

♦ Give preventive interventions – immunization, vitamin A supplementation, counselling on feeding of children, tetanus immunization, and family planning advice for mothers

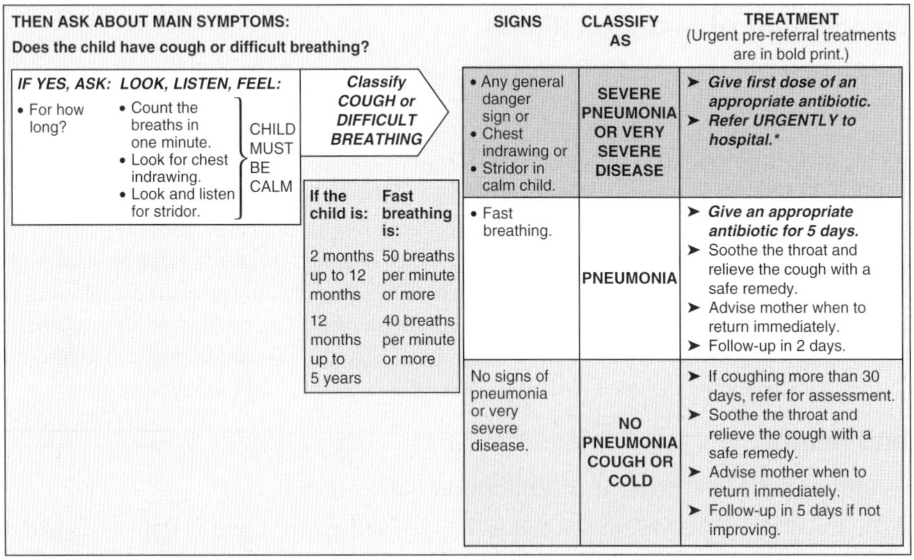

Fig. 11.7 IMCI case management.

This approach is more efficient and economizes on training and supervision. The health worker requires only seven essential drugs: oral re-hydration solution, an oral antibiotic (such as cotrimoxazole), an antimalarial, an antihelminthic, vitamin A drops, iron tablets, and paracetamol. The only equipment needed is a watch or timer for the counting of the respiratory rate.

There is a training course called 'Management of Childhood Illness'. The course package includes a set of six training modules and facilitators' guides, including videos and slides. Hands-on practice of the skills is included, with observation of the clinical signs of sick children in health facilities. [To order the materials write to the World Health Organization, Division of Child and Adolescent Health or www.who.int/healthtopics/childhealth/imci or for all documents www.who.int/child_adolescent_health/imci/en/index.html Fax: +41(22)791– 4853 or E-mail: CAH@who.ch]

The details of case management should be adapted according to the local situation. Guidelines for adaptation are available from the World Health Organization, as are guidelines for hospital management of the sick child. Care needs to be given to developing local case definitions on which treatments will be based. Modifications include those for the diagnosis and treatment of children with fever. This will be different where malaria is endemic (present for most of the year) than from where it occurs as seasonal epidemics.

The approach covers the five major illnesses in childhood. It does not, for example, include the management of asthma or meningitis. However, in countries where meningitis epidemics are common this could be added. In each country, based on available research, it is necessary to adapt the content and words used for how to manage malnutrition and feeding problems. Clinical management in first-level health facilities and the reasons why families do not seek health care for sick children also need to be investigated locally.

Health workers need to appreciate the crucial role of mothers, as **diagnosticians** of the signs of illness and deterioration and as **carers** giving food, fluids, and drugs correctly. Health workers should not view the mother as only the passive recipient of instructions. Following the IMCI approach will improve communication between health workers and parents. Each contact with the health facility should help the mother improve her skills in the care of her children, and empower the parents to care for their child.

The IMCI interventions

IMCI integrates the assessment and management of common clinical problems with prevention (Table 9.1). The most effective preventive interventions (vaccinations, vitamin A supplementation, health and nutrition messages) have been included. The messages of information are brief, clear, and adapted in-country to the local language, such that they are practical within the time limitations of a consultation. Related messages should be given in the community, such as through community health workers working with women's groups.

IMCI interventions

IMCI has three main areas of intervention:

1 IMCI case management of cough and difficult breathing, diarrhoea, fever (malaria), ear problems, malnutrition (and where particularly prevalent, other illnesses such as HIV or asthma are added).

2 IMCI treats the presenting illness, but then goes on to promote growth and prevent disease through interventions in the family and community as well as the health service (see Table 11.1).

Table 11.1 How messages given to the family and community health services can work together in IMCI

	Promotion of growth/prevention of disease	Response to sickness
Family and Community Health services	◆ Community/home-based interventions to improve nutrition ◆ Insecticide-treated bednets ◆ Vaccination ◆ Complementary feeding and breastfeeding counselling ◆ Vitamin A and mebendazole (de-worming) supplementation	◆ Early case management ◆ Appropriate care-seeking ◆ Compliance with treatment ◆ Case management of ARI, diarrhoea, measles, malaria, malnutrition, other serious infection ◆ Complementary feeding and breastfeeding counselling ◆ Iron treatment ◆ Antihelminthic treatment

3 IMCI goes further still, in that it recognizes the need for strengthening the district health facilities (component 2 of IMCI; see below). What is more, it is recognized that these are general health service development issues and are best addressed in coordination with the district and provincial health/medical officers, as well as with the other health programmes such as those for reproductive health, STIs etc. IMCI also recognizes the need to utilize opportunities to work with various groups in the community, in order to get across essential health and nutrition messages (component 3 below).

The three components used to achieve these aims are:
1 Improvement of the skills of health workers.
- ◆ Case management guidelines and standards
- ◆ Training of health providers in the public and non-government sector
- ◆ IMCI roles for private providers
- ◆ Maintenance of competence among trained health workers
2 The improvement of health systems
- ◆ District planning and management
- ◆ Availability of IMCI drugs and organization of work at health facilities
- ◆ Quality of improvement and supervision at health facilities
- ◆ Referral pathways and services
- ◆ Health information system (HIS)
- ◆ Adapting IMCI within health sector reforms
3 The improvement of family and community practices
- ◆ Care-seeking
- ◆ Nutrition
- ◆ Home case management and adherence to recommended treatment
- ◆ Community involvement in health services and supporting community health workers

Component 3 aims to promote key health and nutrition messages, for example the promotion of exclusive breastfeeding of young infants, then continuing breastfeeding with frequent meals, how to give fluids to a child with diarrhoea, and the signs of a sick child who should be brought to the health facility.

The role of community groups in achieving IMCI aims

Groups may include church groups, women's groups, preschool, or feeding centres as well as community health workers. It is important to find out which groups already exist and to go and talk to them about how they can improve the health of children in the community by communicating information to parents. Health workers need to involve community leaders in the planning and monitoring of primary and community services.

The improvement of health systems

The second component mentioned above is about improving the health facility and district systems. This includes ensuring a reliable supply of the essential drugs, the referral and use of health information systems. Supervisors need to ensure that staff can carry out care and prevention tasks properly according to their training (component 1). There is a need to decide locally how best to ensure that the health facilities are organized efficiently. Supervisors will need to work with the staff to arrange clear roles for each health worker, to arrange better patient flow to avoid unnecessary waiting or crowding, and to make sure that preventive interventions such as vaccination and health education are provided. Regular supervision visits will need to include observing (sitting in the rooms and watching) and talking to the health workers to find out how well the service is functioning, followed by a discussion with the health workers and community leaders about the good and not so good points of the service, and agreeing what should be improved before the next visit (**quality improvement**).

Overcoming constraints to integrated care

Within the health centre, IMCI includes improving the case management of the presenting illness and counselling of the parents. The health worker should assess requirements and provide immunization and interventions for under-nutrition. Finally, preventative interventions for the mother such as tetanus immunization and family planning should be offered. All of this is very important but also time-consuming. Health workers may take between 10 and 20 minutes to complete this process. However, existing consultations may average less than 5 minutes—even where sick children are also routinely assessed for immunization and growth monitored. This is because often the existing practice is to treat on the basis of the presenting symptoms (without further questions or examination) and there is limited communication with the mother. The time demands of the IMCI programme are therefore such that consultations will take considerably longer than with the current practice. See Box 11.1 for a description of how to provide integrated MNCH primary care service.

Health workers find it difficult to implement a new service if it involves different procedures from those they are used to. They need to see and practise the new procedures, to be able to carry out a new approach. It may be possible to include sessions on clinic organization in the IMCI training course. Course participants could first look at the existing organizational problems in the clinic. Then they could practise reorganization of the clinic procedures. They could learn to maximize efficient use of staff, rooms, and equipment and to improve patient flow. Soon after the course they would implement the organizational changes, making time available for better patient care. This would then be followed up by their supervisors.

Expanded programme of immunization

The expanded programme of immunization (EPI) with the standard six childhood vaccines is well established in most countries. Many countries give BCG, polio, and hepatitis soon after birth,

Box 11.1 Deliver an integrated 'supermarket' MNCH service

An integrated daily curative and preventive MNCH service is practised in health centres and hospital outpatients in many countries. All the essential interventions are available on the same visit – as in a supermarket where all products are available in the one shop – a 'one-stop shop' service. This includes treatment of illness based on guidelines such as IMCI (which *do not* just treat the presenting symptom, but *do* check for the relevant symptoms and signs). The mother is counselled on the treatment to give her child and the signs of deterioration to look out for. She is given a review appointment, e.g. in 2 days time. Preventive interventions are given at the same visit, i.e, the child's weight is monitored, immunizations are given, and these are recorded on the child health card record. Pre-natal care and family planning are available as a daily service. The mother is asked about pregnancy and given an ante-natal check, or if she does not want a pregnancy yet, is offered family planning. Women of reproductive age can be offered tetanus immunization.

Quality curative care and offering preventive interventions take longer than just treating the presenting symptom. To make time, make efficient use of the available health workers, rooms and equipment, so more staff are busy seeing patients. Give follow-up and chronic care (e.g. TB, HIV, and epilepsy) appointments in the afternoon, when staff are less busy.

then three monthly doses of diphtheria, pertussis (whooping cough), and tetanus (DPT), polio, Hib and hepatitis, and measles at 9 months. The *Haemophilus influenzae* or Hib vaccine protects against some forms of pneumonia and ear infections. Countries may add vaccines against locally endemic diseases such as yellow fever. A pneumococcus vaccine is effective but expensive. Fortunately in 2008, the GAVI Alliance (UNICEF, WHO, and many other agencies committed to EPI) has committed funds to introduce pneumococcal vaccine, When available these should reduce the incidence of pneumonia and meningitis. The new vaccines add little additional cost to delivering the service, only the cost of buying the vaccine. Because the benefits are high, the addition of new vaccines may increase cost-effectiveness of the immunization program. Vitamin A capsules can also be added to the EPI schedule with similar benefits and at low cost.

Generally, EPI is well-integrated with MNCH services at health facilities, though in some countries EPI is still carried out by specific staff separate from other MNCH services. Operating EPI separately may be easier to manage, but there will be missed opportunities to vaccinate when children attend for other MNCH services. False contraindications to vaccination, such as the presence of mild illnesses, need to be avoided.

Outreach services, by vehicle or bicycle, are a useful way of extending the coverage of EPI to places distant from health facilities. Other MNCH services such as health and nutrition education and family planning services should also be added where possible.

Globally, EPI has made much progress increasing coverage from about 5% of infants under 12 months fully immunized in 1970 to 79% by 2007. However, immunization coverage is still too low in much of sub-Saharan Africa and in some other developing countries. In some countries, coverage is low due to failure to maintain services and extend coverage to all areas. The strengthening and maintaining of routine facility and outreach EPI services is sometimes called 'keep-up' – keeping up coverage. The districts and localities where coverage is low need to be given extra inputs to improve access and, acceptability (Technical problems, such as breakdowns in the cold chain and delayed ordering of vaccines and supplies, must be avoided through competent administration). These 'catch-up' efforts require adequate resources, competent administration, and effective targeting of 'hard-to-reach' populations. Hard-to-reach populations include groups living in remote places, or groups marginalized by their occupation or ethnicity. Some are hard to reach due to their being members of religious groups that resist vaccination. All these groups require special activities to promote and deliver services appropriately.

Older children who were missed in previous years, when vaccination coverage of under 1-year children was low, can be protected in 'mopping-up' campaigns. These campaigns commonly vaccinate these children in primary schools. In this case the children are vaccinated unless they have a written record of previous vaccination.

Because EPI is so dependent on the general health system, the GAVI alliance also supports investments in strengthening human resources and other health system components.

Nutrition

Malnutrition is **directly** responsible for fewer than 4% of deaths of children under 5 years of age, through kwashiorkor and marasmus. However, more than a third of child deaths are associated with malnutrition as one of the **underlying** causes. Inadequate food intake and repeated infections are part of a vicious cycle causing malnutrition (Box 11.2). In addition, about 40% of women of reproductive age in developing countries, especially in South Asia, are underweight and have low birth weight babies (under 2.5 kg) who are particularly vulnerable to illness and death.

Growth monitoring and promotion

Growth monitoring involves screening all children in order to identify those who are underweight. It is an established part of MNCH services. Often, however, the intervention – growth

---

Box 11.2 Malnutrition: Hunger is only half the story

Inadequate intake of food results in a condition called protein-energy malnutrition. This may not be clinically apparent, but can be detected by growth monitoring.

In sick children, malnutrition occurs for several reasons:

- Loss of appetite
- Well-meaning carers withhold food
- Absorption of nutrients is impaired
- Energy requirements are increased
- Diarrhoea leads to direct loss of nutrients
- Inadequate food and micronutrients leads to reduced mucosal immunity, increasing the risk of infections.

Children who are starving clearly need more food, but for children with a barely adequate diet, the treatment of infections has an important effect on weight and growth. Surprisingly, there is little difference in growth in children up to three years of age, despite significant differences in energy intake, unless there is control of infections and diarrhoea. Intestinal worm infestation is a problem in children and mass treatment for worms has been shown to lead to weight gain.

There is therefore a complicated interaction between malnutrition and infection. Both inadequate food intake and infection lead to malnutrition.

Adapted from Investing in health research and development, WHO, Geneva, 1996.

promotion – is not carried out effectively. There is much more to it than just regular weighing. A common scenario of ineffective use of growth monitoring is where an auxiliary health worker does the weighing. The nurse or doctor in the consultation room is meant to look at the chart, but is busy and doesn't remember to do so. The mother is not involved and does not understand the process. The opportunity to counsel her on child feeding is lost. In these circumstances a decision needs to be made, either to do growth monitoring properly, or not to do it if staff are completely overloaded. It can be argued that, if the majority of children in a community are under-weight (mostly due to poverty and repeated infections), it is very time consuming to weigh and counsel every individual. It may be preferable to take a group approach, by organizing group discussions with the mothers about child feeding. In Bangladesh, children who were well-grown (the right height and weight for their age) were used as examples to discuss the kind of care and local food that led to their healthy growth, as a guide to the mothers whose children were underweight or small for their age.

Effective growth monitoring and promotion requires staff to be trained and supervised to do each of the following steps properly:

1 Involve the mother while weighing and correctly recording the weight on the child health card.
2 Identify those children whose growth is faltering, i.e. the weight line is either static or going down.
3 Check for the presence of illness in the child and treat accordingly. (Growth faltering is often due to illness)
4 Ask the mother about food given and food available.
5 Provide specific feeding advice which is feasible given her circumstances. Commonly, this is to increase meals for young children to five times a day. The mother should include locally available vegetables, beans and oil together with the staple cereal (and eggs, if available), the main aim being to increase the energy content of the food. This is because young children have small stomachs and high energy needs. Cereal porridge alone is too bulky to provide sufficient energy content for young children.

If done properly growth monitoring with nutrition education is a powerful tool for improving child health. It is important to involve fathers in this as well, as they are decision-makers in household spending including on food and health care.

Food supplementation and food aid

What should be done when there are absolute shortages of food? There are a number of situations when food may be provided in the form of food supplementation or food aid. But each approach has potential problems which need to be carefully considered before starting.

Food supplementation can be targeted at under-weight children or pregnant women. During famine periods, food can be given out to all attending at MNCH clinics or preschools. At other times, food may be targeted only at those children whose growth is found to be faltering. Health workers feel useful, as they are doing more than just giving advice to needy families with underweight children. However, this may lead to dependency, and when supplies end, attendance often declines.

Food aid is essential during famines. Distribution must be targeted to those most in need. Free food may depress the local market price for food, reducing the incentive to grow food for sale. For these reasons food aid is sometimes given as 'food for work' for those participating in community projects such as road building. Phasing out the food aid should be done as soon as possible, but with care.

In the recent past, many governments controlled the prices of staple foods to keep them low. This was popular, especially amongst the urban population. But recent reforms have removed these controls so as to increase the incentive for farmers to produce more food for sale.

Though important, interventions within the health sector are not sufficient to end malnutrition. Interventions are needed to tackle the underlying social and economic factors leading to under-nutrition. Long-term solutions are required. Inter-sectoral approaches, involving departments of education, water and sanitation (promoting health and hygiene), and agriculture are needed, for example, promoting the production of protein-rich, high-energy (oil-containing) crops such as beans and groundnuts.

Micronutrients

Vitamin A deficiency causes night blindness and xeropthalmia, and might result in blindness, especially following measles. Deficiency of vitamin A also increases susceptibility to ARI, diarrhoea, and other common childhood illnesses. Communities can be encouraged to grow and eat dark green leafy vegetables – cassava leaves for example are rich in vitamin A. But changing dietary practice is a long-term task. Simply telling people, as part of a top-down health education talk, is rarely effective. Communities need to be involved in analysing the problem (see 'Assessing health needs', Chapter 3) and participating in improving their own health. To achieve this requires health workers to have a change of approach and to acquire new skills. It will also take time.

Supplementation with regular vitamin A capsules and zinc is effective. Where vitamin A deficiency is a problem, capsules should be given to children with night blindness and those suffering from measles. Supplementation with capsules can be a routine for all young children. One approach is to give capsules together with immunizations, although further doses will also be required after immunizations are completed. Zinc should be given, together with oral rehydration therapy, for diarrhoea.

Fortification is where a vitamin or mineral is added to a food. For example, in Indonesia vitamin A has been added to monosodium glutamate (MSG), a popular flavour enhancer. A more common example of fortification is adding iodine to salt. This can be a highly effective example of health promotion through legislation. Effective regulation is essential, with analysis of samples to ensure that the correct amount of iodine has been added. Manufacturers may attempt to save money by not adding iodine. However, excessive iodine can also be harmful.

Interventions to reduce under-nutrition

Effective interventions are available to reduce stunting, micronutrient deficiencies, and child deaths. If implemented on a sufficient scale, they would reduce child deaths and disability by about a quarter in the short term. These include:

- Counselling on breastfeeding, fortification and/or supplementation with vitamin A and zinc – these have the greatest potential to reduce the burden of child morbidity and mortality

- Improved complementary feeding (through intervention strategies such as counselling about nutrition for food-secure populations and nutrition counselling, food supplements, conditional cash transfers, or a combination of these, in food-insecure populations) could substantially reduce stunting and related burden of disease

- Maternal nutrition interventions (supplements of iron folate, multiple micronutrients, calcium and balanced energy and protein diet) can improve outcomes for maternal health and infants

These available interventions can make a clear difference in the short term. Elimination of stunting will also require long-term investments to improve education, economic status, and empowerment of women. See Bhutta et al. (2008) in further reading.

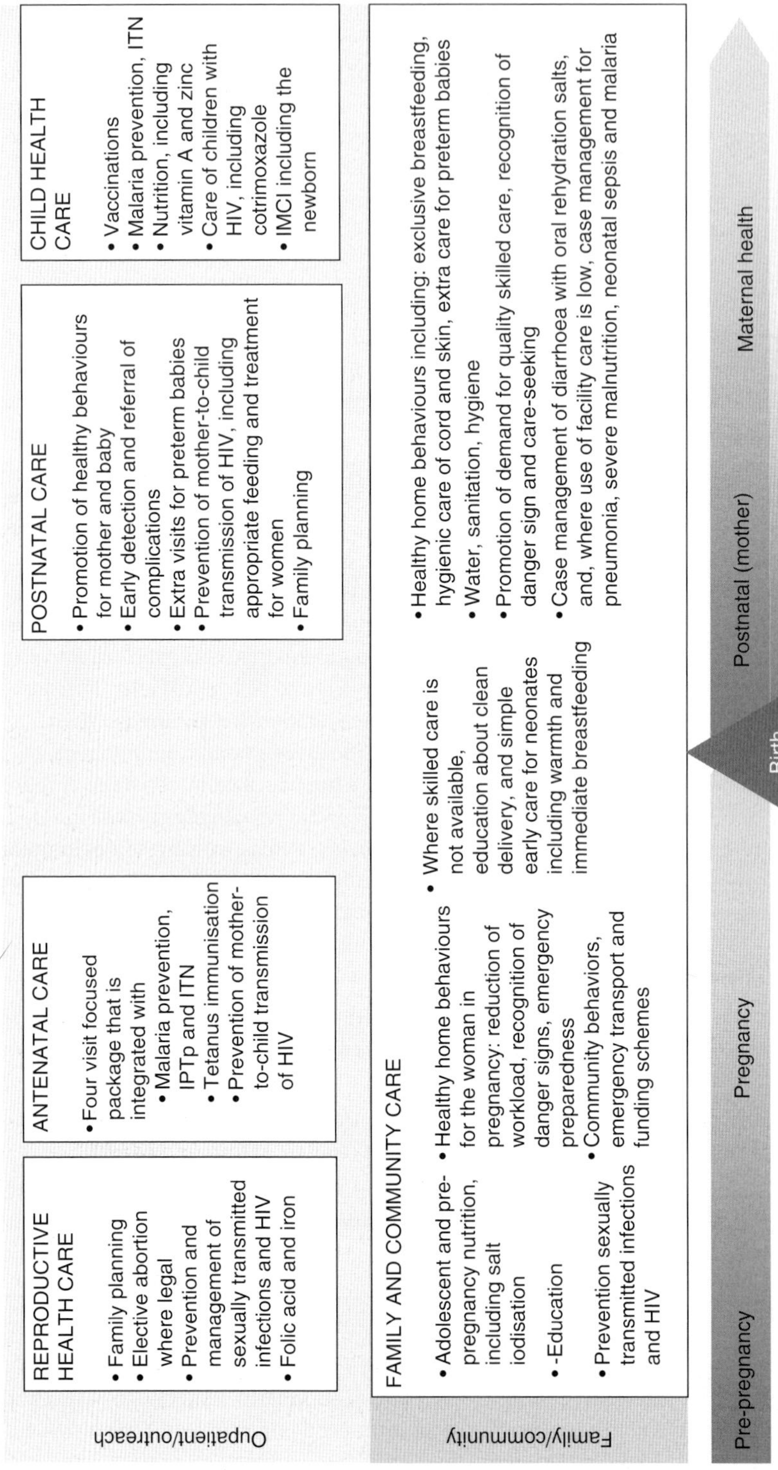

Fig. 11.8 Recommended Packages for continuum of care in PHC settings.
(Bhutta ZA Lancet 2008, adapted from Kerber et al. Lancet 2007.)

School education and health

School education curricula and books in many countries include health and family life (including sex education). This is very important to improve MNCH (see also Chapter 8, 'Health promotion'). In some countries nurses regularly visit schools to treat minor ailments and treat children for contagious diseases such as head lice and scabies. The schools health service is an opportunity to provide age-appropriate health education on various issues, from nutrition to sexual health. Children may pass on their knowledge to their parents and to younger siblings. In the **child-to-child** programme, booklets designed for reading practice health and hygiene topics also include. Children are encouraged to talk about this information to their brothers and sisters (and parents!). The national curriculum should include health topics and health material should be integrated into the course books. Children can be trained as **peer educators** on sexual health issues in countries with HIV. They can be encouraged to form health or anti-AIDS clubs.

The 'safe talk' programme of Uganda distributes newspapers to schools. These incorporate sexual, reproductive, and general health information. They include letters sent in by the children and adolescent readers. As a result they are highly popular and informative.

Nursery and primary school age children have the highest levels of worm infestation. Heavy infestations contribute to under-nutrition and reduce learning potential. Mass treatment, often done in schools, has been shown to be effective in reducing worm loads. The drugs albendazole and praziquantel are very safe and can be given to all children on a regular basis. Mass treatment should be combined with hygiene education, and ensuring the adequate provision of toilets, water, and soap.

Health promotion

Health promotion should be based on an analysis of the existing situation. The health-promotion intervention should specify the target group, and the setting (such as households, communities, schools, or health facilities). The content may include information about exclusive breastfeeding, weaning practices, good eating during pregnancy, and lactation and other MNCH/ family planning issues. The health promotion plan should specify the communication methods, such as the mass media, community groups, or health workers (see Chapter 8). As with other components of MNCH, the health promotion interventions should be monitored and evaluated.

Setting priorities according to the local situation

The process of setting priorities for MNCH and family planning starts from a review of the existing situation. This review should take into account the needs and demands of the community and the limitations of the existing services. Then, options for intervention strategies can be reviewed and decisions made on the best course of action in the circumstances. That is, the priority interventions for MNCH and family planning depend on the existing setting (see Chapter 4). For example, in an **isolated setting**, such as in much of South Asia, sub-Saharan Africa, and the Andean region of South America, there is no care or information available for many women. The priority in that case will be to expand delivery of MNCH/family planning services, as well as to ensure that hospitals are able to provide emergency obstetric care such as blood transfusion and caesarean sections.

Where there are **existing services** in health centres and hospitals with trained staff, as is the case for much of southern Africa, Central America, and Southeast Asia, the priority is to coordinate primary and secondary services in order to deliver improved quality of MNCH/family planning and emergency obstetric care services.

In **urban and peri-urban** areas with quite well developed but overloaded public and private health facilities, the priority is to decentralize MNCH/family planning and to redirect women to the appropriate level of care. It is also important to ensure that primary-care services are available in the peri-urban slums.

Community-based family planning and maternity services

Projects in several developing countries have contributed to our knowledge of strategies for effective (or ineffective) safe motherhood programmes. As an example we describe here the findings of such a project in a rural sub-district of Bangladesh:

It was found that the maternal mortality had declined substantially over the past 10 years. This was due to effective community-based **family planning** services which reduced the maternal mortality rate by about one-third (primarily by decreasing the total number of pregnancies) and an effective community-based **maternity care** intervention which reduced the risk of dying once pregnant by two-thirds. Midwives, backed up by a referral system, assisted women during pregnancy and with delivery in their homes, if requested. They provided prenatal care, carried supplies to stabilize or treat women with complications (for example antibiotics, sedatives, infusions and plasma expanders and pitocin to be administered intranasally), and had access to transport and referral services in cases which they were unable to manage.

Such results show that we need to ensure women's access to:

◆ Family planning services and appropriate abortion management (appropriate treatment for complications of unsafe abortion and, where legal, safe services for termination of pregnancy)

◆ Skilled assistance available quickly during pregnancy, labour, delivery, and the post-partum period

◆ Referral services and transport for pregnancy-related complications and emergencies

◆ Communication to promote positive health, nutrition and family planning practices, and especially to recognize danger signs during pregnancy, labour, delivery, and post-natally, and to respond with utilization of the appropriate services.

Population and family planning

Family planning is one of the most effective interventions for health. Providing family planning services is the easiest way to reduce maternal mortality.

Pregnancy is more risky for older women, where they have had many previous pregnancies. Pregnancy is more risky for teenage women who are are more likely to resort to induced abortion, or if they have the child, are likely to lose out on their educational opportunities. For these reasons, services must be provided to all people who are sexually active, including the young and the unmarried. Reproductive health (including family planning services and information) is recognized internationally as a right for all couples. But for a large part of the developing world these rights have yet to become a reality. Though most countries have positive population and family planning policies, in practice, for many, these services are not very accessible or acceptable. The result is an *unmet need* for family planning. Unmet need is defined as women of fertile age who wish to postpone (space) or stop childbearing, but are not using a contraceptive method, as a percent of all fertile age women. Using this definition, around 25% of women in developing countries have an unmet need for family planning.

Demographic change

Over the past century, improvements in agriculture, health, and hygiene have caused death rates to reduce dramatically. All populations have seen reductions in their fertility rates, but in some countries, rates remain relatively high. Populations in most developing countries have risen hugely in the last century. In western countries and newly industrialized countries such as South Korea, people now have small families and the proportion of children in the population is much less compared to the working adult population. With further demographic change, population sizes in these countries are stabilizing. In western countries, such as in Europe, the number of children per couple is on average around 1.5. The number of births now roughly equals the number of deaths. See Chapter 1, for the effects of the demographic transition and epidemiological transition. An increasingly elderly population puts pressure on social and health services (not forgetting that high numbers of children put pressure on education, health, and social services).

Population pressure

In developing countries the population is growing less quickly than a few decades ago, but is still growing rapidly. In many low-income countries, such as in sub-Saharan Africa and South Asia, much of the land is dry or regularly suffers droughts. In these countries most of the available potential agricultural land is already being farmed. People are forced by pressure of population to clear and plant in dry and marginal land, which was previously used for grazing. This land suffers drought and soil is blown away. Sometimes there are conflicts between agricultural and pastoral peoples in these countries, and this can contribute to civil unrest and conflict. Food production seems to have peaked globally and food prices have risen.

Where population rises and land pressure is high, the 'surplus' population either migrate across borders (though the opportunity to do so is increasingly limited by governments), or migrate to the cities. Some get formal paid jobs, but in most low-income countries the growth of the economy hasn't absorbed the increasing numbers looking for a job. In the cities most people survive day-to-day in informal and insecure work. Most live in the peri-urban slums. Levels of malnutrition in rural and urban areas may be very high. Food aid is provided for a few, with supplies targeted to people 'internally displaced' or refugees due to conflict. As populations rise, the risk of hunger increases, especially in dry years.

Population pressure is also contributing to climate change. Human activities such as energy production, transport, cattle production, and rice growing have increased the levels of greenhouse gases (for example, carbon dioxide and methane) in the atmosphere. The sun warms the earth and heat is reflected back into the sky. But increasing levels of greenhouse gases reflects and 'traps' this heat. Though there is a small change in the temperature, there is a larger change in the climate. A major effect in much of the world is that the rains have become unpredictable making it difficult for farmers. There are more frequent drought years.

In some countries, such as Malawi, where populations continue to rise, land pressure is high, industrial growth is slow and people are less able to migrate to other countries for work, they may become demographically 'trapped'. Dry-land countries with an even higher population growth rate, such as Niger, are in a more dangerous situation (Cleland 2007). Even agricultural productive countries, where fertility remains high, such as Uganda, are threatened (see Box 11.3). In contrast, due to commitment to their population policy and family planning efforts, Kenya's fertility has decreased by 40% in recent decades.

Demand for family planning

As mentioned above, the unmet need for family planning is sizeable in many developing countries. Unmet need includes women who either wish to postpone their next birth (spacers) or wish to stop childbearing altogether (limiters) but are not using a contraceptive method.

Our first responsibility is to reduce unmet need of family planning by providing family-planning services alongside health services. In addition there is a need to make information available about

Box 11.3 Unmet need and population pressure in Uganda

In Uganda:

- There is a lack of government commitment to family planning
- Over half of married women report an unmet need for family planning
- Only 14% of married women use a modern method
- 50% of pregnancies in Uganda are unplanned
- Women say the reason is they lack access to facilities and supplies
- Medical stores and health workers do not prioritize family planning
- Stockouts of contraceptives in health facilities are common
- Women average 7 children, but want 'only' 5 (their husbands want 5 or 6)
- Abortion is illegal, but around 300 000 (mainly unsafe) occur annually
- Maternal mortality is one of the highest in the world at 500–1200 per 100 000 live births
- Population growth continues at 3.3% per annum
- Population is doubling in less than two decades
- Land is in increasingly short supply in much of the country
- Malnutrition is very common and child mortality is very high.

family planning. Many people know about the existence of some methods, but not others. They may have heard of a method, but don't know how it works. For example, they may have limited understanding of their own anatomy, and fear that an 'Intrauterine contraceptive device (IUCD) can get lost inside themselves. They may believe misinformed rumours that condoms don't work (they are close to 100% effective both in preventing pregnancy and HIV/ STIs – if consistently and properly used). They may not understand 'emergency contraception', which are hormone pills, containing the same hormones as oral contraceptive pills.

There are various health-promotion approaches that apply to family planning as for other health interventions, (see Chapter 8). Behaviour change communication is most likely to be effective if there are various approaches used. These include:

- Family life education in the schools, including on sexuality, contraception etc.
- Peer education for in-school and out-of-school youth
- Radio and TV information, best including family-planning issues and messages within drama series
- Newspapers, posters, bill board messages
- Health worker group or individual health education

> Couples should have 'children by choice rather than by chance'.

Contraceptive methods

A major element of quality in family planning is the availability of a range of contraceptive methods, the method mix. A mix of methods should be made available so that couples can choose the method that suits them best.

Oral contraceptive pills, condoms, injectables, and longer acting methods such as IUCD (sometimes called a coil') are examples of methods that are suitable for couples who want to *space* their children. Spacing gives the woman time to recover from her previous pregnancy, and gives time enough for the physical care and emotional development of the existing child.

Method mix

Permanent methods such as vasectomy and tubal ligation are ideal for when a couple have reached their desired family size. That is, they allow a couple to *limit* their family size. In some, e.g. African countries men need to be reassured that vasectomy will not affect their masculinity.

Short Acting Methods include condoms and the combined oestrogen and progesterone (combined) pills, which are the most effective. Also progesterone only pills which are less effective but are especially useful for women who are breast feeding.

Longer acting reversible contraceptive methods are suitable for most women and popular when made widely available. These include:

- IUCDs; including copper or progesterone containing IUCDs which are more effective than regular IUCDs.
- Injections of progesterone, such as depo-provera (DMPA) or NET-EN
- Implants of progesterone (e.g. implanor)

Any progesterone contraceptive methods may give irregular bleeding, no bleeding or persistent bleeding. Advice that if these occur they usually settle down after a few months. They cause low mood or sex drive in some women. If side effects persist or are a problem, then change to another method. IUCDs can cause also pain in some women.

Counselling

Counselling is a two-way discussion between the provider and the clients, and is a very important skill. This combines providing information e.g. about the advantages and disadvantages of a range of contraceptive methods, together with helping clients to make *their* own **informed choice** about which method suits them at their stage of life. In this way family planning counselling leads to more satisfaction and less discontinuation of use. Clients will know about the possible side-effects of their chosen method, and will not be afraid and stop use unnecessarily. For example, if they choose an injectable contraceptive such as Depo-Provera they will know about the possibility of irregular or absent periods or a delay in return of fertility. However if side effects are a problem or she wishes to switch for other reasons, then discuss, choose and start another method without delay.

Emergency contraception contain a progesterone called levonorgestrel. This can be as a special pack with pills containing 1.5g to be taken at once or by taking levonorgestrel contraceptive pills with a total dose of 1.5mg pills can work for up to five days after unprotected sex because the sperm are in the woman's body for a number of days before it reaches and fertilizes the ovum ('egg'). It is best taken within these three days, when the hormones in emergency contraception will usually stop the ovum from being fertilized by the sperm. The earlier the emergency contraception is taken, the more likely it is to be effective. Because speed is so important, the method should be easily accessible. The method is very safe. For these reasons, in countries such as the UK, emergency contraceptives are being made available 'over-the-counter' in pharmacies (drug shops), as well as from all health centres.

Introducing new methods

Introducing new methods improve choice. Furthermore, the well publicized introduction of a new method will increase demand for contraception.

Currently there is wide variation in which contraceptives are known, trusted and used, largely due to the emphasis given by family programmes in the past. For example, in Africa, commonly oral contraceptive pills and condoms are the best known and used methods, whereas in Vietnam the IUD is the most used method. In South Asia and the UK, vasectomy is common, while in Africa it is currently rarely prompted or accepted. However, it is possible to introduce and promote new methods, as has occurred with injectables e.g. Depo-provera, which are now popular in most countries.

New methods should be introduced where choice is currently limited. For example, community health worker programmes usually provide oral contraceptive pills and condoms, and refer for other methods. But other methods can be added for community-based distribution by CHWs. For example, the Lady Health Workers of Pakistan have been trained to give injectables, so improving access in the rural areas and slums to this popular method.

Delivery of family planning services

Together with other MNCH services family planning need to be delivered in a number of ways in order to meet the needs of different urban, rural, rich, poor and other groups. The family planning services which are delivered should be accessible, acceptable, affordable and of good quality. Contraceptive methods and family planning services are commonly oriented towards women. However, the needs of men may require particular attention. Special services may be needed to reach minority and hard to reach groups and organizations such as the military. In addition, 'youth-friendly' services are provided where they are most accessible to young women and men. They are informal and non-medicalized (no white uniforms) so as to be less 'off-putting'. They are provided in confidence (young people are encouraged but not required to inform their parents). Because these young people are already sexually active, contraception helps prevent pregnancy, and avoid interruption of a girl's education.

Approaches to service delivery include the following:

- General health centre and hospital services
- Specialist family planning clinics
- Community-based distribution
- Social marketing
- Private practitioners

General health centre and hospital services

Family planning may be provided separately, or even on a different day from other MNCH services. However, family planning is more accessible and acceptable if provided as part of an integrated MNCH service — as in the integrated 'supermarket' approach described in Box 11.1 above. Provision through integrated daily MNCH clinics requires adaptation of procedures and additional training. However, this will increase access and will help avoid missed opportunities to provide family planning information and contraceptives to women attending for other reasons. For example, in a region of Ethiopia, family planning was made available as part of a daily integrated MNCH service in all health centres. Within a year, the level of contraceptive use had increased by 260 percent.

Governmental and non-governmental organizations (NGOs) provide these services. Access, however, is variable depending on the geographical distance to the facility from a woman's home and waiting times. Acceptability varies according to factors such as privacy and the sympathetic manner of the health worker trained in counselling. This should be a two-way dialogue, which helps the couple to choose the method, and informs them about the method. A problem with MNCH facilities is that they do not reach men as easily as women, whereas research shows that counselling the husband and wife together results in a more sustained use of family-planning methods. Services need to be made accessible and be promoted to men as well as women.

Specialist family planning clinics

Specialist family planning clinics are operated separately from the general health services. Commonly this is by national family planning associations or NGOs such as affiliates of Marie Stopes International. They have the disadvantage that women have to visit these clinics separately from other MNCH services and the clinics are usually available only in the towns. On the other hand, they often provide a high-quality service with a wide choice of methods, privacy, and individual counselling. They may also provide safe abortion services. For example, the Bangladesh Women's Coalition is a local NGO which operates clinics in the capital Dhaka. They provide abortion, contraception and other MNCH services. The clinic stresses individual and couple counselling and informed choice. Three out of four women who have an abortion leave with contraceptives. Some organizations, such as Marie Stopes, provide similar services, together with tubal ligation and vasectomy services. These may be "franchised" to private providers to provide a form of public–private partnership.

Community-based distribution

Community-based distributors (CBDs)are local residents who have a few days' training to distribute contraceptives (usually condoms and oral contraceptives) within communities. Distributors may or may not get a fixed salary. If not, they may be allowed to retain a percentage of their sales and often receive various non-monetary incentives. In Zimbabwe and Colombia, for example, there has been extensive coverage using community-based distribution which contributed to a high prevalence of contraceptive use. Various studies have shown that community-based distribution does not introduce additional health risks. However, community-based distribution requires well-organized supervision systems, and on-going training of new distributors. The CBDs may be trained to give emergency contraceptive pills and/or injectables. They refer clients to other family-planning providers for permanent methods such as vasectomy and tubal ligation. Some countries have community health worker programmes, where the trained women provide family planning as well as other MNCH and preventive and promotive services (see Chapter 10, 'District health services').

Social marketing

Social marketing uses commercial channels and techniques such as market research and advertising to distribute subsidized contraceptives (and other health products such as bednets). Sponsoring agencies may be the ministry of health, donors, and non-profit agencies, such as the family planning association. Condoms and oral contraceptive pills are sold. This implementation strategy is used in the more extensive programmes in Bangladesh, Colombia, and Egypt and serves more than 30% of current users. Pharmacies are the major outlet, but small convenience shops and even market traders have been effective in Ghana, Nigeria, and Peru. Social marketing is the cheapest of the approaches, at about US$2 per couple year of protection.

Social marketing of condoms is a major strategy for control of HIV. A well-known example is in the Congo, where condoms are widely available through shops and vendors. The condom brand name is 'Prudence' and the logo on the packet is a black panther. In Pakistan they are called "Sathi" meaning "Shield". Social marketing also used for other health products such as bednets, however, cannot supply methods such as IUDs or sterilization, which require the skills of health workers.

Private practitioners

Private practitioners (for-profit providers) provide curative services that are accessible and credible to customers. Doctors and other practitioners, can provide family-planning services. In Indonesia, for example, the government has encouraged contraceptive supply through private practitioners by training them, and actively promoting these services through the media. However, because of fees, the service may not be affordable to the very poor.

A mix of these service delivery strategies will be required to ensure coverage of the various demographic and socio-economic groups in both urban and rural areas.

Ensure quality of MNCH services

The most comprehensive and perhaps the simplest definition of quality is 'doing the right thing in the right way, right away'.

Quality control of MNCH services, as for other components of the health service, requires a periodic review of the situation. The structure, process, and outcomes of services can be assessed to identify problems and solutions. Improvements in the structure and process will then lead to improved outcomes as shown in Table 11.2, and also the quality control section in Chapter 16. This may identify missed opportunities for prevention if for example, adult and children's curative and preventive services are provided separately. As a result, the mother has to walk long distances to obtain treatment for a child sick with a respiratory infection, only to be told to come back on another day for vaccination, pre-natal care, or family planning.

Improvements in staff competence and performance in facilities and in the process of care will lead to, client satisfaction (feeling happy with the service), and attendance (utilization of services), as well as contributing to better physical and mental health.

MNCH services are commonly provided by multi-purpose health workers, who also provide care for children, adults and pregnant women. Quality care is facilitated through the use of evidence-based guidelines. For MNCH the WHO packages of integrated care include IMCI, IMAI, and the 'pregnancy, childbirth, post-partum and newborn care' guide.

New interventions, such as 'emergency contraception,' may need to be introduced. The review and choice of the best interventions is covered in Chapter 5. New delivery strategies may need to be piloted initially in one health facility and then replicated. (The MNCH continuum of care is part of the district health system. See Chapter 10, which describes the roles of community health workers, health centres and hospitals as part of district health services).

Good planning and management is required to implement and maintain the quality of MNCH services. See Chapter 6, which includes sections on training, supervision and a case study on the implementation of integrated MNCH services in Ethiopia. Changing the health-seeking

Table 11.2 Structure, process, and outcome: The way to improve service

Structure	Process	Outcome
Range of services	Information Given	Patient attendance
Human resources	Competence	Health status
Physical facilities	Client-provider interaction	Client satisfaction
Supervision	Continuity of care	
Record-keeping	Access	

behaviour and care practices of pregnant women and those with sick children requires effective health promotion (Chapter 8).

Conclusion

MNCH services, including family planning, have the potential to reduce by one-third the overall burden of disease in developing countries. Child health includes vaccination, nutrition, interventions and the IMCI package. Maternal and neonatal health depends on the provision of essential obstetric care and avoiding delays in seeking care, reaching skilled care and receiving quality care. There are both technical and organizational issues to consider when developing MNCH services. IMCI is key to the quality of diagnosis and treatment of illness and counselling of parents. If attention is also given to the organizational efficiency of clinics, then time will be available for providing essential preventative interventions, including offering family planning. The strengthening of MNCH delivery provides the foundation for other district health activities.

Further reading

Bhutta, Z.A., Ahmed, T., Black, R.E. et al. (2008) 'What works? Interventions for maternal and child undernutrition and survival' *Lancet*, **361(9351)**, 2226–34.

Bhutta, Z.A., Ali, S., Cousens, S. et al. (2008) Interventions to address maternal, newborn and child survival: What difference can integrated primary health care strategies make? *Lancet*, **372**, 972–89.

Bulatao, R. (1993). *Effective family planning programmes*. World Bank: Washington.

UNICEF (2008). *The state of the world's children* 2008. ISBN 978-92 806-4192-2. www.unicef.org. http://www.unicef.org/sowc08/docs/sowc08.pdf

UNICEF (2008). 'Countdown to 2015' *Maternal, neonatal and child survival: tracking progress in maternal, newborn and child survival*. http://www.childinfo.org/countdown.html

WHO (1994). *Contraceptive method mix: guidelines for policy and service delivery*. Geneva: World Health Organization.

WHO/ RH/ 08.17. Medical Eligibility Criteria for Contraceptive use. http://www.who.int/reproductive-health/publications/mec/mec_update_2008.pdf

WHO (2002). *Selective Practice Recommendations for Contraceptive use,* 2002, second edition 2004, and update 2008 http://www.who.int/reproductive-health/publications/spr/spr_2008_update.pdf

WHO (1999). IMCI *information: information sheets on integrated management of childhood illness*, WHO/CHS/CAH/98.1A to M. Geneva: World Health Organization.

WHO (2003) *Kangaroo Mother Care a practical guide*. WHO Geneva. http://www.who.int/reproductive-health/publications/kmc/

WHO, United Nations Population Fund, UNICEF, The World Bank (2003) *Managing complications in pregnancy and childbirth*. WHO Geneva http://www.who.int/making_pregnancy_safer/documents/9241545879/en/index.html

WHO 2005. *World Health Report 2005 - make every woman and child count'*. WHO: Geneva. http://www.who.int/whr/2005/en/index.html

World Health Organization, United Nations Population Fund, UNICEF, The World Bank (2006) *Pregnancy, childbirth, postpartum and newborn care A guide for essential practice*. WHO Geneva http://www.who.int/making_pregnancy_safer/documents/924159084x/en/index.html

WHO and John Hopkins INFO project. Family planning: a global handbook for providers www.infohealth.org/globalhandbook

WHO child health information and documents including IMCI and pocketbook of hospital care for children. www.int/topics/child_health/en

Chapter 12

Essential drugs

Kathleen Holloway

This chapter gives an overview of the following topics:

◆ The Essential Medicines Concept and its practical implications

◆ Medicine supply and access to medicines

◆ Promoting the rational use of medicines

◆ Medicine regulation and ensuring the quality of medicines

◆ The role of government in the pharmaceutical sector

Introduction: How medicines fit into public health – a responsibility at all levels

This chapter has been written because the efficient management of essential medicines is a condition for the successful functioning of health systems at all levels. Despite spending about 20% of their limited overall health budgets on medicines, many developing countries are unable to deliver health services for their people. Safe, effective, and affordable pharmaceutical products are fundamental to public health, yet at present at least a third of the world's population lacks access to even the most basic medicines.

Where medicines are available they may be poorly managed, so that scarce resources are wasted. In addition, medicines are frequently mis-prescribed, dispensed without adequate information, and improperly used, so that they cannot contribute to good health outcomes. Finally, the quality of medicines in many countries too often fails to meet international standards.

As threats to global public health continue to evolve, national strategies to cope with the resurgence of tuberculosis, the widening impact of malaria, and HIV/AIDS and its related conditions depend on organized health and pharmaceutical services. Disease organisms are increasingly resistant to affordable, simple antibiotics, and treatments for the common infections, including pneumonia and *shigella*, are often no longer effective. Public health has reached crisis point in many countries. Never has it been more important, or more difficult, to concentrate scarce resources on a list of medicines that meet national needs, and to manage and use these well.

For more than two decades WHO has provided leadership, technical support and a conceptual framework – the essential medicines concept (EMC) – to help governments and health institutions to manage medicines in their health services. In 1977 the first Model List of Essential Medicines (Drugs) was produced, enabling governments to match their medicine needs to the prevailing health priorities with available resources. By the end of 2003, 113 countries had national lists, and where these had been implemented, they had been shown to reduce costs and to lead to safer medicine use.

Health professionals at all levels need to understand and implement the general principles which govern the management and rational use of medicines. These principles include the following core components:

- Medicine selection and the essential medicines (drug) concept
- Access
- Appropriate prescribing and use
- Quality and regulation
- Government policy

Medicine selection and the essential medicines concept

Advantages of using fewer medicines

The core premise of the essential medicines concept is that a limited range of carefully selected medicines leads to a better supply of medicines, more rational prescribing and lower costs. Essential medicines are defined by WHO in 2003 as:

> those medicines that satisfy the priority health care needs of the population. They are selected with due regard to disease prevalence, evidence of efficacy, safety and comparative cost-effectiveness. They are intended to be available within the context of functioning health systems at all times in adequate amounts, in the appropriate dosage forms, with assured quality and adequate information, and at a price the individual and the community can afford. The implementation of the concept of essential medicines is intended to be adaptable to many different situations; exactly which medicines are regarded as essential remains a national responsibility.

The advantages of reducing the number of medicines in a pharmaceutical system may be summarized as follows:

Medicine supply

- easier procurement, storage and distribution
- more focussed, and hence better, quality assurance
- better dispensing, since dispensers can gain greater familiarity with fewer medicine items.

Prescribing

- fewer products to be taught and learnt
- better quality prescribing with fewer medicines
- improved medicine information, better used
- easier recognition of adverse medicine (drug) reactions
- less use of irrational alternative medicines

Patient use

- more focused education strategies leading to increased patient understanding
- better adherence since patients may benefit from fewer medicine items and more helpful guidance from those in charge of dispensing

Costs

- cheaper medicines: Essential medicines are usually available in generic form, from multiple suppliers, so allowing increased competition and negotiation of lower prices
- economies of scale since fewer items can be procured in greater bulk

- reduced storage and distribution costs
- reduced costs of providing medicine information when fewer items are involved

Practical implications of the Essential Medicines Concept (EMC)

Fundamental to the adoption of the EMC is the development of a limited list of essential medicines. In order for any list to be credible and accepted by prescribers and other health workers, explicit criteria must be defined and published. The experience of hospital formulary committees has shown that involving prescribers and others in the process of selection will help to increase acceptability.

In 1995 WHO defined the following criteria for including a medicine in an essential medicines list:

- Relevance to the pattern of prevalent diseases, the treatment facilities and the training of personnel
- Proven quality (including bioavailability and stability in the anticipated storage conditions), efficacy, and safety
- Evidence of performance in a variety of settings
- Relative effectiveness: When two medicines appear to be similar, the choice between them should be made in terms of their relative quality, safety, efficacy, price and availability
- Evidence of cost effectiveness in a variety of settings
- Relative cost benefit: When comparing the costs between two medicines, what is the cost of total treatment, not just the unit cost of the medicine
- Preference for medicines that are well known, with desirable pharmacokinetic properties and possibilities for local manufacture
- Single compounds except in defined circumstances, such as the use of combination medicines in TB, HIV/AIDS, malaria and leprosy
- Generic (International Non-proprietary Name – INN) name, not the brand name chosen by the specific manufacturer

Within all health care systems facilities exist at different levels. These include pharmacy shops, primary health care facilities, district hospitals and tertiary referral hospitals. The medicines lists for each of these different facilities must be appropriate to the training of the staff working in them. Figure 12.1 illustrates this principle.

No country has all the medicines in the world freely available in its domestic market. Thus it must be decided which medicines will be (1) registered for use, (2) available over-the-counter or with prescription, (3) available for use in the public sector (often known as the national essential medicine list in developing countries or the reimbursement list in developed countries), and (4) available in different types of facility. Within these lists, individual facilities and hospitals may agree to choose their own more limited lists.

It is important to note that graded lists of essential medicines are not an end in themselves. In addition other management tools such as standard treatment guidelines and formularies, consistent with the essential medicine lists, will be needed to reinforce the correct use of those medicines which have been identified and included.

Medicine information and the formulary process

The procedures to develop an essential medicines list, a formulary and standard treatment guidelines are together called the formulary process. As with an essential medicine list, standard treatment

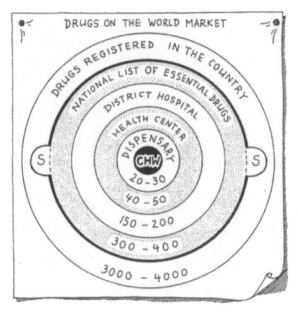

Fig. 12.1 The essential medicines target Legend: CHW means Community Health Worker.
Source: Managing Drug Supply, 1997, Kumarian Press, ISBN: 1-56549-047-9.

guidelines and formularies may be targeted to the different levels of health care. It can often be difficult to get all those involved to agree on the most appropriate treatments for specific clinical conditions, and consequently on which medicines should be included in an essential medicine list. Basing decisions upon medical evidence can help to overcome this problem.

Standard treatment guidelines are disease-oriented and include information on diagnostic criteria, treatment of first choice, important side-effects, contraindications, referral criteria, and also medicine information for the patient. Sometimes, if there are alternatives and the guidelines are regularly updated, they may include information on the cost of treatment. Standard treatment guidelines, protocols and prescribing policies are all terms used to indicate 'systematically developed statements to help practitioners or prescribers to make decisions about appropriate treatments for specific clinical conditions.' (Managing Drug Supply 1997).

Evaluations of treatment guidelines have found that clinical guidelines are significantly associated with improvements in the process of care and patient outcomes if accompanied by other measures, such as training, to improve the use of medicines.

Formularies contain summary medicine information on a selection of medicines. They are medicine-orientated and information is usually organized in therapeutic groups. Formularies include information about each medicine (generic name, dosage forms, indications, pharmacological information, contraindications, precautions, side-effects, dosage schedule, instructions and warnings, and medicine interactions). Other information may include price, level of use, whether it is available over-the-counter or by prescription, storage guidelines, patient counselling information, brand names, rational prescribing, dispensing guidelines and special requirements for controlled medicine prescriptions (narcotics). The British National Formulary is an example of a comprehensive medicine formulary that also contains clinical advice.

Figure 12.2 summarizes how an essential medicines list, standard treatment guidelines and formularies should run parallel, contributing to improved availability and more rational use of medicines.

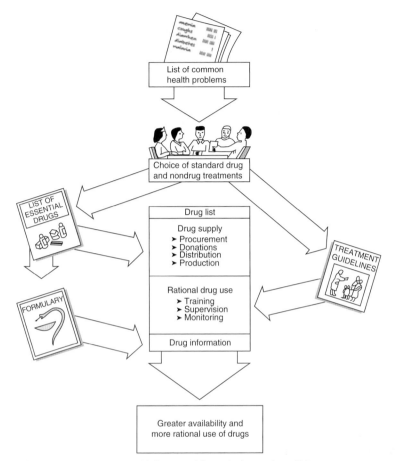

Fig. 12.2 Medicine lists, treatment guidelines and formularies and medicine use.

Source: Managing Drug Supply, 1997, Kumarian Press, ISBN: 1-56549-047-9.

The advantages of rational medicine use and greater availability will only be realized if the medicine lists, treatment guidelines, and formularies are, in fact, used by health professionals. Distribution of these documents alone will not achieve the required goals. Training and supervision, together with support from the regulatory authorities, are necessary in order to achieve change (see Box 12.1).

Objective medicine information is provided in standard treatment guidelines and formularies. Other sources of unbiased information include technical journals (medical and therapeutic, pharmacology, specialist medical), medicine and toxicology information and medicine bulletins. Medicine information centres supported by government and academic institutions have a critical role to play in providing up-to-date, unbiased and comparative information to providers, and sometimes also for consumers. Often, however, the only information available about a particular medicine is produced by the medicine company itself, and thus, by definition, is non-comparative. Prescribers and other users should be aware that manufacturers' promotional medicine information may not be approved by the country's regulatory authority; may not include references to the literature, or comparisons of cost, efficacy or safety with other medicines; and may underplay side-effects and over-play efficacy and safety. In many countries the

Box 12.1 Impact of treatment guidelines in Uganda 1996

A randomized controlled trial to test the impact of standard treatment guidelines plus training and supervision on rational prescribing was carried out in Uganda.

Prescribing quality, as judged by the percentage of prescriptions conforming to standard treatment guidelines, did not improve when only guidelines were disseminated, but greatly improved if dissemination of the guidelines was accompanied by training and supervision.

Group	Percantage Pxs conforming to STG
1. Control group	24.8→ 29.9% (+5.1%)
2. Dissemination of STG	24.8→ 32.3% (+7.5%)
3. STG + on-site training in therapeutic problems	24.0→ 52.0% (+28.0%)
4. STG + on-site training in therapeutic problems + 4 supervisory visits in 6 months	21.4→ 55.2% (+33.8%)
STG = standard treatment guidelines	Pxs = prescriptions

Source: Kafuko J, Zirabumuzale C, Bagenda D, (1994) UNICEF Uganda 1996.

only source of information that prescribers receive is from the pharmaceutical industry who spent nearly 20 billion US$ in 2004 in the USA alone on promotional activities. This is more than many poor countries spent on their entire health budget.

Access

Access to essential medicines has been defined as 'a basic range of essential medicines available at an affordable price within one hour's travelling time.'

Whether essential (as opposed to non-essential) medicines are physically present in the various medicine outlets (Fig. 12.3) such as health facilities and pharmacies, (geographic or supply access), is dependent upon four factors.

1 Rational Selection of medicines (see above)

2 Affordable Prices (financial access)

Can patients afford to pay for medicines from facilities? It may be that, though medicines are physically present, the patients cannot afford the fees charged for the medicines they need, or that patients lack the resources to attend facilities which are situated too far from their homes.

3 Sustainable Financing (financial access)

Is the money available within the health system sufficient to cover the cost of the medicines? This will depend on the system of health financing: the proportion of money paid by governments from taxes, and by patients in fees. Insufficient contribution of funding from governments will result in overly high prices for patients or non-availability of medicines.

4 Reliable health and supply systems (supply access)

Are medicines reliably supplied to health facilities and are there sufficient trained staff and diagnostic equipment to use the medicines safely and effectively? This will depend on medicine supply and distribution systems and also whether there are sufficient finances for procurement, storage, distribution, equipment, and health personnel.

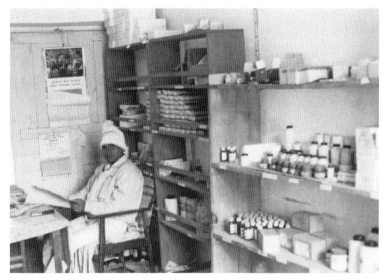

Fig. 12.3 A district drug store.

Access and the management of medicine supply

Procurement – encompasses quantification of medicine requirements, inventory management, the tender process, contracting for medicines and services, quality assurance, small-scale local production, and medicine donations.

Distribution – encompasses importation and port clearance, medical stores management, the management of medicines for health facilities, planning and building storage facilities, transport management and kit system management.

Medicine procurement

Procurement is the process of acquiring supplies from private or public suppliers, or through purchasing directly from manufacturers, distributors or international agencies, or through bilateral aid programmes.

Procurement in both public and private sectors includes most of the decisions and actions that determine which medicines are purchased in what quantities, how much is paid for them, and whether they are of satisfactory quality.

Medicine procurement is an important factor in determining total medicine costs. It is necessary to have policies in place to ensure efficient procurement in the public sector, and policies can also be beneficial in the private sector.

The major procurement methods are open tender, restricted tender, competitive negotiation, and direct procurement. The training and experience of staff in the procurement office may dictate which of these methods is used, and the choice of procurement method may affect the price and delivery times.

In the public sector, systematic tendering procedures with pre-qualification of suppliers have been found to be successful. Supplier pre-qualification is a process whereby product quality, service reliability – including delivery time – and financial viability are considered. The process of evaluating new suppliers can include formal registration, reference checks with past clients and international agencies, and test purchases of small quantities of the products required.

Effective medicine procurement ensures the availability of the most cost-effective medicines in the right quantities, at high quality standards, and at the lowest possible total cost. (see Box 12.2)

The main principles of good medicine procurement are:

- Procurement by generic name
- Procurement based on an essential medicines list or reimbursement list or formulary list
- Reliable methods of quantification of medicine needs
- procurement in bulk
- Formal supplier qualification and monitoring
- Product quality assurance
- Competitive procurement
- Transparency and annual audit
- Reporting based on performance indicators
- Reliable payment and good financial management
- System to recall defective products.

Once tenders have come in and have been compared and suppliers selected, attention should also be paid to the management of the rest of the procurement process. This includes:

- Specifying contract terms
- Monitoring order status
- Receiving the delivery, provision of receipts and inspection of medicines
- Making payments.

It is very important that the procurement process is managed efficiently and transparently, 'different functions and responsibilities (selection, quantification, product specification, pre-selection of suppliers and adjudication of tenders) should be divided among different offices, committees and individuals, each with the appropriate expertise and resources for the specific function' (WHO 1999).

Medicine storage and distribution

Storage and distribution include the activities needed to ensure that medicines arrive at all levels of the health care system in good condition, at the right time and with minimal wastage. In order to reach this goal technical staff must be trained in medicine identification, packing, store maintenance, stock-keeping and quality control. They must also competently undertake inventory control and the provision of information on consumption rates which are necessary to accurately forecast future medicine needs and budgets. A combination of public and private initiatives may be the most effective means of distributing medicines to meet the needs of the majority of the population, including those in remote areas.

An effective storage and distribution system will:

- Maintain supplies of all necessary medicines
- Keep medicines in good condition
- Minimize under and overstocking
- Minimize losses due to expiry
- Minimize losses due to theft
- Provide information on consumption to forecast future requirements
- Ensure the timely delivery of consignments.

Medicine donations

Medicines are frequently donated by international organizations as a response to an emergency situation or as part of a development project. Inappropriate medicine donations – sometimes in very large quantities – have caused problems, particularly in emergency situations. To promote beneficial medicine donations and to minimize problems with donations, interagency guidelines have been published by WHO to guide donors and recipients. The guidelines set out four core principles which should govern all medicine donations:

◆ Maximum benefit to the recipient country

◆ Respect wishes and authority of the recipient country

◆ No double standards in medicines quality

◆ Effective communication between donor and recipient country.

Box 12.2 Medicine procurement in India

Delhi state (population 14 million) in India launched a comprehensive rational medicine policy in 1995, which included a change in medicine procurement practices. Prior to the introduction of the change of policy, individual hospitals procured some medicines from the government procurement agency and some from the local market. After the policy change, hospitals grouped together to procure medicines, using selective tender and supervised by a special purchase committee. Doctors were asked to prescribe only those medicines on the procurement list. An evaluation showed that where the rational medicine policy operated, medicine prices were 30–40% lower and significantly more essential medicines were actually available to patients at facilities.

Medicine prices (Indian Rupees)	Previous government medicine procurement agency	Newly developed rational medicine policy, using pooled procurement and selective tender
Amoxycillin syrup (125 mg)	11.4	7.5
Cloxacillin injection (500 mg)	13.5	4.7
Erythromycin tab.250 mg	0.57	0.15
Erythromycin syrup (125 mg)	20.8	9.8
Amikacin injection 500 mg	92.8	23.6
Ciprofloxacin tab.500 mg	0.29	0.14
Atenolol tab.50 mg	0.02	0.05
Ranitidine injection 150 mg	4.25	1.63
Medicine availability		
Percentage of prescribed medicines available at five hospitals	5–22%	60–98%

Source: Roy Chaudhury, (1999), Essential Drugs Monitor, 27:2–4; and Roy Chaudhury et al., (2005), Health Policy and Planning, 20(2): 124–136.

Table 12.1 Private and government per capita expenditure on pharmaceuticals, 1990–2000 in US$

Income clusters	1990			2000		
	Private	Government	Total	Private	Government	Total
WHO member states	28	21 (43%)	49	45	29 (39%)	74
High-income	130	110 (46%)	240	229	167 (42%)	396
Middle-income	13	5 (28%)	18	22	8 (27%)	30
Low-income	2.6	1 (28%)	3.6	3.2	1.1 (25%)	4.4

Source: The World Medicines Situation, WHO/EDM/PAR/2004.5.

Access and finance for the pharmaceutical system

The financial resources available for running a sustainable pharmaceutical system will depend on the government's expenditure on health and pharmaceuticals and the health financing system. Table 12.1 summarizes government and private expenditure on pharmaceuticals in different regions of the world and shows that while expenditure on pharmaceuticals has increased between 1990 and 2000, the proportion funded by the government has reduced from 43% to 39%. In addition, comparison of developing with developed countries shows that in developing countries per capita expenditure on health and pharmaceuticals is much less, and that a greater proportion of expenditure is from private sources, and a lesser proportion from governments.

The pharmaceutical market is not a perfect market where supply perfectly balances demand. The market for pharmaceuticals fails for several reasons.

Firstly consumers have much less knowledge about the quality, efficacy, safety, and appropriateness of medicine products than do health care providers. Secondly, little competition exists, since there are many consumers (patients) but relatively few providers (health care providers, purchasers and manufacturers). Thirdly, manufacturers create a monopoly through patent protection of medicines and manufacturing processes, brand loyalty due to intensive marketing, market segmentation through the introduction of therapeutic subclasses and price-fixing by producer cartels. Fourthly, the demand for health care and its provision are not the same for all patients. For example, at one extreme some patients may require paracetamol for mild headaches, whereas others may require hip replacements for crippling arthritis. Finally, externalities exist within the pharmaceutical sector, for example treatment of sexually transmitted diseases or tuberculosis and the provision of immunization provide benefit not only to those treated but also to others who will have less likelihood of contracting disease.

Therefore, if it is accepted by society that health is a fundamental right to which all sections of the population should have access, it is necessary that governments play an active role in the financing and regulation of the pharmaceutical and health sectors to ensure equitable access to care.

Financing of medicines

Although almost all governments world-wide play some role in financing health and pharmaceuticals, the amounts they contribute and the mechanisms by which they do so vary enormously. It should be remembered that the private sector is often a major source of health care in developing countries and that the poor often have no alternative but to pay a high proportion of their incomes out of pocket in order to gain access to treatment.

Whichever health or medicine financing system is used, medicine costs can be contained by:

1 Adhering to selection procedures, for example national essential or reimbursement medicine lists and focussing on cost-effective medicines;

2 Increasing market competition through the use of:

- ◆ Generic medicines, including generic substitution by pharmacists and promotion of the generic market.
- ◆ Therapeutic substitution.
- ◆ Medicine pricing policies, whereby governments (1) negotiate prices with manufacturers either on the basis of the manufacturers' costs or profits, or on the basis of comparison with other similar medicines on the market, and (2) regulate the type and level of dispensing fee and distributors' profit margins.
- ◆ Parallel imports, whereby patented medicines are purchased and imported from countries where the negotiated price is lower; parallel importing is not specifically covered under the TRIPS agreement, which leaves the issue to be dealt with under national legislation.
- ◆ Compulsory licensing, whereby government may license a local manufacturer to produce a product that is still under patent in order to obtain that product at a lower price; compulsory licensing is permitted under the World Trade Organization's Agreement on Trade Related Aspects of Intellectual Property Rights (TRIPS) under certain conditions if 'justified by the public interest'.

It is important that any financing system is feasible in terms of financial sustainability, administrative requirements and acceptability and that it promotes equity, efficiency and rational medicine use. The various health financing systems are described in Chapter 7 on health financing. The different issues concerned with managing medicines in association with different financing mechanisms are discussed below.

Public financing

Public financing through centralized revenues (raised through taxes or social insurance) occurs to some degree in many countries, particularly developed countries where the degree of public expenditure on medicines is greater. It has the following advantages:

- ◆ Medicine supplies may be better selected and targeted to those most in need
- ◆ Medicine quality can be better controlled by the government
- ◆ Economies of scale may be achieved in medicine procurement
- ◆ The burden of payment for medicines may be shifted from (1) the sick to the healthy because everybody pays, and (2) the poor to the rich through payment structures such as income tax or insurance premiums based on income.

Health insurance

Health insurance is a mechanism whereby the risk and burden of paying for illness is shared among a community or a society. Health insurance may be funded by both the public and the private sectors and may be in the form of compulsory social health insurance, private voluntary insurance or community pre-paid schemes. Community schemes are usually voluntary; they occur often in rural areas and may be administered through cooperative structures. Almost all developed countries, with the exception of the USA, operate health insurance systems which cover most of the population, cover all or part of the cost of medicines and which improve affordability and equity. In contrast, only a minority of the population has insurance coverage in developing countries and few of the systems cover the cost of medicines. Since medicines account for a large share of total household expenses for health in many developing countries, including medicine costs in insurance schemes would make these more readily acceptable. However, utilization and cost control measures (e.g. reimbursable medicine lists) must be in place to ensure that any scheme is not bankrupted through over-prescription, abuse and fraud. Low coverage in very poor countries may be due to the lack of capacity in record keeping, and of experience in operating insurance systems and the cost control measures necessary.

User fees

User fees for medicines in developing countries usually account for over two-thirds of all medicine spending, mostly in the private sector but also in the public sector. Most commonly, medicines are sold from private vendors. However, user fees may also be charged in cost-recovery health schemes, either run by the government on a national basis, or by individual communities. User fees, or co-payments, are also charged in many insurance schemes. In cost-recovery schemes, money collected through user fees is used to fund recurrent costs, either of health services in general, or of medicines in particular. User fees are often justified on the basis that they will improve medicine availability and efficiency, reduce over-consumption and allow public funds to be more targeted to those in need – so increasing equity. In reality many of these objectives are often unmet and use by the very poor is decreased. User fee systems will only be successful if accompanied by perceived quality improvement in services, especially medicine availability, and there are safety mechanisms e.g. low fee levels, exemption criteria, to ensure that the poor are not excluded from use. Improved availability of medicines is only likely to be achieved through user fees if business-like arrangements are made concerning personnel and financial and supply management with strict measures to ensure accountability including financial audit.

Fees may be charged per patient visit or prescription, or per medicine item (single standard fee or multiple standard fees covering a full course of treatment), or per medicine unit (fee per tablet varying according to the medicine), or per course of standard treatment according to the disease. The various fees have different advantages and disadvantages. For example, the fee per prescription may be easy to manage but is known to stimulate over-prescription (see Box 12.3). Variable fees may be administratively difficult, and fees per course of treatment may stimulate health workers to make multiple diagnoses per patient.

Other financing mechanisms for medicines

Voluntary Financing Schemes are usually locally operated community pre-paid schemes run by charitable organizations often in rural areas. In Sub-Saharan Africa and low-income Asian countries, as much as 50% of curative services may be provided by NGOs.

Donor Financing is important for many developing countries and may be in the form of money or medicines (medicine donations). In some very poor countries of sub-Saharan Africa, donor support may account for as much as 30% of medicine expenditure.

Development Loans are often used to purchase medicines. This is not the best option since expenditure for medicines is recurrent and all loans require re-payment with interest.

Rational use of medicines

Rational use of medicines has been defined by WHO as requiring that patients receive medications appropriate to their clinical needs, in doses that meet their own individual requirements, for an adequate period of time, and at the lowest cost to them and their community.

In addition, it is necessary that the patient adheres to treatment. Irrational use of medicines not only wastes resources, but may harm patients through therapeutic failure, side-effects, and toxicity. Over use of antibiotics is contributing to increasing antimicrobial resistance. It has been estimated that more than half of all medicines in low and middle-income countries are used in an irrational or inappropriate way and that 50% people worldwide fail to take their medicines correctly.

It has been reported in various parts of the world that 25–75% of antibiotic prescriptions are inappropriate (results from teaching hospitals in ten countries) and that in many countries over two thirds of antibiotics are used without a prescription and 90% of antibiotics are bought in amounts lasting 3 days or less. Some 2-year-old children have experienced more than 20 injections and over-use has led to the spread of HIV and hepatitis B due to poor sterile technique. It has been found that private providers use up to 80 different tuberculosis regimes. In 2002, it was found that outpatient antibiotic consumption in France was three times that in the Netherlands. Cost savings of up to 50% could be made if all prescriptions conformed to standard treatment guidelines.

Irrational behaviour of providers encompasses:

♦ Polypharmacy (the prescription of unnecessary medicines)

♦ The prescription or dispensing of wrong medicines, dosage or duration (Fig. 12.4)

♦ Non-adherence to treatment guidelines

♦ Use of brand names instead of generic names

♦ Insufficient information to the patient.

Irrational use of medicines by consumers involves inappropriate self-medication and non adherence to dosing schedules.

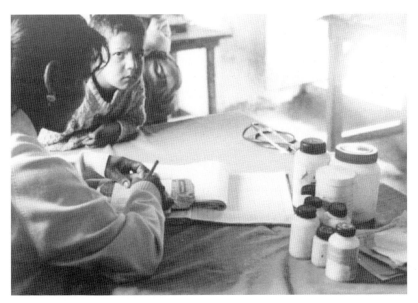

Fig. 12.4 A primary health care consultation.

Investigating the irrational use of medicines

In order to promote the rational use of medicines it is necessary to:

1 Measure the size of the problem, using quantitative indicators, so that the impact of any strategies to improve medicine use may be scientifically established

2 Understand the problem, using qualitative methodologies, so that effective interventions may be designed.

The quality of prescribing and dispensing may be assessed by examination of facility records, e.g. patient registers, dispensing registers, supply depot records, or by structured observation. A number of different kinds of quantitative indicators to monitor provider use, at facility level, have been developed and are summarized in Table 12.2.

The WHO indicators, together with a methodology for collection, were developed in association with the International Network for the Rational Use of Drugs (INRUD) specifically for use in situations where facilities and infrastructure are lacking, as in many developing countries. Aggregate medicine consumption data collected from other sources such as warehouse records, medicine manufacturers or importers, may also be useful to assess use in terms of, for example, per capita consumption or the proportion of budget spent on different medicine items.

The quantitative indicators so far described can be used to monitor prescribing. However, they cannot be used to identify appropriate interventions – for this, qualitative methods such as in-depth interviews or focus group discussions with prescribers and health workers are necessary. People often have very rational reasons for using medicines irrationally and these must be understood in order to develop and implement interventions that are likely to be effective in changing behaviour. Causes of irrational use include lack of knowledge, skills, or independent information, unrestricted availability of medicines, overwork of health personnel, inappropriate promotion of medicines, and profit-motives from selling medicines.

Investigation of medicine use by consumers is more complex and traditionally has used anthropological and sociological qualitative methodologies. WHO has developed a simplified methodology to investigate medicine use in communities using household surveys, surveys of various medicine outlets, for example medicine stores, and qualitative investigation by focus group discussion or in-depth interview.

Table 12.2 Medicine use indicators for use in out-patient facilities

WHO drug use indicators

- ♦ core prescribing indicators suitable for rapid appraisal
  - number of medicine items per prescription
  - percentage prescriptions with antibiotics
  - percentage prescriptions with injections
  - percentage medicines prescribed from Essential Medicine Lists

- ♦ supplementary prescribing indicators requiring more complex data collection
  - average cost per prescription
  - percentage prescriptions conforming to Standard Treatment Guidelines
  - percentage medicine costs spent on antibiotics
  - percentage medicine costs spent on injections

- ♦ patient care indicators
  - average consultation time
  - average dispensing time
  - percentage prescribed medicines that are dispensed
  - percentage dispensed medicines that are adequately labelled
  - patient's knowledge of correct dosage

- ♦ Health facility indicators
  - availability of essential medicine list, formulary
  - availability of standard treatment guidelines
  - availability of key medicines

Source: 1993 WHO/DAP/93.1.

Responsibility for monitoring medicine use, and review of unbiased medicine information for prescribers, varies according to the level of health facility and between countries. In hospitals, such responsibility often lies with the pharmacy and therapeutics committees, which may be responsible for developing guidelines, introducing prescribing restrictions, pharmacist monitoring, audit with feedback and medicine (drug) bulletins. At the primary health care level, monitoring may be done by public health authorities. In the UK the audit of general practitioners' prescribing is undertaken locally, but the data is stored and processed centrally by the Prescription Pricing Authority. Each prescriber receives a monthly and annual statement of costs to compare with the previous year and with the national pattern. In many countries no monitoring of medicines use is undertaken at all.

Promoting rational medicine use

There are four kinds of strategy to improve medicine use – regulatory, economic, managerial and educational.

Regulatory strategies

These are based on limiting prescriber/consumer decisions (for example banning unsafe medicines, or regulating the use of different medicines to different levels of the health sector). Enforcement of regulations requires political will and a functioning infrastructure, which are

---

Box 12.3 Nepal 1997

A pre–post control study of the effects of different kinds of user fees on prescribing quality was conducted in rural Nepal. The fees were priced so that the total cost to the patient would be similar for all fee types at about 25% of the average daily household income. In 1992 all three study districts charged the same flat fee per prescription but in 1995 the control district charged the same fee, one district charged a single fee per medicine item and a second district charged a higher fee per expensive item and a lower fee per cheap item. The item fees covered a complete course for each item. It was found that prescribing quality was significantly poorer ($p < 0.001$ for the number of items prescribed per patient and $p < 0.01$ for antibiotic use and the percentage of prescriptions conforming to standard treatment guidelines) with a fee per prescription than with either type of item fee.

Group	Control flat prescription fee	1-band fee per medicine item	2-band fee per medicine item
1 Av. No. items per prescription	2.9→ 2.9 (0%)	2.9→2.0 (−31%)	2.8→2.2 (−21%)
2 Percentage prescriptions with antibiotics	66.7→67.5 (+0.8%)	63.5→54.8 (−8.7%)	60.7→54.3 (−6.4%)
3 Percentage prescriptions with injections	23.4→20.0 (−3.4%)	19.8→16.1 (−3.7%)	21.8→14.9 (−6.9%)
4 Percentage prescriptions conforming to STGs	23.5→26.3 (+2.8%)	31.5→45.0 (+13.5%)	31.2→47.7 (+16.5%)
STG = Standard Treatment Guidelines			

Source: Holloway KA, Gautam BR, Reeves BC, *J. Clinical Epidemiology, 2001;* 54(1):1065–1071.

often lacking in developing countries. Thus in most developing countries, despite regulation to the contrary, prescription-only medicines are freely available without prescription. Sometimes unforeseen negative consequences may result. It has been reported in a number of countries that the banning of certain unsafe medicines has resulted in the inappropriate substitution of other medicines by prescribers.

Economic strategies

These are based on incentives to providers (prescribers, dispensers and institutions) and consumers to behave in a certain way. One of the commonest disincentives to rational use of medicines concerns prescribers (e.g. dispensing doctors and drug retailers) who themselves sell medicines. Allowing the same person to both prescribe and sell medicines has been shown repeatedly to encourage over-prescribing. Reimbursement policies can deter the use of non-essential medicines by reimbursing only essential medicines and not non-essential ones. User fees, though frequently implemented to raise funds, have rarely been evaluated for their effects on medicine use. Charging the same amount, irrespective of the number or quantity of medicines prescribed, for example a flat fee per prescription, may lead to over-prescribing as found in Nepal (see country example 12.3).

Managerial strategies

These are based on improving the decision-making process, for example by medicine selection (essential medicine list), procurement (morbidity-based quantification), distribution (kit systems), prescribing (standard treatment guidelines) and dispensing (course of treatment packaging). Although many management strategies have been implemented, evaluations of their effects are few. In Yemen (Box 12.4), significantly better medicine availability and more rational prescribing

Box 12.4 Yemen 1990

In Yemen, the prescribing was compared in health facilities where no essential medicine programme was operating and in those where an essential medicines programme was operating. The essential medicines programme consisted of supplying essential medicines in kits, supplying standard treatment guidelines and providing a 1-week training in the use of the standard treatment guidelines and kits. It was found that the quality of prescribing was significantly better ($p < 0.001$ for all indicators) where the essential medicine programme operated.

Group	No.items per Px	Perecentage Px with antibiotics	Percentage Px with injections
1 Control	2.4	67%	58%
2 Kit supply system + Standard Treatment Guidelines + 1-week training	1.5	46%	25%
3 Expected results if all Px conformed to Standard Treatment Guidelines	1.4	23%	17%
Px = prescription			

Source: Walker et al., (1990) Social Science and Medicine, 31(7), 61–67 and Hogerzeil et al., (1989), *Lancet*, **333**(1), 141–42.

were observed in health facilities where an essential medicine kit supply system operated together with concurrent health worker seminars, as compared to facilities where the kit system did not operate and there were no health worker seminars. Many management strategies such as the use of an essential medicine list alone or arbitrary limits on the number or quantity of medicines per prescription have been shown to be ineffective in promoting rational medicine use.

Educational strategies

These are based on information and persuasion, for example health worker training and public health education, and are the methods most commonly used to promote rational prescribing. Educational strategies include formal pre-service training and continuing in-service training and may include pharmacology, therapeutics and problem-based pharmacotherapy. The use of printed materials alone is ineffective. Educational strategies appear to be effective in changing prescriber behaviour, as opposed to knowledge, only if they are face-to-face and/or include follow-up, or are very targeted, as in Indonesia (Box 12.5), are combined with management strategies such as the introduction of standard treatment guidelines, or involve a change in behaviour of an opinion leader such as the head of an academic department.

However, regular face-to-face contact is expensive – possibly beyond the reach of many developing countries, while targeted training only addresses one area of irrational medicine use at a time. The problem of consumer behaviour and demand for medicines has not been addressed by most educational strategies, which require the prescriber to change his prescribing behaviour in a way which may be unpopular with his patients on whom he may be dependent for his living. In Indonesia, the effect of consumer demand on prescribers was addressed through the use of facilitated interactive group discussions between patients and prescribers, resulting in a significant reduction in the proportion of patients receiving injections (see Box 12.5).

Public Health Education interventions to promote more rational use of medicines by consumers have been infrequently done and even more infrequently evaluated for impact. Very few indeed have demonstrated any change in consumer behaviour.

Box 12.5 Indonesia 1996

A randomized control trial of a group process intervention to reduce injection use was conducted in Indonesia. The group process involved a facilitated 2-hour discussion between health workers and the community concerning the use of injections. In the group discussion, staff beliefs that patients demanded injections and patients beliefs that they did not demand injections, were shared. This intervention resulted in a significant reduction in injection use ($p < 0.025$) and the number of items prescribed per patient ($p < 0.025$).

	Group	Control	Facilitated discussion
1	No. items/prescription	3.97→3.88 (−2.3%)	4.03→3.67 (−8.9%)
2	Percentage prescriptions with injections	75.6→67.1 (−8.5%)	69.5→42.3 (−27.2%)

Source: Hadiyono et al, (1996), Social Science and Medicine, 42(8), pp.1177–1183.

Most public health education interventions have used the mass media – radio, television, newspapers and printed materials such as posters, leaflets and books. Using the mass media has the advantage of reaching a large number of people in a short time, with a low cost per person reached, but also has the disadvantage of a high total cost and of lacking immediate feedback. Person-to-person interventions, such as community and school talks, phone-ins and street theatre, have the advantage of reaching specific target audiences and providing immediate feedback, but they require trained field staff, take longer and have a higher initial cost per person reached.

Person-to-person strategies are more likely to change consumer behaviour than mass media campaigns. However, the best approach is to combine both approaches (see Box 12.6), although this is often difficult due to lack of funding and a supportive infrastructure, and sometimes due to organized opposition from groups with vested interests.

Public education campaigns are likely to be more successful if combined with strategies aimed at prescribers (Fig. 12.5), with the same message being given to both groups. Thus, a number of European countries have succeeded in reducing consumption of antibiotics for coughs and colds in recent years through mass education campaigns aimed at both prescribers and consumers.

Much of the evidence concerning what interventions are effective in promoting rational use of medicines was presented at the first and second international conferences for improving the use of medicines held in Chiang Mai Thailand in 1997 and 2004 respectively (URL: http://www.icium.org). On the basis of this evidence the second conference issued a major recommendation for countries to have national programmes to promote rational use of medicines. The conference further recommended that such programmes should be based on coordinated implementation of sustainable multi-faceted interventions, scaled up to the national level and with in-built systems for monitoring medicines use in order to evaluate progress.

Box 12.6 Peru 1996

A study was conducted in Peru whereby an intensive community intervention focussed on diarrhoea was introduced in one area and comparison made with a control area concerning medicine use in cases of diarrhoea. The intervention involved video, market broadcasts, printed materials, face-to-face visits, booklets and prescription pads for prescribers. There was some reduction in the prescription of medicines and antibiotics for cases of diarrhoea in the intervention area.

	Cases of diarrhoea	Control	Community intervention
1	Percent all cases prescribed medicines	48.8→41.9 (−6.9%)	43.1→33.3 (−9.8%)
2	Percent cases seeing a medical doctor who were prescribed medicines	92.4→91.9 (−0.5%)	94.6→84.9 (−9.7%)
3	Percent all cases prescribed antibiotics	29.3→21.4 (−8.9%)	25.5→17.9 (−7.6%)

Source: Paredes et al. (1996), Applied Diarrhoeal Research Project, Lima, Peru, also presented at the 1st conference for improving the use of medicines in 1997, http://www.icium.org, and reprinted in How to improve the use of medicines by consumers, WHO Geneva, 2007.

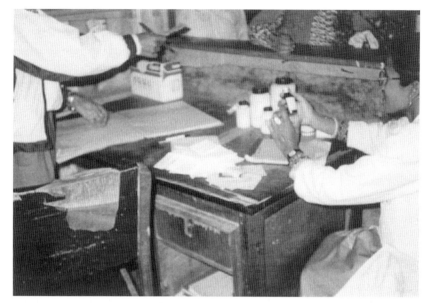

Fig. 12.5 A district hospital dispensary.

Medicine quality and medicine regulation

Medicine quality

The quality of medicines is of equal importance to questions of access and rational use of medicines, and the purpose of quality assurance is to make certain that all medicines reaching patients are safe, effective and of standard quality. Accepted quality standards are published in various pharmacopoeias, for example the US Pharmacopoeia or the British Pharmacopoeia. The main quality criteria are purity, potency, uniformity of dosage form, bioavailability and stability. All these aspects of quality may be affected by the manufacturing process, packaging, storage and other factors and lack of quality may result in lack of therapeutic effect, and adverse or toxic reactions, all of which may result in patient harm through prolonged or medicine-induced illness and waste of limited resources.

Product quality is ensured through three basic processes – quality assurance, good manufacturing practice and quality control. Brief definitions are given below, courtesy of Managing Drug Supply, 1997, Kumarian Press.

- *Quality Assurance* is the sum of the activities and responsibilities intended to ensure that medicines reaching patients are safe, effective and acceptable to the patient.
- *Good Manufacturing Practices (GMP)* are part of the quality assurance that ensure that products are consistently produced and controlled to the quality standards appropriate to their intended use and required by medicine regulatory authorities.
- *Quality Control* is the part of GMP where medicine samples are tested against specific standards of quality.

Medicine regulation

Medicine regulation is critical to ensuring that quality assurance is carried out and, in turn, quality assurance is critical to maintaining medicine quality. Medicine regulation is not confined only to quality assurance, but in fact consists of all the legal, administrative and technical arrangements made by governments to ensure that:

- All premises, persons and practices engaged in the development, manufacture, importation, exportation, wholesale, supply, dispensing and promotion of medicines comply with approved standards, norms, procedures, and regulatory requirements
- Medicine products are safe, effective, and of adequate quality
- Product information is unbiased, accurate and appropriate
- Medicines are available and used rationally.

In order to meet the above objectives, the following basic functions must be undertaken:

1 Licensing and inspection of manufacturers, importers, distributors, wholesale, and retail outlets, with regard to the premises, persons, and practices involved;

2 Assessing the safety, efficacy and quality of medicines and issuing market authorization or registration (for which a fee is usually charged) for medicine products;

3 Quality control laboratory testing to monitor the quality of medicines on the market;

4 Provision of objective medicine information and monitoring of medicine promotion and advertising. WHO has developed ethical criteria for medicine promotion, which should be based on truthfulness, apply to all prescription, over-the-counter or traditional medicines, and refer to all informational and persuasive activities;

5 Adverse medicine (drug) reaction monitoring (pharmacovigilance);

6 Application of sanctions to organizations and persons who do not adhere to the regulations;

7 Authorization of clinical trials;

8 Setting educational standards for pharmacists, doctors, and other health professionals, licensing these health professionals and developing and enforcing codes of conduct.

A medicine regulatory authority is the central body that coordinates the complex set of medicine regulatory activities which involve many different players – manufacturers, distributors, experts, prescribers, patients, consumers, and government. Activities vary from country to country but generally include most of the above although licensing of health professionals is often undertaken by separate legal bodies, for example the General Medical Council in the UK. In order for a medicine regulatory authority to function properly, it must have adequate human resources and a sustainable financing mechanism, and there must be political commitment and comprehensive legislation and regulations, which can be enforced through a functional independent judicial system. Effective medicine regulation depends on the society and political system within which it exists. Factors which enhance effectiveness include:

- Coordination of activities by an adequately resourced central independent body that is accountable to the public, the government, and agencies to which regulations apply
- A transparent regulation process with the regular application of appropriate sanctions
- Freedom of information and association, together with organized consumer pressure groups
- A political system that gives adequate priority to the public health value of medicines.

The consequences of weak medicine regulatory capacity include the manufacture, distribution and trading of medicines that are often of inadequate safety, quality, or efficacy, prescribing and dispensing by unqualified personnel, and the distribution of misleading inappropriate product information. This in turn leads to (1) the irrational prescription and consumption of medicines, including the sale of prescription-only medicines without prescription, and (2) the sale of medicines

Box 12.7 Counterfeit and substandard medicines

♦ A WHO study conducted in 2003 in seven sub-Saharan African countries on the quality of chloroquine tablets showed that only 58% had an acceptable level of chloroquine and only 25% had acceptable dissolution properties. The use of such medicine results in low bio-availability and under-dosage so promoting the development of resistance.

♦ In 2001, in South-East Asia, a Wellcome Trust study revealed that 38% of 104 anti-malarial drugs on sale in pharmacies did not contain any active ingredients.

♦ During a meningitis epidemic in Niger in 1995, more than 50 000 people were inoculated with fake vaccines resulting in 2500 deaths. The vaccines were received as a gift from a country which thought they were safe.

♦ 89 children died in Haiti in 1995 and 30 infants died in India in 1998 due to the consumption of paracetamol cough syrup prepared with diethylene glycol (a toxic chemical used in antifreeze).

♦ In Cambodia, in 1999, at least 30 people died after taking counterfeit anti-malarials prepared with sulphadoxine-pyrimethamine (an older, less effective anti-malarial) which were sold as artesunate.

Source: WHO Fact sheet no.275 on counterfeit medicines,
URL: http://www.who.int/mediacentre/factsheets/fs275/en/print.html

that are substandard, counterfeit, harmful and useless. At present, about 20% of countries have adequate regulation. Of the rest, about half have partial regulation, and 30% have virtually no capacity to regulate medicines. Furthermore, many developing countries do not have a quality assurance laboratory with quality assurance mechanisms.

It is presently estimated that of all medicines sold, 1% in developed countries and 10–30% in developing countries are counterfeit. Medicines purchased over the Internet from sites that conceal their physical address are counterfeit in over 50% of cases. The US based Centre for Medicines in the Public Interest predicts that counterfeit drug sales will reach US$ 75 billion globally in 2010, an increase of more than 90% from 2005. country example 12.7 shows what has happened around the word with regard to counterfeit and substandard medicines as a result of inadequate medicine regulation.

National medicine policy

A national medicine policy expresses the goals and objectives set by the government for the pharmaceutical sector (involving private and public sectors and all stakeholders) and identifies the main strategies for achieving them. In other words it is framework within which the activities of the pharmaceutical sector are prioritized and coordinated. However, in order to be effective it is important that national medicine policy is developed in a consultative way involving all stakeholders and that the process and results are documented. Without a consultative process and documentation, different parts of the policy may be conflicting, goals and responsibilities may not be understood by stakeholders and there may be less commitment to action. Finally, the national medicine policy document should be endorsed by the Ministry of Health, the Cabinet or Parliament. Industrialized countries may not have one all-embracing formal policy document, but they all have defined goals, and have identified and documented strategies for reaching those goals.

A national medicine policy must:

◆ Ensure access to essential medicines by making them both available and affordable, and

◆ Ensure that all medicines available in the country are safe, effective and of adequate quality and

◆ Promote rational use of medicines.

There are a number of different components to any national medicine policy and the absence of any component may undermine the effectiveness of others. A national medicine policy should contain the following components:

1 Legislation, regulation, and guidelines
   Government defines what is permissible and the roles, rights and responsibilities of the various actors

2 Medicine regulation and quality assurance
   A regulatory system to ensure that all medicines are of adequate quality is defined

3 Medicine selection
   National medicine policies should be based on the essential medicines concept, which implies the existence of an up-to-date list of essential medicines. This will set priorities, and lead to improved access and more rational use of medicines

4 Access to essential medicines
   (i) Medicine supply
       Effective coordinated policies on production, procurement, storage and distribution are needed to ensure good quality medicines are available at a reasonable price; without such policies there may be shortages, or medicines may expire and be wasted
   (ii) Financing strategies
       Decisions are made concerning appropriate financing mechanisms to ensure equitable medicine availability, the balance between the public and private sectors and how to regulate the pharmaceutical market in order to avoid excessive profit margins or other adverse manipulation by key players in the pharmaceutical sector.

5 Rational use of medicines
   Decisions are made concerning how to promote the rational use of medicines. Key policy issues include establishing a national mandated multi-disciplinary body to coordinate medicines use policies; and the implementation of policies concerning the training and supervision of health professionals, public education about medicines and the avoidance of perverse financial incentives to prescribers and dispensers.

6 Research and development
   Strategies to encourage national research and development of both medicines and health systems should be consistent with national capacity and the priorities identified in the policy document.

7 Human resource development
   Policy decisions concerning training are needed to ensure that there are sufficient personnel with adequate expertise. This includes defining the minimum education and training needed for each category of health professional.

Box 12.8 Implementation of national medicine policies in 12 countries

A study was conducted in 12 countries (Bulgaria, Chad, Colombia, Guinea, India, Mali, Philippines, Sri Lanka, Thailand, Vietnam, Zambia and Zimbabwe) to evaluate the effectiveness of their national medicine policies. It was found that:

- All countries had medicine regulatory authorities with mandates which included medicine registration and inspection;
- Most countries had established structures, but implementation was not always working and monitoring and evaluation were rarely done;
- It was much easier to improve medicine availability than to change medicine use behaviour;
- Generic policies resulted in lower cost of treatment in the public sector;
- Withdrawal of irrational medicines led to less irrational use;
- Good quality assurance led to better acceptance of generics, prescribing and dispensing;
- Good registration had a positive impact on medicine use;
- An appropriate financing system led to better prescribing;
- Procurement through tender led to better availability of medicines;
- Public sector training led to better prescribing in the public sector as compared to the private sector.

Source: Comparative analysis of national drug policies, WHO/DAP/97.6

8 Monitoring and evaluation

Monitoring of each component of the policy, including the use and availability of medicines, is essential to assess progress, and provision for it (adequate staff and budget) should be built into the policy itself.

WHO has developed a number of indicators, based on these components, to monitor what national medicine policies are being implemented (see Box 12.8).

A survey was done in 2003 (WHO 2006) to assess what pharmaceutical policies and structures were in place by sending a questionnaire to all Ministries of Health. It was found that less than half of all Member States were implementing basic policies to promote rational use of medicines. Such policies include regular monitoring of use; the presence of Pharmacy and Therapeutics Committees in hospitals to oversee the use of medicines; updated essential medicines list and standard treatment guidelines; use of reimbursement lists based on the essential medicines list; presence of a medicine information centre for prescribers; obligatory continuing medical education; and enforcement of policy concerning the availability of prescription-only medicines only with prescription.

The role of government in the pharmaceutical sector

Government involvement in the health and pharmaceutical sectors is much more extensive than in other sectors and markets because the pharmaceutical sector operates in an imperfect market, as discussed previously, and because society demands that governments take responsibility for ensuring minimum health services. Laws and regulations are needed because:

- Pharmaceuticals affect the whole population
- Pharmaceuticals involve many parties (e.g. patients, providers, manufacturers, sales people)
- There are serious consequences from the lack or misuse of medicines and
- Informal controls are insufficient.

The role of government is to develop and implement national medicines policy, medicines regulation, professional standards and to adopt other strategies to ensure access to and rational use of essential good quality medicines. All these various components are described above. Box 12.9 shows the far reaching negative consequences that occurred when government 'liberalized' the pharmaceutical sector in China in 1983.

Box 12.9 When government let go of the reins in China

The context

During the period 1960–1983 China established a 'Cooperative Medical System' which brought at least basic health care services to almost the entire population. Rural doctors were paid on a work points system by the local commune. The commune also purchased some care from higher-level facilities for its population.

As the system of communal agriculture in China broke down; so did the old ways of financing and providing health care. By the end of the 1980s the Cooperative Medical System had collapsed in about 90% of Chinese villages. About three-quarters of finance for health care in China came from user fees. Rural doctors generally no longer saw themselves as government employees but as independent private practitioners. At the same time, government controls on higher-level facilities were relaxed; hospitals were given greater managerial autonomy and control over their own finances.

The impact on health and welfare

The reforms in China have had a negative effect on access to health care services, particularly in rural areas. It is now estimated that 700 million Chinese have no prepayment or insurance coverage and must thus pay out-of-pocket for virtually all health services. Household surveys have documented a large number of untreated sick people. For example, a national household survey in 1988 showed that 25% of the rural population who needed referral to a hospital were not admitted, largely due to financial problems. Health care expenditures also appear to be a major factor in causing poverty. In a survey of 1013 poor households, nearly 50% of them cited illness as the principal cause of poverty.

The declining financial accessibility of health care services has also affected health status. Immunization coverage began to decline towards the end of the 1980s and there have been several recent unexpected outbreaks of immunizable diseases. Both child and infant mortality declined steadily until the 1980s, but the decline in these indicators then stopped and even showed a slight upward drift. This is despite recent rapid macroeconomic growth.

> **Box 12.9 When government let go of the reins in China** *(continued)*
>
> ## The impact on the pharmaceutical sector
>
> Prior to 1980 health stations stocked only a small number of essential medicines. Since that time, rural doctors have been granted the right to prescribe all medicines except narcotics and major tranquillizers. They have not been provided with extra training to match these new powers.
>
> Health stations in poorer counties often appear to stock more medicines than those in wealthy ones. This probably reflects economic necessity; medicine sales are the easiest way to make money. Health facilities have the right to manufacture medicines, and an increasing number of small health stations are producing traditional remedies in order to generate revenue.
>
> Inappropriate medicine use has been reported, such as the use of injectables rather than oral preparations and the over-prescription and use of medicines.
>
> Source: WHO 1997, Public-Private roles in the pharmaceutical sector.
> Implications for equitable access and rational use, DAP series no.5, WHO/DAP/97.12.

Summary

Essential medicines are one of the most cost-effective ways of preventing, treating or alleviating disease. This chapter provides a summary of what we know should be done concerning the management of medicines to ensure that everyone receives good quality medicines appropriate to their clinical needs, in doses that meet their own individual requirements, for an adequate period of time and at the lowest cost to them and their community. Despite our present knowledge about medicine management, millions of people in developing countries have no access to medicines. Furthermore, millions of people in both rich and poor countries are given medicines inappropriately – either the wrong medicine or the wrong dose or duration. The challenge of the future is to implement what we know, and find out what we do not know, in order to ensure that nobody need suffer from lack of appropriate medicine treatment.

Further reading

Chaudhury R. (1999) 'Rational use of drugs: Delhi's change in policy changes lives', *Essential Drugs Monitor*, **27**, 2–4.

Chaudhury R., Paremeswar R., Gupta U., Sharma S., Teku U., Bapna J. (2005) 'Quality of medicines for the poor: experience of the Delhi programme on rational use of drugs', *Health Policy and Planning*, **20(2)**, 124–36.

Hadiyono J.E., Suryawati S., Danu S., Sunartono, Santoso B. (1996) 'Interactional group discussion: results of a controlled trial using behavioural intervention to reduce the useof injections in public health facilities', *Social Science and Medicine*, **42(8)**, 1177–83.

Hogerzeil H.V. (1995) 'Promoting rational prescribing: an international perspective', *British Journal of Clinical Pharmacology*, **39**, 1–6.

Hogerzeil H.V., Walker J.A., Sallami A.O., Fernando G. (1989) 'Impact of an Essential drugs programme on the availability and rational use of drugs', *The Lancet*, **333(1)**, 141–2.

Holloway K.A, Gautam B.R, Reeves B.C. (2001) 'The Effects of Different Kinds of User Fee on Prescribing Quality in Rural Nepal', *Journal Clinical Epidemiology*, **54(1)**, 1065–71.

Laing R.O., Hogerzeil H.V, Ross-Degnan D. (2001) 'Ten recommendations to improve use of medicines in developing countries', *Health Policy and Planning*, **16(1)**, 13–20.

Management Sciences for Health (1997) Managing Drug Supply, eds: Quick J, Rankin J, Laing R, O'Connor R, Hogerzeil H, Dukes M, Garnett A, *Management sciences of health in collaboration with the World Health Organisation*, Kumarian Press, USA, ISBN: 1-56549-047-9.

Paredes et al. (1996) *Applied Diarrhoeal Research Project*, Lima, Peru.

Sauwakon R., Wondemagegnehu E. (2002) *Effective drug regulation: a multi-country study*; World Health Organization, Geneva, ISBN 92 4 156206 4.

Walker et al. (1990) 'Evaluation of rational drug prescribing in Democratic Yemen', *Social Science and Medicine*, **31(7)**, 61–7.

World Health Organization. (1997) *Comparative analysis of national drug policies*, WHO/DAP/97.6.

World Health Organization (1993) *How to investigate drug use in health facilities, selected drug use indicators*, WHO/DAP/93.1.

World Health Organization (1995) *The use of essential drugs, sixth report of the WHO expert committee*; WHO Technical Report Series 850, ISBN 92 4 120850 0, Geneva.

World Health Organization (1997) *Public-private roles in the pharmaceutical sector: implications for equitable access and rational use*, WHO/DAP/97.12.

World Health Organization (1999) *Operational principles for good pharmaceutical procurement*, WHO/EDM/PAR/99.5.

World Health Organization (2002) *Promoting rational use of medicines: core components*, WHO Policy Perspectives on Medicines no.5, WHO/EDM/2002.3.

World Health Organization (2003) *The selection and use of essential medicines: Report of the WHO expert committee 2002 (including 12th model list of essential medicines)*; WHO Technical Report Series 914, ISBN 92 4 120914 3, Geneva.

World Health Organization (2003) *Effective medicines regulation: ensuring safety, efficacy and quality*, WHO Policy Perspectives on Medicines no.7, WHO/EDM/2003.2.

World Health Organization (2004) *Drug and Therapeutic Committees: a practical guide*, WHO/EDM/PAR/2004.1.

World Health Organization (2004) *The World Medicines Situation*, WHO/EDM/PAR/2004.5.

World Health Organization (2004) *How to investigate the use of medicines by consumers*, WHO/EDM/PAR/2004.2.

World Health Organization (2006) *Using indicators to measure country pharmaceutical situations: fact book on WHO level I and level II monitoring indicators*, WHO/TCM/2006.2.

World Health Organization (2007) *How to improve the use of medicines by consumers*, WHO/PSM/PAR/2007.2.

Chapter 13

Communicable disease control principles and toolkit

Martin Schweiger

This chapter gives an overview of the following topics:

- ◆ Control communicable diseases;
- ◆ Prevent them from occurring, if possible;
- ◆ Limit their spread when they do occur;
- ◆ Reduce harm to individuals and communities from communicable diseases;
- ◆ Manage outbreaks in a competent way;
- ◆ And try to stop them from happening again.

Communicable diseases can occur in any community, but they are particularly common in poor communities, adding to the burden of poverty. The prevention of communicable diseases is an important element in any strategy of poverty reduction.

The control of a communicable disease is a way of reducing the number and severity of cases to a tolerable level. It is generally easier to achieve control than the elimination of a communicable disease.

Those responsible for communicable disease control have different responsibilities depending on where they work. People working at a national level, within a Ministry of Health have a strategic role and need to ensure that policies are agreed and resources found from the national budget to implement them. Other people work at a regional level with a tactical role and have responsibilities for ensuring that training, supply lines, manpower levels, and other resources are adequate. Most people working in communicable disease control work at local level, with an operational role that brings them into direct contact with individuals and communities affected by the diseases they are seeking to control. Whatever organizational level you work at, it is important to understand the roles and remit of the other levels and ensure that there is good communication between levels. In some areas, particularly those with sparse populations, individuals may have to take on both the tactical and the operational role (Table 13.1).

Major killers

Morbidity and mortality

Communicable diseases account for considerable sickness and disability (morbidity) and have killed and continue to kill (mortality) more people than war. The control of communicable disease is essential if a community is to be able to live with any level of security.

Smallpox has been defeated, with the last recorded case being reported from Somalia in 1979. The eradication of smallpox was achieved at a great cost in money and effort, but it demonstrates that

Table 13.1 The different organizational roles in communicable disease control

Work location	Organizational role	Responsibilities
National	Strategic	Policy development, co-ordination and overall budgeting. National surveillance.
Regional	Tactical	Staff development, training, manpower placement, resource logistics, data collection.
Local	Operational	Local surveillance, implementing prevention programmes within communities and responding to incidents of infection.

communicable diseases can be controlled and eradicated, if the conditions are right. It is reasonable to expect that other diseases will be eradicated, with polio being well on its way to eradication.

While some diseases are being controlled and eradicated, others are emerging into our awareness for the first time and others are returning. The last decade alone has seen the emergence of hepatitis C and various antibiotic resistant strains of bacteria. The collapse of communism was associated with a breakdown in the child health programmes of Russia and Eastern Europe and the rapid rise of diphtheria (Fig. 13.1).

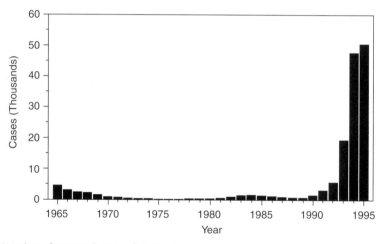

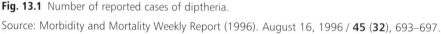

Fig. 13.1 Number of reported cases of diptheria.

Source: Morbidity and Mortality Weekly Report (1996). August 16, 1996 / **45** (**32**), 693–697.

Relationship between individual health and the health of the community

Local beliefs and understandings

An important key to the control of communicable diseases is knowing what people believe about the illness. Where does the illness come from, what does it do to the person and their family, and why has it affected that person? These are important to the patient and those around them, any advice you give will be interpreted in terms of these beliefs.

Understanding local beliefs make it possible to give advice that people will act on. In an example from Northern Bangladesh, it was possible to explain that measles vaccine was such a kind and strong spirit that it would protect children against measles even if someone had done something wrong. Injections are popular; some people also believe that the metal in the needle adds to the strength of the measles vaccine spirit.

Good practice point: Take the time and trouble to learn what local people believe about the cause of common diseases.

Stigma can be worse than the disease

Misunderstanding about a communicable disease can cause considerable fear and anxiety. This may lead to cases being hidden, or afraid to come forward for treatment. The patient may also be rejected by family and friends. Patients with tuberculosis, leprosy, and HIV may need special help to prevent them being cast out by their family and friends. Special care needs to be taken when contact tracing (looking for other cases of infection) to prevent someone being blamed for spreading or causing the disease. The situation is made worse when health care workers adopt inappropriate precautions to protect themselves from infection.

Good practice point: Take time to make sure patients understand the routes by which their infection may be spread and teach them the appropriate methods to stop infection spreading.

Changes over time

Changes in the physical and social environment which occur over time may allow some infections to become more common and even facilitate the appearance of new communicable diseases. The development of dams has lead to considerable spread of schistosomiasis and the introduction of air conditioning equipment has resulted in several outbreaks of Legionnaires' Disease, a disease not recognized until 1976. The opening of new transport routes and the migration of people have been important means of spreading communicable diseases into areas that previously have been free of them. The spread of HIV infection in Africa has followed major road transport routes. In 2002 SARS was able to spread rapidly from continent to continent when patients were able to fly long distances without any sign of illness because they were still incubating the disease.

Putting other people at risk

For any communicable disease to spread, three things are required – a source of infection, a route of transmission, and people to be susceptible to that particular infection. If any one of these is missing, the disease cannot spread. On the other hand, it only requires one person to introduce a communicable disease into a susceptible population for it to spread if there is a suitable route of transmission. For example, it only takes one refugee to come to enter a camp while suffering from cholera to cause this waterborne infection to spread to many of the other refugees in the camp within a few days.

Balance between the host and the invader

There is always a balance between the capacity of communicable disease organisms to cause illness and the capacity of the human body to resist infection. The balance is a dynamic one, changing all the time. The higher the infecting dose (the more organisms are present) the more likely it is that illness will occur. On the other hand existing good health, good nutrition and a high level of immunity to the specific infection will all help the body to resist infection and reduce the level of any illness subsequently suffered. Access to prompt diagnosis and treatment are also important factors in resisting infection.

Good practice point: Seek to promote the health of the whole community in order to protect the health of all individuals within it.

Host factors

General health

While being in good general health is not a guarantee of protection from infection it certainly reduces the risk. People at the extremes of age are both more likely to acquire infections and to suffer them more seriously than the rest of the population. Some illnesses, such as diabetes, make the individual particularly prone to a wide range of infections. Immunity can also be damaged by diseases such as HIV or treatments with steroids and anticancer treatments.

Nutrition

Diet plays an essential role in developing protection against infection. A variety of substances known as vitamins are essential for maintaining human health. Different foods contain different types and amounts of vitamins. Nutritional deficiencies in children and elderly people are recognized as a risk factor for infection.

An adequate fluid intake is an important part of nutrition. People who become dehydrated or who are regularly even mildly dehydrated are more prone to many types of infection.

Good practice point: Always enquire about the diet of your patients and encourage the consumption of a diet that contains plenty of fruit and vegetables.

Breast-feeding

Breast milk, especially colostrum, is known to be rich in antibodies, many of which can be absorbed by the neonatal gut, providing passive immunological protection for the new-born. The incidence of gastrointestinal disease is lower in breast-fed children than in bottle fed children living in the same communities. There is less evidence but protective effects can also be demonstrated with respiratory infections. The protection afforded by breast-feeding diminishes over time, but if breast-feeding is continued after the introduction of other foods (weaning) the infant will be helped to survive the most critical period for serious childhood infections.

The encouragement and support of breast-feeding is a major public health measure in the control of communicable disease.

Good practice point: Always enquire about breast-feeding whenever infants are seen in clinic or other health settings.

Immunity, natural, and administered

Disease specific immunity is developed before birth by exposure to circulating maternal antigens. Tetanus specific maternal antibodies are generated by immunizing pregnant women with tetanus toxoid. Their infants are born immune to tetanus and protected from neonatal tetanus. The environment around a new-born infant is kept clean, not sterile. This means the child will be exposed from birth to a wide variety of pathogens, but in doses too small to cause disease. The exposures will however prime the immune system so that later exposures to larger doses do not cause disease either. Careful observation of this process led to the discovery that deliberate immunization was possible. An antigen is a substance that produces an immune response, usually the production of antibodies. Antibodies provide protection by attaching themselves to antigens and inactivating them, often by sufficiently damaging them so that they can be destroyed and removed by special white cells called macrophages.

UNICEF, WHO and other partners in the GAVI Alliance support the Expanded Programme of Immunization, which is a programme of childhood immunization, which makes use of vaccines that are known to be safe and effective against a range of serious infections (see also Chapter 11. MNCH).

Good practice point: At every opportunity check that children are up to date with their immunizations.

Portals of entry

There are only a limited number of ways that invading organisms can enter the body. Particular organisms use particular routes to gain entry. Knowledge about which route of entry is used by a particular organism allows rational control strategies to be developed. Some infections are only known to use one route of entry, for example measles is only thought to be acquired through the airways, entering through the mouth and nose. Other infections such as Hepatitis B may be blood-borne or sexually acquired. Blood-borne infections may be the result of medical treatment with blood or blood products containing the virus. The virus may also be carried from an infected person to someone who is not infected by reusing needles that are not adequately sterilized.

Genetic makeup

Understanding the ways in which our genetic inheritance protects us from or makes us vulnerable to infection is at an early stage. It has been known for several decades that sickle cell trait was protective against malaria. This means that inheriting sickle cell trait is a definite advantage for people living in those parts of Africa with a high incidence of malaria. Cystic fibrosis, a condition in which the lungs are very vulnerable to serious infection is known to be an inherited condition. The enormous amount of work being done on understanding human genetics means that we will soon know more about how our genetic make up affects our vulnerability to infection.

The invaders

Bacteria, viruses, and parasites

A wide variety of organisms are responsible for causing disease. Many organisms can enter the human body and successfully survive and multiply. The common feature of pathogenic (disease causing) organisms is that they not only multiply within the body they have invaded but in doing so they cause a degree of damage to the host. If the damage is too severe the host may die and in doing so the organism will also perish, unless it has found a way of spreading to another host before death occurs.

1 Bacteria are cellular organisms
2 Viruses are composed of strands of DNA or RNA, often encapsulated in a protein coat.
3 Parasites are organisms that depend on another species in order to survive, obtaining all their nourishment from that host. They range in size and complexity from single cells (e.g. the protozoan parasite causing malaria) to sophisticated multi-cellular organisms with differentiated parts adapted for life inside the human body (e.g. tape worm). In order for the species to survive, parasites have lifecycle stages outside the body. Understanding the lifecycle of an infectious disease makes it possible to develop control strategies.

Infecting dose

Most infections require a minimum number of organisms to cause disease, the precise number being related to the host's capacity to with stand the invasion. For salmonella to cause illness in an otherwise healthy person several thousand bacteria are required, numbers that will not be reached if good food hygiene is observed. Many of the strategies involved in the control of communicable disease are based on lowering the number of organisms to which susceptible people are exposed, so the infecting dose is not reached. Control by containing the number of organisms is more achievable than trying to eliminate them altogether. It is essential that control measures are repeated at regular intervals to keep the number of pathogenic organisms below those required for an infecting dose. The lower the number of organisms required to cause illness the more virulent the pathogen is said to be. When outbreaks of measles occur, those infected in the later stages of the outbreak tend to be sicker and are more likely to die than the initial cases. This is probably because they will have been exposed to very large numbers of viral particles when they acquired their infection.

Time scales

Pathogenic organisms are a diverse group, with a wide variation in many of their characteristics. One characteristic that needs to be considered if control is to be achieved is the time taken for the organism to reproduce it self. Salmonella can reproduce itself in about 20 minutes at room temperature, while the tuberculous bacilli may take months to do so. The speed with which reproduction takes place determines the time taken for a small number of organisms to reach an infecting dose and the incubation period of a disease once infection has occurred. It will also influence the speed with which treatment needs to be arranged, ranging from an immediate need when dealing with a meningococcal septicaemia to a more measured response when treating tuberculosis.

Control measures usually need to be implemented promptly if they are to protect others at risk of infection. It is helpful to have plans agreed and ready before incidents occur.

Natural history of the disease in the local setting

One of the keys to managing communicable disease is knowledge of the natural history of the disease in your area. The epidemiology and presentation may be different in a number of ways from textbook descriptions.

Good practice point: Get to know the common diseases in your area. How do they present? Do they reflect text book descriptions or even the way they present in other areas of the country?

Nosocomial infection

Nosocomial infection is infection transmitted or acquired in a health care setting.

Hospital and health care worker transmitted infection

Hospitals present particular problems for infection control. They are a place in which vulnerable people are placed together with those who suffer from communicable diseases. During time in hospital a patient is likely to be in close and often clinically intimate contact with health care staff. Staff can bring infections into hospitals with them, from other hospitals or even from home. They may then infect patients and/or other staff. It is also very easy for health staff to act as carriers of infection from one patient to another. It is a paradox that health care staff are often highly motivated to care for their patients and yet may act as the vector of a serious infection.

Hand-washing

One of the most basic controls of infection procedures is washing hands properly before and after any clinical contact with a patient. Knowledge that hand-washing is important is well known to health care staff who advocate it, but are likely themselves to often forget to practice washing their own hands. The thumb is that part of the hand most often missed when hands are washed.

It is important that all members of the clinical team wash their hands regularly and certainly before and after any significant clinical contact. Hand-washing is certainly more likely to occur if there is easy access to wash basins, soap, and hand drying facilities.

Some people have problems with dermatitis from frequent hand-washing and may need special types of soap. Soaps with scents or perfumes are more likely to cause dermatitis than soaps without scents or perfume. Mixtures of alcohol and glycerol can be a satisfactory alternative to simple hand-washing and have the advantage that they evaporate quickly, so there is no need for hand drying facilities. Alcohol and glycerol mixtures are not good at cleaning away dirt, so this method can only be used to disinfect hands that already look clean.

Good practice point: Encourage colleagues to remind each other to wash their hands before touching patients.

Sharps

Needles and other sharp instruments need to be handled with care. Increased awareness of blood-borne infections, including hepatitis B and HIV, has focussed attention on the dangers of accidental penetration of the skin with contaminated instruments.

Proper disposal arrangements should be planned to prevent accidental injury. A suitable disposal container should be next to the area in which any injection or operative procedure is carried out. The commonest time for needlestick injuries to occur is when needles are being put back into the plastic needle cover (or sheath). It is safest not to try and put the needle back into its cover. Needles should be dropped straight into the disposal container with a minimum of handling after use. Working when tired is also a recognized risk factor for accidental injuries.

If needlestick or other accidental injuries do occur the following steps should be undertaken without delay:

1 Encourage the wound to bleed for a few minutes, this can be done by the application of warm cloths or placing the injured part in warm water if that is practical. This will help to wash out any contamination.

2 Clean and dress the wound.

3 Record details of the injury in a permanent record book.

4 Determine, if possible, the infection status of the patient on whom the instrument was previously used. If the patient is suffering from Hepatitis B or HIV infection it may be appropriate to take some specific treatment. A decision about specific treatment needs to be made as soon as possible; otherwise any treatment offered may be too late.

5 Discuss with colleagues if there are ways in which such injuries could be avoided in future.

It is safest not to reuse scalpel blades or needles. If they, or other sharps, must be reused plan how to handle and store them safely and make sure that they are cleaned and properly sterilized before their next use.

Laundry

Gastrointestinal infections and some skin infections can be transmitted through contaminated sheets and clothing. If contamination has taken place the laundry should be removed with care, seeking to avoid contaminating anything else. Ideally contaminated cloths and sheets should be put into special bags that open by themselves when in contact with warm water. This allows them to be placed into a washing machine with a minimal amount of handling. Traditional methods of sluicing faecally soiled linen may only serve to contaminate a wider area.

If you are working in a situation without special laundry bags and maybe without washing machines there is a need to limit the number of people in contact with soiled linen. Good quality, waterproof aprons will afford some protection and it is essential that hands are washed well after contact with any soiled clothing.

A special problem for laundry staff is injuries from sharps mixed into cloths coming from operating theatres. If injuries do occur they should be treated as described in the section on sharps. It is also worthwhile regularly reminding operating theatre staff to be careful to ensure that all laundry is free of sharps.

Control of infection teams

A valuable tool in the control of infections in all health care premises is the Control of Infection Team. Small health centres and mobile clinics can be visited by members of the Infection Control Team; larger hospitals should have their own permanent team. A microbiologist, backed up by a specialist nurse and adequate administrative support can do a lot to recognize infection risk areas and provide advice on how to deal with them. It is essential that the Control of Infection Team have access to the senior management, so that advice is implemented as soon as possible.

When dealing with serious infections, such as Ebola fever, which spread easily to health care staff it is worthwhile deputing one member of staff to spend all their working time carefully observing other staff and prompting them to stop any actions that put themselves, other staff, or patients at risk.

Communicable disease toolbox

There are a number of ways of tackling communicable disease; these can be regarded as the tools required for communicable disease control. For some problems only one tool is required, other problems will need a combination of tools. Among the available tools are:

◆ Surveillance
◆ Epidemiology
◆ Diagnosis
◆ Treatment
◆ Antibiotics
◆ Immunization
◆ Chemoprophylaxis
◆ Education
◆ Environmental change
◆ Vector control
◆ Legislation

Surveillance

The most essential tool in the toolbox is surveillance, without it no action can be sensibly taken. Unfortunately, surveillance is often regarded as of little importance and is not developed to the point of usefulness. A lot of work is undertaken to collect data that is then simply stored away. The result is that much valuable effort to control communicable disease is wasted.

Surveillance is a process of detecting the incidence of disease, trends in incidence or geographical spread of infection. From collected data it should be possible to determine the background incidence of an infection. If the incidence is above the background rate it is reasonable to consider if an outbreak or epidemic is occurring.

The nature of the surveillance system used depends on the expected frequency of the disease, how serious a threat to the public health a single case represents and the difficulty of detecting cases.

Good practice point: Nominate and support one member of the team to be responsible for surveillance. They need to be given proper training and listened to promptly when they report events or changes in the incidence of diseases.

Passive systems

Passive surveillance systems are the most widespread. They rely on events being reported, such as visits to a health clinic or admissions to a hospital. The data is collected and passed on to those managing the surveillance system at agreed intervals. In addition to clinical events being recorded, surveillance systems can monitor laboratory findings of particular organisms or their characteristics, such as antibiotic resistance. Patterns observed can be used to plan or adjust control programmes. Endemic diseases, such as tuberculosis, that have a long natural history can be followed with passive surveillance systems.

Active systems

Active surveillance systems are based on a process of seeking out cases that are of particular interest. It is needed when particular conditions become less common as a result of previously introduced control measures. A small number of undetected cases may undermine a lot of work done previously, so active surveillance is required to detect them. An example would be taking malaria slides from cases of fever in a community that now has a low incidence of malaria. After flooding or some other major environmental disaster it would be wise to set up an active surveillance system for diarrhoeal disease.

Case definitions

It is important that all concerned with the control of a particular disease have the same understanding of what it is that they are dealing with. If every child with a fever and a rash is considered to be a case of measles, it will be difficult to detect other conditions which present with fever and a rash! Equally not all cases of illness caused by the measles virus will have a fever and a rash. It is useful to think of three levels of case definition, possible, probable and confirmed. E.g.

- possible measles, a case presenting with a fever and a rash.
- probable measles, a case presenting with a fever, rash, Koplick spots, and a history of contact with other known cases.
- confirmed measles, a case with the clinical presentation of a probable case, and positive virological findings for measles.

One problem with confirmed cases is that all laboratories have some errors, with false positive and false negative results. Hopefully these are few and quality control measures should keep them to a minimum.

Whatever case definitions are used it is very important that all those using them agree to use them in the same way.

Local feed back and relevance

Surveillance systems are only as good as the information put into them. If those supplying the data do not know what the information will be used for and get no feed back the accuracy of the reporting will deteriorate. It is well worth taking the time to keep all those who are meant to report informed about the value of the work. It is also worthwhile asking them to send in 'nil returns' when there are no cases. This ensures that the system remains alert, even when there are no cases.

Maps

The use of maps has been of great assistance in the control of communicable disease. Dr John Snow managed to identify the source of cholera in London in 1854, by plotting cases on a map. The cases clustered around a water pump in Broad Street, Soho. Removal of the handle of the pump was associated with a rapid decline in the number of cholera cases. Plotting individual cases in this way is still useful for investigating outbreaks.

Maps can also be useful in monitoring trends of disease. This is done by dividing the map into recognizable areas with known populations. The rate of disease (e.g. cases per 10,000 people per year) is then calculated and areas of the map shaded to show which areas have particular rates of disease. The information gained by studying these maps can help to focus control strategies.

Epidemiology

Epidemiology is the practice of studying the distribution of disease. This allows the disease to be understood so that control measures can be developed and monitored. People who practice epidemiology are called epidemiologists. Trained epidemiologists have a responsibility to support surveillance systems and to ensure that data collected is analysed correctly and acted on when required.

Laboratory diagnosis

A key element in the control of communicable disease is laboratory-based information. Laboratory findings are usually required to confirm a case of a particular disease. Laboratories can help to detect the presence of particular pathogenic organisms and their characteristics such as their appearance on an agar plate, antibiotic resistance, or ability to ferment different sugars. By collecting data the laboratory can also act as a source of information on the presence and distribution of particular communicable diseases.

Treatment of cases

While some communicable diseases are passed from the environment to man (e.g. tetanus) or from animals to man (also called zoonotic infection) (e.g. salmonella) most communicable diseases are communicable from one person to another. Reducing the capacity of a case to transmit the infection is one of the keys to controlling the disease. Treatment is one of the ways of reducing capacity to transmit an infection that has the added advantage of helping the person with the disease. It is important to give treatments that are appropriate and effective, otherwise the capacity to infect other people will not be reduced and the patient's health may become worse. A serious complication is the development of antibiotic resistant strains of the infection, as a result of inadequate dosage of the antibiotic. This may require that not only is the correct antibiotic made available to the patient, but steps may also need to be taken to ensure that the patient takes it properly. For example in TB, it is important to help the patient choose a treatment supporter who will help them take the antituberculous therapy, so the right dose is taken at the right time.

Antibiotics

Antibiotics are a range of drugs that work against bacterial infection by either destroying the invading bacteria (bacteriocidal) or by stopping them from multiplying (bacteriostatic). Different antibiotics are effective against different organisms. Some are effective against only a small range of bacteria and are said to be narrow spectrum antibiotics, while others are effective against more types of bacteria and are said to be broad spectrum antibiotics. Many infections will resolve of their own accord, so prescribing antibiotics is not always required. Sore throats do not require antibiotics unless there is reason to believe that they are streptococcal in origin. Many cases of diarrhoea will not be helped and may be made worse by antibiotics, so attention should be focussed on urgent rehydration and preventing spread of infection, which will save lives. Treating viral infections with antibiotics is a waste of time, money, and drugs. Far from curing the patient it may only be the unwanted side effects of the antibiotics that remain when treatment is complete.

Need for proper choices

There are only a limited number of antibiotics available, even if different companies choose to call them by different names. It is worthwhile knowing the effective range of antibiotics that you are likely to use, so that if they are used they are likely to be used correctly. If local laboratories can test for antibiotic sensitivity that information should be sought, preferably before starting treatment if the patients' condition can cope with the delay. For acute infections there is rarely any need to give more than one type of antibiotic at a time.

Need for adequate supplies

If antibiotics are to be used they must be used in quantities adequate to eradicate the infection. If antibiotics are used in too low a dose or stopped too early the result may be a recurrence of the infection, possibly in a form resistant to antibiotics. Apart from supplying sufficient antibiotics to the patient it is essential that they know how often to taken them and that they realize the need to continue after symptomatic improvement.

Need for good storage

Antibiotics that are stored in too warm a place or simply kept beyond their expiry date may no longer be effective. Antibiotics that are made up to a liquid form when dispensed usually only have a short shelf life and must be kept in a refrigerator. Poorly stored tetracyclines have caused renal damage and must not be used after their expiry date.

Recognition of side effects

All drugs can have side effects and antibiotics are no exception. Because they have an effect on living organisms they can kill the good organisms as well as the bad organisms. Antibiotics taken by mouth will disturb the organisms living in the gut, so episodes of diarrhoea are common after antibiotics. In elderly people, or those who are frail, a course of antibiotics may so alter the balance of organisms in the gut that an organism called clostridium difficle can invade and cause a very serious inflammatory condition. Nausea and occasional vomiting may also take place. Skin rashes and allergic reactions can take place and allergy to penicillin is well known. The allergic reactions are usually mild, but can be life threatening on occasion. Any health care staff giving intramuscular or intravenous penicillin should be alert for the rare anaphylactic response and be trained and equipped to deal with it.

Some antibiotics are known to have particular side effects; streptomycin can cause eighth cranial nerve damage leading to a loss of balance and deafness. Ampicillin is associated with a distinctive rash in people suffering from glandular fever (infectious mononucleosis).

Recognition of resistance problems

If a course of antibiotics has failed to have the expected effect it may be that the course was not taken correctly, the course was too short or the organism is resistant to that antibiotic. Before taking another course of the same antibiotic, it is worthwhile considering resistance. Have similar cases failed to respond? Is there any local laboratory evidence to show the presence of antibiotic resistant organisms of the type responsible for the infection? Can an appropriate sample be taken from the patient to look for antibiotic sensitivities? If antibiotic resistance appears to be a problem it is worthwhile taking advice from a microbiologist and a pharmacist, if they are available, before proceeding.

Multi-drug resistant tuberculosis is becoming a global problem, with second line drugs being both more expensive and less effective than first line drugs. There are concerns that some pathogenic enterococci are becoming resistant to all available antibiotics.

Extended spectrum beta lactamase (ESBL) producing organisms are a newly recognized problem; they are of many different types and can resist a wide range of antibiotics.

Individual protection

Protecting individuals from infection is a well-established means of controlling communicable disease. An individual who is protected from infection cannot later transmit the infection to others. If a sufficient proportion of people are protected from infection, transmission of that particular infection is prevented within a community. Protecting enough people from smallpox infection eventually enabled smallpox to be eradicated. This would have been more difficult if the smallpox virus had affected animals or could survive in the environment for any length of time.

Immunization

Immunization is a natural process. It is the means by which the body's defence systems learn to recognize foreign proteins (antigens) and to produce antibodies which destroy or neutralize them in some way. Short-term protection can also be obtained from being given ready-made antibodies, this is called passive immunization. Immunization occurs before birth with exposure to antigens across the placenta and the acceptance of some maternal antigens which give passive immunity. This process is boosted after birth by antigens and antibodies in colostrum and subsequently in breast milk.

Natural infections also induce immunity, which is often long lasting. Babies cannot be kept in a totally sterile world; they develop immunity in response to the organisms to which they are exposed. The problem with natural infections is that they may also cause illness. With most infections a low infecting dose will allow the development of immunity, while a higher dose will cause disease. Medically administered vaccines are prepared in such a way that they should not cause illness, because:

- The organisms have been killed (pertussis),
- Or do not contain whole organisms (modern Hepatitis B vaccines),
- Or are developed from products of the organism rather than the organism itself (tetanus toxoid).
- Or the organism is a live one, but has been modified to be non-pathogenic (measles).

The success of the smallpox eradication campaign of the 1970s has boosted confidence in the safety and effectiveness of immunization. The Expanded Programme of Immunization (EPI) has provided a framework for immunization, particularly for children. The World Health Organization has supported immunization of children around the world as a major contribution to improving health and reducing childhood mortality. The diseases for which vaccines are generally used are measles, whooping cough (pertussis), tetanus, diphtheria, tuberculosis (BCG) and polio. In recent years the value of including immunization with other measures such as Growth Monitoring, Oral Rehydration and Breast-Feeding has formed the basis of a significant international programme called GOBI, saving millions of children's lives. More recently the integrated management of childhood diseases (IMCI) care guideline and training course has been developed by WHO (see Chapter 9 Maternal and child health). IMCI guidelines include that after assessing and treating the child, to check the child health card and either give any vaccinations that are due, or if the child is very ill to give an appointment when they should return for vaccination. This avoids missed opportunities to vaccinate the child.

The timing of immunization is worked out from a balance of the age at which the child is likely to be (immunologically) mature enough to be able to produce antibodies and before they are exposed to the infection.

Some vaccines have to be given several times to develop a sufficient level of immunity, these are usually not live vaccines. Live vaccines give long-lasting immunity after a single dose. An exception to this is polio which does need to be given in multiple doses.

Vaccines exist for many other infections, the decision as to which ones to use are based on the efficacy of the vaccine, the prevalence of the disease and its associated morbidity, the side effect profile of the vaccine, its cost and availability.

Vaccines are the subject of much research. Many developing countries have already added vaccines to the original six (EPI plus) such as Hepatitis B, as this is common in many developing countries. Also vaccines against locally endemic diseases may be added, such as yellow fever in West Africa. New vaccines such as the Hib vaccine for *haemophillus influenzae* have also been added. Vaccines against *pneumococcus* are also available, but remain expensive. The number of new and useful vaccines continues to increase and as the price tends to fall over time making them worth considering for inclusion in schedule. Because the same staff and cold chain which already exists for EPI, the extra cost is only that of the vaccine. Economists call this a 'marginal' cost. For this reason, adding new vaccines against high prevalence diseases, such as hepatitis B, can be very cost effective. Most of the vaccines available today need careful handling and must be kept between 2°C and 8°C or they loose their effectiveness. It is also important to remember that the injection technique should be right. Most vaccines need to be given into the muscle rather than subcutaneously, so use a long enough needle and be sure to push it in far enough to reach the muscle.

Chemoprophylaxis

There are some serious infections for which there are no vaccines, such as malaria, for which specific agents are available that can prevent infections becoming established. To be effective, chemoprophylaxis has to be taken before exposure or very early in the course of the infection. Malaria prophylaxis is generally started a week prior to exposure and should continue for about 4 weeks after the last exposure. Chemoprophylaxis is not normally recommended for those living long term in malarious areas because of the cumulative side effects of the drugs used. It would also be difficult to maintain regular chemoprophylaxis over a lifetime. There may be times when long term residents of malarious areas should be advised to take chemoprophylaxis, such as during pregnancy or for some months after a period time living away from the area when any acquired immunity may be lost. Chemoprophylaxis has been used for a long time in protecting those exposed, such as infants of mothers with TB. More recently WHO has recommended chemoprophylaxis with 6 months of isoniazid to people who are infected with HIV and TB. Between a third and a half of adults living in developing countries are infected with TB and if also infected with HIV about 1 in 10 become ill with TB per year. Chemoprophylaxis with 6 months of isoniazid clears this latent infection and prevents them becoming ill when the body's immunity level drops due to HIV, (however only long term chemoprophylaxis would prevent reinfection with TB).

Chemoprophylaxis has been used for a long time in protecting those exposed to tuberculosis. It is also used in connection with meningococcal infections when its purpose is to reduce carriage of a pathogenic strain of meningococci rather than to treat early disease. The possible protective benefits of chemoprophylaxis in any individual must always be balanced against side effects from the agents being used.

Education

Information about communicable diseases is a valuable tool in its control. It is not, however, enough to simply give people the information, they must be able to understand it and able to do something about it. Information about the risk of drinking contaminated water is only going to be helpful if safe water supplies can be made available.

Health worker

Health workers have a particular role in education about communicable diseases. By the nature of their work they may be more exposed to infection than the rest of the population. They need to be educated about the communicable diseases they are likely to encounter, so that they can recognize them and take appropriate steps to protect themselves and other staff. The health worker is usually respected by his or her patients and is well placed to educate them about communicable diseases to them. Education takes time and needs skills, not all health workers are natural teachers. Simply instructing patients what they should do is not the same as educating them. The person who has been educated about the problem can make informed judgements about the risks and will be able to work out ways of minimizing them.

Patient

Patients with communicable diseases need to be educated about their illnesses. If the patient can understand how they may have been infected they may be able to prevent later re-infection. If they know how it is spread they and their carers can take rational precautions to prevent the spread of infection. The patient may be able to motivate other people to take sensible precautions.

Public

Public education about communicable disease is a major contribution to public safety. It enables the population to behave in such a way as to reduce risks. However like the education to individual patients, educating the public requires more than the simple passing of information. Achieving positive behaviour change requires a lot of effort and considerable patience. This is either because the activity recommended is unexciting, like hand washing, or an activity discouraged is seen as enjoyable, such as sex or intravenous drug use.

Environmental change

The environment in which people live is a major determinant in the likely level of exposure to pathogenic organisms. In simple terms, if it is dirty, it is dangerous! The environment is a complex entity, with many different things in it, many of which will change over even quite short periods of time. Those changes affect the balance between human beings and the organisms that can harm us. The control of communicable disease demands that we pay attention to the physical surfaces of the ground, plants, animals, and buildings as well as air and water. Because it is a complex area it is useful to know where to turn for additional information and advice. The people with particular responsibilities for maintaining a healthy environment may not work for the Government Health Service, being employed instead by local councils and authorities. The working environment also needs to be considered as infections may be occupationally acquired.

Water, sanitation, and hygiene education

According to WHO, 80% of the illness in the world is linked to water, every year more than 5 million people die each year from unsafe water, 450 million people in Africa do not have safe drinking water. There are four kinds of water-related disease

> *Waterborne disease*: Included all those disease which can be transmitted through drinking water including cholera and typhoid.

Water-washed diseases: where the main source of infection comes from contact with faeces and lack of hygiene such as trachoma, diarrhoea, and soil-transmitted helminths (worms).

Water based infections: where water plays a role in host/parasite lifecycle, e.g. schistosomiasis and guinea worm

Water related insect vector: where water forms the breeding ground for an insect vector, e.g. malaria, dengue, onchocerciasis, and filiariasis.

See Chapter 14 (Control of major Comm Diseases) for more detail on epidemiology and control interventions.

The most basic need is to provide good quality water to communities, but more needs to be done. In many cases the problem is not contamination of water but insufficient quantity for adequate hygiene. Much of the disease transmission was taking place through the water-washed routes and it was realized that provision of water needs to be accompanied by the promotion of latrine use and simple hygiene measures including washing of hands and clean storage of water in the home. Community trials have demonstrated that simple interventions such as hand-washing with soap or an abrasive such as ashes can have an impact on diarrhoeal disease. Low cost latrines have been developed such as the ventilated improved pit latrine and pour flush latrine which represent major improvements over traditional pit latrines.

However, the need for sanitation and hygiene is not always recognized. One of the challenges is to ensure that programmes for improving water supply include a strong health education and communication component. This helps to ensure that the water systems are maintained and used properly, that water is collected and stored in clean containers, that latrines are used and hygiene behaviours such as washing of hands are regularly practised. See also Chapter 8, 'Health promotion'.

Ventilation

Air-borne infections are difficult to control, since breathing is something we all have to do. However it is possible to reduce individual risk of infection by adequate ventilation, because it reduces the concentration of organisms present in the air. If the concentration is low enough the infecting dose is not reached. Improved ventilation as part of better housing is important in reducing measles, tuberculosis and other diseases spread by coughing and aerosols. In health facilities where people with chronic cough and TB are managed it is important to ensure good cross-flow of air through large open windows on opposite sides of the room. Air that contains cigarette smoke is associated with an increased risk of airborne infections, probably because of the action of nicotine on the airways. Passive smoking is associated with an increased incidence of meningococcal infections, so it not just the smoker who is at risk.

Cleanable surfaces

One of the main contributions to improved hygiene in recent years has been the development and use of cleanable surfaces. The capacity to clean and disinfect surfaces is essential in the control of food-borne infections and many hospital acquired infections.

Vector control

Some organisms causing communicable diseases have complicated life cycles. During the life of the organism it requires more than one species of host. If one of the species is not available the disease will not be present. If we regard the human as the potential patient, the other species is called the vector. From the other species point of view it is the human that is the vector! The vector is often an insect, although for schistosomiasis the vector is a snail which can release thousands of cercariae, a form of the parasite that penetrates the intact skin of the human host to cause infection. Control of the vector is essential if the communicable disease is to be controlled.

In the control of communicable diseases it is important to interrupt the cycle of transmission. Which interventions to use will depend on the epidemiology of the disease.

Helminths such as roundworm (ascaris) contribute to malnutrition, and hookworm to anaemia. Transmission is by faeces contaminating the soil with eggs which then contaminate water or food and gets into the mouth. These soil-transmitted helminths are therefore oral-faecal transmitted diseases (as are bacteria and viruses causing of diarrhoea and dysentery). They are prevented by education for better hygiene, especially washing hands before eating and after defaecating and by access to clean water and sanitation.

Neglected tropical diseases control

In schistosomiasis and soil transmitted helminths, multiple interventions are recommended including yearly mass drug administration together with improved water and sanitation and education. Together these should maintain low levels of transmission and hence control the disease. What to do in your context depends on your review of the situation and interventions (see Chapter 5, 'Choosing the best interventions'). Other 'neglected diseases' caused by worms in the tropics include onchocerciasis (river blindness) and lymphatic filariasis both of which can also be controlled by mass drug administration.

While generally the drugs are supplied free, the community may be concerned about side effects to the treatment. There may be existing cultural beliefs about the diseases (e.g. onchocerciasis). Health promotion has a vital part to play in encouraging affected communities to participate and play an active role in the decision to go for treatment and return for follow-up. One of the most successful strategies has been to train members of affected communities as village level distributors for ivermectin and provide on-going support. This intervention strategy is called community-directed distribution, with drug distribution by community volunteers linked to existing primary health care infrastructures.

Mosquito control programmes

Large mosquito control programmes have been established as a way of limiting mosquito-borne diseases. It is not only malaria that is spread by mosquitos. Filaria, yellow fever, dengue, and Japanese encephalitis are also mosquito-borne diseases, causing substantial morbidity. See Chapter 14, 'Controlling major communicable diseases'.

Legislation

Most people will cooperate with communicable disease control programmes out of enlightened self-interest. Unfortunately, there are times when an individual or a group of individuals refuses to do so. The first response must be to try and educate them and encourage co-operation. If this fails it may be necessary to resort to legal sanctions. Most countries have some relevant legislation, empowering those responsible for public health to prohibit movement, examine people, take samples, admit to hospital or to keep some one in hospital. It is sensible to find out what legislation exists in your country and how it works, both in theory and in practice.

The successful control of communicable diseases may also require the authority to act in a particular way. Sometimes special measures are required, such as needle exchange schemes or the supply of condoms. Resources are required, of people with skills, of equipment, of money, and time. Above all, control of communicable disease requires effective teamwork.

Outbreaks

Many people and most health organizations only think about communicable disease when an outbreak occurs. Communicable disease control is often only given a low priority in management of time and resources. Outbreaks provide a sudden focus on the communicable disease. However, outbreaks really demonstrate a failure to prevent the spread of infection! Having outbreak plans ready makes the control of outbreaks when they do occur much more straightforward.

Objectives

There are four objectives in the management of any outbreak:

1 Reduction in the number of primary cases

   Primary cases are those people who become ill following exposure to the original source of the outbreak. This usually requires identifying the source of the outbreak and controlling it. The earlier you know about the outbreak the more chance you have of finding it before even more people are exposed.

   If the source is polluted water, providing a safe alternative and preventing access to the polluted water will prevent any more primary cases. In the same way, a restaurant or other food outlet may need to be closed.

2 Reduction in the number of secondary cases

   Secondary cases are those people who acquire their infections from those who were infected from the primary source. They are often family or social contacts. It is important to find those who have a greater chance of spreading the infection because of the work they do, for example a cook with an acute salmonella infection could infect a lot of people.

3 Reducing the harm from the outbreak

   Communicable diseases can be very serious, causing significant morbidity and mortality. Ensuring that those made ill by the outbreak receive proper care is an essential element in managing the outbreak. There may be other harm consequent on the outbreak, for example hospitals may have to close because too many staff are sick to provide care to others, or in situations perceived to be serious people may flee from the area. Clear and accurate information to the newspapers and any local radio may help. Outbreak management includes paying attention to all the harm that may result from it.

4 Preventing a recurrence

   If an outbreak has occurred once it can happen again. Seek to understand what caused the outbreak and see what can be done to prevent it happening again.

   All actions following an outbreak should address one or more of these objectives.

Managing an outbreak

It is always easier to manage an outbreak if you have made plans in advance. For example, planning for a meningitis outbreak in sub-Saharan region of Africa, see Box 13.1.

Time taken to write down a plan before you have problems will be time well spent. Before you start to prepare your outbreak plan you may to check if a suitable plan already exists, or there is an old one that simply needs to be brought up to date. Failure to plan is planning to fail!

If you have a prepared outbreak plan, read it carefully. Does it reflect the situation?

Can you verify the facts, what is happening, to whom, where, and when did it start? Obtaining this information is crucial to your investigation and management of the outbreak. Consider who else needs to know about the outbreak and see that they are informed.

You may want to call an urgent meeting of people who can help. This is often called an Outbreak Control Meeting. The people who need to be there are those with skills or responsibilities relevant to the situation. They are likely to include local environmental health officers, microbiologists, doctors, and nurses looking after the patients, managers, or people with access to more resources, clerical support, and an epidemiologist.

Box 13.1 'Planning' for outbreaks – meningitis epidemics in Africa

Planning for meningitis epidemics in the sub-Sahara 'sahel' countries, is very important. These epidemics tend to come in cycles of 10–14 years, though this varies from country to country. The frequency of epidemics is moderated by several factors, including the spread of new strains, the extent and frequency of previous vaccination campaigns, and climatic and environmental factors.

The WHO intervention strategies are (i) reactive vaccination to halt the outbreak and (ii) effective case management through antibiotic treatment to reduce the lethality of the disease. For this to be effective, a system of early detection and rapid laboratory confirmation is required. This would then help to determine predefined alert and epidemic thresholds and distinguish between a seasonal rise and an emerging epidemic. For instance, for a population of more than 30 000, the epidemic threshold is an incidence of 15 cases per 100 000 population per week (WHO World Health Statistics, 2008).

The Outbreak Control Meeting will:

- ◆ Want to review the facts that are known about the outbreak;
- ◆ Wish to confirm that there really is an outbreak;
- ◆ Decide what other information is required and how to obtain it;
- ◆ Agree a case definition for someone affected by the outbreak. What signs and symptoms or laboratory results are required for possible, probable and confirmed cases?
- ◆ Decide on the most appropriate form(s) of investigation and control;
- ◆ Wish to ensure that the investigation is proceeding and sick people are being treated;
- ◆ Decide who else needs to know, this is particularly important if the outbreak involves people in more than one district or will attract a lot of publicity;
- ◆ Decide what is said to the media and who will say it;
- ◆ Decide on the form of documentation to be kept. Individual patient forms and log books for the different elements of the investigation need to contain an agreed minimum amount of information;
- ◆ Review the outbreak plan to ensure that it is appropriate for this outbreak;
- ◆ Determine if adequate resources are available to manage the outbreak;
- ◆ Determine what else needs to be done and who should do it;
- ◆ Assess the risk associated with the outbreak. Risk can be considered in terms of the seriousness of the disease, how easily it spreads, the level of confidence in knowing exactly what has happened, ability to the intervene and the level of community concern about the outbreak.
- ◆ Agree a frequency for Outbreak Control Meetings.

At the first opportunity decide if there are others who should also be called to join the Outbreak Control Meetings. Ensure that all decisions are recorded and agree who will do what and by when. At the end of the outbreak all records should be reviewed and a final report prepared to serve as a record of what has occurred.

Like so much else in communicable disease control, managing outbreaks is a team effort. Good teams have members that respect and trust each other; they also talk and share their learning (Table 13.2).

Table 13.2 To show some of the responsibilites of those responsible for communicable disease control at national, regional, and local level before, during, and after major outbreaks

	Well before	Shortly before	During an outbreak	Shortly after an outbreak	Some time after an outbreak
National (strategic)	Develop national polices. Plan national resources	Ensure adequate surveillance programmes in place	Advise central government and pass information to relevant government departments Maintain contact with WHO	Check that policies have been followed	Review the event to see if there are lessons to be learnt
Regional (Tactical)	Develop and deliver training programmes, staffing and other resources	Ensure that data is collected from all parts of the region and collected in a timely manner	Ensure that there are adequate resources of staff, transport, medicines etc are available to affected areas. Maintain good communication local area and national government	Consider what actions should now be taken to prevent a recurrence. Do resources now need to be redeployed? Was staff training adequate?	Review what actions need to be modified next time. Has the local outbreak report been received and receiwed?
Local (Organisational)	Routine surveillance. Health promotion programmes including immunization	Look out for indications that some infections are increasing in frequency	Co-ordinate local response. Maintain good data collection and deploy staff and other resources to the best effect	Check that all local actions that should have been taken are complete Write report of the outbreak	Review the outbreak with all local frontline staff involved. Are there any local lessons to be learnt?

Conclusion

There are many factors contributing to the spread of communicable diseases. In public health we seek to promote the health of the whole community in order to protect the health of all individuals within it. Understanding the lifecycle of an infectious disease, and reviewing the national policy, local service delivery situation, and health beliefs are all essential to knowing how to control the disease.

The tools for communicable disease control include: surveillance, epidemiology, diagnosis, treatment, antibiotics, immunization, chemoprophylaxis, education, environmental change, vector control, and legislation.

Further reading

Kassambara, M., Poudiougo, P., Philippon, B., Samba, E.M., Zerbo, D.G. (1986) Village community participation in onchocerciasis vector control. *World Health Forum*, **7**(**1**), 57–61.

Ngoumou, P., Essomba, R.O., Godin, C. (1996) Ivermectin-based onchocerciasis control in Cameroon. *World Health Forum*, **17**, 25–8.

Richards F., Jr., Gonzales-Peralta C., Jallah E., Miri E. (1996) Community-based ivermectin distributors: onchocerciasis control at the village level in Plateau State, Nigeria. *Acta Tropica*, **61(2)**, 137–44.

Whitworth J.G., Alexander N.D.E., Seed P., Thomas W., Abiose A., Jones B.R. (1996) Maintaining compliance to ivermectin in communities in two West African countries. *Health Policy and Planning*, **11(3)**, 299–307.

Jamison D. et al. *Disease control priorities in developing countries*, 2nd edition (DCP2). http://www.dcp2.org/main/Home.html

Heymann David (2004) *Communicable diseases manual*, 18th edition. APHA. ISBN 0-87553-242-X.

Hawker J., Begg N., Blair I., Reintjes R., Weinberg J. (2005) *Communicable disease control handbook*, 2nd edition. Blackwell.

Webber R. (2004) *Communicable disease epidemiology and control*, 2nd edition, Oxford: CABI Publishing. (new edition due 2009).

Internet

Morbidity & Mortality Weekly Report (MMWR of CDC) at www.cdc.gov/mmwr/

Weekly Epidemiology Report (WHO) at www.who.int/wer/en

PROMED at www.promedmail.org

CDC at www.cdc.gov

Eurosurveillance at www.eurosurveillance.org

HPA at www.hpa.org.uk

Chapter 14

Controlling major communicable diseases

John Walley, Roger Webber, and Andrew Collins

This chapter gives an overview of the following topics:

◆ Water, sanitation, and hygiene related diseases

◆ Tuberculosis, and other respiratory diseases

◆ Malaria and other vector borne diseases

◆ HIV and other sexually transmitted diseases

Interventions need to be based on an understanding of the epidemiology of the disease and review of the context in which it occurs (Chapters 3 and 4). The best intervention need to be chosen according to their relative effectiveness and feasibility in a given situation. For each intervention the delivery strategy and related activities need to be chosen (Chapter 5).

Ideally interventions should be integrated within Primary Health Care and the district health system (Chapter 10). They need to be designed to be sustainable and replicable in all affected communities.

Transmission, control, and classification

Communicable diseases are numerous and vary considerably in their resulting clinical presentation, but the key to their control lies in understanding the method by which they are transmitted. The point of transmission, whether by the aerosol droplet spread of respiratory tract infections or the use of a vector such as mosquitoes in malaria transmission is the point at which they are most vulnerable. Targeting interventions at this part of the infection cycle usually has the greatest chance of success.

There are many methods of classifying communicable diseases but if a transmission based classification is used they can be divided into 10 groups as follows:

◆ Water-washed diseases

◆ Faecal-oral diseases

◆ Food-borne diseases

◆ Skin infections

◆ Diseases of soil contact

◆ Diseases of water contact

- ◆ Airborne transmitted infections
- ◆ Diseases transmitted via body fluids
- ◆ Vector-borne diseases
- ◆ Zoonoses

It is beyond the scope of this book to cover the epidemiology and control of all these disease groups. However, at the end of the chapter other books and online resources are recommended. Instead, the emphasis in this chapter will be on the epidemiology and control of major communicable diseases accounting for the greatest burden of disease in low-middle income settings.

Water, sanitation, and hygiene-related diseases

Diarrhoea and other water, sanitation and hygiene related diseases are the biggest cause of the burden of disease in low income countries e.g. Sub Saharan Africa and Southeast Asia. Elsewhere, even though the burden is less, they remain the 'best buy' in terms of cost-effective interventions (see Chapters 1, 2, and 7). The routes of transmission of the water and sanitation-related diseases are illustrated in Fig. 14.1.

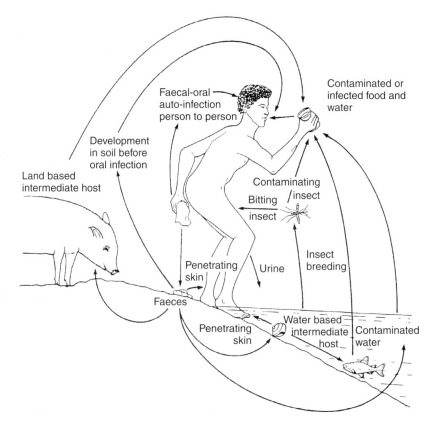

Fig. 14.1 'Routes of transmission of the water and sanitation related diseases'.

Water-washed diseases

This group includes many diarrhoeal diseases and eye diseases such as trachoma, the major cause of blindness in the world. The main intervention is the provision of water in sufficient **quantity** to allow for adequate washing. Daily face washing has been shown to significantly reduce the risk of developing trachoma. So the long-term strategy will be the provision of water supplies and proper sanitation. Simple hand washing will help to reduce infection from some 90 (bacterial, viral, protozoa, and worm) infectious agents.

Faecal-oral diseases

This large group of infections includes many of the diseases that present as diarrhoea such as gastroenteritis and cholera. The main cause of death, especially in children, is through dehydration. The deaths are due to child loss and dehydration. Their management is with the replacement of fluid through oral rehydration, and their prevention by the provision of adequate water supplies. The essential feature is the improvement of the **quality** of water because it is the contamination of water supplies that mainly leads to these infections. In an emergency this can be by boiling the water, but the long-term aim should be to find a good water supply and protect it from contamination. The provision of sanitation and proper disposal of rubbish (to control flies) are additional methods.

The main diseases in this group are: cryptosporidiosis, cholera, shigellosis, *Giardia*, amoebiasis, typhoid, paratyphoid, Hepatitis A, Hepatitis E, *Enterobius*, and poliomyelitis. The main control measures are water, sanitation and hygiene promotion. Also hepatitis B can be orally faecally transmitted, though more commonly through blood. While, hepatitis B vaccination has been included in Expanded Programme on Immunization (EPI) in many low income countries, ensuring that only new or sterilized needles are used for injections is important to prevent hepatitis B and C.

Food-borne diseases

Many infections are transmitted by food, such as food poisoning (*Salmonella, Campylobacter)* or are transmitted by specific foods such as the beef tapeworms. This is one of the most specific groups of diseases and adequate cooking and proper storage is required.

The main diseases in this group are Salmonella, *Campylobacter*, beef and pork tapeworms, Trichinosis and *Fasciolopsis,* the sheep liver fluke, the fish-transmitted, liver flukes, and the lung fluke.

Skin infections

The skin is a common site for several communicable diseases, presenting with rashes of various kinds. Infection is often transmitted from person to person directly by skin contact or indirectly by the airborne route.

Examples of skin infections caused by direct contact include streptococcal infections and examples of airborne infections include chickenpox/shingles, measles, rubella, mumps, and leprosy. Control is by the avoidance of contact with infected individuals and, where available, the use of vaccines. Measles vaccine is part of EPI, while in high income countries measles is combined together with mumps and rubella vaccine. The BCG vaccine helps prevent leprosy as well as the worst forms of childhood TB, while multi-drug treatment of leprosy and TB cases prevents onward transmission to others and so is important for control of these diseases.

Diseases of soil contact

Soil can be a source of infection for several diseases, particularly those caused by nematode worms and the bacterial infection, tetanus. Transmission can either be ***direct*** from contamination of wounds with soil and by swallowing worm eggs, or **indirect** through the penetration of the skin by hookworm larvae when it comes into contact with the soil.

Since there is a common mode of transmission for the three main infections (e.g. *Round worms, threadworms*, and the *hookworms*), they nearly always go together, so if the person is infected with one they are likely to have all three. *Roundworms and threadworms* contribute to malnutrition, while hookworms contribute to anaemia, especially affecting children. The promotion of personal hygiene and preventing contamination of soil through sanitation are the main methods of control. Additionally, mass drug administration (MDA) in schools and villages is also effective.

Tetanus bacillus is found naturally in the soil but is controlled by vaccination through the EPI programme.

Diseases of water contact

Water is an important medium for the transmission of diseases. Normally, infection occurs through drinking water that has become contaminated by faecal material, or using this contaminated water to wash food prior to consumption (as described above). Water also it serves as a medium for intermediate hosts such as the snails which are the intermediate host for schistosomiasis. These snails can release thousands of cercariae, a form of the parasite that penetrates the intact skin of the human host to cause infection. See Fig. 14.1 above (routes of transmission of the water and sanitation-related diseases).

Diseases this category also includes Guinea worm (dracunuliasis) which by the simple strategy of making wells safe and protecting all water sources is being eradicated.

Water, sanitation, and hygiene interventions

As with the control of any communicable diseases it is important to interrupt the cycle of transmission. Transmission of certain types of helminths (worms) occurs when faeces containing their eggs contaminates the soil, which in turn contaminates water and food and subsequently enters the gastrointestinal tract on ingestion. Most soil transmitted helminths are therefore oral-faecal transmitted diseases (together with the bacteria and viruses causing of diarrhoea and dysentery). An exception is hookworm which directly penetrates the skin of the foot (and so wearing shoes helps to prevent it). These diseases are controlled by water, sanitation, and hygiene promotion interventions.

According To UNICEF (2008) in low-middle income (LMIC) countries:

70% of people use improved drinking **water** sources (87% urban and 56% rural).

43% of people use improved **sanitation** facilities (urban 60% and rural 32%).

These figures show that a large percentage of people live in the absence of improved water and sanitation. There is also a huge variation in coverage between the rich and poor within any LIMC countries. Large variations in coverage also occur between various low-middle income countries. Individual countries range from 22–100% for improved drinking water, and from 10–86% for access to improved sanitation.

Water

Water of sufficient quantity and quality are critical to the control of these diseases. In addition, there is a need to make safe water more easily accessible to households with the resulting major benefits to women who no longer need to walk long distances to collect water. Thus, they expend less energy and have more time to care for their children, carry out farming activities, and do their other work. In rural situations local communities can be helped to protect wells, fit hand-pumps and carry out basic maintenance. This may be facilitated by outreach workers such as health assistants or environmental technicians employed by the ministry of health. Communities are

Box 14.1 Promoting sanitation and water in Zimbabwe

The building of ventilated improved pit (VIP) toilets was promoted throughout the Mashona-land Central province by training local builders and educating the villagers.

◆ Local builders built VIP toilets, under the guidance of Environmental Health Assistants at local schools

◆ School children were shown the toilets and told about their importance as part of hygiene

◆ Parents were invited to the school and were shown the toilets by the builders. They there-fore knew who the trained local builders are, and many families later paid them to con-struct toilets for the family.

The provincial health department paid for the building of toilets at schools, but in doing so promoted toilets and hygiene for the whole community, thus helping to reduce diarrhoeal disease, schistosomiasis, and helminth transmission.

generally willing to support efforts to improve their water and sanitation through protection of wells and springs, sinking boreholes, digging wells and are willing to contribute labour and resources. See Box 14.1 above for an example of a community-based approach with local com-mercial builders to support improved sanitation at schools in Zimababwe.

In urban areas (and preferably in rural areas also) piped water supplies must be provided. Typically these large-scale water schemes are the responsibility of the ministry of water and the local government. Usually this is done by contracting private companies to develop and maintain water supplies. It is important to advocate for and assist in planning for water supply schemes. Priorities may include urban slums and peri-urban areas where water supplies are not yet within reach of all households. Hand washing with soap is very effective in interrupting oral-faecal transmission.

Hygiene promotion

Health promotion of hand washing after the toilet and before cooking or eating helps to prevent diarrhoeal diseases and some respiratory infection spreaded by oral-faecal transmission. This can be part of mass media, social mobilization, and community health worker messages to groups or individuals (see Chapter 8, 'Health promotion').

Water purification. Many people in low income countries do not have piped tap water. They may have to purify their water themselves – by boiling, chlorinating, or by filtering the water. In the 'solar method' users take a clear plastic bottle with a maximum size of three litres, fill it with water and put it on the roof or a corrugated iron sheet to soak up the sun's rays. Between 6 hours and 2 days later, depending on the strength of the sun, the water should be purified. The sun's heat and UV-A rays kill all the organisms that can potentially cause diarrhoea.

Promotion can be to particular groups, such as school students, or to the whole community. The messages may be through health workers e.g. CHWs, and the mass media e.g. local radio. Provision of soap and promotion of hand washing after using the toilet and before cooking or eating meals has been shown to interrupt transmission of diarrhoeal diseases, e.g. in refugee camps. Promotion of hand washing also helps control other diseases such as soil transmitted helminths (worms) and a disease of the eyes called trachoma. Promotion of hand washing with soap should be included with other water and sanitation interventions.

Health promotion for better hygiene is an essential to the mix of interventions used to control these diseases. This can be through community mobilization, with orientation of local community and religious leaders who then put up posters and pass on messages during community and religious meetings. These community or 'interpersonal' approaches may be used together with mass media, approaches such as programmes or advertisements on local radio in the local language. In the Zimbabwe example below, (see Box 14.2) this included poster and drama competitions within and between local schools. Also see Chapter 8 (Health promotion).

Sanitation

While in high income settings flush toilets are the norm, low income settings require other methods of sanitation. These structure use locally available building materials, are low cost, and are appropriate to the culture in that country or local area. Generally in Africa and Latin America people use paper or leaves to wipe after the toilet, and so dry systems such as improved pit toilets are appropriate. However, in Asia people generally water wash after the toilet, and so wet systems such as the pour-flush toilets are more appropriate (see Fig. 14.2).

There are various approaches to promoting sanitation. In higher income settings, building standards legislation can specify standards for sanitation. In rural areas, health assistants employed by the ministry of health can advise and assist with toilet building as well as protection of wells. One can use a public–private mix approach to promote improved water and sanitation. Government funds may be used to train commercial builders, who practice latrine construction while constructing toilets in public places. This can either be in large scale urban settings, or with rural commercial builders as in the example below from Zimbabwe for building improved pit latrines, illustrated in Fig. 14.2 (see also Box 14.2).

Box 14.2 Control of schistosomiasis with multiple interventions in Zimbabwe

The provincial health office and the national communicable disease (Blair) institute implemented surveys and multiple control interventions with good results.

The surveys used were:

- A survey showing that the majority of school children are excreting schistosomiasis, both *S. haematobium* in the urine and *S. mansoni* in their faeces
- A survey mapping the transmission points at streams and lakes, where water is collected, children swim and urinate and defecate in or near the water

The interventions used initially to reduce transmission were:

- Mass treatment of school children, with the safe drug praziquantel, to reduce worm load and eggs contaminating water
- A single dose of a molluscicide killing snails at water contact points helping to reduce the amount of transmission (but it is too expensive to use repeatedly)

The interventions to maintain lower transmission were:

- Health education by school teachers in all schools, reinforced by school children competing in a drama and posters competition
- Health education for adults with posters and films followed by a discussion led by a health worker
- Constructing ventilated improved pit toilets to reduce contamination with eggs, and construction
- Protecting wells with a cover slab and a hand pump, so there is less need to collect water from streams

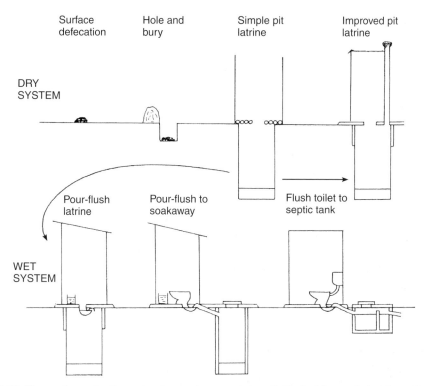

Fig. 14.2 'Types of excreta disposal systems – incremental sanitation' with permission from Roger Webber, *Epidemiology and Control of Communicable Diseases*, CABI, second edition, 2004.

Mass Drug Administration (**MDA**) is a key strategy in the control of a number of communicable diseases (see the further reading and the web link to WHO 'Preventive chemotherapy in human helminthiasis'). MDA involving 'community-directed treatment' is where community volunteers distribute medication(s) to fellow villagers. This delivery approach has been used in the annual distribution of the drug ivermectin for onchocerciasis (river blindness) in West Africa for many years. Where lymphatic filariasis co-exists with onchocerciasis, ivermectin will control both infections. If lymphatic filariasis does not co-exist, then yearly doses of DEC *and* albendazole can be given using the same strategy.

Similarly, soil transmitted helminths such as roundworm, threadworm, and hookworm can be treated with regular doses of albendazole *or* mebendazole. Also, MDA with prazequantal is an intervention for the control of schistosomiasis. For soil transmitted helminths and schistosomiasis, doses may be given annually or less frequently. Where prevalence is of helminths very high, all members of the community need to be treated, and where it is not so high, MDA can be targeted at schools and pre-schools, as children are the most affected.

Trachoma, the eye infection caused by a small bacteria called *Chlamydia*, which can lead to inflammation, scarring, and is the commonest cause of worldwide blindness, can also be managed using the MDA approach. In this case, yearly doses of the antibiotic azithromycin are administered. See also examples of MDA delivery strategies Chapter 5, Box 5.4.

Multiple interventions

Multiple interventions are often used in controlling infections such as schistosomiasis and soil transmitted helminths. Mass treatment is used to bring down the level of transmission, and then yearly mass treatment helps to maintain reduced transmission. Mass treatment can only be done if drugs used are safe and not too expensive. Improved water and sanitation and health education also help to maintain low levels of transmission and hence control the disease. In addition, in some settings where women wash clothes in the river, washing slabs have been built next to water pumps thus avoiding exposure to infections. The method of control to be employed in a specific context depends on a review of the situation and analysis of the effectiveness and feasibility of interventions in that context (see Chapter 5, 'Choose the best intervention').

Respiratory and other airborne infections

The respiratory apparatus is a common site by which the person can become infected. This is normally through the nose or mouth and the lungs.

Respiratory infections are transmitted directly from one person to another and, generally, the closer the contact, the greater the chance of spread. Vast amounts of microorganisms may be discharged in a coughing episode, yet only a few individuals manifest the disease. It is the infecting dose and host response which determine whether infection will occur. Environmental factors that can increase the infecting dose (e.g. overcrowding) or reduce the host resistance (e.g. malnutrition) can determine whether the disease will develop or not.

Some airborne-respiratory infections present predominantly with respiratory disease, e.g. influenza, but other diseases, such as meningitis and leprosy present with non-respiratory symptoms. One of the major diseases in this group and responsible for a large proportion of mortality and morbidity in the world is tuberculosis.

Tuberculosis

Tuberculosis is one of the commonest causes of death in adults in developing countries. Between a quarter and a third of all people in developing countries are infected with TB but do not have the disease (i.e. they have live TB bacteria in their chest, but their immune system is keeping them in check). Over their lifetime, about one in ten of these will go on to get active TB which, if left untreated, is often fatal. When an infected person develops the disease and has the bacilli in their sputum, the period of infectiousness is usually prolonged, permitting transmission of the infection to an average of ten other people. In countries with an endemic balance or constant prevalence, the number of cases that no longer have TB (e.g. through spontaneous resolution, cured by medical treatment, or death), is replaced by an equal number of new cases entering the pool of tuberculosis. In countries with good TB programmes whereby TB is effectively identified and cured, the rates of TB are decreasing. However, in others, HIV infection has added to the likelihood of people developing tuberculosis, so that TB is increasing, e.g. in sub-Saharan Africa. Worldwide, 8 million persons develop tuberculosis every year and 2 million die from it.

Health workers have to be alert to the possibility of TB in anyone with a cough lasting 2–3 or more weeks, coughing up blood, weight loss, fever or night sweats. Such individuals should have three sputum smear samples taken for examination to screen for TB. If two or more are positive, the patient should be diagnosed as having TB and receive antituberculous medication. If only one positive smear this may be a false positive. However, one positive sputum is enough to diagnose TB also in a patient co-infected with HIV. If sputum is not positive for bacilli, complete a course of broad spectrum antibiotics and arrange a follow-up appointment. If they still have symptoms repeat the sputum smears and do a chest X-ray. The medical officer may diagnose sputum negative TB if there are persistent clinical symptoms and X-ray appearances suggestive of TB. Younger children present a diagnostic challenge as they may have particular difficulty in generating sputum for examination (see further reading, Clinical TB).

TB-HIV

Around half of people in developing countries with both HIV and TB infection will develop active TB disease. People with HIV are also more susceptible to new TB infections or to re-infection. TB is a major cause of death in people with HIV/AIDS. Conversely tuberculosis patients are more likely to rapidly progress to full blown AIDS when infected with the HIV virus. All HIV positive cases should regularly be asked about the presence of cough and other TB symptoms and all tuberculosis cases tested for HIV.

All people infected with HIV should receive long-term cotrimoxazole preventive treatment, including TB patients to prevent pneumonia and some other infections common in people with HIV.

TB Control

The four main strategies for the control and prevention of tuberculosis are as follows:

- ◆ Improvement of social and living conditions.
- ◆ BCG vaccination.
- ◆ Identification and treatment of all cases, especially those who are sputum positive.
- ◆ Contact tracing.

Improvement in living conditions   As highlighted previously, respiratory infections, such as TB, measles, and pneumonia, are transmitted through aerosols containing the causative micro-organisms which are coughed out by ill people. The transmission of *infection* is highest where there is crowding of people in rooms and where ventilation is poor. It is important therefore to promote improved housing and in particular to improve ventilation within houses (e.g. in warm countries, adding more windows).

Furthermore, people are more susceptible to progress from infection to *disease* where people have reduced immunity due to under-nutrition and other diseases such as diabetes. In general about 1 in 10 people infected with TB later develop TB disease. However, for those who are infected with TB and HIV, around half will get active TB during their lifetime.

The socio-economic development of formerly poor countries such as China and India will have an effect in reducing TB and other respiratory diseases over time. Indeed TB was very common in Europe and rates declined greatly before the discovery of BCG or antituberculosis medications. The main reason rates came down was due to the improvement in housing and nutrition – though identification and treatment accelerated its decline. Tobacco smoking increases the risk of TB (and chronic bronchitis etc.) and efforts to control tobacco will help reduce TB.

BCG vaccination   BCG vaccination alerts the body's white blood cell defences rather than inducing antibody formation (other vaccines directly induce antibodies). After a BCG vaccination a primary infection may still take place among exposed individuals, but the risk of disseminated infection will be greatly reduced. For these reasons BCG protects against the worst kinds of childhood TB, which are miliary TB and TB meningitis (and against leprosy as well). But BCG does not have a very big effect on reduction of adult TB cases, which are the main source of transmission. BCG should be given in developing countries at birth or as soon after as possible. As it is a live vaccine, it should not be given to children who are known to be HIV positive, or to pregnant women. BCG is given as part of the expanded programme of immunization (EPI).

Identification and treatment   The main focus of TB programmes is ensuring the early identification, diagnosis, and treatment of all cases. All patients presenting with cough of more than 2 or 3 weeks duration need to be screened for TB by sputum microscopy. Also, all contacts of a confirmed case should have two sputum smears taken. Microscopy slides should be kept in boxes ready for sampling for external quality assurance (EQA). EQA is where a higher level laboratory re-checks the slides taken at lower level facilities and gives a report on the percentage of slides that agree (concordant) or disagree (discordant) with their result. If many of the sample slides are discordant slides, then supervision and in-service training is given. TB slides should not be re-used because of the risk of false positives.

The treatment of TB cases reduces onward transmission. The earlier the TB treatment starts the better it reduces the number and period of infectious cases. Good TB programmes help prevent the emergence of resistant strains. Unfortunately, due to poor implementation of TB care in the past, many countries already have a significant percentage of cases that are multi-drug resistant (MDR). MDR is when the TB infected individual does not respond or is resistant to the two most important first line drugs called isoniazid and rifampicin. These people need to be put on the MDR regimens which contain more drugs, are more expensive and need to be taken for pro-longed periods of up to 2 years. This is especially the case in South Africa among HIV positive persons. There is also an increasing emergence of extreme drug resistant (XDR) TB. These strains of TB are resistant to all the drugs available in low-middle income countries. For all these reasons, it is very important to implement TB care systematically and with standardized procedures.

The term 'DOTS' is the 'brand name' for the WHO package of care for TB. Until recently WHO Stop TB recommended that all cases should have directly observed therapy (DOT) to ensure compliance. However, trial evidence has shown that DOT does not improve cure rates. So now WHO only recommends DOT for cases such as prisoners, mentally ill people and for retreatment cases. Ensuring compliance (adherence) to treatment is done through education. It is very impor-tant that all patients should have a **treatment supporter**, as well as supervision of treatment at the monthly follow-up at their local health centre. The treatment supporter is chosen by the patient in discussion with the health worker, and should be someone who is accessible, concerned and reliable, such as a community health worker (CHW) or family member. The same approach is good for HIV/antiretroviral treatment where a treatment supporter is sometimes called a 'treatment buddy'. The treatment supporter encourages the patient when they are feeling de-motivated. This encouragement includes keeping to follow-up appointments and taking the right number of tablets consistently (Fig. 14.3).

A newly diagnosed case of TB should be treated with a four-drug regimen for 2 months, preferably as a fixed-dose combination tablets which encourages adherence. The WHO approved regimen consists of isoniazid, rifampicin, pyrazinamide, and ethambutol. This is followed by isoniazid and rifampicin, which are taken daily for a further 4 months. Alternatively, isoniazid and ethambutol may be taken daily for a follow-up period of 6 months. Recent trials have shown that replacing ethambutol with gatifloxin is more effective and will allow the total period of treatment to be reduced to 4 months. In retreatment cases the initial four drug treatment is extended by a third month, and for the first 2 months streptomycin injections are given daily.

The TB programme includes standardized diagnosis, treatment, follow-up care, and monitor-ing. This model of case management provides an example to other programmes such as HIV and could be used for other chronic cases such as diabetes and mental health patients who also require long-term follow-up. The TB programme requires the following activities by the health worker and clinic:

- Record patient diagnosis and treatment details on the TB card.
- Register the case in the unit TB register on diagnosis.
- Ensure the patient receives regular follow-up treatment or go and find the patient if they default.

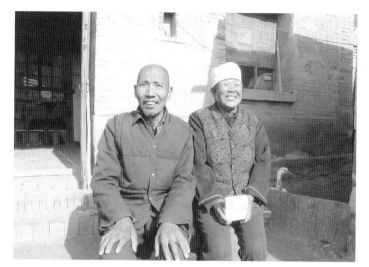

Fig. 14.3 A cured TB patient and his treatment supporter (his wife) in China.

- When the patient is discharged, record the treatment outcome, e.g. cured or treatment completed in the register.
- The TB coordinator visits on a regular basis and checks the TB card records and copies the record into the district TB register, and ensures that other aspects of quality care are happening properly.

To *not* follow-up a partially treated patient is a waste of expensive hospital treatment, encourages the development of resistant organisms, and increases the risk to the community. Follow-up is always cheaper than re-diagnosis and treatment.

Management of Contacts When a new case is diagnosed, the patient and accompanying relatives are asked about whether there are any other family members with a cough. Close contacts of the case are people who live in the same house. If they have a cough they should have sputum examined for TB. Child contacts, who do not have a BCG scar already, should be given the BCG vaccination. Chemoprophylaxis is given to children under 6 years old with no sign of active TB, and they are followed up at regular intervals.

Preventive treatment (prophylaxis) with 6 months of daily Isoniazid is given for contacts of smear positive TB cases, if they have no sign of active TB. Similarly, prophylaxis is given to HIV and TB co-infected people who no sign of TB. This clears the TB bacilli and prevents progression to TB disease (though they may get re-infected, especially if they have HIV). If HIV/TB co-infected individuals present with signs of TB they are given a TB (multi-drug) treatment.

Programme monitoring Evaluation of tuberculosis control programmes is by measuring the proportion of new smear positive cases that are cured or are certified to have completed treatment. The WHO target is 85%. The other main target is to achieve is to find at least 70% of TB cases. This means diagnosing and registering at least 70% of the estimated incidence of new smear positive TB cases. Commonly the rate is lower than this because health workers don't think to screen for TB by requesting sputum smears for people with a cough lasting more than 2–3 weeks (high burden countries, especially where there is a high HIV prevalence would state a cough lasting more than 2 weeks) or other symptoms which are suggestive of TB. Also many patients attend private practitioners who may not think of TB or do not register the patients. The registration of cases in the TB register is very important. This may be held at the hospital or other TB unit, or by the district TB coordinator. Every 3 months the TB coordinator reports on the number of patients added to the register during that quarter (a quarterly 'cohort'). This number, divided by the expected number × 100 gives the percentage case finding rate (the expected number is an estimate based on the population and the national TB incidence rates). In addition, for the quarter ending a year earlier, the TB coordinator calculates the treatment outcomes. The outcomes are the numbers and percent which are:

- Cured (originally sputum smear positive, now remaining sputum smear negative),
- Completed treatment (originally sputum smear positive but no final sputum smear was examined, or were originally sputum negative),
- Defaulted (not collected drugs for 2 or more months)
- Failed (still sputum positive after 5 or more months of treatment) or
- Dead.

TB programmes use these treatment outcomes to monitor whether the programme is improving (in that district, province, or country). Some other programmes, such as HIV/antiretroviral treatment, are now using similar registers and outcome measures (except there is no cure for HIV).

In the future, programmes are likely to use new drugs such as moxifloxacin instead of ethambutol, in order to reduce the length of treatment to 4 months. WHO aims to minimize the delay between licensing, availability, and adoption of new drugs and tests in high burden countries.

In order to share experiences between programmes and other international and country agencies involved in TB WHO has established a Stop TB Partnership http://www.stoptb.org/.

Other respiratory diseases

Other important diseases in this group are Acute Respiratory Infections (ARI), influenza, whooping cough (pertussis), diphtheria, meningococcal meningitis, *Haemophilus influenzae,* pneumococcal disease, otitis media, and acute rheumatic fever.

The diagnosis and treatment of acute respiratory diseases and otitis media are part of the WHO integrated management of childhood illness (IMCI) and Integrated management of adolescent and adult illness (IMAI). Vaccination against Pertussis (whooping cough) and diphtheria are part of the trivalent diphtheria, pertussis and tetanus (DPT) vaccine, and in many countries *Haemophilus influenzae* has also been included within routine EPI, see Chapter 11 (MNCH).

A world pandemic of influenza may occur some time in the future. This will occur when the H5N1 virus present in wild birds and chickens (and which causes severe pneumonia in people in close contact with birds) further adapts so it can more easily spread from person to person. Vaccines are being developed, some antiretroviral drugs reduce symptoms. For more information see www.who.int/healthtopics (influenza).

HIV and sexually transmitted diseases

STIs such as HIV and syphilis are transmitted from one person to another by the body fluids; blood, semen etc. Transmission is normally by direct contact. Sexual transmission accounts for the largest number of persons affected by these diseases.

As well as HIV, other diseases transmitted by sex are syphilis, gonorrhoea, Chlamydia, trichomonas vaginalis, lymphogranuloma venereum, granuloma inguinale, chancroid, genital herpes, and human papilloma virus.

They are social diseases, determined by the habits and attitude of people and it is only by effecting change in these behaviours that any permanent improvement will occur. Not all sexual activity is voluntary (rape). Sexual behaviour is disinhibited by alcohol, with risky sexual behaviour. People with high risk behaviours include sex workers, truck drivers, and men who have sex with men.

HIV infection can pass from an infected mother to her child, before or during delivery, or through breastfeeding. Syphilis can also be congenital, and gonorrhoea can infect the babies' eyes during delivery.

STIs prevention

STI diagnosis and treatment need to be made available in all health facilities, thus providing early and adequate treatment and preventing further transmission. Health workers should be trained and supervised to use the STI syndromic management guidelines or the IMAI guidelines, which include a section on STIs (see Further reading).

Health promotion to high risk behaviour groups and the general population is essential (see Chapter 8 and below for HIV).

Condom promotion and distribution is also the key to prevention of STIs. Delivery strategies include:

- Free provision of condoms in brothels, bars, and other opportunities to reach high risk groups
- Peer education about condoms and STIs
- Condom distribution through social marketing (using commercial marketing and distribution through shops, see Chapter 5)

See further reading for details on STIs. However, elements of the control of HIV, below, are also relevant to other STIs.

HIV epidemiology

HIV has a worldwide occurrence, with nearly 40 million people affected in 2007. An estimated 4.1 million become newly infected with HIV each year and nearly 3 million die from it. The worst affected area is sub-Saharan Africa, particularly Southern Africa, whereas improvement has taken place in other parts of the continent. In Africa, the HIV prevalence among young women is three times that of young men, indicating the associated gender inequality, and the fact that women are under pressure to have sex at an earlier age getting infected earlier. Many women lack socio-economic independence, education, access to health information, and health services, making it difficult for them to avoid exposure to the virus.

Infection has now spread to most countries of the world. The prevalence is increasing in Indonesia, Papua New Guinea, southern China and Vietnam, while transmission is currently low in Pakistan and Bangladesh. There are estimated to be 8.3 million people with HIV in Asia, two-thirds of them in India. Some states of India have more than 1% of ante-natal women HIV positive, and so meet the WHO definition of a generalized epidemic. The annual number of new HIV cases diagnosed continues to rise in Russia and the Ukraine, while the Caribbean remains the second most affected area in the world.

Immune deficiency and opportunistic infections

HIV infection leads to a disruption of specific T lymphocytes that bear the CD4 receptor (CD4+). This leads to a disruption of the cell-mediated immune mechanisms, resulting in an increased susceptibility to opportunistic infections. The breakdown of the body's defence system and the range of symptoms produced are called Acquired Immunodeficiency Syndrome (AIDS). The clinical presentation of AIDS is generally determined by the symptoms of opportunistic infections, which can be many and varied.

These include common infections that occur in normally immune people, but in AIDS these occur more frequently. For example pneumonia is eight times more common in HIV positive people and so are other bacterial infections, while 50% of people with HIV develop active TB in their lifetime. Additional to these common infections are opportunistic infections, which occur because of immune deficiency (and are rare in people with a normal immune system). These include:

♦ Candidiasis – Oral, vulvo-vaginal, oesophageal

♦ Tuberculosis – Pulmonary or extrapulmonary tuberculosis (see above)

♦ Pneumonia and other severe bacterial infections

♦ *Pneumocystis carinii* pneumonia

♦ Non-typhoid *Salmonella* septicaemia

♦ Shingles – reactivated varicella zoster virus

♦ Cytomegalovirus

♦ Cryptococcosis

♦ Cryptosporidiosis and isosporiasis with diarrhoea

♦ Toxoplasmosis of the brain

♦ Lymphoma and Kaposi's sarcoma

Any process that stresses the immune mechanism such as repeat infections will accelerate progression to AIDS. Persons with tuberculosis who contract HIV infection will progress more rapidly to AIDS.

The WHO case definition for HIV infection is:

Adults and children 18 months or older

A positive HIV antibody test (rapid or laboratory-based enzyme immunoassay). This is confirmed by a second HIV antibody test (rapid or laboratory-based enzyme immunoassay).

Children younger than 18 months:

Positive virological test for HIV or its components (HIV-RNA or ultra sensitive HIV p24 antigen), confirmed by a second test taken more than 4 weeks after birth.

HIV transmission

Unprotected sexual contact whether heterosexual or homosexual, is the commonest method of HIV transmission. The important epidemiological factor is the number of sexual contacts, especially concurrent partners. Anal intercourse carries a higher risk of infection than vaginal intercourse. There is no evidence of increased risk while having sexual intercourse during menstruation.

In many countries the incidence of HIV (e.g. in ante-natal women) has come down, but has then levelled off, and remained roughly consistent – becoming an endemic. In these countries, the number of people becoming infected with HIV equals those dying. The incidence level (of being infected) depends on the numbers of partners (especially concurrent partners) the risk of transmission (negligible if condoms consistently used) and the degree of sexual mixing between high risk e.g. sex workers, and lower risk, e.g. men and their wives.

Male circumcision provides about 50% protection against acquiring HIV. An individual's risk of acquiring HIV is increased in the presences of other sexually transmitted infections, particularly genital herpes simplex virus type 2 and ulcerating conditions such as chancroid. Non-ulcerating STIs may also potentiate infection to a lesser extent.

Blood transfusion of infected blood will almost always transmit HIV. Syringes and needles if they are not properly cleaned and sterilized can contain small quantities of infected blood sufficient to transmit infection. Hepatitis B and C and other infections are also transmitted this way. Examples of this type of transmission include by informal practitioners using non sterile needles or knives for scarification and intravenous drug abusers sharing needles. Transmission by needle stick injury can occur, but is uncommon.

An infected mother can pass on infection to her child. Infection can be transmitted congenitally, but it is more likely to occur from a mixing of the mother's and infant's blood at the time of delivery. HIV is found in breast milk and breast-feeding by an infected mother accounts for almost 50% of childhood infections. Therefore, in countries with significant HIV, all pregnant women should be counselled and tested for HIV. The risk to the child is reduced by treating the HIV positive mother with antiretroviral therapy, such as a single-dose nevirapine around the time of delivery and also treating the new born baby. The mother's sexual partner should also be counselled and tested for HIV. HIV positive parents, if they otherwise qualify, should be started on antiretroviral treatment.

Serological tests may not become positive for up to 3 months after the person becomes infected so it is possible for a person to transmit infection before they are shown to be positive.

The time from infection to becoming HIV positive is 1–3 months. The development of full blown AIDS can range from 1–18 years after HIV infection, with a mean of 10 years. In perinatal infection the incubation period to AIDS is often shorter than 12 months.

Infectiousness is highest during initial infection. It then remains steady and increases again as immunity becomes suppressed. People treated with an effective antiviral therapy regime and taking tablets regularly can achieve undetectable viral loads but it has not been shown to completely eliminate the risk of transferring infection. Therefore, condoms and other precautionary measures should continue to be utilized.

Control of HIV

Control and prevention are aimed at the three routes of transmission: sexual, blood and perinatal. The search for a vaccine has been a major priority, but none have progressed beyond stage II of clinical trials. The problem with all the vaccine candidates so far developed has been the rapid rate at which the HIV virus alters its antigenic make-up. So until a vaccine has been developed, other control measures are required.

To prevent **sexual** spread.

- Limit the number of sexual partners, encouraging monogamous relationships. (B, behaviour change)
- Avoid sexual contact with persons at high risk, such as commercial sex workers and bisexuals.
- Encourage male and female condom use. (C, condom use)
- Provide adequate facilities for the detection and treatment of STIs.
- Make HIV testing and counselling available, both at specialized and general clinics.
- Provide sex education to both boys and girls.
- Initiate lifestyle training (how to say 'no') to adolescents learning how to negotiate e.g. to start sex when they want, not when pressurised into sex prematurely. (A, abstinence)

To prevent **blood** spread.

- Screen all blood for transfusions.
- Test donors before they give blood.
- Restrict blood transfusions only to essential cases.
- Discontinue paid blood donors.
- Use disposable syringes, needles, giving sets, lancets etc.

- ◆ Inform injecting drug users about the risks of sharing equipment and set up needle exchange schemes (giving equal numbers of new needles for used ones).
- ◆ Medical workers should always wear gloves when in contact with blood, e.g. at delivery and in the laboratory.

To prevent **perinatal** spread.

- ◆ All mothers attending ante-natal clinic should be encouraged to have an HIV test.
- ◆ Advise HIV infected pregnant women about the risk to their infant and themselves during and after pregnancy.
- ◆ Ensure good obstetric practice
  - reduce trauma and minimize procedures such as artificial rupture of membranes.
  - only cut the umbilical cord when it has stopped pulsating.
- ◆ Give antiretroviral therapy to HIV positive pregnant women and to the newborn infant.
- ◆ Provide information on exclusive breast-feeding

Exclusive breast-feeding, which means breast milk only (with no water or food given in the first 6 months) is the best method of breast feeding to prevent HIV transmission. Exclusive breast-feeding reduces the risk of HIV transmission whilst reducing the risk of diarrhoea with its associated high mortality among infants in developing countries. Exclusive breast-feeding carries a similar risk for HIV transmission as artificial feeding. Artificial feeding is only feasible for women with higher incomes and who can access clean piped water.

WHO recommends that no change should be made in the vaccination programme to mothers and children even though they may be infected with HIV. The exception to this are infants known to be infected with HIV, who should not be given the live BCG vaccine.

Communication on HIV

The main method of control is health promotion and should involve community leaders, religious organizations, and NGOs. This can be aimed towards the general public by supplying them with information, or towards specific high risk groups. The most cost-effective health education will be aimed at people with high risk behaviours such as commercial sex workers, homosexuals, truck drivers, etc. Criminalization of sex workers and homosexuals only drives the practice underground. Thailand has had much success with its promotion of condoms, including close to 100% condom use in brothels. This is a model being tried in other countries.

Peer distribution of condoms was found to be very effective in Mumbai in reaching these disadvantaged groups. Such a strategy requires identifying good communicators from amongst a particular peer group (e.g. of sex workers), training them, and supplying them with condoms to distribute to their peers. Similarly peer education works well with men who have sex with men, such as (some) truck and rickshaw drivers. Remember that these men often have sex with women as well, making the women vulnerable to infection, so programmes to reach these women also need to be developed. Needle and syringe exchange programmes in a number of countries have helped reduce the risk of infection in drug users. Prisons have been termed 'incubators of HIV', due to male-to-male transmission and injecting drug use in a high prevalence population. On the other hand, prisoner populations are captive audiences so much more could be done to reach this highly vulnerable group.

Education of the general population is also important, using various mass media approaches, such as newspapers, posters, radio, and TV. Drama is a particularly attractive and potentially effective health promotion approach. This can be live drama in a village or town, by amateur or professional actors. It can be drama on the TV or radio, as local radio often reaches most rural areas. An example of this is Makutano Junction, a TV drama set in the slums of Nairobi, which is highly entertaining but also includes dialogue educating about TB and HIV prevention and care.

Girls should have equal opportunity for education as boys, with sex education an integral part of the school curriculum. News sheets are written and distributed to school children by organizations such as 'Straight Talk', Uganda, which contain girls and boy's letters, questions and answers about safe sex and other issues of concern to them. Straight Talk also include discussion and information on the local radio.

Counselling

Counselling and testing facilities need to be made readily available as a preventive intervention as well as being an entry point to treatment and prevention of mother-to-child transmission. Voluntary counselling and testing (VCT) should be made available to all the public with the aim of everyone being tested in countries with a generalized epidemic of HIV (greater than 1% of the ante-natal women testing positive). These VCT services can be in stand-alone centres and outreach services, and be promoted through attractive media messages. VCT is an example where 'well' people 'opt-in' to HIV testing. Alternatively, ill people, in countries with HIV, who go to health facilities need 'HIV counselling and testing' (HCT). HCT stresses the advantages of a test for better diagnosis and care, recommends the test and this is done unless the patient 'opts-out' of the test. All health workers should briefly counsel and test people who present with infections known to be associated with HIV such as candidiasis, pneumonia or chronic diarrhoea and other conditions listed above. Guidelines such as the WHO 'Integrated management of childhood Illness (IMCI) and the adult-adolescent version called IMAI make clear which conditions are associated with HIV, and give details of counselling, testing and care. In countries with high HIV, such as east and southern Africa, all patients attending health facilities should be tested (unless they have been recently tested). This form of HCT is called 'provider initiated counselling and testing' as health workers such as nurses on the wards and in each outpatient department need to briefly discuss, recommend and (unless the patient opts-out) take blood for an HIV test. Knowing the HIV status will help provide the best treatment and follow-up care.

Condoms and information on the treatment should be given to the patients together with a partner notification letter. This letter is to be given by the client to their partners requesting them to come in for treatment.

All persons with HIV, including those under treatment, are at risk of passing on infection to others and should be counselled about preventive measures to be taken including consistent use of condoms.

Condoms can be dispensed free at clinics and in bars, hotels and brothels. Social marketing is an important intervention strategy to reach the general public. This form of marketing is through the media with messages and images that appeal to a good life-style. Messages are developed and promoted using the same methods large commercial companies promoting products such as soft drinks (e.g. coca cola™), detergents and other products. These methods may include advertising posters, songs on the radio and messages written into the popular dramas on the television. Condoms are attractively packaged, distributed and sold all over the country in shops and by street vendors. They may be subsidized by the government/donor so that the price is acceptable. The 'social' in social marketing is the fact that it is a healthy product. This implementation strategy (or service delivery approach) is also used for increasing coverage with other healthy products such as mosquito nets and contraceptive pills (see also choosing the best interventions Chapter 5).

Preventive treatment

Cotrimoxazole prophylaxis can be given to HIV positive persons to prevent *C. carinii* pneumonia, some forms of diarrhoea and also (partially) protecting against malaria too. People with dual TB and HIV infection should have long-term cotrimoxazole preventive treatment – reducing the death rate in TB patients by 20% in a Zambia trial.

All HIV positive persons should be tuberculin skin tested for TB and isoniazid prophylaxis for 6 months if positive, providing they have no symptoms or signs of active TB. If the tuberculin ('mantoux') testing is not available, then give isoniazid prophylaxis to any HIV positive person. Any opportunistic infection must receive specific treatment for the condition, preferably referring to nationally adapted case management guidelines for adults and children such as IMAI and IMCI.

Antiretroviral treatment

There has been a strong movement to increase the availability of ART in developing countries, although by 2008, ART was only reaching one in five people who need it. It is hoped that ARV therapy will reduce the stigma of AIDS and allow preventive programmes to be more effective. Both preventive and treatment strategies need to proceed concurrently so as to reduce the numbers of people needing to start ART.

Initiation of ART

The CD4+ T cell count is used to decide when to start first-line ART treatment – for example people below a CD4 count of 350. ART regimens include a combination of three drugs, preferably in a fixed dose combination (FDC) tablet, for example containing stavudine, lamivudine, and nevirapine (or efavirenz if the patient is taking rifampicin for TB). There are other first line drug combinations containing for example zidovudine (previously called AZT) or tenofavir. Second line drug regimens include other drugs from the same group and a protease inhibitor. Second line drugs are used when there is evidence of clinical failure on the first line drugs – for example, weight loss, new opportunistic infections, and/or rising CD4 count.

Adherence

ART clinical failure and drug resistance is caused by poor adherence to treatment. Poor adherence to treatment is due, to a large extent, to poor education and follow-up by health workers.

It is important that people are counselled individually or in groups before starting ART. It is important that they disclose their HIV positive status to a family member or friend, and bring this person to the ART clinic to be informed on how to be a 'treatment supporter'. The patient and treatment supporter need to understand the importance of attending appointments and taking the tablets **at the same time** every morning and evening. As few as three missed doses in a month can lead to the viral load rising, risking drug resistance, and treatment failure. Information leaflets, treatment diaries, and other aids to better adherence are needed. In addition, during follow up appointments, there should be careful questioning about adherence, and pill counts should be monitored. ART patient cards and clinic registers should be for monitoring treatment, similar to how they are used in TB programmes.

Other diseases spread through blood and body fluids

The STIs have been mentioned at the beginning of this HIV and STI section.

In addition, hepatitis B, hepatitis C, hepatitis delta, ebola haemorrhagic fever, and Malburg haemorrhagic fever are spread through blood and body fluids. The prevention of these diseases is by infection control measures such as care with used needles, sharps containers, gloves, gowns in health facilities etc. Vaccination for hepatitis B is given at birth as part of EPI. See further reading, especially www.who.int/healthtopics, and the books by Heymann and Webber.

Insect-borne diseases

Among the various modes of disease transmission, those transmitted by vectors are by far the most numerous, with 160 at the last count. Of these, 76 are transmitted by mosquitoes alone. Some of the diseases transmitted by mosquitoes contribute to a disproportionately large burden of disease. Malaria, for example, affects 3.3 billion in 109 countries giving rise to 350–500 million cases with 2 million deaths annually in 2008. On the other hand, other mosquito borne diseases such as dengue, yellow fever or rift valley fever occur in more epidemic fashion in scattered smaller geographical locations in the tropics and subtropics.

Therefore, vector control is one of the most important intervention methods for interrupting disease transmission. The vector is an essential stage in the transmission of many parasitic diseases, so targetting the vector with interventions achieves the greatest success.

The most common disease vectors include mosquitoes and flies (e.g. *Simulium*, sandflies, and the Tsetse), Reduviid bugs, ticks, lice, and fleas. Insecticides are the main substances used to attack these vectors, as well as other methods – such as traps for Tsetse flies. See further reading and www.who.int/healthtopics. The most important disease in this group, and a good model for the control of most of the vector-borne diseases, is malaria.

Malaria

There are four malaria parasites that can infect humans, namely: *Plasmodium falciparum*, *P. vivax*, *P. malariae*, and *P. ovale*. Of these, *P. falciparum* causes the most serious disease and is the commonest parasite in tropical regions, but differs from *P. vivax* and *P. ovale* in having no persistent liver stage (the hypnozoite). *P. vivax* has the widest geographical range, being found in temperate and sub-tropical zones as well as the tropics.

The malaria parasite shares its cycle between two hosts, the human and the female anopheline mosquito. It reproduces asexually in the human and sexually in the mosquito.

Following human inoculation by an infected mosquito during a blood meal, sporozoites travel from the salivary glands of the mosquito via the bloodstream and make their way rapidly to the human liver. Here, they undergo division and multiplication within the liver cells (tissue schizonts) over a period of one or more weeks. In *P. vivax* and *P. ovale*, a persistent liver stage called a hypnozoite is formed. These forms persist despite the clearance of blood parasites and allow relapses to occur, often continuing for many years after the initial infection, unless radical treatment is given.

Parasites released from the liver are taken up by red blood cells. Once in the RBCs, the parasites periodically divide asexually, rupturing the cells entering other RBCs.

When red blood cells rupture, toxins are released which produce the clinical symptoms such as fever, headache, muscle, and joint pains. Some parasites go on to form a stage of the parasite called 'gametocytes' which are taken up and multiply in the stomach of a female anopheline mosquito after it has taken a blood meal from an infected individual.

Malaria vector

The efficiency of the malaria vector will depend upon the species of *Anopheles*, its feeding habits and the environmental conditions. This varies widely, with *A. gambiae* being the most efficient and common of all the malaria vectors. The efficiency of the vector is determined by a number of factors, such as the preferred food source (man or animal), the time of biting (easier in the middle of the night when people are sleeping), and whether it lives inside the house or outside.

One of the most important factors in the successful transmission of malaria is the mosquito's length of life. 50% of a population of *A. gambiae* will live longer than 12 days. It can take between 7–21 days after taking an infected blood meal for an anopheline mosquito to complete the sexual cycle and become infective to humans. Therefore, the longer female mosquitoes survive, the more opportunity they have to transmit malaria parasites.

Apart from mosquito vectors, malaria can also be transmitted by blood transfusion, but this accounts for a very small percentage of infections.

Incubation period depends upon the species and strain of the parasite, for *P. falciparum* it is 9–14 days and for *P. vivax* 12–17 days (But it may take up to 9 months in temperate countries before symptoms appear).

In a non-immune population, children and adults of both sexes are affected equally. In areas of stable transmission (or continuous infection) with *P. falciparum,* malaria is predominantly an infection of younger children in whom mortality can be considerable. The survivors acquire immunity, which is only preserved by the maintenance of parasites in the body, through re-infection. Should the individual leave an area of stable malaria transmission, immunity may be reduced. The other time when immunity is reduced is during pregnancy and severe malaria can occur in the pregnant woman, even one that has lived in an endemic area. This is worse in the first pregnancy than subsequent pregnancies.

Malaria is found in the tropics and sub-tropical parts of the world and is predominantly due to *P. falciparum*, although *P. vivax* is the predominant species in the Indian sub-continent. Malaria used to be more extensive, with seasonal malaria in temperate regions, but extensive control programmes have confined it to its present limits. However, due to problems, such as the development of drug and insecticide resistance, malaria still causes and estimated 300 million cases and two million deaths annually.

Global climatic change is leading to an increase in epidemic malaria (infecting new or infrequently involved areas). Highland areas such as Harare and Nairobi, which were protected by their lower temperatures, are increasingly affected by malaria as climate change progresses (due to carbon dioxide released with burning of oil, gas and coal).

Early diagnosis and treatment

Early diagnosis and treatment of malaria is one of the important interventions for malaria. Early treatment, ideally within 24 hours of developing fever, is particularly important for young children in settings with stable *P. falciparum* malaria.

Uncomplicated malaria infection may present with fever, chills, sweats, headache, joint pains, muscle aches and, particularly in the very young, with refusal to feed, lethargy and vomiting. These clinical features are quite non-specific and are shared by a number of other conditions. Severe malaria (Falciparum malaria) can present in many different forms including cerebral malaria (encephalopathy and coma), confusion, recurrent seizures, severe anaemia, acute shock, haematuria (blackwater fever) and jaundice.

Diagnosis of malaria may be made by clinical or parasitological means. The most common means of diagnosing uncomplicated malaria in developing countries is by clinical diagnosis. All those presenting with fever and some of the clinical features listed above are assumed to have malaria and are treated with a first line medicine, such as artemisinin combination therapy for *P. falciparum*, or chloroquine in the case of *P.vivax*.

Increasingly, parasitological diagnosis of malaria using light microscopy or rapid diagnostic tests (RDT), is being used. A slide for microscopy is prepared by smearing a finger prick sample

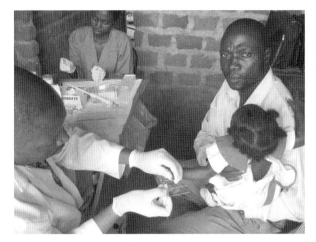

Fig. 14.4 Rapid diagnostic test for malaria [is done] in a child with fever in Uganda (photo reproduced with permission from the Malaria Consortium, Africa).

of blood on a glass slide. The slide is then specially stained and viewed under a microscope which uses electricity or reflected sunlight as a light source. Microscopy requires skilled laboratory personnel, laboratory reagents and good care and maintenance of light microscopes as well as a light source. In recent years, malaria rapid diagnostic tests (RDT) have been increasingly employed to diagnose malaria. These are dipsticks or cassette devices on which a finger prick sample of blood is placed. The presence of parasites is shown as lines on the strip somewhat like a home pregnancy kit. RDTs can be used effectively by less skilled health workers and even community health workers. This is making the detection of *P. falciparum* malaria simpler (though currently the RDTs for vivax are not as sensitive or specific, and do not replace the need for microscopy). RDTs are improving access to malaria diagnosis, especially in health centres where microscopy isn't available. The results from RDTs are similar to microscopy done in peripheral health facilities. The cost of the RDT is similar to the cost of a course of the first line artemesinin combination therapy (ACT). Therefore RDTs are particularly useful in settings where P. *falciparum* exists, microscopy isn't available, and where ACTs are recommended as first line treatment (Fig. 14.4).

Testing for malaria by microscopy or an RDT is highly preferable to a diagnosis based upon clinical presentation. However, in highly endemic malaria areas such as in tropical Africa, and where the cheaper drugs are still effective, it is reasonable to treat 'presumptively' people ill with fever with antimalarials. Especially so in children, who are at higher risk and have a higher prevalence of malaria parasites among fever cases. Therefore, the health worker needs to look for and treat other causes of fever, such as possible pneumonia if rapid breathing is a feature of the presentation. This more syndromic approach is employed by Integrated Management of Childhood Illness (IMCI) and Integrated Management of Adult Illness guidelines, which need to be adapted to the specific epidemiology of malaria in each country.

Malaria treatment

ACTs are recommended as the first line treatment for malaria in areas where there are significant levels of resistance to the commonly used cheaper drugs such as chloroquine and sulpfadoxine-pyrimethamine (SP, Fansidar) which now includes most of Africa, South East Asia and, increasingly, large parts of in South America. Intramuscular or intravenous quinine is still employed for the management of severe cases of malaria. However, newer approaches, including the use of parenteral artemisinin derivatives and the use of rectal artemisinin derivatives, are increasingly being used.

Home-based treatment of malaria is a strategy to make malaria accessible to those living further away from health facilities. In endemic malaria countries community health workers are trained and supplied with antimalarials. In countries such as Uganda 'community-based medicine distributors' (who may or may not be general community health workers) are trained. The aim is that every village has someone trained to give antimalarials to children who present with fever, so that they are treated within 24 hours of the onset of the fever. The drugs are best pre-packaged in blister packs and with an illustrated leaflet to improve adherence.

The various control methods for malaria are illustrated in Fig. 14.5

Personal protection

They include insecticide treated mosquito nets, repellents, and covering up with clothing. Clothing may be treated with repellents, or repellents can be applied directly to the skin. Of these various methods of prevention, insecticide treated mosquito nets and indoor residual spraying have been employed by malaria control programmes. Larviciding is used to a limited extent in certain countries.

Mosquito nets   Mosquito nets are the most effective means of personal protection, if used properly. Treating the nets with synthetic pyrethroid insecticides, such as permethrin, is the main method used in the control of malaria. Malaria carrying mosquitoes in many parts of the world

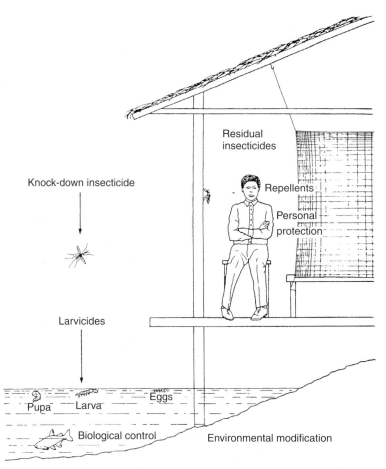

Fig. 14.5 Techniques for mosquito control.

have a preference for taking a blood meal late in the night when most people are asleep. The net provides a physical barrier to the mosquito while the insecticide repels mosquitoes and kills those which come into contact with the net. When used on a community scale the concentration of insecticide treated nets (ITN) can produce a mass effect reducing the mosquito population and the sporozoite rate. An improved though more expensive technology, is the manufacture of mosquito nets with the insecticide already in the net fibres, known as long-lasting insecticidal nets (LLIN). These retain activity for at least 4 years and avoid the regular and programmatically expensive, re-treatment of nets. They hold considerable potential as the main method of malaria control.

There are various strategies for promoting and distributing ITNs. These include mass free distribution, targeting of vulnerable groups with subsidized or free nets using vouchers, social marketing, and private sector distribution. In addition, the insecticide treatment may be distributed by these means for those who have already purchased an untreated mosquito net.

It is important to choose the best delivery strategies to increase mosquito net, coverage, as explained in Chapter 5. Because pregnant women and young children are particularly vulnerable, nets can be given free to women attending ante-natal care. Alternatively vouchers can be given, which can be used to purchase nets from shops. Nets or vouchers may also be given to parents of young children attending health centres. Giving vouchers works better where there is an established market with a variety of makes of ITNs. In many countries nets (preferably LLIN) are promoted through social marketing. (Social marketing is also a delivery strategy for condoms, contraceptive pills and other health products). Marketing includes posters and as well as messages, songs and drama in the TV and radio. Quite often, the nets are subsidized to make them more accessible to the poor. Providing a subsidy is particularly helpful in places where nets have been little used and the market needs to be stimulated. However, it can be expensive delivery strategy and can undermine the private sector if only one particular subsidized brand is used.

ITNs can also offer effective protection against the mosquitoes that carry filariasis against sand flies, the vectors as well as for leishmaniasis. Where either of these and malaria co-exist then bed-nets can contribute to the prevention of both diseases.

In many countries a high proportion of people have already purchased mosquitonets but not the insecticide treated ones. Insecticides can be applied to these untreated nets. Health workers can arrange a date with villages a date when they will come and dip all the (non-impregnated) nets. This 'campaign' approach is to make sure all existing nets are impregnated, while also promoting LLIN which are a better long-term solution. Where this service isn't provided, then families can purchase packets of insecticide (e.g. KO-tab is just one example of a brand name in Uganda) which have clear directions on how to treat the net. Usually, the contents of the packet are poured into a set quantity of water in a bucket. Items such as coca cola bottles or local plastic mugs can be used as measures for the water. The net is dipped in the insecticide and then laid out on the ground to dry. This procedure needs to be repeated every six month or a year (depending on how many months malaria is present in that setting). More recently, long lasting insecticide treatments have become available which can be used to turn untreated nets into LLIN.

Mosquito bednets are more effective and cheaper to maintain than putting screens on the doors and windows of the whole house, which is only recommended for people with a high standard of living. A small hole in one area of screening can render the rest of the screening ineffective. A knockdown spray can be used to kill mosquitoes that have entered a screened house but lasts for a limited duration.

Other methods of malaria control, including bush clearance from around homes, smoke from mosquito coils or vaporizing mats, or the addition of certain plants to fires to produce a repellent smoke, have not been shown to be cost effective means of malaria control.

Indoor residual spraying of insecticides (IRS)   These insecticides are applied to the inside surfaces of the walls and roofs of houses so that the resting mosquito (after it has taken its blood meal), absorbs a lethal dose of insecticide and dies before the parasites it has taken up in the blood can complete development. This was the main method of the malaria eradication programmes used in many countries of the world during the sixties and seventies. Unfortunately, insecticide resistance, organizational breakdown, and reluctance by people to have their houses sprayed resulted in an abandonment of the goal of eradication. Most recently, the Global Action Plan for malaria 2007 has once more stated the potential of elimination and eradication. This optimistic goal is based on the recent early successes of new interventions, combined with a substantial global investment in malaria interventions such as ITNs, IRS, and ACTs. Therefore, interest in IRS has been revived.

The insecticides may be DDT (dichlorodiphenyltrichloroethane) or pyrethroids. DDT is cheap, easy to use, and has a high residual effect necessitating only one spray operation per year, unlike many of the pyrethroids which require two rounds of spraying per year. In the past there have been problems of environmental contamination with DDT but this was due to agricultural spraying with DDT rather than spraying of walls for malaria control. However, because of the environmental concerns or because of resistance to DDT, most countries use pyrethroids – despite their being more expensive. In recent times, some manufacturers are developing pyrethroid insecticides with longer residual effects. Indoor residual spraying is particularly useful in epidemic malaria settings where malaria transmission is less stable, such as parts of Asia and in highland and dry-land areas of Africa. Malaria programmes recommend indoor residual spraying, the promotion of bednets, and other measures in order to control malaria. Combinations of effective treatment and prevention methods have led to impressive progress in malaria control. The islands of Zanzibar have seen massive reductions in malaria cases and malaria fatalities since the initiation of ACT for treatment, almost universal coverage with ITNs and higher than 90% coverage of households with IRS. Parasite prevalences in young children have seen reductions from over 70% to less than 1% on average between 2003 and 2007.

Larviciding, drainage and biological control   Larvicidal substances include oils that spread over the surface and asphyxiate the larvae or substances that have insecticidal properties but these are rarely feasible or effective.

Drainage or filling-in potential breeding sites is often promoted by community leaders as a cheap means of effective malaria control. This may contribute to malaria control in densely populated areas where there are well defined breeding sites. However, in most rural areas the mosquito vector can breed in the many small puddles, including those caused by animal hoof prints – making this approach an expensive and impractical undertaking.

Drainage can be feasible in flood irrigation areas. An example ot this is, in South Asia and elsewhere where wheat, rice and other crops are grown by flooding 'paddy' fields with water. Malaria can be controlled by farmers draining the fields of water periodically – not giving time for the adult malaria mosquito to hatch.

Biological control with particular species of fish or bacilli will reduce mosquito larvae to a certain extent, but is rarely feasible. The release of sterile male mosquitoes is another technique, but has not been successful.

In epidemic malaria using a fogging machine or ULV spray from aircraft can rapidly reduce adult mosquito density. This will cut short the epidemic by killing off flying adults, but needs to be repeated regularly as new adults will continually be produced from larvae that are not affected by the knockdown sprays. In addition, the malaria carrying mosquitoes in many areas like to rest indoors and may not be exposed to the insecticide. It is rarely used for malaria control apart from epidemics in refugee camps. It may also be used in urban areas or refugee camps to control *Aedes egyptii* the mosquito vector responsible for dengue and Yellow fever epidemics.

Vaccination against malaria is likely to become a reality in the coming decade, and there are (in 2008) nine candidate vaccines being tested. To date a vaccine RTS S has been shown to be effective in a trial in Mozambique. This was a small trial, where the vaccine was given in three injected doses to infants under 1 year old, and reduced the risk of catching malaria by 65%. Larger trials are currently being carried out, and if successful, a vaccine will be prepared for general use.

Preventive chemotherapy

Intermittent preventive treatment during pregnancy (IPTp)   Pregnant women and their unborn infants are particularly at risk of malaria. In areas of low transmission, this gives rise to a high incidence of premature abortion during pregnancy in areas of high transmission, whereas malaria results in a high incidence of low birth weight babies as well as severe maternal anaemia. IPTp consists of giving an antimalarial such as *sulpfadoxine-pyrimethamine* (SP) to pregnant women during ante-natal visits. The drug is given two or three times during pregnancy. A first dose is given once after foetal quickening and again after no less than a one month interval but before the last month of pregnancy. Three doses of antimalarial are given where the prevalence of HIV is high. It should be a routine part of ante-natal care for all pregnant women in highly endemic malaria areas. IPTp clears or substantially reduces the load of malaria parasites in the placenta and so prevents illness, anaemia, and death of the mother, and anaemia or stillbirth of the infant. In addition to IPT, all pregnant women and young children priority in the distribution of mosquitonets (preferably LLIN) has been shown to reduce malaria in pregnancy.

Intermittent preventive treatment for infants (IPTi) has been found to significantly reduce the incidence of clinical malaria in trials in Africa. Three or four doses of an antimalarial such as SP are given at the time of the routine vaccinations as part of EPI. This intervention may become routinely recommended in the coming years.

Chemoprophylaxis should be given to persons at particular risk such as non-immune immigrants or migrant workers coming from non-endemic malaria areas-together with advice on personal protective measures including the use of mosquitonets.

Global Malaria Control   In the past decade, substantial progress has been made in bringing malaria control to the top of the global agenda with references to it in the Millennium Development Goals, with the creation of a strong global partnership to fight malaria in the form of Roll Back Malaria, and by setting Global targets to scale up effective interventions, halve malaria deaths by 2010 and move towards elimination of malaria. Most importantly, funding for malaria control has increased substantially with the establishment of a number of global initiatives such as the Global Funds to fight AIDs, TB and Malaria, the US presidential malaria initiative, the World Bank Booster programme and others.

Since 2005, countries such as Rwanda, Eritrea, Zanzibar, and Togo in Africa, as well as Thailand, Laos, Cambodia and Vietnam in South East Asia have shown impressive reductions in malaria burden through the scaling up of cost-effective interventions such as ACTs, ITNs, IPT, and more recently, IRS. While initial successes have been reported in Ethiopia and Zambia among others, it remains to be seen if these continue and are sustained.

Other insect vector diseases

Other important diseases transmitted by mosquito vectors are lymphatic filariasis and arbovirus diseases such as dengue and yellow fever (also transmitted by mosquitoes so the same method of control can be used). For dengue and yellow fever the vector is *Aedes egyptii,* a mosquito that breeds in clean water containers. Vaccination is the main intervention to control the spread of yellow fever. For dengue, an important control measure is education of the public to use well covered containers for water; with environmental workers visiting homes to check for open water containers; and 'source reduction' of other breeding sites such as dumped car tyres and cans. Other flying insect-borne diseases include leishmaniasis, spread by the sandfly; onchocerciasis spread by the simulium fly (see above for mass drug administration) and trypanasomiasis the cause of African sleeping sickness spread by the tsetse fly.

An important group of vector-borne diseases in a complex cycle with reservoir animals, can affect humans when they accidentally enter the zoonotic cycle. The vectors are non-flying ectoparasites such as fleas and ticks. The main diseases in this group are: plague, typhus, relapsing fever (louse-borne or tick-borne), tick typhus, Rocky Mountain spotted fever, and lyme disease.

Zoonoses

A zoonosis is an infection that is naturally transmitted between vertebrate animals and humans. Several zoonoses have already been mentioned, such as the beef tapeworm and plague, but there remains an important group of infections in which control of the animal is the main method of preventing infection. It includes animals that are livestock or pets, such as cows and dogs, or those animals that are closely associated with humans, but are not wanted, such as rats. The main diseases in this group are: Rabies, hydatid disease, toxocariasis, toxoplasmosis, brucellosis, anthrax, leptospirosis, and lassa fever (which also can be transmitted via body fluids).

See 'Fruther reading' and www.who.int/healthtopics for more details of the epidemiology and control of communicable these diseases.

Integration within district health systems

The challenge is to scale-up programmes of effective preventive and curative interventions for all communicable diseases. The best delivery strategies and related activities need to be selected and applied (Chapter 5). Many interventions will require intersectoral collaboration, such as between agencies responsible health and water, sanitation and housing. Many communicable disease interventions such as, mosquitonets and IRS will require some degree of community participation. This may include local decision-making on outreach services, volunteers' time (for mass drug administration against helminths, or home based treatment of fever), cooperation of households on the use of mosquito nets or allowing their houses to be sprayed with insecticide or maintenance of water pumps.

The design of interventions should ensure that they will be sustainable, and replicable in all affected communities. Often the delivery of interventions against one disease can be combined in the same community health interventions. They can become part of the work of CHWs. These issues are covered in many other chapters of this book.

The programme interventions will be technically guided and supplied by the national programmes, e.g. malaria control programme. At sub-national levels countries vary in how malaria and other control programmes are managed. In China they are part of the communicable disease control departments, at each level from national to county levels, managed separately from hospitals. In other countries the clinical and preventive services are together within the provincial and district health system. At district level, malaria/vector control is commonly the responsibility of an environmental health officer while community doctors or nurses supervise treatment and personal preventive interventions (such as IPT) conducted within the general health services. These officers are often members of the district health team (Chapter 10).

Conclusion

Water, sanitation and hygiene, TB, HIV, and malaria and some other major communicable diseases can be controlled with cost-effective interventions. Effective control depends on knowledge of the epidemiology and control interventions as well as knowledge of the local situation. Commonly a combination of preventive and treatment interventions is needed. The interventions fit within PHC, and often intersectoral collaboration and community participation will be required. This is a rapidly developing field, and new diagnostic tests, vaccines and drugs are becoming increasingly available. The effectiveness and feasibility of these need to be reviewed, adapted and incorporated into country health systems and programmes. The challenges are considerable but the potential benefits are huge.

Further reading

Jamison D. et al. Disease Control Priorities in developing countries, 2nd edition (DCP2). http://www.dcp2.org/main/Home.html

Heymann David. Communicable Diseases Manual. 18th edition, 2004, APHA. ISBN 0-87553-242-X.

UNICEF 2008. 'Countdown to 2015' *Maternal, neonatal and child survival: tracking progress in maternal, newborn and child survival.* http://www.childinfo.org/countdown.html

Webber R. *Communicable disease epidemiology and control* CABI Publishing. Oxford, 2nd edition, 2004 (a third edition due in 2009).

Weekly epidemiological record. www.who.int/wer/en. And specifically for soil transmitted see, www.who.int/wer/2008/en

WHO information on specific diseases, either google WHO health topics (HIV, TB, malaria or leishmaniasis etc.) or search www.who.int/healthtopics

WHO. *Preventive chemotherapy in human helminthiasis.* WHO Geneva. 2006. http://whqlibdoc.who.int/publications/2006/9241547103_eng.pdf See also

WHO. *Guidelines for the evaluation of soil-transmitted helminthiasis and schistosomiasis at community level: a guide for managers of country programmes.* WHO/CTD/SIP/98.1.

WHO. IMAI/ IMCI home page. http://www.who.int/hiv/pub/imai/en/

WHO. 2004. *Monitoring and evaluation toolkit: HIV/AIDS, tuberculosis, and malaria* ISBN 92-9224-001-3, http://www.who.int/hiv/pub/me/me_toolkit2004/en/

WHO. *Towards universal access Scaling up priority HIV/AIDS interventions in the health sector,* WHO Geneva, 2007 http://www.who.int/hiv/mediacentre/2008progressreport/en/index.html

WHO. *Sexually Transmitted Diseases home page, including provider initiated HIV counselling and testing.* http://www.who.int/hiv/pub/sti/en/

WHO. *Training modules on the syndromic management of STI's.* http://www.who.int/reproductive-health/stis/training.htm

WHO. *Publications on water, sanitation and health.* (available online).http://www.who.int/water_sanitation_health/publications/en/index.html

WHO/CDS/TB/2003.313. *Treatment of tuberculosis: guidelines for national programmes.* Geneva. http://www.who.int/tb/publications/cds_tb_2003_313/en/

WHO/HTM/TB/2004.329 *TB/HIV A clinical manual.* 2nd edition, 2004. Geneva. ISBN-13 97892411546348. http://www.who.int/child_adolescent_health/documents/9241546344/en/

Clinical tuberculosis (2nd edition) J. Crofton, N. Horne, F. Miller. London and Basingstoke: MacMillan Education, 1999. ISBN 0-333-72430-5

Bruce-Chwatt. *Essential malariology.* 3rd edition, edited by Herbert Gilles. Hodder Arnold. 2002. ISBN - 9780340740644

Malaria Consortium resources. http://www.malariaconsortium.org/resources.php

Chapter 15

Non-communicable diseases

Kamran Siddiqi

This chapter gives an overview of the following topics:

◆ Global impact of non-communicable disease;

◆ Causes and determinants;

◆ Prevention and control;

◆ Interventions targeted at high risk individuals and settings.

Introduction

'We cannot afford to say 'we must tackle the other diseases first – HIV/AIDS, malaria, tuberculosis – then we will deal with chronic disease'. If we wait even 10 years we will find that the problem is even larger and more expensive to address.'

(President Olusegun Obasanjo of Nigeria)

Chronic conditions not caused by an infectious agent, are generally classified as non-communicable diseases. These include a long list of conditions some of which are of global importance including cardiovascular diseases, cancers, alcohol, and substance misuse, neuropsychiatry conditions, and injuries as result of violence and road traffic accidents. They are usually a consequence of prolonged exposure to certain environmental, lifestyle, or socio-economic factors. These conditions develop often over prolonged periods and lead to premature death, disability, and poor quality of life. Countries with high prevalence of non-communicable diseases bear the economic consequences in terms of loss of productivity and constant drain on services. Low- and middle-income countries face the dual challenge of controlling communicable and non-communicable diseases.

International agencies have been warning against the recent global rise in non-communicable diseases. This is considered as a major threat to future development and efforts to reduce world poverty. Governments have been urged to place due emphasis on the control of non-communicable diseases through healthy public policies and investment in their prevention. This is considered as an imminent global epidemic. Due to a wide range of determinants of non-communicable diseases, only a multi-sectoral approach is likely to succeed in controlling it. However, this chapter, with the help of few useful examples, illustrates an approach, which can be applied to understand and deal with several non-communicable diseases.

Global impact of non-communicable diseases

Chapter 1 describes ways to estimate the global burden of disease. These estimates help us to understand the current health gap, observe disease patterns, predict future trends, and set disease control priorities. Chapter 1 also illustrates how most of the global burden of disease is attributable to non-communicable diseases and injuries.

Mortality

Two out of every three deaths worldwide are due to either non-communicable diseases or injuries. In 2005, 35 million people died of non-communicable diseases including many young people and those in their middle ages. Eighty percent of these were living in low- and middle-income countries and half of them were women (Fig. 15.1). In these countries, 56% of all deaths are secondary to non-communicable diseases. Cardiovascular diseases (ischaemic heart disease and stroke) remain the top leading cause of death responsible for a quarter of deaths globally (Figs 15.1 and 15.2).

Economic consequences

There are two major economic consequences of non-communicable diseases, i.e. loss of productivity and cost of illness. Both factors are an enormous strain on the already weak economies of many low- and middle-income countries. These are also major impediments to their development. In developing countries, adults in working age have a much higher share of chronic disease burden compared to developed countries. In low-income countries, 44% of adults' deaths due to non-communicable diseases occur below the age of 60. In middle income countries, such as South Africa and India 41% and 35% of all cardiovascular deaths occur in adults below 65 years of age respectively. Tobacco itself kills a quarter of its users in their productive years. Consequently, countries lose out substantial proportion of potential national income as a result. In 2005, the loss in national income from cardiovascular diseases and diabetes was estimated around $18 billion dollars in China, $11 billion dollars in the Russia, $9 billion dollars in India, and $ 2.7 billion dollars in Brazil. Therefore, the notion that non-communicable diseases are merely a disease of the elderly is not true, especially in the developing world (Box 15.1 and Fig. 15.3).

The cost of non-communicable diseases (excluding neuropsychiatry conditions) account for a sizeable proportion (0.02–6.77%) of a country's GDP. Majority of individuals and families are

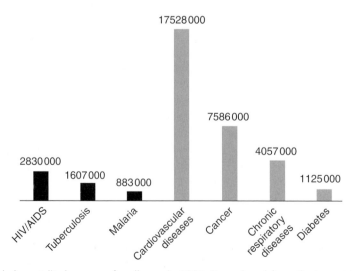

Fig. 15.1 Global mortality by causes for all ages in 2005. Reproduced from the Lancet, Fuster & Voute (2005), with permission from Elsevier.

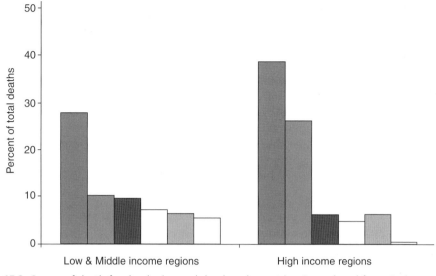

Fig. 15.2 Causes of death for developing and developed countries. Reproduced from Gaziano (2007) with permission.

not insured for health care in low- and middle-income countries. Expenditure on the treatments for chronic disease is likely to impose a significant economic burden. In addition, smoking tobacco that is costly, as well as leading to a number of such conditions is for poor people less money to spent on food, education, and housing (Box 15.2).

Common mental disorders and primary care

Mental disorders are common. Worldwide, more than one in four people suffer from mental or behavioural disorder at some point in their life. Globally these disorders are the leading cause of disability, accounting for almost one-third of morbidity (years lived with disability) and over one tenth of total Disability Adjusted Life Years lost (DALYs). Depression is predicted to become the second most important cause of DALYs lost by 2020. Prevalence in LMIC is at least as high. However, in LMIC, because of continuing high burden of communicable diseases, the *proportion* from mental health is less – depression contributing 9% of all disability and 3% of all DALYs. Common mental disorders (CMD) have a considerable economic impact. However, in LMIC patients present with physical symptoms, the cause is often not recognized and so the high burden not recognized.

Reducing the burden of CMD requires a multi-sectoral approach, with wide-ranging measures to address the wider determinants of health. Primary care can play an important role, by providing cost-effective care. This includes long-term treatment e.g. anti-depressants or major tranquilizers (for schizophrenia), together with psychosocial interventions. The majority of patients with mental illness present to health services do so in primary care. A population-level analysis estimated a potential reduction of 10–30% in the global disease-burden by implementing evidence-based interventions for depression in primary care at low cost. CMD are prevalent in primary care in all LMIC studied. Though most people present to primary care services, they commonly mention the physical symptoms (somatic) associated with mental illness, such as abdominal pains and headache. However, approximately two-thirds of cases go undetected, and

Box 15.1 Case of diabetes

Diabetes currently affects 194 million people worldwide and is expected to affect 333 million by 2025 (Fig. 15.3). In 2007, the three countries with the largest numbers of people with diabetes are India (40.9 million), China (39.8 million) and the United States (19.2 million). In 2007, the three countries with the highest diabetes prevalence are Nauru (30.7%), United Arab Emirates (19.5%) and Saudi Arabia (16.7%). By 2025, the number of people with diabetes is expected to rise by 20% in Europe, 50% in North America, 75% in the Western Pacific and 85% in South and Central America. For developing countries, there will be a projected increase of a 170% of cases; for developed countries, there will be a projected rise of 42%. Diabetes is the fourth main cause of death in most developed countries. Key determinants of this trend are:

♦ Ageing populations

♦ Rapid increases in urbanization and associated changes leading to increased smoking, obesity, physical inactivity, high blood fats, hypertension

♦ Obesity and physical inactivity in particular are associated with future risk of diabetes

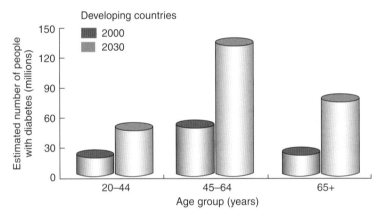

Fig. 15.3 Predicted trends in diabetes for low- and middle-income countries. Data from International Diabetes Federation (2003).

Box 15.2 Case of double burden of disease

Double burden of disease is used to describe those populations who are facing rise of non-communicable diseases while communicable and nutritional diseases still persist among the poorest sections of the society. There is a rise in many risk factors, such as obesity, alcohol, and tobacco use among poor populations in low- and middle-income countries. This can lead to a double burden of diseases which is not only concentrated in the poorest regions and poorest populations. In the early period of economic growth and income, as recently in China and parts of India, there is a rise in overweight and cholesterol. Later this rise in these risk factors levels off and then declines. In addition, urbanization is also directly correlated to high levels of obesity. This highlights that low- and middle-income countries need to take prevention of non-communicable diseases into consideration much earlier on in the economic development.

there are large variations in treatment. Depression is commonly treated with ineffective treatments and few patients receive antidepressants or psychological therapies.

There is growing evidence for interventions for mental illness in LMIC. Implementation should be accompanied, however, by robust evaluation. The WHO has long advocated integrating mental health services in primary care in order to achieve this, particularly in resource-constrained settings.

Causes and determinants

Common modifiable risk factors

Future burden of non-communicable diseases is going to be determined by current population exposures to risk factors. Smoking, hypertension, and alcohol use are three of seven identified top 10 risk factors to non-communicable diseases that make the most significant contribution to burden of disease in low- and middle-income countries (Fig. 15.4).

According to a WHO report on non-communicable diseases, each year at least:

- Tobacco use kills 4.9 million people;
- Physical inactivity takes 1.9 million lives;
- 2.7 million people die as a result of low fruit and vegetable consumption;
- Obesity results in 2.6 million deaths;
- Raised blood pressure takes 7.1 million lives; and
- High cholesterol levels become responsible for 4.4 million deaths.

Diet and physical activity

Socio-economic transition in many countries is shifting population to move from rural to urban settings resulting in dramatic changes in their lifestyles and health behaviour. These changes include a shift toward more 'Western diets' and a drop in physical activity resulting in high levels

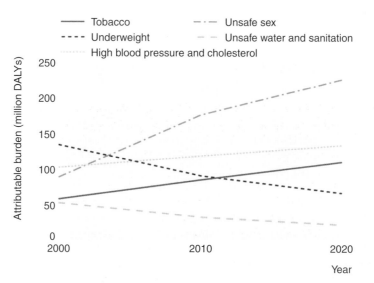

Fig. 15.4 Projected burden of disease attributable to the leading risk factors. Reproduced from Shibuya et al (2003) with permission.

of obesity. Urban diets are generally different from rural diets. There are more processed grains (e.g. rice, wheat); food with high fat content; more animal products; high sugar, and increasingly more food prepared away from the home.

The contrast between urban and rural diet is more marked in low-income countries compared to middle-income countries. Economic transition has shifted consumption of food mainly based on agriculture towards food mostly manufactured and processed in industry. Therefore, more industrialized countries are seeing a rapid growth of food service industry compared to less industrialized nations where reliance is still on agriculture. One of the most unavoidable changes with the socio-economic transition is the reduced use of physical labour to produce goods and services. The inevitable result is a shift in the levels of physical activity and adoption of a much more sedentary lifestyle. As expected, there is a much higher level of obesity in urban than in rural areas in low- and middle-income countries.

Tobacco

Nearly 1.25 billion people in the world use tobacco regularly and every year 5.4 million people die of it. Prevalence among men is reaching almost 50% in low- and middle-income countries. Rates of tobacco use among women is around 9% in low- and middle-income countries but peaks as high as 30% among south Asian populations due to tobacco chewing. As populations go through transition, more poor and uneducated people are affected by the use of tobacco.

Most tobacco growth and cigarette manufacturing is now taking place in developing countries. Free tobacco trade is becoming one of International Monetary Fund's conditions for loans in Eastern Europe and Asia. Such trade liberalization is making cigarette cheaper, easily accessible, and better marketed. Populations in low- and middle-income countries are highly vulnerable as law and taxation has little control on tobacco industry there. It is no surprise that in 2030, the number of deaths attributable to tobacco worldwide will rise from 5.4 million in 2005 to 8.3 million. In 2015, tobacco will be responsible for 10% of global deaths, which will be more than the deaths due to HIV/AIDS.

Tobacco puts enormous burden on a country's economy through high health care costs, absenteeism, loss of productive life years, fires, loss of agricultural land and loss of foreign exchange to purchase imported cigarettes. The cost of an imported brand of cigarette is more than half a day's average salary in many low- and middle-income countries, cost of 10 litres of milk in Algeria and the cost of one kilogram of rice in India.

Globalization

Globalization is defined as the increasing interconnectedness of countries and the openness of borders to ideas, people, commerce and financial capital. Globalization in theory can make trade work for countries to improve their national incomes and eventually public health. However, international power imbalances, trade rules, and lack of national expertise have not allowed all countries to reap these benefits. On the other hand, public health in many poorest countries has suffered due to production and marketing campaigns of the tobacco and alcohol industries. Therefore, globalization has now become an important determinant of non-communicable diseases due to its direct effects on risk factors and indirect effects on national incomes and health infrastructure.

As a direct results of subsides granted to the agriculture sector in Europe and US many developing countries have been unable to sell their food produce in global markets at a competitive rates. This has reduced their national incomes and bankrupted their farming industry in many places resulting in increased reliance on imported and often more processed food. Globalization has also allowed international companies taking advantage of weak regulatory environments in many low- and middle-income countries to market their more fatty and sugary foods. These marketing

campaigns are often targeted at children below 15 yea
purchasing behaviour and shifting it more towards ur

Expansion of tobacco industry in many low- and mi
of the ill effects of globalization. Facing stricter laws and
companies have focussed their marketing towards ch
income countries. These companies are expanding at a p
mainly due to: (a) variable political will to implement to
public awareness about the economic and health effects
many young people to be seen as more 'westernized'.

Poverty

In many countries, non-communicable diseases affect poc
Poverty affects poor people by exposing them to increased ris.   .. prevention less accessible. The association between poverty and risk   ... non-communicable diseases is inconsistent in different regions. Tobacco use is mostly concentrated among the poor in
many low-income countries. Tobacco use leads to further economic downshift by loss of jobs due
to ill health, health care costs, and substituting it for food and other essential items. For other poor
health factors such as obesity, the risk quickly shifts from rich to poor within countries. On the other
hand, diabetes is more common in affluent sections of societies in both rich and poor countries.
These findings are partly explained by the different stages of transition that different countries are at
in these regions as rich taking up new unhealthy behaviours and then discarding them quickly while
poor taking these up later. There is sufficient evidence to reject the traditional notion that non-
communicable diseases and their risk factors are significant only in the most affluent societies.

Epidemiologic transition

The rise of non-communicable diseases in low- and middle-income countries can be explained by
epidemiological transition (Fig. 15.5). As societies progress, infant mortality generally declines,

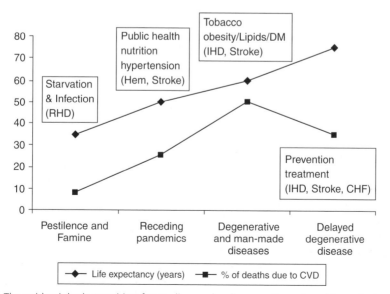

Fig. 15.5 The epidemiologic transition for cardiovascular diseases. Reproduced from Gaziano TA
(2007) with permission.

ancy increases, and the causes of death shift from communicable disease
eases to chronic conditions. Four phases have been described in the literature:
pestilence and famine; (b) the age of receding pandemics; (c) the age of degenera-
n-made diseases; and (d) the age of delayed degenerative diseases. Countries enter the
ologic transition at different times but they move through these phases in a predictable
nner. This is often in parallel with other transitions such as economic (increasing per capita
income), social (industrialization, urbanization, improved access to health care and health
technologies) and demographic (reduced fertility and age specific death rates and increase life
expectancy and ageing population).

Age of pestilence and famine

This phase is characterized by high infant mortality rates and low life expectancy mainly due to
high incidence of communicable and nutritional diseases. Many developed nations came out of
this phase in late 18th or 19th century. However, people living in most of sub-Saharan Africa and
parts of South Asia are still in this age.

The age of receding pandemics

Increasing wealth results in better availability of food leading to a decrease in nutritional diseases
and susceptibility to infections. Better public health infrastructure also helps in curbing communicable diseases. Life expectancy improves and infant mortality rates decreases. Examples include
modern day China and early 20th century USA.

The age of degenerative and man-made diseases

Increasing urbanization and shift in work patterns results in dramatic changes in activity level,
diet and mental stresses. This leads to readily and cheaply available high fat diets, obesity, tobacco,
and alcohol use. As the life expectancy increases beyond 50 years, non-communicable diseases
mainly cardiovascular diseases become the leading causes of death. Many eastern European and
central Asian countries are currently going through these stages.

The age of delayed degenerative disease

In many high-income countries, cancer and cardiovascular diseases are still the main causes of death.
However, due to primary and secondary prevention and improved access to health technologies, life
expectancy has improved further and age specific mortality has declined (Box 15.3 and Fig 15.6).

Prevention and control

There have been many recent advances in health behaviour management, therapeutics, and
organization of care. This provides us the opportunity to effectively prevent and control the
non-communicable diseases and achieve rapid results in many cases. If the current advances are
fully applied, 80% of cardiovascular diseases and 40% of cancers can be prevented. Even a
small reduction in exposure to tobacco use, unhealthy diet, and physical inactivity can achieve
significant reduction in the prevalence of obesity, high blood pressure, blood glucose, and cholesterol at population level. In addition, major international initiatives such as WHO's Global
Strategy for Diet, Physical Activity, and Health and the WHO's Framework Convention for
Tobacco Control also provide a basis for developing and implementing such strategies. Despite
this evidence, little attention has been given to develop cost-effective integrated approaches to
deal with such conditions in majority of low- and middle-income countries. This is partly due
to competing priorities for limited resources and the fact that many of such countries are facing
the dual burden of diseases.

Box 15.3 China: Example of a country in transition

China is currently facing a major non-communicable diseases epidemic. 70% of all deaths and 80% of total burden of diseases is due to non-communicable diseases mainly cardiovascular conditions, cancer and chronic obstructive pulmonary diseases. This epidemiologic transition is a direct result of the demographic and socio-economic transition in Chinese population. In 2000, nearly 7% of Chinese population is 65 years or older. This proportion may reach up to 20% in 2040 if the current trend continues. There has been phenomenal sustained economic growth (over 10%) in the last two decades in China, which has also increased urbanization from 26% to 36%. If the current trend of moving towards cities continues, this may reach up to 45% by 2010 and 60% by 2030. Such changes have also resulted in dramatic changes in Chinese lifestyle, health behaviours, and physical activity levels. Almost one-third of world's cigarettes are consumed in China and 57% of Chinese men smoke. Hypertension (blood pressure 140/90 or higher) in adults is 19% which is a 30% increase over a 10-year period. Prevalence of obesity (7%) and overweight (23%) also went up since 1991, which is an increase of 39% and 97% respectively (Fig. 15.9). This has economic consequences as in the year 2000 China lost 6.7 million of productive life years at a cost of US$30 billion due to cardiovascular disease alone.

A public health approach – population and individual

A unified public health approach that combines individual and population level interventions is required to tackle the problem of preventing and controlling non-communicable diseases. This is best illustrated in the case of cardiovascular diseases. The individual approach includes interventions that identify and manage people with high risk of cardiovascular diseases. On the other hand, population approach includes other interventions that work to reduce the population exposure to these risk factors. Individual level interventions range from providing smoking

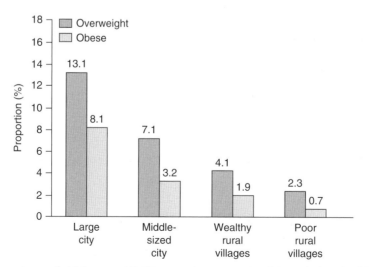

Fig. 15.6 Percentages of children aged 7–17 years who were overweight and obese in China, 2002. Reproduced from Wang L et al (2005) with permission.

cessation and dietary advice to facilitate increased physical activity and healthy eating habits. Several pharmacological interventions have also proven effective in improving outcomes for individuals at high risk of cardiovascular events, including treatment of hypertension, aspirin, beta-blockers in patients with established ischaemic heart disease, and treating high levels of cholesterol. Similarly, several population level interventions aimed at preventing and controlling risk factors have been shown to be effective. These include reducing the risk of hypertension by reducing salt intake, increased physical activity, and high intake of fruit and vegetables. Similarly, improved diets and increased physical activity in populations have been shown to reduce type 2 diabetes.

Setting targets

In a recent Lancet series, there was a call to set a global target to reduce mortality rates due to non-communicable diseases by a modest 2% per year. This is likely to avert 36 million deaths by 2015. In addition, there will be a gain of about 500 million years of life over a period of 10 years between 2006 and 2015. Most of these health gains will be in low- and middle-income countries. There are also potential economic gains. By achieving this target, there can be an economic growth of $36 billion for China and $15 billion for India in the following ten years.

In addition to the aim of reducing mortality, reduction of morbidity due to non-communicable diseases can also be used as an achievable goal. Healthy ageing has been successfully achieved in many developed nations through interventions aimed at reducing morbidity. Given that in low- and middle-income countries such interventions are generally not available, there is even higher health and economic gains if policy makers have a dual objective of reducing mortality as well as morbidity.

Box 15.4 points towards cost-effective solutions to assist policy makers and health providers in achieving the above target giving examples where such interventions have been successful. These interventions will include two basic categories:

1 Population-based interventions
2 Interventions applied to high-risk individuals and settings

Population-based interventions

Interventions in this category are generally applied in non-clinical settings to reduce population exposure to risk factors and address wider determinants of non-communicable diseases. Some examples are as follows:

Laws and regulations

Influencing laws and regulations has been one of the most effective ways to improve health through public health policy. Examples include prevention of dental caries through water fluoridation; harm reduction after a road traffic accident by making wearing seat belts mandatory; and encouraging smokers to give up smoking through compulsory placement of health warning on cigarette packets.

Seat belt legislation

Seat belt legislation is a law that requires the fitting of seat belts to motor vehicles and/or the wearing of seat belts by motor vehicle occupants. Seat belts have been shown to be effective in reducing the severity of injuries. The UK government estimated that since seat belt wearing was made compulsory in 1983 the casualties have been reduced by at least 440 deaths and 8000 serious injuries per year. Seat belt legislation has been introduced in some middle-income countries such as India. However, enforcement of legislation has been slow.

Box 15.4 WHO global strategy for diet, physical activity, and health

This strategy seeks commitment from WHO member states on the following actions:

- To develop a national action plan on diet and physical activity with clear milestones, identified resources, national centres for collaboration, and broader partnership to develop and implement wider public policies

- To establish national guidelines on physical activity and diet

- To provide a sound and consistent source of information to allow consumers to make healthy choices. This should be provided through awareness raising education and media campaigns. Government should also ensure that food labelling provides accurate information and should tackle false health claims associated with certain products. Governments should work with industry to ensure responsible advertising, e.g. unhealthy snacks advertising targeted at children.

- To make national food, agricultural, and fiscal policies consistent with promoting healthy diet

- To ensure that multi-sectoral policies are developed to promote increased physical activity

- To ensure that school policies and programmes enable children to have a healthy diet and opportunities for physical activity

- To make prevention part of health service in order to exploit every clinical encounter as an opportunity for health improvement

Water fluoridation   Water fluoridation through community water sources is one the most equitable and cost-effective methods of providing fluoride to all members of most communities. Water fluoridation is highly effective in preventing dental caries among children and adults. Water fluoridation is especially beneficial and relevant for deprived communities with a high burden of dental caries and poor access to dental-care services than higher income communities. Therefore, water fluoridation is an effective way to reduce health inequalities.

Tobacco control and legislation   Laws and regulations play a major role in controlling tobacco use and the fight against the influence of tobacco industry on younger people. There are a number of ways to exert the influence of legislation:

- Smoke-free places: Legislation to ban smoking in enclosed public places and workplaces has been introduced in several countries. The evidence of its effectiveness in controlling tobacco use is gathering pace.

- Prohibition of tobacco advertising is strongly associated with a decrease in smoking levels. A comprehensive ban on advertising tobacco products is now in place in many countries in Europe. It is estimated that in the UK, a ban on advertising tobacco products will result in a 2.5% fall in smoking levels.

- Governments in western countries are now legislating for bigger, hard-hitting health warnings on tobacco products. Such regulation should also include prohibition of the use of misleading terms such as low-tar, mild, and light on tobacco packs. Studies from Canada suggest that graphic picture warnings are even more effective in encouraging people to stop smoking compared to mere textual messages.

- ◆ A high minimum age for sale of tobacco products along with sanctions against the retailers breaking the law is another effective way of protecting children from the influence and harmful effects of smoking.

In Philippines since 1999, a number of legislations and ordnances have helped in reducing the prevalence of smoking especially amongst their youth. In 1999, smoking was restricted to confined areas all over Philippines and was subsequently banned in public places in many cities. In addition, smoking was also banned in educational institutions and age restriction regulations were strictly implemented. The prices also went up due to increased taxation. This and other interventions resulted in a decline of smoking prevalence in young people by almost a third.

Taxation and price regulation

Taxation and price is an important tool to influence behaviour related to risk factors for non-communicable diseases.

Taxation and cigarette sales Taxation increase on cigarette sales results in reduced consumption especially among young people. Increases in cigarette taxes discourage children from smoking and raise funds that can pay for other tobacco control initiatives, such as stop-smoking campaigns. An increase in taxation on the cigarette sales in South Africa in 1994 resulted in a 33% reduction in cigarette consumption.

Taxation and alcohol use Taxation is rarely used as an alcohol control measure. However, there is strong evidence to suggest that increasing the price of alcohol can reduce secondary road accidents and casualties, workplace injuries, and deaths from secondary liver diseases. High prices also results in less number of alcohol related crimes, domestic violence, and child abuse. Alcohol lessens self-control and is related to risky sexual behaviour, for example non-use of condoms with casual partners and sex workers. A example to show the link between taxation, price and public health was recently provided by Finland. In 2004, the Government reduced alcohol excise duty by 33% immediately resulting in 17% increase in alcohol-related deaths.

Subsidizing healthy food Subsidized healthy food and reduced subsidies and increased taxation on unhealthy food and drink can have a positive influence on dietary behaviour. Poland saw a dramatic decline in the mortality rates secondary to ischaemic heart disease in recent years. Between 1990 and 2002, mortality rates fell by 38% for men and 42% for women in the age range of 45–64 years. One of key change attributed to this was a decline in the use of saturated fat (7%) and a sharp rise in the consumption of polyunsaturated fat (57%). This was accompanied by per head increased fruit consumption of up to four times. This change in dietary habits was a result of changing subsidies to food industries.

Promoting physical activity through taxation Canada has recently introduced measures to remove sales taxes on sport and recreation equipment. Taxation also allows subsidized sport and recreation activities by providing tax credits to people taking a proactive approach to increase their physical activity (gym membership, fitness classes, etc.)

Improving physical environment

In traditional public health teaching, improving physical environment meant improving housing, and reducing overcrowding and pollution. For countries with double burden of diseases, the above notions are still valid. In addition, they are also required to consider environmental factors such as built environment that are crucial to encourage and make it easier for people to be active in their daily lives.

Built environment is generally defined as all of the buildings, spaces, and transportation systems created by people. The measures within built environment that encourages people to increase their physical and prevent obesity activity are as follows:

- Town planning that ensures that pedestrians and cyclists are prioritized when developing streets and roads.
- Building design that ensures that staircases are designed and positioned to encourage people to use them.
- Staircases that are clearly sign-posted and are well-lit to make them more attractive to use.
- Schools with play areas designed to encourage children to take part in varied physical play.
- Workplaces, libraries, schools, shopping centres, and hospitals linked on the walking and cycling routes.
- Walking and cycling routes that are well-maintained and provide access to public and work-places.
- Open spaces and public paths that are accessible by public transport, encourage people to walk, cycle, and use other modes of transport that encourages physical activity.

In many western countries, improving access to physical activity by building cycle ways, footpaths and opening green spaces has shown to increase physical activity levels among their population. Compact town planning and availability of exercise facilities has shown similar effects. Similarly, use of stairs has been encouraged by placing signposts in strategic places. There are also some good examples from low- and middle-income countries e.g. opening up public footpaths and creating open leisure spaces in the city of Bogota in Columbia resulted in an increase in the levels of physical activity among its residents.

Advocacy

Advocacy, generally defined in this context as an act of arguing on behalf of a particular public health issue, has been used very effectively in changing public and policy makers' perception in a number of areas. This can take many forms such as face-to-face meetings, wider public education and media campaign. The aim is to gather wider public support for a specific public health issue. This may concern a marginalized group within society and focus decision makers to have a strategic focus on the issue. A historic example is when John Snow successfully persuaded London's civic authorities to remove the handle from the Broad Street pump that was connected to a faecally polluted water source to interrupt cholera transmission. The art of public health advocacy remains the same but the challenges are different. There are several contemporary examples of this in gathering momentum towards banning cigarette advertisements and use in public places in many countries. Other examples include use of advocacy to reduce salt intake in many western countries.

The objective of advocacy is to change 'upstream' influences on health (policy) rather than efforts focussed on encourage individuals to change health-related behaviours. Australia with one the most successful tobacco control programmes has successfully used public health advocacy to get prohibition on smoking in indoor public places and advertisement of tobacco products. The advocacy was mainly driven by health NGOs and policy-oriented researchers. The key to their success in Australia was the ability to frame and present a public health issue successfully to attract public, media, and political support.

Community-based programmes

Such programmes rely on community participation and mobilization to deliver a health promotion intervention in specific settings. These include population-based approaches but often targeted towards a high-risk section of the society in one particular setting. These are often led by community-based organizations in partnership with statutory and other similar bodies. Here are some examples:

Reducing salt intake in China   A community-based programme in China led an educational campaign to reduce the salt intake. This was done by distributing leaflets using media and community groups to disseminate education about salt intake among a targeted population. The programme also provided information on food content and worked with local industry and shops to provide low salt food. This resulted in significant reduction in salt intake over a period of three years compared to the reference population. Subsequent surveys suggested a reduction in blood pressure as well as number of deaths secondary to stroke and cardiovascular diseases. This led the Chinese government to replicate this programme in a number of other sites in the country.

Five–a-day scheme   In the UK, a national campaign to encourage children to eat at least five portions of fruit and vegetables a day backed by a fruit and vegetable scheme in schools has shown an increase of 13% children achieving their five-a-day target. The scheme worked in a number of regions in the UK with local schools encouraging children to eat more fruit and vegetables using creative methods. Scheme also ensured that a free portion of fruit is provided every day to all children between four and six.

Smoke free workplaces   The evidence to support smoke free workplaces comes mainly from USA and Europe. However, it suggests that such schemes can not only reduce the risk to non-smoker but also encourage smokers to quit smoking. The overall benefit in making workplaces smoke free is in the order of 29% reduction in cigarette consumption. The approaches to promote smoking cessation ranges from giving information on local stop smoking cessation services to the provision of such services in the workplace itself.

Promoting physical activity in the workplace   Workplace can encourage their employees to walk, cycle, or use other modes of transport that involves physical activity to travel in relation to work. This includes provision of information on how to become more physically active and its health benefits. Employers can encourage their staff by: (a) Putting up signs at critical points and distributing prompts to use the stairs rather than lifts, (b) inform them about walking and cycling routes, and (c) address any health and safety issues in relation to their work.

Population screening

Screening is defined as the systematic application of a test to identify individuals at risk of a specific disease. The objective is to ensure that people who are unlikely to seek medical attention due to the absence of symptoms benefit from the further investigation and preventive action. In situations, where a sensitive and specific test can distinguish individuals at risk who could benefit from early intervention, screening can potentially save lives and lead to healthy ageing. Screening has been developed for a number of cardiovascular and other non-communicable diseases. However, population screening has shown to be most effective in certain cancers, for example cervical and breast cancer. Population screening for cervical screening has been shown to be highly cost-effective in five low- and middle-income countries in reducing deaths due to cervical cancer. However, screening programmes require organization to the scale of immunization programmes and access to marginalized groups remain an issue even in developed countries.

Interventions targeted at high-risk individuals and settings

People with high risk of developing a non-communicable disease or a related clinical event can benefit from identification and appropriate intervention either in the community or in health service setting. Vulnerable groups who are at high risk of specific health problems often benefit from a targeted approach in community settings. These are applicable in health care settings however, most interventions identify high-risk individuals. These prevent disease onset and progression to reduce subsequent mortality and morbidity. Similarly, people with established disease also benefit from interventions to stop disease progression and prevent disability and death. Therefore, such interventions can prevent premature deaths and promote healthy ageing. Some examples are as follows:

Community-based interventions to reduce substance misuse among vulnerable children

Marginalized and disadvantaged children and young people are at risk of substance misuse in many societies. It is a major problem in many rapidly growing economies particularly cities. Substance misuse leads to health risks including psychiatric problems, accidental injury, hepatitis, HIV infection, coma, and death. It can also lead to an increased risk of sexually transmitted infections. There is evidence to suggest that early identification of children who are vulnerable to substance misuse benefit from early identification by schools, social workers, health professionals, etc. and early intervention. The intervention is generally community based, involving parent or guardian of the child and consists of an individual behavioural support programme consisting of motivational interviews and support services. Group behavioural therapies are also effective in such circumstances.

Reducing the risk of disease onset (primary prevention)

Brief interventions in primary care to encourage physical activity

Primary and community care professionals can help in encouraging people to become physically active through providing them with opportunistic advice, discussion, negotiation, and encouragement. The interventions may vary from basic advice to more extended, individualized attempts to identify and change factors that influence activity level. In general, identification of individuals who are relatively physically inactive using a standardized tool and encouraging them to do moderate exercise for at least 30 minutes on most days of the week is an effective intervention. However, such advice should be tailored to individual circumstances and needs.

Weight management programmes and primary care

Obesity remains the single most important risk factor for developing type 2 diabetes. Therefore, weight management is the best strategy to prevent the development of type 2 diabetes. Even small amounts of weight loss (5–10%) can prevent or delay the development of type 2 diabetes in individuals with a high risk of the disease. Lifestyle interventions, including diet and moderate physical activity (for example, walking 25 minutes per day, six times per week) can reduce the risk of diabetes by as much as 40–60%. Primary care is well suited to help and advice individuals who are at a high risk of diabetes due to their weight, and are willing to lose and then maintain their weight. Weight management advice offered by health professionals in such settings need to be multi-component and must consist of both lifestyle changes and behaviour modification in relation to physical activity and diet. Weight loss drugs also have a role in individuals in whom lifestyle changes are either insufficient to produce the required weight control or are impossible to achieve because of physical incapacity.

tion advice

...able evidence that brief smoking cessation advice given by any health profes-
...ntist, or nurse) increases the likelihood of quitting. There is also overwhelming
...ffectiveness and cost-effectiveness of a number of psychological and pharmacological treatments for tobacco dependence. In low- and middle-income countries, spontaneous
quit rates are lower suggesting an even greater need for supporting people who wish to quit, and
an opportunity to have a higher health benefit.

Preventing cardiovascular diseases

Changes in risk factors, such as a reduction in cholesterol or blood pressure, or quitting smoking,
can rapidly reduce the risk of developing cardiovascular diseases. Individuals with no clinical
symptoms or signs of cardiovascular diseases can be assessed for the overall risk for developing
those conditions. An overall risk assessment taking account of person's age, lifestyle, blood pressure, weight, and cholesterol level can accurately predict the likelihood of a cardiovascular event
in the next 5–10 years. Psychological interventions to modify lifestyle and therapies such as aspirin, lipid lowering agents and anti-hypertensive agents can reduce this risk substantially.

Reducing the risk of complications in people with established disease (secondary prevention)

Non-communicable diseases often result in complications and non-fatal events, which lead
to subsequent disability, poor quality of life, and hasten death. Nevertheless, intervention at
early stages of the disease can still stop or delay disease progression and prevent onset of such
complications.

Secondary prevention in coronary heart disease

Practice nurses often deliver secondary prevention for patients with established cardiovascular
conditions in primary care in the UK. This includes a risk assessment, lifestyle advice, therapeutic
review, and further investigations. People with ischaemic heart disease are at high risk of developing
heart attacks and such interventions have been shown to be effective in preventing both fatal and
non-fatal cardiovascular events.

Keeping type 2 diabetes under control

In people with diabetes, maintaining near-normal levels of blood glucose and blood pressure
significantly decreases the risk of complications in people with diabetes. Regular eye examination
with a slit-lamp and phototherapy can prevent blindness secondary to diabetes. Similarly, regular
foot examination and treatment of early sores can reduce need for amputation. Checking of urine
for proteins and subsequent treatment can prevent renal failure.

Delivering non-communicable diseases services in poorly resourced health systems

Above discussion points towards a number of cost-effective interventions to prevent and control
non-communicable diseases. However, in many low- and middle-income countries the health
systems are often too fragile and fragmented to deliver these interventions. Historically, many
public health programmes (EPI, TB, malaria etc.) have been disease-specific and vertical in their
mode of delivery. This approach has further weakened health systems in many instances.
Strengthening health systems (health workforce, drug supply, health financing, and information
systems) whilst delivering public health programmes appears to be a key challenge. The Alma

Ata declaration emphasizes that a 'bottom-up approach' through primary health care can strengthen systems. As a result, many countries have focussed on providing a comprehensive primary health care. Other recent strategies have also advocated delivery of cost-effective solutions in priority areas with an integrated approach (IMCI and IMAI). Such a systems-wide approach can potentially cope with constraints (systems barriers) better and help in developing longer-term solutions, without losing the focus on priority areas. An integrated approach to deliver non-communicable diseases services is required which does not lead to further fragmentation of poorly resourced health systems that currently exist in many low- and middle-income countries. International agencies and academic community need to support low- and middle-income countries in this endeavour through operational research and enhancing capacity in health systems expertise.

Chronic disease management models

A number of service delivery models have been established in developed countries. Not all of these are applicable in low- and middle-income countries. However, some can be applicable in poorly resourced health systems.

Chapter 10 describes how to provide chronic care in primary care health centres with referral support from hospital doctors (and specialist psychiatrists if available). Chronic care is required for all long-term diseases including diabetes, epilepsy, and mental health. This model of chronic care is similar to the TB DOTS programme (see Chapter 14) – which provides standardized care and systematic follow-up. For TB and depression this is for six or more months until cure, for diabetes (and HIV/ART care) follow-up care is for life. It is important for education of the patient and a relative (acting as a treatment supporter) on their illness, treatment and follow-up care is important. Once well and over time patient's become 'experts' on their own condition. Experienced diabetics can recognize the effects of low blood glucose, check their urine for glucose, and adjust their diet, insulin, or drugs within a limited range agreed with their doctors, see 'self help' below. This is a long-term relationship of on-going education and support provided by (preferably the same) health worker. That is, continuity of care, which is an advantage of primary care. In primary or hospital outpatient care, quality care depends on clinical information. A chronic disease record card is essential on which the treatment and key clinical indicators are summarized. A card may remain with the patient, as facility records are often not accessible in LMIC facilities. This information makes it possible to monitor patient progress or deterioration – which may require increased dosage or prompt referral for specialist opinion. In hypertension cases recording the BP and in epilepsy recording the presence or absence of seizures in the previous month, which is a good indicator of control (as in a chronic care programme in Swaziland). Monitor the overall facility and district programme performance. Record each patient in a facility or district register. From each quarter the percentage remaining well on treatment, percentage late attending or percentage defaulting from treatment etc. are calculated. Trends in this give an indication of the performance of the programme, as the results will reflect how well patients are educated, supported, and follow-up.

Another model is known as Kaiser Permanente. Fig. 15.7 illustrates how this model can be adapted in low- and middle-income countries. The three tiers on top of the population-wide prevention and health promotion programmes represent health service delivery to people with chronic conditions. It is envisaged that in the majority (70–80%) of people with non-communicable diseases supported self-care is the key to maintaining health and is less resource intense. 10–20% of patients with chronic conditions can be managed within primary care. This in case of diabetes and cardiovascular conditions often involve risk identification and management to prevent progression of disease and development of complications. Only a minority, 5% of cases require

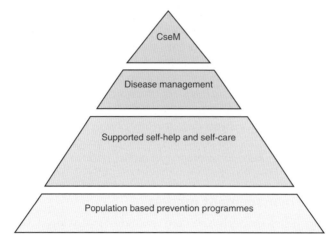

Fig. 15.7 Chronic disease management model.

specialist management in which case a specialist input may complement a case management (CseM) approach.

Self-help and self-care

People with non-communicable diseases and other chronic conditions rely on self-care especially where organized care is less accessible. Self-care needs to be supported by health care as it empowers people, helps them to understand and manage their conditions better and makes them less reliant on the organized care. One of the best ways of supporting self-care is providing people with appropriate skills and information. In China, a successful self-help programme has been rolled out in a number of places. This programme recruits lay people as health trainers who then in turn work in the community to equip people with chronic conditions with life-coping skills. Significant improvement was observed among participants' health behaviour and status. This also reduced the number of secondary hospital admissions. A similar programme in the UK known as the Expert Patient Programme recruited people with chronic conditions as trainers and supported them in running training courses with other people with chronic conditions empowering them to take more control of their lives. This programme has been successful in improving the self-confidence of people with chronic conditions and reducing their reliance on organized care.

Rehabilitation and palliative care

People with many non-communicable diseases are disabled secondary to their condition. These disabilities vary from blindness, inability to walk secondary to amputation, and lack of physical ability to perform routine daily activities due to stroke and heart failure. There is sufficient evidence to support people with disabling conditions and helping them in returning to normality through rehabilitation. Evidence is particularly strong to support rehabilitation after a heart attack and a stroke. However, it is often not possible to provide a multi-disciplinary rehabilitation service to such people in poorly resourced health systems where specialist staff is rare. In such situations, community based rehabilitation programmes utilizing social networks and community support have been successful. There is evidence from many countries including India and Pakistan to suggest that community based approaches can be very useful in helping people with disabilities to return to their social functions.

Palliative care is there to help people with terminal illnesses (most notably cancers but also include other conditions such as heart failure) in coping with the last phases of their illness. The aim of palliative care is to improve the quality of life of people at the end of their existence. The care may take many forms including counselling for depression, pain relief, and stoma-care. There is little evidence from low- and middle-income countries to suggest useful models of palliative care. However, organized care that considers peoples' religious and cultural values and brings families and other social contacts into it is likely to be more useful.

Stepwise action to prevent and control non-communicable diseases

Figure 15.8 illustrates a WHO framework for action to help decision-makers in planning strategies for tackling non-communicable diseases. Following are some principles that underpin this framework:

1 A national framework for action for prevention and control of non-communicable diseases that provides a coherence to actions at all levels

2 An inter-sectoral action as majority of determinants of non-communicable diseases are outside health sector

3 Focus on common risk factors that cut across many specific diseases

4 A comprehensive public health approach combining population and individual level approaches

5 A stepwise approach to implement policies and plans starting with the most feasible and cost-effective ones

6 A set of explicit milestones to monitor stepwise activities and interventions

The first measure in planning according to this WHO recommended stepwise framework is to assess the national burden of non-communicable diseases and develop a profile of their risk factors. Taking this first step was instrumental in establishing a national policy and strategy to deal with non-communicable diseases in Indonesia in 2004. Surveys conducted during the planning phase revealed that the proportion of deaths due to non-communicable diseases has doubled since 1980 from 25% to 49% in 2001. This concerned government and stakeholders and what followed was the establishment of an integrated prevention platform involving all stakeholders at different levels. One useful tool in this regard is the stepwise approach to chronic disease risk factor surveillance developed by WHO. This tool provides a starting point to establish surveillance for risk factors for non-communicable diseases for poorly resourced health systems.

How can globalization assist in achieving global targets for non-communicable diseases?

The previous section discussed how globalization is a key determinant of non-communicable diseases especially in low- and middle-income countries. Here some approaches are presented which can help in reducing the global burden of diseases utilizing globalization as follows.

Global advocacy

Advocacy is generally scarce and fragmented at a global level. A wider and stronger alliance is required between professional bodies, academic community, consumer associations and industries to focus on reducing the global exposure to major risk factors common for many non-communicable diseases. One such example is World No Tobacco Day, which receives wide media coverage.

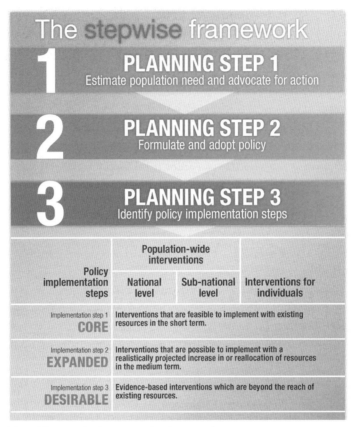

Fig. 15.8 World Health Organization's stepwise framework.

Partnerships

Partnerships and cooperation need to extend beyond national governments and international agencies. In relation to tackling obesity, work is underway to develop a common understanding between multi-national food industry, consumer associations, UN agencies and national governments. Similar work has started around alcohol to safeguard young people against its use and harmful consequences.

Capacity and resources

National response in many low- and middle-income countries has been slow to the epidemiological transition partly because of lack of capacity to plan and implement cost-effective interventions. Donor agencies have been reluctant so far to invest into non-communicable diseases often due to other competing priorities. Recently an alliance consisting of several international donor agencies has launched a strategy to fund five non-communicable diseases centres of excellence around the globe to help national governments to build their technical capacity to deal with the non-communicable diseases epidemic.

Global standards and international treaties

The transition health effects of globalization justify the establishment of global norms and international treaties in order to reach consensus on key policy issues and balance the sphere often

Box 15.5 WHO Framework Convention on Tobacco Control (FTCT)

FTCT is one of the few examples where a legal instrument can be used to influence international health by setting global norms to deal with shared problems. The framework convention is a legal approach to make international law used often in dealing with environmental threats shared globally. This treaty is an acceptance that tobacco control is a global issue requiring an international standardized approach. This framework shows how international public health problems can be dealt with an international legal approach binding governments to follow an evidence-base led strategy. The Convention has the potential to have a major positive influence on global health and provides a test case for proactive involvement of public health bodies in international law making. This treaty primarily focussed on demand reduction, provides a coherent approach to introduce various tobacco control measures. Tobacco control measures aimed at reducing demand include tobacco taxation policies, control policies such as antismoking media campaigns and advertising bans, smoke free public places and smoking cessation strategies.

dominated by other uncontrolled international players. One such example is the Framework Convention on Tobacco Control that has helped many countries in reorienting their policies around tobacco control (Box 15.5).

Reorientation of health services

Globalization also provides opportunity to provide a coordinated response to reduce risk exposure, prevent disease progression and provide better and effective care for non-communicable diseases. Such interventions, e.g. secondary prevention of CVD (although of proven effectiveness) is not even fully implemented in developed countries. Such strategies can prevent early life loss and reduce morbidity in people with such conditions (Box 15.6).

Box 15.6 Building blocks of care for chronic conditions

1 A shift from acute episodic care towards more prolonged and regular care
2 Care based on building consensus among stakeholders and gaining political commitment
3 Organizing care in an integrated fashion to provide an effective, efficient and patient centred service
4 Aligning public policies towards health improvement
5 Using health care workers more effectively by focussing on skills required for chronic care and not on professional boundaries
6 Reorientation of healthcare around patients and their families empowering them to have more control over their lives
7 Care looking beyond clinic and extending to support people with chronic conditions in their living and working environment
8 Prevention should be focus of every clinical encounter with people with chronic conditions

Conclusion

Non-communicable diseases are the leading cause of global burden of disease and contribute significantly to the mortality and morbidity in low- and middle-income countries. These conditions contribute to global poverty and results in significant losses to country's economy. However, cost-effective interventions have been successful in averting the rising tide of non-communicable diseases in many developed countries. Low- and middle-income countries need to prioritize establishing programmes to tackle the rise of non-communicable diseases using public health approaches. These approaches need inter-agency collaboration, political will, and support from international agencies. If implemented, such initiatives have the potential to achieve huge health and economic gains in future.

Further reading

Adeyi O., Robles S. (2007) *Public policy and the challenge of chronic noncommunicable diseases.* Washington DC, World Bank.

Beaglehole R., Yach D. (2003) Globalisation and the prevention and control of non-communicable disease: the neglected chronic disease of adults. *The Lancet,* **362.9387**, 903–08.

Epping-Jordan, JoAnne E., et al. (2005) Preventing chronic diseases: taking stepwise action. *The Lancet,* **366.9497**, 1667–71.

Fuster, Valentin, Janet Voute. (2005) MDGs: chronic diseases are not on the agenda. *The Lancet,* **366.9496,** 1512–14.

Gazino T.A. (2007) Clusters of Excellence for Chronic Diseases. Boston, Ovations.

International Diabetes Federation. (2003). The Diabetes Atlas. Brussels: International Diabetes Federation.

Lenfant, Claude. (2001) Can we prevent cardiovascular diseases in low- and middle-income countries? *Bulletin of the World Health Organisation,* **79**, 980–82.

Shibuya K., Ciecierski C., Guindon E. et al. (2003). WHO Framework Convention on Tobacco Control: development of an evidence based global public health treaty. *BMJ,* **327(7407)**: 154–7.

Wang L., Kong L., Wu F. et al. (2005). Preventing Chronic diseases in China. *The Lancet,* **366(9499)**: 1821–4.

WHO Innovative care for chronic conditions (2002): Building blocks for action. WHO. Geneva, WHO.

WHO Preventing Chronic Diseases: A vital investment. WHO. 2005. Geneva, WHO.

Chapter 16

Quality control, safety, and better practice

John Wright

This chapter gives an overview of the following topics:

Aspects of quality in health;

Quality improvement methods;

Clinical audit;

Patient safety;

Evidence based practice;

Clinical guidelines;

Getting knowledge into practice.

Part 1: Health care quality assurance

Hospitals and health clinics are situated downstream on the river of health. While public health traditionally focuses further upstream on improving health through the prevention of illness, it also has an important role to play in improving health through prevention of poor clinical practice.

Quality in health care

Quality assurance (QA), quality improvement, and quality control tend to be used synonymously in the health care literature. Generally, QA is used as shorthand, catch-all term. Assuring quality stems from several broader QA definitions such as:

- Meeting or exceeding customer's expectations. There are two health care customers:
  (i) Internal – our professional colleagues; and
  (ii) external – the patient.
- Zero defects – getting the service right first time by removing weak links.
- Fit for purpose – services evolve into best practice.
- Conforming to specification – policy and practice is guided by pre-determined standards and guidelines.

Each raises issues for health care professionals but at least they give us a framework in which to think about QA.

Quality of health care has a number of dimensions and it is useful to have a framework that describes these. These dimensions include:

♦ Accessibility – ensuring health care is accessible to patients

♦ Equity – health care should be provided fairly to all patients

♦ Effectiveness – there should be evidence of benefit for improved patient outcomes

♦ Efficiency – resources should not be wasted

♦ Safety – health care should be provided without harming patients

Quality improvement methods

There are different quality improvement methods that have been used in industry and adapted to health care and yet little evidence that any one method is better than others.

Avedis Donabedian, considered a clinical quality assurance founding father, devised three inter-related QA components:

♦ Structure – health care staffing, equipment, policies and procedures, clinical guidelines, etc.

♦ Process – how equipment is used and what procedures are followed.

♦ Outcome – structure and process impact on health and well-being.

Most agree that Donabedian's triad provides a robust framework for measuring and improving health care quality. In recent times, however, QA experts moved from Donabedian's linear approach to cyclical or spiral models. The common feature of these methods is a cycle of learning and action. One example of this is the PDSA cycle.

Plan, Do, Study, Act (PDSA)

The *Plan, Do, Study, and Act* (PDSA) model (Fig. 16.1) involves a cycle of review and planning for improvements (Plan); implementation of small changes (Do); monitoring change through agreed measures (Study) and implementing further change on the basis of early results (Act).

The aim of the model is to encourage constant change, reflection and demonstrable improvement. It recognizes the dynamic nature of quality improvement, and how we learn from experience

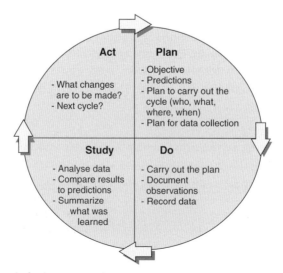

Fig. 16.1 The PDSA cycle for improvement.

and feedback. Most importantly it is a quick and simple model for testing new ideas to improve quality of care. The PDSA cycle provides an achievable stepwise approach to change:

Plan plan the change you intend to introduce to improve patient care. Clarify the aims of the planned change and how you will measure the change. Agree the information necessary to demonstrate change (e.g. waiting times; proportion of patients on an appropriate drug; numbers of drug errors) and the time-scale for measurement of this information. Start with small ideas, but if the planned change is complex, then break it down into bite-size chunks.

Do put the change into practice and measure its impact by collecting the agreed data. Keep this step as short as possible and identify any problems or barriers along the way.

Study review and analyse the data. Has there been change? Could things have been done better?

Act change the plan to focus on what works and change what did not work. Go back to the 'DO' step and measure further change.

The **PDSA** model combines features in the definitions we raised earlier. It provides an easy abbreviation for thinking about, implementing, and evaluating change in real practice settings. It emphasizes that quality improvement is a continuous evolution of small changes rather than a big bang that is too ambitious to ever take place. The cycles of change are small but clever adaptations that can happen tomorrow afternoon rather than large trials that will take years to start. Problems can be quickly identified and changed rather than wasting time waiting for long term outcomes.

Clinical audit

Clinical audit is a well-established variation of a quality improvement cycle. It has been defined as 'the systematic, critical analysis of the quality of clinical care, including the procedures used for diagnosis and treatment, the use of resources and the resulting outcome and quality of life of the patient'. Simply put, it involves looking at what you or your colleagues are doing, learning from it and changing your practice. If we do not examine or review what we are doing in clinical practice, then we will never pick up our mistakes. This review must be structured and systematic if it is going to be accurate and believable.

There are six key steps in undertaking clinical audits (Fig. 16.2):

1 Choose your Topic (e.g. drug administration errors)
2 Define criteria and standards (eliminate errors within 6 months)
3 Collect data on past or current performance (using untoward incident reporting forms)
4 Analyse and present this data to your colleagues (benchmarking meetings)
5 Identify areas of poor performance and implement change (multi-disciplinary workshops)
6 Re-audit performance in the light of change (IT monitoring and alerting systems)

A programme example is TB: e.g. criteria case default rate, standard 5% or less, collecting and analysing data from in the TB register.

Remember that audit works best in improving care when it provides clinicians *with accurate and regular feedback on their own individual performance, compared to their peers*. As we can see in our drug administration error example above, feeding back clinical performance can be a powerful force for promoting change where there is complacency about individual and departmental practice. The feedback should be to the whole department so that open discussion can take place about the results and an honest appraisal of why good and poor performance occurred. Ensure that everybody has the opportunity to attend and participate. Try and involve people by making the session as interactive as possible, not just the same old voices monopolizing the discussion.

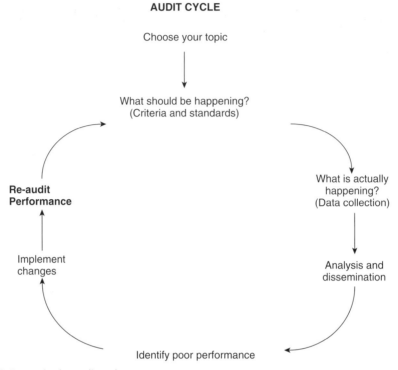

AUDIT CYCLE

Choose your topic

What should be happening?
(Criteria and standards)

What is actually
happening?
(Data collection)

Re-audit
Performance

Analysis and
dissemination

Implement
changes

Identify poor performance

Fig. 16.2 Stages in the audit cycle.

Action taken to improve performance may involve setting up a training session for staff, an induction workshop for new doctors, clinical guidelines, changes to the process of care such as how and where patients are admitted or documentation in records.

Without external assessing our QA policy and practice, there's a risk that motivation wears thin or the business becoming incestuous, so external teams are invited (increasingly compulsorily) to vet QA practice. This so-called accreditation mechanism 'oversees' whatever QA spiral we adopt.

Part 2: Patient safety

Improving patient safety

Until recently, medical errors or adverse events have been a taboo subject for doctors. A culture of blame and shame has prevented any rational attempt to learn from our failures and prevent recurrences. Doctors have for too long been considered as infallible and when mistakes do happen there has been nowhere for them to turn to for support or discussion. The doctor becomes isolated in his or her guilt and defensiveness and the patient becomes angry at the lack of honesty.

It is estimated that about 10% of inpatient episodes will lead to adverse events, half of which are preventable. Common errors (as we saw in our clinical audit example earlier) include prescribing errors – wrong drug, wrong dose (e.g. adult dose given to a child), wrong administration (e.g. intravenous drugs given intramuscularly); communication failures; delays in diagnosis.

Previous approaches to human error have focussed on individuals and blamed their actions on carelessness, tiredness, inattention, or negligence. This is the easy approach, with someone to blame and to shame. However even the best doctors, nurses, and health professionals make

Box 16.1 Examples of medical errors

1 A 3-month-old infant was admitted to hospital with gastroenteritis. She was put on IV fluids, but the nurse failed to check the volume being given. As a result the infant received one litre of fluid over 1 hour and died of heart failure secondary to fluid overload.

2 A 45-year-old man presented with an infected foot. He explained to the doctor in out patients that he was allergic to penicillin. When he was admitted the ward doctor failed to take an allergy history and prescribed IV magnapen. The patient told the nurse on the drug round about his allergy, but she did not realize that magnapen contained penicillin and the patient had an acute anaphylactic reaction and died.

3 A 23-year-old woman was on antituberculosis treatment with four drugs. The pharmacist and the doctor assumed that the other had explained how to take her medicines. As a result she took a sub-optimal dose for 2 months and developed multi-drug resistant TB.

4 A young child was taken to theatre for removal of a foreign body in her left hand. The surgeon checked the X-ray but failed to confirm the correct hand and operated on the right hand.

5 Two different antiretroviral drugs were supplied by a manufacturer in almost identical boxes. As a result the pharmacist ended up dispensing the wrong box to patients who developed side effects from treatment.

mistakes. Errors are not random events, but follow the same patterns. The same adverse events happen over and over again, not only in other hospitals, but also in the same hospital over time.

Individual factors are an important part of clinical practice; however they are only one component. When an adverse mistake occurs, the individual factor may just be the last, but most visible link in a rusting chain of errors that owe more to the context or system within which the health profession is working. These may include poor teamwork and communication, staff shortages, time pressures, lack of experience or inadequate equipment. Everyone makes mistakes every now and then, and adverse events will always occur. However, we can reduce their frequency by learning from them and putting into place defences in the system that will reduce the risk of individual mistakes (see Box 16.1).

Reducing errors

The methods and proposals for reducing medical errors have drawn heavily on experience in other sectors with more experience, particularly the airline industry. Like the health care industry, the airline industry is extremely complex and every error is potentially lethal. However if the airline industry had a similar error rate to the health care industry then we would have aircraft falling out of the sky all over the place. Other sectors such as nuclear power plants also provide examples for risk management. One obvious difference between health care and industry, which complicates health care, is that unlike machinery, patients don't always comply with treatment and care.

A model that industry uses is that of the 'Swiss cheese' (so called because Swiss cheese has holes in it) (Fig. 16.3). There are different layers of defences preventing errors from happening. However, each of these layers can develop holes, and if these holes line up then errors can occur. In medicine, there can be dangerously few protective slices of cheese waiting to line up and cause disaster.

The approach the airline industry took to reduce errors was to ensure that every mistake, and more importantly, every near miss was identified and reported. There will be tens and hundreds

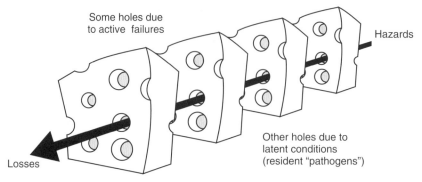
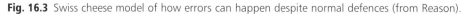

Fig. 16.3 Swiss cheese model of how errors can happen despite normal defences (from Reason).

of near misses for every reported error, and so this is an important stage to identify failure in standards and rectify them before they end up as mistakes (Fig. 16.4).

In 2004 the WHO launched the World Alliance for Patient Safety to cut the number of errors suffered by patients. The lessons for improving patient safety cover a number of common themes:

1 Build a safety culture which is open and fair. Staff should not fear reporting errors

2 Promote reporting of errors and 'near misses' so that staff have good evidence about safety of care

3 Learn from errors by investigating them and understanding the causes.

4 Redesign health care to promote safety and prevent human error.

The problem should not be under-estimated, For example, in the last UK staff survey one in three staff had witnessed potentially harmful incidents.

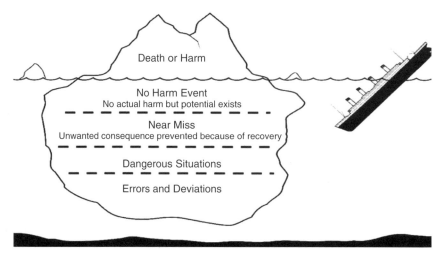

Fig. 16.4 Adverse events can be the tip of a much bigger iceberg.

Part 3: Improving quality and patient safety

Keeping up-to-date: Evidence based practice

We cannot predict what the future holds however we can assume there will be new health challenges and new treatment breakthroughs. This last section of the book deals with how as public health workers we can attempt to keep up to date in a rapidly changing world.

Traditionally training of health workers has relied on trying to transfer a large amount of information to students who are then expected to remember this information for the rest of their lives. Now we know that such information is quickly forgotten and soon out of date. We need to replace the old methods of trying to cram information into people with new strategies of teaching them where to look for the answers. Newly qualified health professionals should not feel that they are expected to know everything, but they must have the confidence to know how to address the problems that they will come across in their work.

This *lifelong learning* encourages staff to admit when they do not know rather than try and bluff their way through ignorance. It encourages them to feel comfortable with uncertainty and equips them with the confidence to look up the answers. There is a huge and exponentially increasing volume of medical knowledge. Over 2 million research papers are published each year and this number is doubling every 16 years. Obviously it is not possible to keep on top of such a tidal wave of information. But we need to know where to go to get the right information, whether this is a colleague, a book, a journal, or increasingly internet and electronic sources.

Distance learning and electronic sources of information (such as those on the worldwide web) hold great promise for developing countries that have traditionally been left out of the information loop and left with the crumbs of out-of-date Western textbooks. New skills will need to be provided for health workers to know not only where and how to look up answers, but also how to assess the information they find. It is important to remember that anyone can spout their opinion on a particular health topic, but many will be biased and wrong. The following stages are required to make sense of research evidence:

(a) Searching – knowing where to track down answers to specific problems. Attempts are currently being made to improve access to research information and effectiveness information using the internet and to ensure high quality, useful information. Some examples of internet sites include:

  ◆ UK Cochrane Centre – http://www.cochrane.co.uk

  ◆ South African Cochrane Centre: http://www.mrc.ac.za/mrcnews/march96/cochrane.htm

  ◆ International Network for the Availability of Scientific Publications – http://oneworld.org/inasp/network.html

  ◆ Global Health Network – http://www.pitt.edu/HOME/GHNet/GHNet.html

  ◆ WHO – www.who.int/healthtopics

(b) Appraising – judging if the information is accurate and applicable to your population. A simple set of questions can address this: does the information focus on the problem at hand? Is it scientifically robust enough to be believable and accurate? Is it relevant to the local population?

Health informatics. In developed countries, and increasingly in LMIC, health information is computerized. Open source software may be used in hospital information systems. Many patients have mobile-cell phones, and appointment reminders can be sent to these. Health workers may use their cell phones for urgent referrals. See Box 16.2

Box 16.2 Health informatics

When Americans feel unwell they Google. Most Europeans and North Americans now use the Internet and tools like Google to find information on the Web. They also communicate via email, text, and telephone via the internet e.g. on 'Skype'. Whole industries are being transformed by commercial applications communicating through the Internet.

In the UK the National Health Service is investing in the largest IT project in the world, an attempt to provide a national integrated digital health care system with patient records, including pathology results and digital images such as x-rays, shared between General Practitioners and hospitals. GPs use computer records and chronic care management systems, e.g. for diabetes care. This IT system will make information available on waiting times, clinical performance, and effectiveness to health managers and for public health surveillance.

The packaged software developed for Europe and North American is expensive and complex, and computing hardware and networks can be expensive to purchase, maintain, and support with trained staff. In addition in LMIC there are IT literacy, language, cultural, operational, and organizational challenges. However, there are the open source (no cost) health applications – such as OpenMRS (www.openmrs.org), an electronic medical record system which has been implemented in east and southern African countries.

Personal computers and mobile phones are increasingly affordable for ordinary individuals and health services in middle income countries of Asia and becoming so in low income countries such as in Africa. Their use is spreading rapidly including that by health workers. It is now possible to send text messages from a computer on the Internet to a mobile phone. For example, a clinician working in a remote area could send details of a critically ill patient or an order for more drugs by text message to a district hospital. Some hospital IT systems in Africa already send appointment reminders by text message.

The challenge and opportunity for LMIC developing countries is to get the benefits of electronic health care while avoiding the high cost of buying over-complex software packages. The Internet will continue to bring new technologies, new opportunities, and a better awareness that there is a huge global market for innovative health systems. Google grew from the ideas of a single PhD student in 1996 to a $23-billion company by 2004. Its innovation and success would have been difficult to foresee in 1996 and it is similarly difficult to foresee how technology will transform health in the future. The one thing you can be sure of is that technology will keep getting cheaper, more powerful, and more pervasive. How you exploit that knowledge is up to you.

Owen Johnson, 2008.

Guidelines

Guidelines, or protocols, can provide an effective method of summarizing research evidence. Good guidelines can provide a simple and concise reminder for health professionals about how to diagnose and treat patients with a particular illness. A number of steps should be considered when developing a guideline:

1 Choose the topic. Concentrate on health priorities where there is evidence of variation in practice and poor quality.

2 Get the right people involved. If you want others to adopt it then you need to make sure the right people are involved – doctors, nurses, managers, community health workers.

Box 16.3 Interventions to promote changes in practice among health professionals

- Educational meetings – small group and interactive sessions for staff
- Audit and feedback – measurement of team or individual performance and feedback of this data on a timely and regular basis
- Opinion leaders – messengers who are respected and trusted by health professionals
- Educational outreach – one-to-one visits to doctors or health teams within their own clinical setting (hospital room or clinic)
- Reminders – posters, guidelines, and prompts that reinforce the message
- Patient involvement – community training sessions and expert patients so that patients are empowered to ensure they receive the best treatment
- Dissemination – circulating the guidance in an accessible format by post or in newsletters

3 Build on good evidence. The guideline should be credible and based on good research evidence rather than personal opinion.

4 Obtain consensus. The process of developing a guideline is just as important as the message that is provides. If it is to be effective then different stakeholders must agree with it.

5 Make it accessible. Try to ensure that the format is clear and attractive and accessible to staff in busy clinical settings.

Knowledge into practice

Public health professionals have an important role in communicating knowledge and trying to change professional behaviour of health staff in a district or country. For example to prescribe certain essential and appropriate drugs, or to effectively monitor and follow up patients with tuberculosis using guidelines, or to diagnose respiratory infections accurately. Simply sending information in the post does not change staff practice. Simply communicating information in a lecture is unlikely to make much impact. Knowledge alone is not enough. If knowledge is to lead to improved performance, then it must be accompanied by training in skills and practical competence.

There are methods of changing practice that have been shown to be effective in producing change (Box 16.2). It is important to consider how to balance these different methods of training and education to get the best result. An hour spent in a local health clinic as an educational outreach may be a worthwhile investment to reduce inappropriate referrals or improve standards of care (Box 16.3).

It is also important to look beyond the mechanisms for change to exploring what the current situation is in a certain area, and what the barriers to change may be (such as lack of resources, or drugs or investigations) prior to implementing change. Broader factors that will enhance the chances of success in producing change include:

1 Having a credible message of importance and relevance to staff
2 Guidance that is evidence based and not too complex to adopt
3 Ensuring close involvement of local staff
4 Good leadership and communication
5 Developing good teamwork in the health organization

The ultimate challenge for public health professionals is not to work in isolation from other health professionals, but to disseminate the skills of good public health practice to all. Only by achieving this will real and sustainable improvements in the health of populations be gained.

Further reading

Hurst K. (2002) *Managing quality*, London: South Bank.

Wright J., Hill P. (2003) *Clinical governance*. Churchill Livingstone.

Donabedian A. (1980) *The definition of quality and approaches to its assessment*, Ann Arbor: Michigan, Health Administration Press.

Chapter 17

Future trends in global public health

John Wright and John Walley

This chapter gives an overview of the following topics:

- ◆ To understand the changing patterns of populations, environments and diseases in the future
- ◆ To appreciate the social and economic factors that will shape future burdens of ill-health
- ◆ To prioritise policies to tackle future ill-health, infectious diseases and health service delivery
- ◆ To review the importance of effective implementation on achieving change and health gain
- ◆ To recognise the major challenges or mega-problems facing the world in the coming years and decades.

Much has been done to improve the health of populations throughout the World over the last century. Public health policies have provided healthier environments with clean water, effective sanitation, and better housing. Public health programmes have increased vaccination coverage as well as provide preventive health services (such as maternal and child health services). Health promotion campaigns have attempted to improve awareness about the factors that cause disease and how they can be avoided, and change individual risk-taking behaviour.

Yet inequalities in income and health continue to widen, not just in developing countries but throughout the World. Over 1.3 billion people live in absolute poverty with incomes of less than $1 per day. Many developing countries are spending more on debt relief for international loans than on health and education combined. In contrast, 80% of the World's wealth is held by less than 20% of its inhabitants (Fig. 17.1)

In this century there are many challenges that still face health professionals everywhere. Some are the same as those we have dealt with in the past such as urbanization and globalization. Some will be new challenges such as climate change. This chapter will outline some of the changes that have been predicted for the next twenty years.

The global burden of disease

Changes in how people live and where people live will change the type of diseases that affect them in the future (as introduced in Chapter 1). Demographic changes will lead to more people living longer, in more urban and industrial environments, with higher incomes, better nutrition and smaller families. The rise and rise of the population and urban living is producing 'megacities' with many millions of inhabitants. With this transition will come reductions in some of the current threats to health as well as new threats to health.

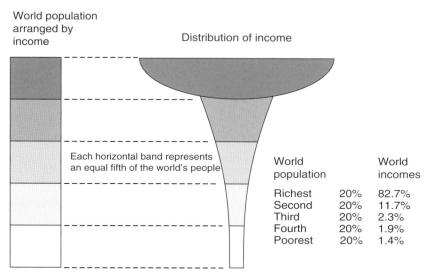

Fig. 17.1 Distribution of the world's wealth.

The threats from urban environments include:

◆ Spread of communicable diseases from poor housing, overcrowding, and poor sanitation;

◆ Spread of AIDS and sexually transmitted diseases from increased casual and commercial sex;

◆ Increased accidents, violence and mental illness from cars and reduced social cohesion and support;

◆ Increased lung disease and asthma from urban pollution;

◆ Increased heart disease from increased fat, less vegetables, and reduced exercise.

Projections and modelling from current health statistics have led to predictions of life and death in the year 2020. These predictions are important to consider in planning health services for the future. Globally we are part way through a trend of demographic and epidemiological change,

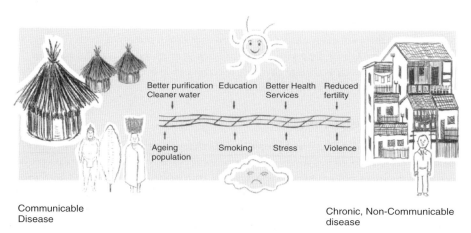

Fig. 17.2 Communicable disease versus chronic, non-communicable disease.

including from more communicable to more non-communicable disease. However, as discussed in Chapter 1, the worlds regions vary greatly with East Asia being further on and sub-Saharan Africa least far along this trend.

Global demographic and mortality changes by 2020:

♦ Increased life expectancy – People will live longer throughout the World. Men in Latin America may have a life expectancy of 71 years in 2020 compared to 65 in 1990. The increase in life expectancy will be greater for men than for women because of the greater prevalence (and anticipated improvements) of risk factors such as smoking and vascular disease.

♦ Fertility – The numbers of children per couple will continue to reduce in many countries (as in Bangladesh). Despite this the population is still rising (though less quickly) and *per capita* economic growth is stagnant or falling in many low income countries. Other countries, such as Uganda and Pakistan are 'trapped' in continuing high fertility. This can lead to conflict over land, hunger and malnutrition. Also health, education, and other services do not keep pace with population growth.

♦ Where there is increased life expectancy and reduced fertility, this leads to an increasing burden of adult ill health relative to childhood ill health. Almost 40% of all deaths in developing countries are in children under 5, and nearly all of these are avoidable. However, nearly 30% of deaths are in adults aged 15–59 years and three-quarters of these are avoidable. The proportion of adult deaths increases as fertility declines. Adult ill health has important implications for communities in terms of impact on family dependants, labour productivity, and consumption of health service resources.

♦ Infectious diseases will become less of a problem. Better living conditions, higher incomes, better education and improved access to health services (immunizations and treatment with antibiotics etc) will probably continue the decline in deaths from infectious diseases. Death rates from HIV have peaked in Africa and will peak in India in around 2010. Newly emerging infectious diseases are potential threats. (Table 17.1)

♦ In contrast, deaths from non-communicable diseases such as accidents, heart disease, stroke and cancers will continue to increase from about 50% of all deaths in 1990 to about 75% of all deaths in 2020. Most of this increase in global deaths will come from developing countries, partly because more people will be living longer and so more at risk of developing vascular disease and cancer, partly because of more people smoking in developing countries. Population growth will also lead to greater numbers of young adults and so greater numbers of deaths from injuries and accidents. (Fig. 17.3)

Changes in the burden of disease 1990–2020

Combining deaths *with* disability, in DALYs as explained in Chapters 1 and 6, the burden of disease shows a much more dramatic change in the developing regions' future patterns of health problems (Fig. 17.3).

Table 17.1 shows how the change in patterns of disease will affect the top 15 commonest causes of ill health. This shows how non-communicable disease and accidents will overtake infectious diseases in global impact.

Not all infectious diseases will decline however. Tuberculosis will remain at a high level of death and disability. HIV has reached the list of top ten causes of ill health globally. Here we are discussing global projections, but remember that there are major variations in the burden of disease in the different regions of the world. Malaria has always been high on the list, and HIV/AIDS has already become high on the list, in sub-Saharan African region – but not so high in the list for

Table 17.1 Disease burden measured in Disability-Adjusted Life Years (DALYs)

1990			2020 (Baseline scenario)
Disease or injury			*Disease or injury*
Lower respiratory infections	1	1	Ischaemic heart disease
Diarrhoeal diseases	2	2	Unipolar major depression
Conditions arising during the perinatal period	3	3	Road traffic accidents
Unipolar major depression	4	4	Cerebrovascular disease
Ischaemic heart disease	5	5	Chronic obstructive pulmonary disease
Cerebrovascular disease	6	6	Lower respiratory infections
Tuberculosis	7	7	Tuberculosis
Measles	8	8	War
Road traffic accidents	9	9	Diarrhoeal diseases
Congenital anomalies	10	10	HIV
Malaria	11	11	Conditions arising during the perinatal period
Chronic obstructive pulmonary disease	12	12	Violence
Falls	13	13	Congenital anomalies
Iron-deficiency anaemia	14	14	Self-inflicted injuries
Protein-energy malnutrition	15	15	Trachea, bronchus and lung cancers

developing countries as a whole as they are less common in some large population countries such as China. Other notable global changes include:

◆ Tobacco will become the biggest single risk factor for ill health in the World. Smoking will become the new global epidemic and its causative effects on heart and lung disease and stroke will create great suffering for individuals and populations.

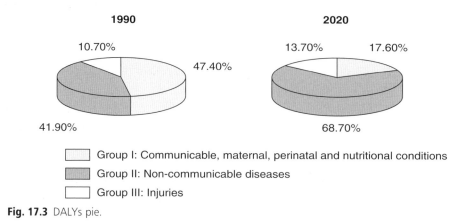

1990

10.70%

47.40%

41.90%

2020

13.70%   17.60%

68.70%

☐ Group I: Communicable, maternal, perinatal and nutritional conditions
▨ Group II: Non-communicable diseases
☐ Group III: Injuries

Fig. 17.3 DALYs pie.

- Mental illness is already a major cause of global ill health and will increase. Depression in particular will increase in prevalence and impact. Suicide will also become a greater problem.

- War, violence, and road traffic accidents are also expected to increase steeply in their impact on the World's health. The increase in violence and road traffic accidents will mostly be due to the increase In the numbers of young men at risk of these events as well as increases in motor vehicles.

The social determinants of health

The underlying cause of death and disability are the social and economic factors.

One depressing finding beyond the control of health workers is the prediction that the rich will continue to grow richer at the expense of the poor. Income in developed countries will rise much faster than in developing countries. Disparities in health that exist in every country will be exaggerated at a global level. Wealth reflects health and until political steps are taken to address this basic cause of ill health, inequalities in health will continue to grow.

Government expenditures on health vary from as little as $20 to $6000 US per year. For people in the low-middle income countries more than half of all health expenditures are through *out-of-pocket* expenditures. According to the WHO report (2008), these expenditures push more than a 100 million people into poverty. There are many approaches to health financing, as explained in Chapter 7. The previous trend towards user fees and privatization of health services is now being reversed. International agencies led by WHO (2008) is calling for user fees should be removed for primary health care (PHC). This should increase utilization of health services, especially by the poor. The lost revenue to health facilities from user fees – though often small – must to be made-up by governments/donors funds. This was done with increased utilization in Uganda. The key to success was increasing salaries (compensating the money health workers received from user fees) and increased essential drug supplies. In addition, social health insurance provision can avoid catastrophic financial stress due to major illness and hospitalization. In social health insurance contributions and benefits are standardized in a national scheme; unlike private insurance the unhealthy pay higher premiums. Middle income countries may move to a *capitation* system, where primary care facilities/practitioners are paid a yearly amount for each person registered. There is a contract specifying the curative and preventive services to be provided, and patients do not need to pay when they attend, as in the UK.

We need a better distribution of wealth – both globally and nationally. For example commitment from rich countries to honour UN pledges to donate 0.7% of Gross Domestic Product to support development in poor countries. This donation will bring no health gain if it spent on highways and guns, so it needs to be matched by commitment from the governments of developing countries to spend 10–15% of their national budget on health.

Primary health care

Thirty years ago in Alma Ata the world's governments called for 'health for all by the year 2000' through PHC. Experience since then has shown that countries that have followed the PHC strategy have a higher level of health for the same investment. PHC is, according to WHO (2008) relevant 'now more than ever'. It is a means to get health development back on track, particularly so in a time of global economic crisis.

WHO proposes reforms that ensure:

- That health systems contribute to health equity, social justice and the end of exclusion, primarily by moving towards universal access and social health protection – *universal coverage reforms*;

- Reforms that reorganize health services as primary care, i.e. around people's needs and expectations, so as to make them more socially relevant and more responsive to the changing world while producing better outcomes – *service delivery reforms*;
- Reforms that secure healthier communities, by integrating public health actions with primary care and by pursuing healthy public policies across sectors – *public policy reforms*;
- Reforms that replace disproportionate reliance on command and control on one hand, and laissez-faire disengagement of the state on the other, by the inclusive, participatory, negotiation-based leadership required by the complexity of contemporary health systems – *leadership reforms*.

An agenda for action

Health priorities

There is a need to prioritize specific programmes and integrating these within health services and budgets. Although changing the pattern of resource expenditure is a very difficult task in any country, it could be argued that any such change is essential if the best use of limited resources is to be achieved. Treatment of cancer or heart disease is expensive and provides only marginal benefit. Such resources may be better spent on treatments that have greater impact or on disease prevention.

Public health professionals in developing countries have a vital role in campaigning for legal change to protect health and for appropriate planning of health services to address ill health. The following steps provide a useful basis for action.

1 Improving child health. Child health programmes and interventions are usually cheap and effective and address some of the major inequalities in health. Promotion of exclusive breast feeding and longer birth intervals is important for child health and development (giving more mother time for existing child).

2 Reduce maternal mortality. Many pregnancies are unplanned and the risk to the woman's health would be prevented if the unmet need for family planning was addressed. Most maternal deaths (from bleeding, infection or eclampsia) are preventable. Maternal health programmes should aim to screen women at high risk of complications; provide tetanus toxoid immunization and iron/folate supplements; monitor weight and blood pressure during pregnancy; provide sterile supplies; and appropriate health worker support during delivery.

3 Improve access to sexual and reproductive health services. Better family planning and contraception are fundamental steps in preventing the poverty and famine that result from excessive population growth.

4 Prevent the rise of smoking. Smoking is the greatest threat to public health in the future. There are effective methods of reducing it and these should be pursued vigorously and persistently. Legislation can limit supply and promotion of tobacco as well as smoking in public places. Taxation is effective at reducing demand for cigarettes and should be supported. Education can prevent young people from starting smoking and encourage smoking cessation.

5 Make road travel safer. Road traffic accidents are an important cause of death and disability in developing countries. A number of factors lie behind this, the main one being that these are not simple accidents but have clear determinants such as: Poor roads (unfenced from animals, no lighting); dangerous driving (too fast, too inexperienced); dangerous vehicles (poorly maintained, overloaded); drink-driving. Interventions to reduce deaths concentrate on enforcement to deter alcohol use, encourage safer cars, a speed limit, and use of seatbelts.

6 Prevention and treatment of HIV/AIDS. All patients with HIV/AIDS should have access to life-saving antiretroviral treatment. Effective strategies to reduce the spread of HIV include provision and promotion of condom use; screening of blood donors; education to reduce unsafe sexual behaviour and promiscuity; treatment of other STDs to reduce HIV transmission.

7 Improve case management for tuberculosis. Tuberculosis is one of the major killers of adults. Treatment is highly cost effective. In TB (as with other e.g. family planning programmes) a public-private partnerships between the national programme coordinate, NGO and private providers is important. In this way involving all providers, promoting adherence and follow-up of treatment.

8 Comprehensive malaria control. There is real potential to eliminate deaths from malaria through comprehensive access to bednets, indoor spraying and effective treatment.

9 Screening for cervical cancer. Cervical cancer is the commonest cancer in developing countries. Although many developing countries have the facilities to undertake the required pathology and surgery, the administration necessary to run an effective screening programme with call-recall of patients is a major barrier even in sophisticated health systems.

10 Relieve cancer pain. Cancer will continue to be a major cause of death and suffering. Palliative care with effective pain relief is simple and cheap, yet most patients in developing countries are neglected. Education of health staff about good care along with greater access to opiate analgesia should be encouraged.

11 Treat diabetes. Diabetes is a serious and under-diagnosed problem in most developing countries. Basic education about diet and foot care is cheap and effective in reducing complications. Also providing long term care involving drug treatment with insulin or oral hypoglycaemic drugs.

12 Vaccinate against hepatitis B. The cost of Hepatitis B vaccine ($3 per jab) is now low enough to be cost-effective to give with other childhood immunization. Other new vaccines such as against pneumococcals are becoming cost effective and can be added to EPI.

Infectious diseases

Infectious diseases will continue to one of the biggest killers, particularly of children and young adults. Most of these deaths will occur in developing countries where poverty, overcrowding, poor housing and sanitation all contribute to breeding grounds for outbreaks and transmission. The leading causes of death and disability from infectious diseases are acute respiratory infections, AIDS, diarrhoeal diseases, TB, and malaria.

New infectious diseases will continue to pose a threat to populations throughout the world. Good surveillance systems are needed to monitor new and changing infectious diseases (Box 17.1).

Investment in the development of diagnostic tools, drugs, and vaccines that can further improve our ability to affordably address the most serious and widespread infectious diseases.

Cheap and effective methods exist to prevent many of these diseases (Box 17.2). The challenge for the future will be to gain the political support necessary to trigger action and provide the administration, training, and skills needed to allow sustainable and effective health service provision. Health programmes to reduce death and disability from these infectious diseases, need to further integrate and help strengthen within the general health services.

Much work remains to be done to promote changes in the day-to-day practice of health workers. They need to use evidence based guidelines such as IMAI, prescribe only the essential drugs, and offer preventive care.

Box 17.1 Priority steps for overcoming the burden of infectious diseases

Political support – particularly money, policies, and multi-sector involvement – is required to overcome the burden of infectious diseases. By mobilizing political support to address the following priorities, much of the death and suffering caused by infectious disease could be prevented.

- ◆ Support for proven, effective, and affordable priority strategies in controlling the most devastating infectious diseases, including:
  - Bednets and treatment strategies for rolling back malaria
  - DOTS the StopTB strategy for stopping TB.
  - Childhood vaccinations against measles and other preventable diseases.
  - IMCI, IMAI, and the 'Pregnancy, childbirth, post-partum and newborn care' – guides for essential practice addressing and common diseases and prevention.
  - HIV prevention strategies such as condom promotion, sex education, STI treatment, male circumcision for reducing the spread of HIV/AIDS.
  - ntibiotics used timely and appropriately for preventing pneumonia.
- ◆ Strengthened health services and delivery systems in developing countries.
- ◆ Intensified efforts to eradicate polio and guinea worm, and eliminate neonatal tetanus, leprosy, lymphatic filariasis, Chagas' disease and onchocerciasis.
- ◆ Expansion of surveillance systems that can alert the world to unexpected outbreaks, the emergence of new diseases and increased drug resistance.

Adapted from WHO – Geneva, Switzerland

Box 17.2 WHO guidelines and training packages

WHO produces guidelines for multi-purpose health workers at the first-level facility. The most widely used of these is the *Integrated Management of Childhood Illness (IMCI)*, greatly improving the management of childhood illnesses at primary level. More recently the *Integrated Management of Adolescent-adult Illness* (IMAI) has been developed. IMAI includes guide-books on acute care (covering the common diseases including STIs), chronic HIV/ART and palliative care. See www.who.int/hiv/pub/imai. *Practical Adult Lung* (PAL) specifically addresses respiratory illnesses in adults. The *Pregnancy, childbirth, post-partum and newborn care: A guide for essential practice* is also available. For these and other WHO guidelines and documents see www.who.int/healthtopics

These clinical care guidelines are very similar in that they are task-oriented, designed in a similar format, the diagnostic process is standardized and symptom-based, and the interventions included are standardized, affordable, and cost-effective. In addition, there is a careful balance between sensitivity (ability of the guide to correctly identify people who are cases) and specificity (ability of the guide to correctly identify people who are not cases). At country level, these guidelines are adapted to suit the epidemiological and operational context.

More importantly there is a need to improve living standards and conditions such as water and sanitation in the urban slums, to reduce the risk of infectious diseases in local populations.

One of the worrying trends of recent years has been the rise in resistance to drugs such as antibiotics, antituberculous therapy, and antimalarials.

Overprescribing, inappropriate prescribing, poor compliance, and lack of drug regulation all contribute to this problem. Better regulation and treatment guidelines (such as Integrated Management of Childhood Illness [IMCI]) are future solutions to reducing drug resistance. New and low-cost drugs are essential if we are to avoid some infectious diseases becoming untreatable, yet less than 10% of research in health is devoted to developing countries and greater priority is needed if solutions are to be found.

While drugs can provide a cure, vaccines provide a method of preventing diseases. New vaccines for diseases such as malaria and HIV/AIDS may offer new opportunities to prevent these serious public health problems. As well as exploring new breakthroughs, it is also important to improve coverage of existing vaccines. While in some African and some Asian countries coverage has fallen as low as 50% of children and here the priority remains to provide vaccination daily as part of an integrated service in all health facilities as well as expand outreach, in order to achieve higher coverage. Even in countries with coverage of more than 80% there are some poor access groups that need to be reached and campaigns to mop up un-vaccinated children may be required. Everywhere there is room for improvement.

Better health services

There is much to be done to improve health services in all countries but particularly in developing countries where major problems prevent the equitable delivery of effective and accessible health services. Some of the solution is through more money, but there is also great scope for improving the effectiveness of health services. Challenges for the future for public health professionals will include:

1 Increasing funding for health services – health budgets in many developing countries have been falling in recent years and this trend must be reversed. While the allocation of resources may be dependent on the wider economic success of the country, all health workers must have more of a role as campaigners and advocates to central governments for greater funding. International advocacy for relief of the debt that currently cripples many developing countries is also vital.

    Donor agencies also have an important role. Around 20% of national health spending in African countries comes from donor agencies. It is essential that such support grows and is invested wisely in sustainable public health programmes

2 Health sector funding – there is great variation in how national health services are funded. Private, whether it be centrally controlled and funded free market private health care holds all the answers in achieving effective health for all. The trend towards new approaches for funding and increased competition, such as separation of purchasers and providers of health care, and the introduction of user charges is likely to continue.

    This trend has in recent years been more due to the pressure of international funding agencies than local need. In recent decades the World Bank has considered public services to be inefficient and even a barrier to the abolition of poverty. This view is, of course, has been supported by the large health industry corporations (insurance, pharmaceutical and service industries) looking for international expansion opportunities. However, international agencies, and the World Bank in particular, have recently been emphasizing to governments the need for more investment in primary health care and education as part of poverty reduction policies.

In recent decades there has been a lot of talk about moving away from large inefficient traditional tertiary care hospitals to supporting good coverage of appropriate primary care service. But there has been little change in resources allocated in government health budgets. This change should become a reality and the hard decisions will need to be made – as have been made by the South African government in limiting hospital budgets, closing hospital wards, and releasing staff and funds to strengthening health centre services. This is essential for improving access for patients to effective treatment. Such primary care must be centred on the patient and the community and provide culturally sensitive services for prevention and care of disease. These primary care centres must be adequately supported by district hospitals providing outreach services and secondary care for the district. However, national governments will maintain core responsibilities in supporting cost effective public health programmes such as immunization, antismoking, condom provision and health education.

3 Tackling the wider determinants of health – clinical health services should be the last resort in tackling disease. Housing, education, employment, environment, all have major roles in causing disease and lifestyle behaviour. Public health professionals of the future will have a much greater role in working with non-health departments and agencies to reduce the root causes of ill health in societies. This new way of working will move away from the narrow focus on health facilities, to develop new partnerships not just with other agencies, but also communities themselves. It is through greater community involvement, ownership and awareness that people will have the confidence to build their own healthy futures.

4 Greater efficiency and effectiveness – there are few health services in the World that can claim to use all their current resources as efficiently as possible, and existing spending should be reviewed to assess value for money. Many current health practices throughout the World owe more to ritual practice than evidence of benefit. As much as 80% of medical interventions are of unproven benefit. Scarce resources should be channelled into treatments that have been shown to be cost-effective in good clinical trials and existing rituals and practices should always be questioned. New technologies such as drugs and scanners also need to be rigorously questioned and appraised before they creep into routine use. Areas such as drug procurement, a major cost for health services, may provide savings of existing resources.

To deal with these issues, better systems for monitoring health trends will be required. Current methods of monitoring diseases and deaths are often bureaucratic, cumbersome and so inaccurate that they provide little information of value. Simple systems to monitor health trends and quality of services (for example access and effectiveness) need to be developed. These systems will allow health gains to be demonstrated and health targets to be established.

The challenge of implementation

The biggest challenge for most health officers and managers is effective implementation *at scale* of PHC and other health services. Over the past decade global funding and activity has focussed especially on MNCH, HIV/AIDS, tuberculosis and malaria. Even for these diseases much still remains to be done – e.g. coverage for HIV prevention interventions is only around 20%. In addition efforts are required to control non-communicable disease (e.g. tobacco control) and provide care for chronic diseases such as diabetes and mental health conditions. There remain many priorities and many possible approaches for effective implementation. These include actions at community, district, national and global levels Box 17.3.

All interventions should be designed so as to be replicable and sustainable with available or realistically attainable human and material resources. Assessment embedded within early district

Box 17.3 Implementation of primary health care services at scale

Community, family and individuals

- Select and support CHWs
- Active participation in community health-promotion activities and development pro-grammes (income generation, water and sanitation)

Health centres, hospitals and practitioners

- Train, supervise, and use packages of care, guidelines, and management methods – e.g. IMCI and IMAI
- Provide outreach activities and links with CHWs and private sector to improve coverage of interventions and strengthen referral
- Support community health promotion
- Plan and budget according to disease burden and related cost-effective packages of care and prevention
- Build CHW, MNCH, and FP delivery, and strengthen referral strategies
- Ensure equitable distribution and quality of health workers

District, sub-district

- Plan and budget according to disease burden and related cost-effective packages of care and prevention
- Build CHW, MNCH, and FP delivery, and strengthen referral strategies
- Ensure equitable distribution and quality of health workers

Nation, state, province

- Integrate health sector plans and use of methods for planning
- Scale-up proven health systems approaches on the basis of evidence
- Coordinate funding with agriculture, food security, climate change, and population policies
- Introduce phased removal of user fees for PHC services

Global

- Prioritize funding by burden of disease, cost-effective interventions, and health systems building over time
- Provide predictable long-term financing for health
- Budget support and sector wide approaches, where good governance allow this approach to donor support
- Increased investment in implementation research for PHC and building local research capacity

Adapted from J Walley, J Lawn and A Tinker et al. Lancet 2008, see Further reading.

implementation can be the basis for refining guidelines and other methods for implementation to ensure effective scale-up nationally and to learn from what works and why, or why not.

Community participation and mobilization approach is important for many interventions, including water, sanitation and HIV prevention. The mobilization of women and other community-based groups in Nepalese villages has been shown to decreases in neonatal and probably maternal mortality. However, the challenge for the community mobilization approach is to effectively replicate it at scale.

Previously, the emphasis has been on rural health services and community mobilization. However, since most of the world's population now live in cities, the need is also to develop primary health facilities and community services for poor people living in urban areas.

Services should be made more equitable, reaching deprived rural and urban areas. Particular attention should be given to women, children, and other disadvantaged and vulnerable groups – such as indigenous people, inmates, elderly people, people with disabilities, refugees and internally displaced populations.

Community health workers (CHW) are an important component of PHC, and provide the link between rural and urban communities with the health services. They need to be on-going training and support by health centre staff. The Pakistan Lady Health Worker Programme provides an example of an effective national CHW programmes. New interventions can be added, e.g. bednet promotion and injectable contraceptives, as in Pakistan. However care should be taken to avoid overloading CHWs with too many tasks. CHWs should be paid. Alternatively they can receive a percentage of the price of health products such as bednets that they promote and sell – as done by CHW of BRAC Bangladesh.

Public, non-governmental, faith-based and private providers need to be linked into a coherent health system under responsible government stewardship. Countries with such frameworks in place are over performing for health outcomes despite major challenges – e.g. Malawi has an essential health package and a national agreement with Christian Health Association of Malawi, which provides 40% of health-care services.

Sufficient numbers of appropriately trained and supported health workers are needed. In addition properly supervised *task-shifting*, from doctors to paramedics and nurses, and from nurses to trained lay health workers is necessary, e.g. for nutrition and HIV counselling. Effective and supportive supervision is the key to improvement of service delivery.

Specialists often do work that could be better managed by general practitioners. Specialist care often restricts access, is inefficient, and fails to provide preventive interventions and health education. Profit-driven care, as in private practice and some public hospitals as in China, leads to unnecessary tests, hospitalization, operations and so higher costs.

Health workers need to give preventive as well as essential curative care. Indeed, better use of existing preventive interventions can reduce the burden of disease by 70% (WHO, 2008).

Good governance has to be fostered and, where it exists, an increased proportion of donor funds should be channelled through budget support and sectorwide approaches as these are more efficient than funding individual health programmes. Furthermore, good governance includes promoting democracy, a free press, tackling corruption, and transparency for the public and private sector finances etc. Also support for civil society organizations and community action, such as for water, nutrition, education and health, as envisioned in PHC.

Future challenges: Mega-problems

The world faces a number of major challenges or mega-problems that will all have a serious impact on health. Global warming is one of the most formidable challenges that the world faces. Human actions are leading to major changes in the world's climate system. The burning of fossil fuels is a major cause of global warming as is excessive population growth with the prediction that the world population will grow to 9 billion people, all consuming goods and carbon-based energy. Risks to health from global warming come from the effects of heat waves, droughts, and famines. The Intergovernmental Panel on Climate Change has warned that the countries that suffer the most from these risks will be the low income countries, and this will further widen global inequalities in health.

Box 17.4 outlines some of the other mega-problems facing the world in the 21st century. All these challenges are multi-national and will require every country to work together to provide solutions. Some of these solutions will be better use of scarce resources (water, fish stocks), some will require political solutions (poverty, health planning) and some will require technological solutions (alternative energy sources).

While these mega-problems may seem daunting, doctors and public health professionals have important roles to play in tackling them. They have particular knowledge and influence both in local communities and wider political networks to promote public awareness about these problems, monitor the impact on health and to develop local, national and international responses. Public health professionals need to be diplomats and champions for promoting change. They need to have passion and advocacy skills to campaign for a healthier global environment as well as campaigning for tobacco bans and cleaner water. A good starting place is by being a good role model and health professionals should act through personal and workplace practices to adopt healthier and greener lifestyles.

Conclusion

There have many problems in recent decades, including insufficient political prioritization of health, structural adjustment policies, poor governance, population growth, inadequate health systems and scarce research on developing country health systems and interventions. The following are priorities for revitalizing PHC and health services in general. Health-service infrastructure, including human resources and essential drugs, needs strengthening; and user fees should be removed for PHC services to improve use. A continuum of care for maternal, neonatal, and child health services, including family planning, is needed. Evidence-based, integrated packages of community and primary curative and preventive care should be adapted to country contexts,

---

Box 17.4 Mega-problems for the 21st century

Global warming – severe climate change leading to droughts, famines, and severe weather events

Population growth – exceeding the capacity of the world to support

Water shortages – rivers and aquifers are drying up leading to shortages for consumption and farming

Loss of fishing stocks – humans have used up over 90% of edible fish in the world's oceans

Shanty cities – the inexorable growth of shanty towns into shanty cities as the home for over 1 billion people, will lead to a vicious cycle of poverty, violence and despair

Spread of deserts – soil erosion and climate change are reducing arable land

Terrorism – extremism and terrorism increase the chances of major nuclear or biological weapons being used

assessed, and scaled up. Community health workers linked to strengthened primary-care facilities and first-referral services should be developed. Community participation and inter-sectoral action linking health and development is necessary, including that for better water, sanitation, nutrition, food security, and HIV control. Non-communicable, chronic diseases, and mental health should be addressed.

Further reading

Disease Control Priorities in a developing world (DCP2). (2006) World Bank/Oxford University Press, 2nd edition. http://www.dcp2.org/page/main/BrowseDiseases.html

Feachem R.G.A., Kjellstrom T., Murray C.J.L., Over M., Phillips M.A. (1992)*The health of adults in the developing world*. World Bank/Oxford University Press.

WHO. (1999) *Removing obstacles to healthy development*. WHO, Geneva.

Walley, J., Lawn J., Tinker A, et al. Primary health care: making Alma-Ata a reality. *Lancet* 2008, **372**, 1001–08.

WHO/IER/CSDH/08.1 Closing the gap in a generation: Health equity through action on the social determinants of health.

WHO. World Health Report 2008. http://www.who.int/whr/2008/en/

Glossary

Absolute Poverty Line The percentage of people in a country whose income is less than a specific cut-off point, such as US$1 per day.

Acceptability The intervention strategy fits within the cultural and social expectations of the community.

Access Living within reasonable distance of health services.

Activity Action to implement a strategy, e.g. doing training, a supervision visit, or ordering supplies.

Adequate coverage Indicator used to monitor and evaluate the progress of health unit activities or services. It is the percentage of the target population receiving the activity or service according to standard guidelines. For example, adequate coverage for prenatal care can be defined as the percentage of pregnant women who made at least three prenatal visits, including one during the last month of pregnancy.

Adverse selection A situation where individuals are able to purchase insurance at rates which are below actuarially fair rates, because information known to them is not available to insurers (see *asymmetric information*).

Advocacy for health A combination of individual and social actions designed to gain political commitment, policy support, social acceptance and systems support for a particular health goal or policy.

Aetiology The causes of disease

Affordability Extent to which the intended clients of a service can pay for it. This will depend on their income distribution, the cost of services and the financing mechanism (e.g. whether risks are pooled; whether exemptions exist for the low-paid etc.).

Allocation (of costs) Deciding how much of different inputs are involved in producing a given output, such as a specific treatment or diagnostic test. The purpose is usually to produce a realistic estimate of the full cost of providing the service, so that managers can identify efficiency improvements and prioritize between services or different delivery strategies.

Ante-natal The period between conception and birth (also called prenatal)

Antibody A protein produced in blood on exposure to an antigen. It binds specifically to the antibody and can lead to its destruction by the immune system.

Antigen A protein that brings about an immune response.

Average cost Average cost equals total cost divided by the quantity of output. Total cost represents the sum of all *fixed costs* and *variable costs.*

Assessment A study of inputs, process, outputs of a project or programme, conducted to measure performance and ascertain readiness and capacity to perform roles and responsibilities or achieve objectives. It is linked to policies and systems under which the programme operates.

Barriers Conditions that prevent people from doing something. For example, lack of time, money, equipment, authority, or supplies might be barriers to doing a job correctly.

Basic Essential Obstetric Care These services include assisted vaginal delivery, manual removal of the placenta and retained products to prevent infection, and administration of antibiotics to treat infection and drugs to prevent or treat bleeding, convulsions and high blood pressure.

Basic Obstetric Care This includes the provision of ante-natal and post-natal care and normal delivery services.

Behaviour Actions and practices by individuals that may affect their health

Bias The deviation of results from the truth, due to the way(s) in which the study is conducted.

Burden of disease (studies) Measurement of premature mortality (deaths) and morbidity (non-fatal illness) in a given area. The aim of the study is usually to define which illnesses or risk factors are most significant in causing death and disability and hence to inform decisions about which services should receive priority. On its own, however, it is inadequate as a decision tool as it omits the issue of effectiveness of prevention or treatment strategies and the cost of implementing them.

Capital costs Expenditure on goods which last longer than one year, such as investment in equipment or infrastructure.

Capitation A method of reimbursement under which a provider is paid a fixed amount per person, regardless of the volume of services rendered.

Carrier A person who is infected but has no symptoms of disease.

Case finding Screening a group of people who have certain risk factors; for example, people with cough more than 2–3 weeks screened with sputum microscopy to detect TB or growth monitoring young children to detect growth faltering (low weight for age).

Case-mix A measure of the assortment of patient cases treated by a given hospital, indicating the degree of complexity of the cases.

Chemoprophylaxis Drug treatment designed to prevent future occurrences of disease.

Cochrane Collaboration This is an international endeavour in which people from many different countries systematically find, appraise and review available evidence from RCTs. The Collaboration aims to develop and maintain systematic, up-to-date reviews of RCTs of all forms of health care and to make this information readily available to clinicians and other decision-makers at all levels of health care systems.

Cohort A group in the community that share some features, e.g. women giving birth in a particular year.

Cohort study Study of a cohort of people over time used to determine incidence and causes of disease – also called a longitudinal study.

Community based distribution A delivery implementation strategy which involves community groups and CHW in promoting and supplying health products such as contraceptives.

Community based distributors Community members chosen and trained to distribute a health product such as contraceptive pills, condoms or supply malaria treatment to children with fever.

Community financing A wide variety of risk pooling and prepayment schemes introduced in developing countries to fill in gaps in the financing of health care. See also *Bamako Initiative*.

Comprehensive essential obstetric care This encompasses basic essential obstetric care, and the ability to perform surgery (Caesarean section under anaesthesia), to manage obstructed labour and to provide safe blood transfusion to respond to haemorrhages.

Compulsory health insurance Health insurance under an obligatory public scheme. Payment for such an insurance amounts to a tax. Employers may have to pay contributions on behalf of their employees. Contributions are usually income-related. CHI is usually, but not always, administered by a public body.

Contract A legal agreement between purchaser and provider, usually specifying which services are to be provided, at what cost and with what minimum quality. See also *performance contracts, block contracts, cost and volume contracts,* and *cost per case contracts.*

Contracting out The process by which work which was previously carried out by public sector employees is shifted to the private sector, but with the state continuing to finance it and to lay down specifications about the type, quantity and quality of the service being provided. Commonly it is the non-clinical services which are easiest to contract out, but clinical contracts are becoming more common too.

Copayment Amounts paid by the insurance beneficiary as a result of *coinsurance* and *deductibles.*

Cost minimization study This assumes that two strategies or interventions achieve exactly the same effect. The study therefore focuses on costing each option in order to find out which one is the least costly. This will identify the most desirable option, assuming that important alternatives have not been omitted and that the benefits are indeed identical.

Cost-benefit analysis (CBA) A method of comparing the monetary value of all benefits of a project with all costs of that project.

Cost-utility analysis (CUA) A method of comparing the costs of a social project with the benefits, measured in terms of an overall index of both quantity and quality of life gained (see, for example, *QALYs*). This avoids the need to convert social benefits into monetary terms, but at the same time allows for comparisons between programmes with differing social objectives. However, collecting reliable information on changes to quality of life is relatively difficult.

Coverage (rates) The proportion of the estimated target population which has been reached. These are often used in relation to preventive programmes, where target populations can be more easily estimated.

Cross-sectional study Study of a section of the community at a specific point in time – used to determine prevalence.

Crude Birth Rate (CBR) This is the number of live births per 1000 total population per year. The denominator includes men, children and women.

Crude Death Rate (CDR) This is the number of deaths occurring per 1000 total population year.

Culture Behaviours, beliefs and values that are shared by the whole community or by a small section (sub-culture). They may have been recently acquired or traditions that have been held for a long time.

Debt Servicing The total of repayments plus interest paid in goods, services or foreign currency on debts to the international creditors such as the International Monetary Fund or rich country governments and banks.

Decentralization Shift of power and/or of functions from the centre to the local level, however defined. This policy, which can have many different motivations and forms, is commonly thought to increase the effectiveness and accountability of services.

Delivery strategy The means to achieve high coverage of an intervention (for the relevant target group), e.g. social marketing of bednets.

Demand The quantity of a good purchased at any given price.

Diagnosis-related Groups (DRGs) A set of case types established under the *prospective payment system*, identifying patients with similar conditions and processes of care. Used for setting charges for different health care interventions.

Direct costs This term is used slightly differently in different contexts. In allocating costs in hospitals, direct costs are the costs which are incurred by patient departments (producing final outcomes), as opposed to the paraclinic, support and overhead departments (which produce intermediary goods). In evaluations, however, the distinction is being made between costs which are actually paid by the health service or patients, as opposed to the *opportunity costs* of time and production lost as a result of treatment (termed *indirect costs*), which are also real but are often omitted from consideration.

Disability-adjusted life year (DALY) Concept developed by the World Bank and WHO to measure the burden of disease, in terms of both premature death and disability. With adequate data, it can be used to compare potential health gain from different disease control programmes and thus to prioritize resource allocation according to cost effectiveness principles.

Discounting/Discount rate The process of converting sums to be received at a future date to a present value. The interest rate which is used is called the discount rate.

Drop-out rate A comparison of the number of children or women who start receiving immunization and the number who do not receive later doses for full immunization.

Economic evaluation Systematic comparison of all relevant costs and benefits of a programme to inform decision-making and maximize technical and allocative efficiency.

Economics The study of how a society with limited resources decides what goods to produce, how to produce them, and how to distribute them among its members.

Effectiveness The degree to which desired outcomes are achieved.

Efficiency The maximum possible sustained output from a given set of inputs this is known as technical efficiency. By contrast, allocative efficiency is used to describe a situation in which either inputs or outputs are put to their best possible uses.

Elimination The reduction of the global prevalence to a negligible amount, as is being attempted for leprosy. Or it is the reduction of an infectious disease's prevalence in the population of a global region to zero; and this has occurred or is underway in malaria, lymphatic filariasis, measles, mumps and rubella, onchocerciasis and yaws.

Empowerment The process through which individuals or communities gain greater control over decisions and actions affecting their health.

Endemic A disease which is continually present in a community.

Epidemic A rapid increase in the levels of a disease

Epidemiology Study of the health and disease in the community and the application of this information to promote health. Descriptive epidemiology is concerned with measurement of health and disease and analytical epidemiology is concerned with determination of risk factors and cause of disease

Equity Access to health care and resources according to needs without discrimination by gender, income, religion and race.

Eradication The reduction of an infectious disease's prevalence in the global human population to zero. Smallpox has been eradicated, and is underway with Polio and Dracunculiasis (guinea worm).

Essential (or basic) package Given the shortage of resources for health in developing countries and the high burden of disease, it suggested that public funds be concentrated on a defined range of highly cost-effective services. These are often called 'essential packages'.

Essential drugs Those drugs that satisfy the health care needs of the majority of the population; they should therefore be available at all times in adequate amounts and in the appropriate dosage forms.

Evaluation The process of determining whether progress has been made toward reaching objectives set in a work-plan, identifying problems or bottlenecks and corrective actions to take.

Externality A case in which someone affects the utility (costs) of another person, through actions which lie outside the price system. In public health a positive externality is present for example when treating a TB patient not only cures sick person but as well reduces transmission to others.

Feedback Information provided by others on the way a person is acting or is doing something.

Fee-for-service (FFS) A method of payment under which the provider is paid for each procedure or service that is provided to a patient.

Fixed budget Budget which is set in advance for a period. Traditionally health budgets were based on historical precedent and were not only fixed in total but also in their internal breakdown by line item. This is likely to lead to inequity and technical inefficiency.

Fixed costs Costs which do not vary with output. They are expressed either as total fixed cost (TFC) or average fixed cost (AFC).

Fortification Is adding a micronutrient(s) into foods consumed by the majority of the population. For example, legislation and monitoring of iodine addition to salt to prevent cretinism, or vitamin A in sugar to prevent blindness.

GATS Agreement The general agreement on trade in services. This agreement of the World Trade Organization was made in 1995. It seeks to liberalize international trade in services, including health care.

Gross Domestic Product (GDP) The total output of goods and services for final use produced by an economy.

Gross National Product (GNP) GDP plus net income from abroad (for example, profits from its multinationals and money being sent back from residents from overseas) minus payments made to foreign firms and workers in the domestic economy.

General Fertility Rate (GFR) This is the number of live births per 1000 women of child-bearing age (between the ages of 15–44) per year.

Goal The broad aim of a programme addressed to a particular health status or health problem.

Health A state of complete physical, social, and mental well-being (World Health Organization constitution, 1947).

Health behaviour Any activity undertaken by an individual for the purpose of promoting, protecting or maintaining their health.

Health centre A primary level health facility which provides outpatient basic clinical and preventive services to people within its catchment area. It may have a few observation and maternity beds, but does not have an operating theatre or general inpatient services. Other names include a health post, (a small health centre) a dispensary, clinic or polyclinic.

Health economics The study of the value of health and how it can be produced most efficiently and distributed to maximize social welfare.

Health education The communication/educational component of health promotion defined by Lawrence Green (1981) as 'Any combination of learning experiences designed to promote voluntary adaptation of behaviour conducive to health'.

Health literacy The cognitive and social skills that are required to gain access to, understand and make use of information in ways which promote and maintain good health.

Health needs assessment Methods for describing ill-health in local communities and defining what people want and need out of the local health services.

Health promotion The process of enabling people to increase control over, and to improve their health (Ottawa Charter, 1986), see above for health education.

Health sector reform A substantial change to the structure or processes of health services, with the intention of improving outcomes.

Home-based care When ill patients, such as people with AIDS, are cared for at home by family carers with support by visiting community volunteers and/or nurses, who may refer them to clinic-based services when required.

Home-based lifesaving skills These are a set of behaviour-change interventions that promote increased knowledge and the acquisition of skills to keep a pregnant woman healthy, to recognize life-threatening maternal and newborn problems and/or complications, and to foster the adoption of health care and health-seeking behaviours at the individual and community levels, to prevent maternal and neonatal deaths.

Horizontal integration Providing clinical and personal preventive interventions at the same place and time so as to avoid missed opportunities for prevention.

Human Development Index (HDI) This index, created by the United Nations Development Programme, ranks all countries according to indicators of wealth (GDP per capita), health (life expectancy) and education (literacy), producing a ranking of development. This is updated each year.

Immunity   A state in which a host is not susceptible to infection or disease they contact.

Implementation   The act of actually undertaking an intended and planned course of action.

Incidence   The number of new cases of a disease in a specified period of time per total population.

Indicator   A measure of progress towards objectives (e.g. impact on mortality or morbidity), strategies (e.g. coverage of vaccination) or activities (numbers of health workers trained).

Indirect costs   Distinguished from *direct costs* and *intangible costs*. **The** opportunity costs **of work, house work or child care.**

Infant Mortality Rate (IMR)   This is the number of infants (children less than 1 year old) who die during a stated year per 1000 live births.

Informal payments   Payments which are not officially set by health providers. These take many forms. They may be money or goods. They may be voluntary or compulsory (i.e. treatment is withheld if they are not paid).

Inputs   The resources used in a programme, such as manpower, money and materials.

International Monetary Fund (IMF)   An international organization set up by governments to monitor and smooth financial exchanges on a global scale. Interventions by the IMF to help countries in difficulty are usually associated with rigorous criteria for financial solvency, including reductions in government spending and encouraging exports. For more information, see 'Structural Adjustment Explained' in the previous elective guide.

Implementation Strategy   Means the same as delivery strategy (or service delivery approach) which is the way to achieve high coverage of an intervention strategy such as ITN. For example the social marketing (of bednets or condoms).

Insurance   Pooling risks with others in order to spread costs of health care (or other commodity) over time and protect against catastrophically expensive illness.

Integrated programme   A programme, such as EPI, which is organized and managed (mainly) within the general health services and management system (c.f. vertical programme).

Intersectoral collaboration   Action in which the health sector and other related sectors (agriculture, education, water and sanitation) work together to achieve a common objective. When an inter-sectoral approach is used, causes of problems are likely to be explored in a more comprehensive way and solutions of problems are likely to be more effective.

Intervention strategies   Intervention strategies (or interventions) are the means to control disease. They are the solutions to health problems. Examples include vaccination, health promotion (e.g. by condom promotion), impregnated bed nets and oral rehydration for diarrhoea.

Legislation (regulation)   Laws controlling personal or companies behaviour so as to improve the lives of the public. In health, for example, laws limiting pollution, tobacco advertising, drinking and driving or making the use of seat belts compulsory.

Life expectancy   Longevity, the average length of life of individuals in a population. In poor communities life expectancy at birth is mainly a reflection of infant and child mortality.

Life expectancy at birth   This is the average number of years that a newborn is expected to live if current mortality rates continue to apply.

Life style   All the behaviours, actions and routines that make up the pattern of living of individuals, families and communities. It includes diet, exercise, work, leisure, housework, caring for family members and use of health services.

Living conditions   The everyday environment of people where they live, play and work. These may be under the control of individuals. However, they are often a result of social, economic and environmental that are outside their control.

Longitudinal study see cohort study. If individuals are followed, this is a study taking place over time.

Marginal cost The increase in total cost resulting from a one unit increase in output. Public health example: the (relatively small) example; increase in cost when a further intervention is added to an existing service; e.g. the cost of hepatitis B vaccine added to the existing cost of the expanding programme of immunization (as the staff, fridges and vehicles etc. are already paid for.)

Mass treatment Giving a (safe) drug to all those at risk, e.g. giving prazequantel to school children in an areas with a high prevalence of schistosomiasis or helminths. Also called mass drug administration (MDA).

Maternal mortality ratio This is the number of maternal deaths per 100 000 live births on an annual basis.

Meta-analysis A statistical technique which summarizes the results of several studies into a single estimate, giving more weight to results from larger studies.

Micronutrients Vitamins such as vitamin A or folic acid, or minerals such as iodine or iron which are essential for health.

Milestone Recognizable achievement toward the accomplishment of an activity.

Millennium Development Goals These were agreed by the United Nations in September 2000. They set targets in poverty, education, access to clean water and sanitation, child mortality, maternal health, HIV/AIDS and other infectious diseases and the environment.

Missed opportunities A missed opportunity for prevention is when preventive interventions such as vaccination, vitamin A capsules and family planning services, are not offered to, for example, a mother attending with a sick child.

Molluscicides Chemical substances which kill snails or other molluscs and used for control of schistosomiasis

Monitoring The process of collecting and analysing information on a regular basis to measure progress of activities.

Non-governmental Organization (NGO) Are private not for profit organizations, just NGO as mission hospitals and health charities e.g. same the children fund(UK)

Objective What you are trying to achieve (and by when) as a result of implementing interventions. An objective should be realistic and measurable.

Odds ratio A comparison of the presence of a risk factor for disease in a sample of diseased subjects and non diseased controls.

Outcome What result has been achieved? In programme implementation what happens as a result of an intervention or activity. The term outcomes may also be used in terms of health status, i.e. morbidity and mortality (but this is more specifically referred to as 'impact').

Outputs A measure of processes conducted in order to achieve better health, e.g. health workers trained, children vaccinated etc.

Pandemic An epidemic spread over many countries, e.g. the AIDS pandemic.

Parasite A disease causing organism – the term is often used for protozoa infections e.g. the malaria parasite.

Passive immunity Immunity which has been acquired through the transfer of maternal or other antibodies.

Pathogen Any organisms which causes disease, e.g. bacteria, virus, protozoa, helminth or prion.

Pathogenicity The degree to which a pathogen causes illness in its host.

Payment systems Way in which medical institutions or staff are paid for their work. These will set certain incentives and encourage certain patterns of health care provision. The most common types are: *Salaries, fee for service, capitation, fixed budgets* and *contracts.*

Performance Level of fulfilment of operational capacity of a programme or person.

Performance measures These can be applied to institutions or individuals. For example, how well is one hospital doing, compared with another? How well is a doctor working, compared with his or her colleagues? These questions call for agreement on what the priorities are. For example, these priorities could be either cost-cutting (a low ratio of inputs to outputs) or through quality of care. In terms of outcomes, is the goal to have low rates of failure, or do you want to maximize health gain? It is a challenge to agree priorities and avoid *perverse incentives* in setting up performance measures.

Perinatal Between the 28th week of pregnancy and the end of the first week of life.

Perinatal Mortality Rate (PMR) This is the number of stillbirths (deaths after the 28th week of pregnancy) plus the number of deaths in the first 7 days after birth, in a stated year per 1000 total births (live births plus stillbirths).

Perverse incentives Where your system of rewards unintentionally encourages behaviour of an undesirable kind (e.g. paying according to the number of patients seen. Its aim may be to increase staff productivity. One result will almost certainly be lower quality treatment for patients.)

Placebo therapy – An inactive treatment often given to controls in trials. The *placebo* is delivered in a form which is apparently identical to the active treatment being tested in the trial, in order to eliminate psychological effects on the outcome.

Plan of action A document defining activities for generating result/product under a specific programme; it defines who does what, when, how and for how much.

Population A group of people sharing a common geographical (e.g. district) boundary or the same age or sex group (children under one year, women of child bearing age) or health risk group (e.g. tobacco smokers).

Post-natal After childbirth up to the end of the first year.

Premium Payment for voluntary insurance. These may be community-rated (averaged across a group of individuals) or risk-rated (tailored to the claims experience or actuarial risk of each individual).

Pre-natal The care before delivery, an alternative word is ante-natal care.

Prevalence The number of people with a disease per total population. This can be at a point in time (point prevalence) or over a defined period (period prevalence).

Primary Health Care The first tier of health care based at the community level defined in the Alma-Ata Declaration of 1978 as 'essential health care made accessible at a cost a country and community can afford, with methods that are practical, scientifically sound and socially acceptable.

Primary level First point of contact, e.g. health centre, services. The primary level may be used to mean both the community and primary level services.

Primary prevention Stopping disease from occurring, e.g. by vaccination or behaviour change (e.g. interventions against tobacco).

Prioritize Putting things in a specific order according to certain reasons. For example, ranking problems according to their seriousness, frequency and concerns for the community.

Priority setting Deciding the relative importance attached to alternative goals or activities in a given setting. It is often connected with resource shortages and the need to *ration* care.

Private sector Usually refers to organizations which are not managed by the state. Covers a wide spectrum of profit and not-for-profit organizations;(see also NGO); formal and informal; competing with public facilities for customers or complementary etc.

Privatization The process of transfer of facilities from public to private management, e.g. by contracting out of catering in a hospital. However in developing country the changes are more passive and bottom-up. Constrained supply and poor quality often leads consumers to turn to the private providers, who may be public health workers moonlighting, drug sellers, traditional healers, mission hospitals or private clinics.

Programme A systematically designed set of interventions and delivery strategies which will achieve high risk group coverage. e.g. the expanded programme of immunization (EPI) includes protocols for child vaccination, modules for training, cold chain equipment and delivery (strategies) through static and outreach health services.

Progress Stage reached towards achievement of an objective or goal.

Project See programme, but time limited.

Promotion See health promotion.

Protocol A step by step description of how something is done, in care may also be called a case management guideline.

Provider An organization which provides health care, such as a primary care doctor or a hospital, and sells its services to purchasers.

Public Health Medicine The science and art of promoting health, preventing disease, and prolonging life through the organized efforts of society.

Purchasing Power Parity (PPP) This allows us to compare international incomes in real terms by adjusting for differences in the costs of goods and services between countries.

QALY Quality-adjusted life year – a measure of health gain which aims to measure life years added but also the quality of life which is achieved in those years. This is one measure used in *cost-utility analysis*. Another is the *DALY* – a narrower definition, but easier to measure.

Quality of care Various process of care factors, more competent staff, consultation time, less waiting time, privacy etc.

Randomized controlled trial (RCT) A trial in which subjects are randomly assigned to two groups: one (the experimental group) receiving the intervention that is being tested, and the other (the comparison group or controls) receiving an alternative treatment. The two groups are then followed up to see if any differences between them result. This helps people assess the effectiveness of the intervention.

Rationing Restricting supply of services according to implicit or explicit criteria, where demand exceeds supply.

Recurrent expenditure Expenditure which has to be incurred during each budget period (usually a year), such as on salaries, drugs, supplies, provision and maintenance.

Referral A patient is referred (sent with a note) for care from one level of the health system to another level. For example a health centre refers to a hospital to diagnose and commence treatment; the hospital then gives the patient a card with the details to take to the health centre for the continuing (follow-up) care.

Referral system The communication, training and supervisory etc. processes which make possible effective referrals and continuity of care.

Regulation Government intervention in the functioning of markets. Such as rules, backed by legal sanctions (may be used more broadly to include economic signals such as subsidies, taxes and incentives).

Replicable The intervention or project can be successfully implemented in other areas.

Resource allocation The system by which recurrent funds (and sometimes staff) are divided between different geographical regions or different programmes. Some kind of population-based formula is preferable to infrastructure-led spending, which tends to perpetuate inequity.

Resources Manpower, money and materials.

Review The study of the situation, including the relevant epidemiology, policies, implementation etc. see also situation analysis, health needs assessment.

Risk behaviour   Specific forms of behaviour which are proven to be associated with increased susceptibility to specific diseases or ill health.

Risk factor   Social, economic or biological status, behaviours or environments which are associated with or cause increased susceptibility to a specific disease, ill health or injury.

Risk ratio   (Odds Ratio or Relative Risk) is one measure of a treatment's clinical effectiveness. If it is equal to 1, then the effects of the treatment are no different from those of the control treatment. If the OR is greater (or lesser than 1, then the effects of the treatment are more (or less) than those of the control treatment. Note that the effects being measured may be adverse (e.g. death, disability) or desirable (e.g. stopping smoking).

Screening   Strategy for detecting a disease in people without symptoms of that disease. That is, screening tests are performed on those without any clinical indication of disease, with the aim of earlier intervention. But there is a risk of misdiagnosis, so the test should be one with a good sensitivity and specificity (especially so if the disease has a low prevalence).

Secondary level   The first referral level hospitals, e.g. district hospital.

Secondary prevention   Identifying disease before it is causing symptoms (screening) or identifying symptomatic disease at an early stage and curing it (treatment).

Sector-wide approaches (SWAPs)   A particular method of collecting and distributing aid money from donors. Rather than funds being earmarked for a specific project, the money is distributed across the whole sector. In this way funds for the health sector, for example, are pooled and the Ministry of Health sets priorities for spending.

Self help   Actions by members of the community to mobilize the necessary resources to promote, maintain or restore their health.

Sensitivity   The ability of a test to detect people who have the disease or are infected.

Service delivery approach   Means the same as Implementation strategy which is the way to achieve high coverage of an intervention strategy such as ITN. For example the social marketing (of ITNs).

Social marketing   The promotion and sale of a socially useful product such as condoms, using methods developed for the marketing of commercial products, such as coca cola; including developing attractive text, pictures, packaging, posters and wide distribution through shops and vendors.

Social mobilisation   A health promotion strategy including the orientation of community leaders, religious leaders, teachers etc. on health issues, who then pass on the key messages to the community/general public.

Specificity   The ability of a test to detect people who do not have the infection.

STD   Sexually transmitted disease also called sexually transmitted infections (STI).

Strategy   The solution to a problem. This may be an intervention (e.g. bed nets as a means to interrupt man-mosquito contact) or a delivery strategy e.g. social marketing as a means to promote and distribute bed nets.

Structural Adjustment Policies (SAPs)   Policies implemented by the World Bank and the International Monetary Fund in the 1980s and 90s. Developing countries' governments made changes to national economic and social policy in order to qualify for debt relief and rescheduling of payments. For more information, see 'structural Adjustment Explained' in the previous pack.

Subsidy   The opposite of a tax: the government funds a portion of the costs of a good. This will benefit producers and/or consumers, depending on how competitive the market is.

Supervision   Working with health workers to help them adapt what they have learnt (e.g. during training) to do a better job. Supervision should be supportive, that is, not threatening, but building peoples confidence.

Sustainability The ability to maintain a system over time, at a reasonable level of operation and using the resources that are likely to be available. Sustainability has various dimensions, including financial, institutional, and social.

Symptom A condition of the body in an individual when suffering from a disease.

Systematic reviews – a scientific method of reviewing published evidence that reduces the bias of traditional reviews.

Target A quantified level of a specific objective to be reached within a given time frame.

Target payments Payments which are made to health care providers once they have exceeded a specified coverage level (e.g. for ante-natal check-ups or other preventive programmes).

Task Something that must be done to carry out an activity, e.g. to arrange a venue for a training course.

Tertiary level The provincial, national and specialist hospitals.

Tertiary prevention Avoiding further complications of an established disease, such as surgery or rehabilitation for paralysis following polio or strokes.

Total fertility rate (TFR) The number of children an average woman would have assuming that she lives her full reproductive lifetime.

TRIPS Agreement The Trade-Related Aspects of Intellectual Property Rights Agreement. This is an agreement on intellectual property rights establishing a standard set of global rules for each of the member states in intellectual property (including drug patents).

User charges Direct payment for services by patients, though not necessarily covering the full costs of that service. These are often introduced to supplement public finance for health services which used to be free. Charges can be officially sanctioned and their levels controlled, but commonly they develop informally and vary between facilities and even members of staff. (See also *informal payments*).

Utilization The percentage of the (relevant) population using the activity or service, e.g. the number of consultations per person (within the catchment area) per year. Utilization reflects the acceptability and affordability of services.

Vaccine A substance intended to induce active immunity against a pathogen.

Validity Refers to the soundness or rigour of a study. A study is valid if the way it is designed and carried out means that the results are unbiased – that is, it gives you a 'true' estimate of clinical effectiveness.

Variable Costs Costs associated with factor(s) of production which change in quantity according to the quantity of output. Often expressed as a total variable cost (TVC) or average variable cost (AVC).

Vector Anything which transmits disease.

Vertical equity The (Aristotelian) principle that those with differing ability to pay for services will contribute different amounts, and similarly that those with different needs will be treated differently. This complements the principle of *horizontal equity*, but is harder to interpret in practice.

Vertical integration The integration of the community, primary and secondary services (see also referral system).

Vertical programme A programme which is organized and managed (mainly) separately from the general health services, e.g. that the staff have different pay, per diem and/or reporting supervision, and planning systems (c.f. integrated programme).

Virulence The case mortality rate of an infection.

Voluntary health insurance Health insurance which is taken up and paid for at the discretion of individuals (whether directly or via their employers). It can be offered by a public or private company.

Weighted capitation Sum of money provided for the services to each resident in a particular locality. The three main factors commonly reflected in the formula are: age structure of the population, its morbidity, and the relative cost of providing services.

World Bank A group of international financial institutions, with its member states as shareholders. The largest shareholder is the USA. The mission of the World Bank is to make grants and loans to improve global economic growth and contribute to a stable world economy.

World Health Organization (WHO) The United Nations specialized agency for health, governed by the United Nations member states through the annual world assembly. Its activities include the setting of global norms and standards in health and stimulating research and development into health issues of international importance.

World Trade Organization A global organization which works to regulate the international trade between member countries.

Further reading

Last J.M. (1988) *A dictionary of epidemiology*, Oxford University Press.

Swinton J. (1998, 1999) *A dictionary of (ecological) epidemiology*, University of Cambridge.

WHO (1984) *Glossary of terms used in health for all*. World Health Organization, Geneva.

WHO (1998) *Health promotion glossary*. World Health Organization, Geneva.

Wikipedia. www.wikipedia.org

Index

Note: page numbers in *italics* refer to Figures and Tables.

abortion 187, 192
   access to 15
acceptability of interventions 2, 126
access to health services 2, 15
access to medicines 218, 233
   medicine procurement 219–20, 221
   storage and distribution 220
action plans 62–3
active surveillance 247
adult ill health, trends 321
adverse events 312–13
   error reduction 313–14
advocacy 130, 299
   framework agreement for tobacco control 131
   global 305
   use of mass media 133
Aedes egyptii 283
age differences 5, *28*
agenda-setting 133
aid 200
   donation of medicines 221
   see also donor financing
aid coordination 91
aims 68
air pollution 15
alcohol consumption 17
   effect of taxation 298
allocating costs 95
Alma Ata declaration 139–40, 143, 170, 302–3, 323
ampicillin, side effects 249
analytical epidemiology 22
anecdotal observations 32
Anopheles mosquitoes 277–8
ante-natal care 188
   service delivery *60*, *61*
antibiotics 248–50
   inappropriate use 225
   TB treatment 268
antimalarials 251
   counterfeit and substandard products 232
   during pregnancy 283
antimicrobial resistance 213, 224, 249–50, 325
   TB 268
antiretroviral treatment 276
appropriateness of health services 3
artemisinin combination therapy (ACT), malaria 279
audit, clinical 311–12
audit cycle *312*

babies *see* maternal, neonatal, and child health
      (MNCH); neonatal care
bacteria 243
Bangladesh Women's Coalition 208
BCG vaccination 18, 261, 267

bednets 280–1
   delivery strategies *60*, 111
behaviours
   determinants 158
   influence on health 121, 122
beliefs 121–2
   about communicable diseases 240–1
BenCost 96
benefits packages, insurance schemes 92
bilateral aid organizations 142
biological control, mosquitoes 282
birth attendants 189
   training 192
blood transfusion
   infection control 273
   transmission of infections 272–3, 278
body mapping 45
booth distribution, MDA 60
breast-feeding 274
   health promotion strategies *118*
   HIV transmission 273
   protective effects 242
budgets 63–4, 69–70, 95
   flexibility 56
built environment, improvement 299
'but why' method 52, *53*

campaigns, MDA 60
cancer, palliative care 325
capital costs 95
capitation payments *108*, 323
cardiovascular diseases
   epidemiologic transition *293*
   mortality *288*
   prevention 295–6, 302
case control studies 22
case definition 22–3, 247
   HIV infection 272
case finding 14
   in TB 25–6
case management guidelines 167–9, 175
case note reviews 42
catastrophic costs 93
'catch-up', EPI 198
causes of death *289*
causes of disease, children 184
cervical cancer screening 324
chairing meetings 79
chappati diagrams 45
chemoprophylaxis 251
   in HIV infection 276
   of malaria 283
   of TB 269
childbirth 189–90

child health indicators 39
child health programmes 17, 324
   see also Integrated Management of Childhood Illness
      (IMCI); maternal, neonatal, and child health
      (MNCH)
childhood obesity, China *295*
child labour, social mobilization project 130
children
   causes of disease 184
   causes of under 5 mortality *183, 184*
   frequency of presenting complaints *182*
child-to-child programme 201, 203
China
   epidemiological transition 295
   impact of health reforms 235–6
   salt intake reduction 300
chloroquine, counterfeit and substandard
      products 232
chronic disease management models 303–*4*
chronic diseases 18–19
   building blocks of care 307
   integrated care 166–7
   see also non-communicable diseases
classification of communicable diseases 259–60
cleanable surfaces 253
climate change 15–16, 144, 205–6, 330, 331
clinical audit 311–12
clinical diagnosis *36*
clinical services 12, 17–19
clinical trials 22
   randomized controlled trials 32–3
clinic records *82*
cluster samples 31
cMYP 96
Cochrane Collaboration 34
coded results, surveys 31
cohort studies 22
collaboration 78
commercial farms, Zimbabwe, community
      appraisals 43
commercial pressures *120*
communicable diseases 17–18, 239
   changes over time 241
   control *240*
      antibiotics 248–50
      chemoprophylaxis 251
      hygiene promotion 263–4
      immunization 250–1
      legislation 254
      mass drug administration 264–5
      multiple interventions 265–6
      sanitation 264
      vector control 253–4
      water provision 262–3
   education 252–3
   epidemiology 248
   future trends 321, 325
   host factors 241–3
   infecting dose 243–4
   insect-borne 277, 283
   integrated services 284
   invading organisms 243
   laboratory diagnosis 248
   local beliefs 240–1

natural history 244
nosocomial infection 244–6
outbreak management 255–7
   objectives 255
priorities 326
respiratory infections 266, 270
sexually transmitted infections (STIs) 270–1
spread 241
stigma 241
surveillance 246–8
time scales 244
transmission based classification 259–62
treatment 248
see also HIV/AIDS; malaria; tuberculosis (TB)
communication 84, 126–7, 129, 169
   advocacy 130–1
   effective 136
   GATHER approach 134
   methods 132–5
   support materials 135–6
communication channels 124–5
communication skills 76
communities
   background information 124
   involvement in decision-making 151
   role in IMCI 196–7
community action 122
community appraisals 40–1
   commercial farms, Zimbabwe 43
   key informants 44
   meningitis 45
   methods 42, 44
   steps 42
   training 42–3
   visually based methods 45
community-based programmes
   bednet provision and maintenance 61
   family planning services 208–9
   prevention of non-communicable diseases 300
community care 157–9
community-delivered treatment 14
   malaria 280
community development 129
community diagnosis *36*
community-directed treatment 60, 254, 264–5
community gathering areas, MDA 60
community health promotion 134–5
community health workers (CHWs) 158–9, 328, 330
   bednet maintenance *60*
   in-service training 175–6
community involvement 9, 78, 170–1, 328
community mapping 45
community views 119
compliance behaviours 122
comprehensive care 166
computer use 316
conditional cash transfers 94
condoms 275
   social marketing 209
consultants, in international support 141–2
contact tracing 241
   TB 269
continuing professional development 173
continuity of care 166, 303

contraceptive methods 206–7
contracting mechanisms 146
contracting out of services 112
control groups 32
control of infection teams 246
Cooperative Medical System, China 235
coordination of activities 77
co-payments 224
CorePlus 96
cost-benefit analysis (CBA) 98
cost-effectiveness analysis (CEA) 97
cost-effectiveness of interventions 19, 47, 56–7
cost-effectiveness ratio (CER) 98
costing services 94–5, 97
  web-based resources 96
cost-minimization 97
cost-recovery schemes 224
costs 69–70
cost utility analysis (CUA) 98
counseling
  on contraceptive methods 207, 208
  on HIV 275
'Countdown to 2015' report, MNCH 185, *186*
counterfeit medicines 232
coverage charts 28–30, *29*
coverage gap, MNCH 182
coverage of health facilities 3
crude birth rate (CBR) *24*
crude death rate (CDR) *24*
crude rates 23
cultural factors, in health promotion 121–3
cultural problems 46
cumulative coverage charts 28–30, *29*

DALYs (disability-adjusted life years) 4, 98, 182
DALYs pie *322*
data collection and handling 83–4
data sources 38–9
DDT 282
death certification, as source of data 38
decentralization 148–*9*, 169–70
decision-making skills 76
delegation 77
demographic transition 7, *8*, 204–5, 319–21
dengue 283
depression 289, 291
  future trends 322
description of disease 27–8
descriptive epidemiology 21
deserts, spreading 331
determinants of disease 5–9, *6*
development loans 224
devolution 148, *149*
diabetes 290, 325
  primary prevention 301
  secondary prevention 302
diagnosis, communicable diseases 248
Diagnosis-Related Groups (DRGs) 108
diarrhoea
  prevention 11
  rational use of medicines 230
  as side effect of antibiotics 249
diet
  effect of food subsidies 298

impact of globalization 292–3
  role in non-communicable diseases 291–2
  see also nutrition
diphtheria, return to Eastern Europe *240*
directly observed treatment (DOT), TB 268
disabilities 304
disasters, health needs assessment 44–6
discounting 98
disease burden 4–*5*
  broad patterns *7*
  future trends 319–22
  leading causes *8*
  MNCH 182–5
disease description 27–8
disease notification, as source of data 38
disease rates 23
distribution of medicines 220
district health systems 156
  civil society participation 170–1
  community care 157–9
  community health workers 158–9
  district health team (DHT) 156–7
  health facilities, role definition 162–6
  in-service training 173–7
  integration of care 166–7, 168
  management 169–70
  management support systems 171–3
  organizational values 177–9
  primary care 159–61
  referral system 167–9
  secondary care 161–2
district hospitals 161–2
  Hlabisa hospital, South Africa 163–4
  role 164–6, *165*
district management teams 150–1
doctors, supervisory work 174–5
donation of medicines 221
donor financing 224, 323, 327
  of non-communicable disease centres 306
DOTS programme, TB 81, 268, 303
double burden of disease 290
draft activities 61–3
drainage, malaria control 282
drug misuse 17
drugs *see* medicines
drug stores *219*

economic evaluation 97–9
  web-based resources 96
education
  health promotion 126–7, 129–35
  HIV 274–5
  patients with chronic conditions 18–19, 303
  in rational medicine use 228–30
  role in communicable disease control 252–3
  see also training
effectiveness of interventions 19, 32, 52, 81, 126
  improvements 328
efficacy of interventions 19
efficiency 81, 105–6
  barriers to 107
  improvements 328
emergency contraception 207
emergency needs assessment 44–6

emergency obstetric care 17
emerging diseases 240
empowerment 121, 129
enabling component, health promotion 125–6
enabling factors, health promotion 123
Entre Nous Jeunes peer education, Cameroon 135
environment, improvement 298–9
environmental factors
    in communicable disease transmission 252
    in health promotion 119–21
environmental health 15–16
environmental variation 39
epidemiological assessment, meningitis 45
epidemiological information 38–9
epidemiological transition 7–8, 293–4
    China 295
epidemiology 248
    definitions 21–2
    evaluative 32
Epi info 31
equity of health services 3, 101
eradication of communicable diseases 240
error reduction 313–14
errors 312–13
essential medicines, access 218
essential medicines concept (EMC) 213
    advantages 214–15
    effect in Yemen 228
    formulary process 215–18
    practical implications 215
    target legend 216
essential services 104, 184
ethics, health economics 99
evaluation 81, 83, 152
    communication of results 84
    data collection methods 82–3
    of health promotion programmes 136–7
    indicators of progress 83–4
    of training 75
evaluative epidemiology 22, 32
evidence-based practice 315
exit interviews 42, 82
expanded programme of immunization (EPI) 13, 198,
    242–3, 250–1
    malaria prophylaxis 283
    review 52–3
Expert Patient Programme 304
'expert' patients 19, 303
explicit rationing 102, 103
extended spectrum beta lactamase (ESBL) producing
    organisms 250
external quality assurance (EQA) 268
extreme drug resistant (XDR) TB 268

facilitation 77
facility-based communication 133
faecal-oral diseases 261
families, care provision 158
family life education 15
family planning 14–15, 17, 324
    community-based services 203–4
    contraceptive methods 206–7
    demand for 206
    service delivery 207–9

unmet need 204, 205
family planning clinics 208
famine relief 46
FamPlan 96
farm health worker scheme, Zimbabwe 159
feedback, clinical audit 311
fertility 14–15
    future trends 320
fertility rate 23
field worker contact sheets 82
financial feasibility 56–7, 61
financing see funding
fishing stocks, depletion 331
five-a-day scheme 300
fleas, as disease vectors 283
flexibility 178
flow diagrams 45
fluoridation of water 297
focus groups 42, 44, 82
food aid 200
food-borne diseases 261
food subsidies 298
food supplementation 14, 200
formularies 216–17
formulary process 215–18
fortification of foods 14, 201
Framework Convention on Tobacco Control 131, 307
functional deconcentration 148, 149
funding 56, 88–90, 327
    future trends 323
    global overview 90
    insurance schemes 91–2
    of medicines 222–4, 233
    policy shifts 141–2
    taxation-based 90
    user charges 93–4
future challenges 330–1

Gantt charts 69, 70
GATHER communication approach 134
gender–cultural feasibility 55, 61, 120
gender differences 5, 28
general fertility rate (GFR) 24
general practitioners 161
genetics, vulnerability to infections 243
geographical resource allocation 100–1
geographical variation 27–8, 39
glandular fever (infectious mononucleosis) 249
globalization
    impact on non-communicable diseases 305–7
    impact on public health 292–3
Global Public Private Partnerships (GPPPs) 141
global warming 15–16, 205–6, 330, 331
GOALS 96
good manufacturing practices, medicines 230
governance 330
    of health systems 148–51
governments, involvement in pharmaceutical
    sector 234–6
greenhouse effect 205–6
Greenstar programme 110
growth monitoring 14, 199–200
guidelines 73, 167–9, 216, 316–17
    impact 216

in-service training 175
  from WHO 326
Guinea worm (dracunuliasis) 262

hand-washing 244–5, 254, 263
health
  influencing factors *37*
  WHO definition 35
health behaviours 122
health care provision, variation 39
health care pyramid *157*
health care systems 145–6
  inputs 146–8
health care workers
  education about communicable diseases 252
  transmission of infections 244
health centres 159–61
  role 164–6, *165*
Health Day promotion, bednets *60*
health economics 87–8, *89*
  project appraisal 99–100
  resource allocation 100–1
  see also funding
health facilities role definition 162–6
Health For All 2000 115
health improvement, methods 145
health informatics 315–16
health insurance 91–2, 223–4
health maintenance organizations 160
Health Management Information Systems 147
health needs, definition 35–6
health needs assessment 36–8, 51, 65–6
  acting on results 46–7
  community appraisals 40–4, 45
  emergency needs assessment 44–6
  identification and analysis of the problem 52–3
  meningitis 45
  routine information 38–9
health outcomes data 51
health promotion 14, 115–16, 203, 254, 263–4
  communication channels 124–5, 126–7, 129–35
  components of interventions 117
  education 126–7, 129–35
  empowerment 121
  enabling component 125–6
  enabling factors 123
  family planning 206
  HIV 274–5
  individual and cultural factors 121–3
  monitoring and evaluation of programmes 136–7
  planning process 117–25
  programme implementation 127–9
  relationship to public health 116–17
  service delivery 126
  service provision 123–4
  socioeconomic and environmental factors 119–21
  special emphases 116
  strategies *118*
  support materials 135–6
health reform policies 140–1, 323
  China 235–6
health sector funding 327
health-seeking behaviour 158
health services

improvement 327–8
  principles 2–3
health surveys 30–1, 37
health systems 139, *144*
  governance 148–51
  purpose 145
helminths 265
  prevention of transmission 254
hepatitis B vaccination 325
  financial feasibility 56
hepatitis prevention 261, 276–7
Hib vaccine 198
HIV/AIDS 16, 18, 324
  antiretroviral treatment 276
  case definition 272
  communication 274–5
  community appraisal 41
  control and prevention 273–4
  counselling and testing 275
  epidemiology 271
  health needs assessment 51
  health promotion *118*, 274–5
  immune deficiency 271
  infectiousness 273
  integrated health care 169
  mother-to-child transmission 96, 273, 274
  opportunistic infections 271–2
  post-natal care 190
  preventive treatment 276
  review of interventions 58, *59*
  TB 267
  TB chemoprophylaxis 251
  transmission 272–3
Hlabisa hospital, South Africa 163–4
holistic services 178–9
hookworm 262
hospital admission 161
hospital records, as source of data 38
hospitals
  district hospitals 161–2
    Hlabisa hospital, South Africa 163–4
    role 164–6, *165*
  health promotion 127
  infection control 244
hospital staff, supervisory work 174–5
host factors, communicable diseases 241–3
household surveys 42
house-to-house MDA 60
housing 15, *16*
human resources *see* staff
hygiene 253, 254, 263–4

illness behaviours 122
immunity 242–3
immunization 250–1
  see also vaccination
implementation 70–1, 86, 328–30
  health promotion programmes 127–9
  phased 72
  piloting 71
  practical elements 73–4
  shortcomings 72
  sustainability 72–3
implementation research 84–6

implicit contracting 111
implicit rationing *102*, 103
incidence 26–7
income, global distribution *320*
income-generation 125
incremental sanitation *264*
India, medicine procurement 221
indicators of progress 83
Indonesia, use of injections 229
inequalities 319
infant mortality rate (IMR) 23, *24*
infecting dose 243–4
infection control teams 246
infections, interaction with malnutrition 199
influences on health *37*
influenza 270
informatics 315–16
information 147
information sources 38–9
injection use, reduction in Indonesia 229
insect-borne diseases 277, 283
   see also malaria
insecticides 282
insecticide treated nets (ITNs) 281
   see also bednets
in-service training 173–7
insurance schemes 91–2, 223–4
intangibles 99
integrated deconcentration 148, *149*
Integrated Management of Adolescent–Adult
      Illness 18, 326
Integrated Management of Childhood Illness
      (IMCI) 185, 193–5, 326
   case management *194*
   constraints upon integrated care 197–8
   interventions 195–6
   role of community groups 196–7
integrated services 85–6, 150, 160, 166–7, 168,
      171, 284
   for non-communicable diseases 303
integrated 'supermarket' approach, MNCH 197
intermittent preventive treatment (IPT), malaria 283
internal markets 109–11
International Network for the Rational Use of Drugs
      (INRUD) 225
international support (aid) 141–2
   donation of medicines 221
   food aid 200
international variation 28
interpersonal communication *132–3*, 134–5
inter-sectoral approach 9
inter-sectoral collaboration 78
interventions 12
   choice 50, 53–4, 68–9
   financial feasibility 56–7
   gender–cultural and political feasibility 55–6
   health promotion 117
   Integrated Management of Childhood Illness 195–6
   MNCH 185–6
   in nutrition 201
   organizational feasibility 55
   review of 57–8, *59*
   technical effectiveness 54–5
interviews 42, 44

iodine fortification of salt 201

job descriptions 67

Kaiser Permanente model 303–*4*
Kangaroo Mother Care 193
'keep-up', EPI 198

laboratory diagnosis
   communicable diseases 248
   of TB 267–8
larvicidal substances 282
laundry, transmission of infections 245–6
leadership 77
   in meetings 79
leadership reforms 323
legislation
   communicable disease control 254
   prevention of non-communicable diseases 296
   supportive 125
   of tobacco use 297–8
leishmaniasis 283
licensing of medicines 223
life expectancy, future trends 320
lifelong learning 315
literature searches 54, 68–9
living conditions, role in TB 267
local variation 28
longitudinal surveys 30
long-term activities 125
low birthweight babies 193
lung cancer, health promotion strategies *118*
lymphatic filariasis 254, 265

malaria 277
   chemoprophylaxis 251, 283
   cost estimation tool 96
   diagnosis 278–9
   effect of sickle cell trait 243
   epidemiology 278
   health promotion strategies *118*
   immunity 278
   treatment 279–80
   vectors 277–8
malaria control *280*, 324
   biological control 282
   drainage 282
   global 283
   insecticides 282
   intervention strategies 54
   larvicidal substances 282
   mosquito nets 280–1
      see also bednets
   vaccination 282
Malawi Anti Child Labour Programme 130
malnutrition 183, 199
   health needs assessment 37–8
management 147
   district teams 150–1, 169–70
   strategies for rational medicine use 227–8
Management of Childhood Illness course 194
management support systems 171–3
managerial technical effectiveness 54
manuals (guidelines) 73

maps, use in communicable disease control 248
marginal budgeting for bottlenecks (MBB) 96
marginal costs 97, 251
Marie Stopes 208
mass drug administration (MDA) 14, 254, 264–6
  delivery strategies 60
  for worm infestation 203
mass media *132*, 133–4
  HIV information communication 274–5
maternal deaths, causes 187
maternal health 187, 324
  access to information and services 187–8
    abortion 192
    childbirth 189
    maternity services 188
    'pathway to survival' *191–2*
    post-natal care 190
    referral system 189–90
    traditional birth attendants 192
  community-based services 203–4
  determinants 6
maternal health information 39
maternal health services 17, 188
maternal, neonatal, and child health (MNCH) 181–2
  burden of disease 182–4
  community-based family planning and maternity
    services 203–4
  family planning 206–9
  health promotion 203
  historical development of services 185
  integrated care delivery 85–6, 197
  interventions 185–6
  nutrition 199–201
  priority setting 203
  programmes and services 184–5
  quality control 209–10
  school education 201, 203
measles
  case definition 247
  infecting dose 244
measurement of disease 23
medical supplies 147
medical technical effectiveness 54
medicines 213–14
  access 218
  counterfeit and substandard products 232
  donation 221
  essential medicines concept 214–15
  financing 222–4
  formulary process 215–18
  governmental involvement in pharmaceutical
    sector 234–6
  national polices 232–4
  per capita expenditure *222*
  pharmaceutical market 222
  procurement 219–20, 221
  quality 230
  rational use 224–30
  regulation 231–2
  storage and distribution 220
medicine use indicators *226*
meetings 78–9, *133*
mega-problems 330–1
meningitis, health needs assessment 45

meningitis outbreaks, intervention strategies 256
mental disorders 289, 291
  future trends 322
micronutrients 200–1
micronutrient supplementation 14, 110, 201
  wheat flour fortification, Pakistan 79
migration 205
millennium development goals (MDGs) 106, 143
minimum clinical packages 104
monitoring 80–1, 83, 152, 328
  data collection methods *82–3*
  health promotion programmes 136–7
  indicators of progress 83–4
  of medicine use 225–6
monitoring trends 28–30
'mopping-up' campaigns, EPI 198
moral hazard 92
morbidity 4, 239–40
mortality 4, 239
mosquito control 254, 283
mosquitoes, malaria transmission 277–8
mother-to-child transmission of HIV 96, 273, 274
multi-donor budget support 91
multi-drug resistance, TB 268
multilateral aid organizations 142
multiple interventions, communicable disease
  control 265–6
multi-sectoral approach 9

national census data 38
national health accounts 92
national medicine policies 232–4
national strategic planning process 151–2
national variation 28
needlestick injuries 245, 273
negative rationing *102*, 103
neonatal care 17, 192–3
  see also maternal, neonatal, and child health
    (MNCH)
neonatal illness 193
neonates, major causes of death *183*
Nepal, user fees, effect on medicine use 227
net present value (NPV) 98
newspapers, communication value *132*
non-communicable diseases 18–19, 287
  diabetes 290
  economic consequences 288–9
  effect of globalization 305–7
  epidemiologic transition 293–4, 295
  in low- and middle-income countries 290
  mental disorders 289, 291
  modifiable risk factors 291–3
  mortality *288*
  palliative care 305
  population screening 300
  prevention and control 294
    advocacy 299
    community-based programmes 300
    improvement of physical environment 298–9
    laws and regulations 296
    primary prevention 301–2
    public health approach 295–6
    secondary prevention 302
    targeted interventions 301

non-communicable diseases *(cont'd)*
  prevention and control *(cont'd)*
    targets 296
    taxation and price regulation 298
    tobacco control 297–8
    water fluoridation 297
    WHO global strategy 297
  rehabilitation 304
  self-care 304
  service delivery 302–3
  stepwise framework 305, *306*
  trends 321
non-governmental organizations (NGOs) 78
  family planning services 208
  service provision 111
norms 122–3
nosocomial infection 244
  control of infection teams 246
  hand-washing 244–5
  laundry 245–6
  sharps 245
nutrition 14
  food supplementation and food aid 200
  growth monitoring and promotion 199–200
  interventions 201
  micronutrients 200–1
  role in resistance to infection 242
  see also diet
nutritional surveillance surveys 39

objective medicine information 217–18
objectives 68
  training *74*
observation bias 33
obstetric care 189–90
occupational risks 15
onchoceriasis 254, 265, 283
operational research (implementation research) 84–6
opportunistic infections, HIV/AIDS 271–2
opportunistic screening 14
opportunities for action 50
opportunity costs 87, 97
organizational feasibility 55, *61*
organization of health systems 148–51
organization of services 105–7
organizational values, district health systems 177–9
Ottowa Charter on Health Promotion (1986) 115, 127
Outbreak Control Meetings 255–6
outcomes, clinical trials 33
outpatient treatment 161–2
  Hlabisa hospital, South Africa 163
outreach services 3, *132*, 160, 171
  EPI 198
ownership of projects 78

palliative care 305, 325
parasites 243
Paris declaration (2005) 91, 142
partographs 192
passive surveillance 247
'pathway to survival', maternal care *191*–2
patient-centred services 178
patient costs 95, 97

patient education 134
  about communicable diseases 252
patient-held health cards 169, 303
patient safety 312
  error reduction 313–14
payment systems 107–9
peer education 135, 203
  HIV 274
people-orientated planning 46
performance contracts 112
perinatal mortality rate (PMR) 23, *24*
period prevalence 25
personal preventive services 12, 184
Peru, rational use of medicines 230
pharmaceutical market 222
  governmental involvement 234–6
pharmacy information 39
phased implementation 72
physical activity
  lack of 292
  promotion through environmental
    improvements 299
  promotion in primary care 301
  promotion through taxation 298
  promotion in the workplace 300
piloting 71
placebo effect 32, 33
Plan, Do, Study, and Act (PDSA) cycle *310*–11
planning 66
  budgeting 69–70
  choice of interventions 68–9
  health needs assessment 65–6
  for health promotion 117–25
  objectives 68
  resources assessment 66
  staff recruitment 67–8
  web-based resources 96
Planning and Budgeting for TB 96
planning process 151–2
PMTCT (preventing mother-to-child
  transmission of HIV) 96
pneumococcal vaccine 198
point prevalence 25
policy 125, 139
  national medicine policies 232–4
policy-making 151–2
policy reforms 323
policy shifts
  Ata Alma declaration 139–40
  funding mechanisms and levels 141–2
  health reforms 140–1
  human resources 142–3
  millennium development goals 143
  on social determinants of health 143–4
political constraints 55–6
pollution 15
population-based interventions 12, 184
  advocacy 299
  community-based programmes 300
  environmental improvements 298–9
  laws and regulations 296
  taxation and price regulation 298
  tobacco control and legislation 297–8

water fluoridation 297
population-based payments *108*
population growth 331
population pressure 205–6
populations
    background information 124
    comparisons 39
    definition 2, 23
    prioritization 94
population screening 300
positive externalities 92
positive rationing *102*, 103
posters, communication value *132*
post-natal care 190
poverty, role in non-communicable diseases 293
practical skills 76
pregnancy
    malaria prevention 283
    see also maternal health; maternal, neonatal, and
        child health
premature babies 193
premiums, insurance schemes 91
prescribing, quality of 225
prescribing policies 216
prescription fees 224
    effect in Nepal 227
prevalence 25
prevalence (cross-sectional) surveys 30
prevalence pool *27*
prevention 117, 330
    levels of 11–12
    of non-communicable diseases 294
        population-based interventions 296–300
        primary prevention 301–2
        screening 300
        secondary prevention 302
        targeted interventions 301
        target setting 296
    versus cure 12
primary care 159–61
    funding 327
    future trends 323
    health promotion 128
    implementation of services 329
    mental health services 289, 291
    role 164–6, *165*
primary cases 255
Primary Health Care (PHC) approach 139–40
primary prevention 11, 117, 301–2
priority setting 20, 94, 101–5, *102*, 323–5
    in MCNH 203
prisons, health promotion 274
private sector 109, 145–6
    family planning services 209
    regulation 152
    subsidies 111–12
problem analysis 57
problem-solving methods 52
problem statements 52–3
procedures (guidelines) 73
process evaluation 81, 83
    data collection methods *82–3*
    of health promotion programmes 137

procurement of medicines 219–20
    India 221
programme coordination 77
programme implementation learning 173
programme monitoring, TB 269–70
project appraisal 99–100
project proposals 61–3
protocols (guidelines) 73, 167–9, 216, 316–17
    impact *216*
    in-service training 175
    from WHO 326
publication 84
public expenditure reviews 99
public financing 109
    of medicines 223
public health
    definition 1–2, 9
    ideals 2–3
    multi-professional nature 3–4
public health education, promotion of rational
        medicine use 229
public health programmes 13–17
public–private partnerships (PPPs) 110
    global (GPPPs) 141
    Marie Stopes 208
pyrethroids 282

QALYs (quality adjusted life years) 98
quality, dimensions of 310
quality assurance (QA) 309
    medicines 230
quality control
    medicines 230
    MNCH 209–10
quality improvement *210*
    IMCI 197
quality improvement methods 310–12
questionnaires 31

radio, communication value *132*
randomization, in implementation research 84–5
randomized controlled trials 22, 32–3
random samples 31
rapid assessments surveys *83*
rapid diagnostic tests (RDTs), malaria 279
rates of disease 23, *24*
rational use of medicines 224–5, 233
    investigation 225–6
    promotion 226–30
rationing 101–5, *102*
record keeping 169
    chronic disease 303
referral 167–9
    information transfer 169
    obstetric care 189–90
regional differences 4–5, 27–8, 39
regulation 112–13, 152
    of medicines 226–7, 231–2
    in prevention of non-communicable diseases 296
rehabilitation 304
rehabilitation behaviours 122
reporting bias 32
reproductive health, peer education 135

research evidence, searching and appraising 315
resource allocation 100–1
Resource Needs Model 96
resources 63, 87–8
  assessment 66
respiratory infections 266, 270
  see also TB
response rate, surveys 31
responsibility 62–3, 178
review of health services 51–2
  choice of interventions 53–4
  detail 57–8
  health needs assessment 51
  health promotion 117, 119–25
  identification and analysis of the problem 52–3
  indications 49–50
  scope 50
  service delivery approach 58–61
reviews of published evidence 33–4
risk factors 21
risk pooling 88, 90
risk-rating, insurance schemes 91
road safety 16, 324
  health promotion strategies *118*
road traffic accidents, trends 322
Roll Back Malaria 283
routes of entry, invading organisms 243

'safe talk' programme, Uganda 203
Salmonella 243, 244
salt intake reduction 300
sampling, surveys 31
sampling frames 31
sanitation 15, 253, 262, 264
  data 39
sanitation-related diseases, transmission *260*
schistosomiasis 262
  transmission control 265
schools, health promotion *128*, 134, 201, 203
screening 13–14, 300
seasonal calendars 45
seasonal variation in disease *27*
seat belt legislation 296
secondary care 161–2
secondary cases 255
secondary prevention 11, 117, 302
Sector Wide Approach (SWAp) 91, 142
self-care 303, 304
self-limiting diseases 32
semi-autonomy 150
semi-structured interviews 44
service based payments *108*
service delivery reforms 323
service delivery strategies 12–13, 54
  bednets *60*
  chronic disease management models 303–*4*
  effectiveness and feasibility *61*
  financial feasibility 56–7
  gender-cultural and political feasibility 55–6
  health promotion 126
  mass drug administration 60
  non-communicable diseases 302–3
  organizational feasibility 55

review 58–61
  technical effectiveness 54–5
service packages 104–5
  design *103*
service provision 123–4
settings approach to health promotion 127–9
sex education 275
sexual activity, prevention of HIV transmission 273
sexually transmitted infections (STIs) 16, 270–1
  see also HIV/AIDS
shanty cities 331
sharps, disposal and reuse 245
short-term activities 125
sickle cell trait 243
side effects of antibiotics 249
situational analysis 117–25
skills 123
  staff training 76
skin infections 261
smallpox 240, 250
SMART targets 68
smoke free workplaces 300
smoking 16–17
  control and legislation 297–8
  Framework Convention on Tobacco Control 131,
    307
  global changes 322
  methods of reduction 324
  role in non-communicable diseases 292
  taxation of tobacco 298
  tobacco industry, globalization 293
smoking cessation advice 302
social determinants of health 143–4
  future trends 322–3, 327–8
  TB 267
social marketing 15, 110, 133–4
  bednets 60, 111, 281
  contraceptives 209, 275
  effectiveness and feasibility *61*
social mobilization 129, 130
social variation 39
socioeconomic factors, in health promotion 119–21
soil, as source of diseases 261–2
specialist care 330
special population group locations, MDA 60
spread of communicable diseases 241
staff 126, 146–7
  payment systems 107–9
  policy shifts 142–3
  recruitment 67–8
  supervision 76–7
  training 73, 74–6
staff turnover 67
stakeholder analysis 152
stakeholders 50
standardized rates 23
stigma, communicable diseases 241
stock records *82*
storage of medicines 220
  antibiotics 249
streptomycin, side effects 249
structured interviews 44
sub-cultures 122

subsidies 111–12
  on healthy food 298
  on sport and recreation 298
substance misuse, targeted interventions 301
suicide 322
supervision 76–7
  district health services 173–7
supervisors, note-taking *82*
supplementation 201
supportive supervision 173, 177
support materials, health promotion 135–6
support systems 171–3
surveillance, communicable diseases 246–8
surveillance systems 46
surveys 30–1, 37, *83*
sustainability 72–3
  assessment 100
SWAps (sector-wide approaches) 91, 142
Swiss cheese model, errors 313, *314*
syndromic approach to disease management 194
systematic reviews 34
systematic sampling 31

Tanzania Essential Health Interventions Project
    (TEHIP) 171
targeted interventions, non-communicable
    diseases 301
targets 68, 83
task-shifting 330
taxation
  health promotion 125
  role in non-communicable disease prevention 298
taxation-based funding 90
TB *see* tuberculosis
teaching methods *75*
teamwork 178
technical effectiveness 54–5, *61*
television, communication value *132*
temporal changes 32
termination of pregnancy 187, 192
  access to 15
terrorism 331
tertiary prevention 11, 117
tetanus, immunity 242
thresholds for intervention, maternal care 191
ticks, as disease vectors 283
time based payments *108*
time charts (Gantt charts) 69, *70*
time management 80
time scales, communicable diseases 244
timing of activities 63
tobacco 16–17
  control and legislation 297–8
  Framework Convention on Tobacco Control 131,
      307
  global changes 322
  methods of smoking reduction 324
  role in non-communicable diseases 292
  smoking cessation advice 302
  taxation 298
tobacco industry, globalization 293
trachoma 265
traditional birth attendants 192

traditional healers 158
traditional leaders 157
training 73, 74–6, 173–7, 315
  of birth attendants 192
    methods of changing practices 317–18
    in rational use of medicines 228–30
transport 80, 171
  obstetric care 190
transport policy 143
transport supervision *172*
Treatment Action Campaign, South Africa 170–1
treatment guidelines 216
  impact *218*
treatment supporters 268, *269*
trends, monitoring 28–30
trypanosomiasis 283
tuberculosis (TB) 324
  case finding 25
  chemoprophylaxis 251, 276
  control 267–70
  DOTS package 81, 268, 303
  health needs assessment 40
  in HIV infection 267
  integrated health care 169
  Planning and Budgeting for TB 96
  prevention 11–12
  programme monitoring 269–70
  public-private partnerships 110
  social mobilization project (YONECO) 130
  technical and support function strengthening 175
  treatment 18, 268–9

Uganda, population pressure 205
UNDP Integrated Health Model 96
universal coverage reforms 323
user charges 93–4, 224
  effect on medicine use 227
utilization behaviours 122

vaccination 13, 250–1, 325, 327
  against malaria 282
  counterfeit products 232
  monitoring using coverage charts 28–30
  see also expanded programme of immunization
      (EPI)
vector control 15, 253–4, 277
Venn diagrams 45
ventilation, role in communicable disease
    control 253
vertical programmes 150, 169
violence 322
viruses 243
vitamin A deficiency 200–1
voluntary counselling and testing (VCT) 16
  HIV 275
voluntary financing schemes 224

waiver systems, user fees 94
war 322
water fluoridation 297
water provision 15, 252–3, 262–3
  data 39
water purification 263

water related disease 262
    transmission *260*
water shortages 331
water-washed diseases 261
wealth, global distribution *320*, 323
weight management 301
wheat flour fortification, Pakistan 79
WHO
    building blocks of care for chronic
        conditions 307
    Choice website 96
    Commission on Macro Economics and
        Health 141
    essential medicines
        criteria 215
        definition 214
    Framework Convention on Tobacco Control 307
    global strategy for diet, physical activity, and
        health 297
    guidelines and training packages 326

stepwise framework for non-communicable
    diseases 305, *306*
World Alliance for Patient Safety 314
working groups 73
workplace, health promotion 127, 134, 300
work plans 69
World Alliance for Patient Safety 314
World Development Report (1993), essential
    service package 104
worm infestation, mass treatment 203

yellow fever 283
Yemen, effect of essential medicine programme 228
Youth Net and Counselling (YONECO) 130

Zimbabwe
    sanitation and water provision 263
    schistosomiasis control 265
zinc supplementation 201
zoonotic infections 248, 284